HEALTH & WELLNESS

SW

Published In 1999
THE SOUTHWESTERN COMPANY
Nashville, TN

Health and Wellness

Manufactured under the direction of FRP™—a division of
Southwestern/Great American, Inc.
Nashville, Tennessee

Sourcing
Sharon Dean
Production Director
Mark Sloan
Production Coordinator
George McAllister
Digital Prepress Coordinator
Donna Bailey
Production
Waller Digital
Sales Directors
Creig Soeder   Roy Loftin
Dave Causer   Fred Prevost
Jeff Hawley

ISBN # 0-87197-4797

Printed in the United States of America.

Library of Congress Cataloging-in-Publication Data
The medical advisor home edition,
by the editors of Time-Life Books.
p. cm.
Includes bibliographical references
and index.
ISBN 0-7835-5250-5 (softcover)
1. Medicine, Popular—Encyclopedias. 2. Alternative medicine
Encyclopedias. I. Time-Life Books.
RC81.A2M38 1997
616—dc21   97-10717 CIP

First printing. Printed in U.S.A.
School and library distribution by
Time-Life Education,
P.O. Box 85026, Richmond,
Virginia 23285-5026.

TIME-LIFE is a trademark of
Time Warner Inc. U.S.A.

**The textual and visual descriptions of medical conditions
and treatment options in this book should be considered
as a reference source only; they are not intended to substitute for a healthcare practitioner's diagnosis, advice,
and treatment. Always consult your physician or a qualified practitioner for proper medical care.
Before using any drug or natural medicine mentioned
in this book, be sure to check with your healthcare practitioner, and check the product packaging or other reliable
source of information for any warnings or cautions. You
should keep in mind that herbal remedies are not as
strictly regulated as drugs.**

TIME
LIFE

By the Editors of
TIME-LIFE BOOKS
Alexandria, VA

PROJECT EDITOR
Robert Somerville
Senior Art Director: Tina Taylor
Deputy Editors:
Kristin Baker Hanneman, Tina S. McDowell
Administrative Editor: Judith W. Shanks

EDITORIAL STAFF
Text Editors: Glen Ruh, Jim Watson
Associate Editors / Research and Writing:
Nancy Blodgett, Kristin Dittman,
Stephanie Summers Henke,
Jennifer I. Vermillion
Technical Art Assistant: Dana R. Magsumbol
Copyeditors:
Mary Beth Oelkers-Keegan (principal),
Claudia S. Bedwell, Donna D. Carey
Editorial Assistant: Katrina Barnes Johnson
Picture Coordinator: Paige Henke

SPECIAL CONTRIBUTORS
Alan H. Anderson, Charlotte Anker,
Adrianne Appel, Jamie Baylis, Celia Beattie,
Angela Burbage, Nancy Cardwell, Leslie Carper,
Lisa Ann Clark, Mary E. Collins,
George Constable, Margery A. duMond,
Juli Duncan, Phyllis A. Friedemann,
Ruth Goldberg , Debra S. Greinke, Peter Gwynne,
Harriet Harvey, Lydia Preston Hicks, Silvia Hines,
Donald E. Holmes, Judith Klein, Sarah Labouisse,
Jeffrey Laign, Amy McGoldrick, Elizabeth Moore,
Narisara Murray, Ann Perry, Susan Perry,
Barbara Fairchild Quarmby,
Eugenia S. Scharf, Jacqueline L. Shaffer,
Colette Stockum, Janet Barnes Syring,
Michael Tenneson, Monika Thayer,
Susan Gregory Thomas, Victoria Valentine,
Mary Weideman, Jayne Rohrich Wood

John Drummond, Robert Herndon (design),
Barbara L. Klein (index)

CORRESPONDENTS
Maria Vincenza Aloisi (Paris),
Christine Hinze (London),
Christina Lieberman (New York)

CONSULTANTS

NEIL BAUM, MD
teaches at Tulane Medical School and serves on the staff of Southern Baptist Hospital. A board-certified urologist, he counsels patients in sexual dysfunction and male infertility and has written extensively in both areas. Dr. Baum is also director of the Impotence Foundation at Touro Infirmary in New Orleans.

HERBERT BENSON, MD
teaches at Harvard Medical School and is chief of the Division of Behavioral Medicine at the Deaconess Hospital. He is also founding president of the Mind/Body Medical Institute, which specializes in the treatment of stress-related illnesses. Dr. Benson has helped draw attention to the field of mind/body medicine through his pioneering work on the relaxation response.

ZOË BRENNER, LAc, Dipl Ac (NCCA), FNAAOM
has practiced acupuncture since 1977 and Chinese herbal medicine since 1984. She teaches oriental medicine and the history and philosophy of Chinese medicine at the Traditional Acupuncture Institute in Bethesda, Maryland.

DWIGHT C. BYERS
began teaching with his aunt, Eunice Ingham, who pioneered and developed the original Ingham method of reflexology. Byers now serves as president of the International Institute of Reflexology in St. Petersburg, Florida.

BARRIE R. CASSILETH, PhD
teaches at the medical schools of Duke University and the University of North Carolina, where she specializes in alternative and psychosocial medicine for cancer patients. Dr. Cassileth is also a member of the Office of Alternative Medicine Program Advisory Council at the National Institutes of Health.

EFFIE CHOW, PhD, RN, CA
is president of the East West Academy of Healing Arts in San Francisco. A registered nurse, certified acupuncturist, and qigong master, Dr. Chow has practiced and taught qigong for more than 30 years.

JOHN G. COLLINS, ND, DHANP
teaches dermatology, gastroenterology, and homeopathy at the National College of Naturopathic Medicine in Portland, Oregon. He also has a private practice in Gresham, Oregon.

STEPHANIE S. COVINGTON, PhD, LCSW
is a psychotherapist and codirector of the Institute for Relational Development in La Jolla, California. She specializes in the areas of addiction, sexuality, families, and relationships. Dr. Covington has taught at the University of Southern California, San Diego State University, and the California School of Professional Psychology. She formerly chaired the Women's Committee of the International Council on Alcoholism and Addiction.

KYLE H. CRONIN, ND
specializes in women's healthcare in her medical practice in Phoenix. Dr. Cronin is also cofounder of Southwest College of Naturopathic Medicine and Health Sciences, where she is dean of Curricular Development.

TIMOTHY B. DEERING, MD
is a board-certified internist and gastroenterologist who practices with Asheville Gastroenterology Associates in North Carolina.

PALI C. DELEVITT, PhD
consults on alternative therapies at the cancer center of the University of Virginia, where she also teaches in the School of Medicine. Dr. Delevitt has consulted on curriculum development for the medical schools of Columbia University, Emory University, and Indiana University.

JAMES A. DUKE, PhD
was an economic botanist with the Agriculture Research Service, United States Department of Agriculture, in Beltsville, Maryland, for much of his career. Dr. Duke consults for many organizations, including the American Botanical Council and the Herb Research Foundation.

KATHLEEN FRY, MD, MD(H)
is a board-certified physician, specializing in obstetrics and gynecology, who practices with A Woman's Place . . . for Healthcare in Scottsdale, Arizona. Dr. Fry is also a licensed classical homeopath.

ADRIANE FUGH-BERMAN, MD
is a medical researcher in the Washington, D.C., area. Currently on the board of the National Women's Health Network, Dr. Fugh-Berman is former head of field investigations at the Office of Alternative Medicine at the National Institutes of Health. She also served as medical director of the Taoist Health Institute and the Green Cross clinic, where she practiced nutritional, herbal, and conventional medicine.

ALAN R. GABY, MD
is president of the American Holistic Medical Association and a member of the Office of Alternative Medicine Program Advisory Council at the National Institutes of Health.

DAVID E. GOLAN, MD, PhD
is an attending physician at Brigham and Women's Hospital in Boston and an associate professor of biological chemistry and molecular pharmacology at Harvard Medical School. A board-certified internist and hematologist, Dr. Golan directs research on blood cell membranes. He has also created a computer-learning program for pharmacology.

CONSTANCE GRAUDS, RPh
is a registered pharmacist, certified herbalist, and registered nutritional consultant. Founder of the Association of Natural Medicine Pharmacists, Grauds consults for companies that make natural products in the areas of herbal and nutritional therapies.

ELLIOT GREENE, MA
is past president of the American Massage Therapy Association and currently maintains a private practice in the Washington, D.C., area. Certified in therapeutic massage by the National Certification Board for Therapeutic Massage and Bodywork, he has spent more than 22 years in the field. He was formerly on the Board of Directors of the National Wellness Coalition.

KEITH S. HECHTMAN, MD, FAAOS, FAOSSM
teaches at the School of Medicine in the Department of Orthopaedics and Sports Medicine at the University of Miami in Florida. Dr. Hechtman is a team physician for the University of Miami, Florida International University, and Saint Thomas University. He is also Medical Director of Dade County High Schools.

VICTOR HERBERT, MD, JD, FACP
teaches medicine at the Mount Sinai Medical Center in New York, where he also chairs the Committee to Strengthen Nutrition. A former president of the American Society for Clinical Nutrition, Dr. Herbert consults in the field of nutrition for many organizations, including the World Health Organization.

DAVID HOFFMANN, MNIMH
is a member of the British National Institute of Medical Herbalists and founding president of the American Herbalist Guild. His writings on therapeutic herbalism were a valuable resource during the preparation of this volume.

MAURITA HOLLAND, MALS
teaches information and library science at the University of Michigan in Ann Arbor. Some of her students provided research for this book and are listed individually in the acknowledgments section.

TORI HUDSON, ND
maintains a private practice, teaches gynecology, and serves as a supervising physician at the National College of Naturopathic Medicine in Portland, Oregon. She specializes in women's healthcare and has advised the Department of Health and Human Services on health reform.

GRACE BROOKE HUFFMAN, MD
serves as a primary care physician at two offices in Maryland and teaches at Georgetown University School of Medicine in Washington, D.C. A board-certified family practitioner, she has additional certification in geriatrics.

STEVEN IDELL, MD, PhD, FACP, FACCP
is chief of the pulmonary division and associate chairman of the Department of Medicine at the University of Texas Health Center at Tyler. His research in pulmonary diseases is sponsored by the National Institutes of Health.

JENNIFER JACOBS, MD, MPH
specializes in homeopathic medicine and has a private practice in family medicine in Edmonds, Washington. She conducts research in the use of homeopathic medicines in primary care at the University of Washington and is a member of the Office of Alternative Medicine Program Advisory Council at the National Institutes of Health.

JOSEPH J. JACOBS, MD, MBA
began his medical career as a pediatrician with the Indian Health Service in Gallup, New Mexico, and has continued working with American Indians throughout his career. Dr. Jacobs was director of the Office of Alternative Medicine at the National Institutes of Health from 1992 to 1994 and is a former president of the Association of American Indian Physicians.

JONATHAN M. KAGAN, MD
teaches ophthalmology at New York Medical College and has a private practice in New York City. He has conducted clinical trials of new drugs for ophthalmic use and is a fellow of the American Academy of Ophthalmology.

STEVEN W. KAIRYS, MD, MPH, FAAP
is associate chair of pediatrics at the Dartmouth-Hitchcock Medical Center, where he directs primary care activities and the Children at Risk Program. He is founder and president of the New Hampshire Alliance for Children and Youth in Concord, New Hampshire.

J. DANIEL KANOFSKY, MD, MPH
teaches psychiatry, epidemiology, and social medicine at the Albert Einstein College of Medicine and at the Bronx Psychiatric Center, both in New York City. A board-certified psychiatrist, Dr. Kanofsky is also a fellow of the American College of Nutrition.

TED KAPTCHUK, OMD, CA
teaches at Boston University School of Public Health and Harvard Medical School and is a research associate at Beth Israel Hospital. As a doctor of Oriental Medicine, Dr. Kaptchuk practices both Chinese herbal medicine and acupuncture.

ROBERT B. KLEIN, MD, FAAP, FAAAI
is chairman of pediatrics at the University of Texas Health Center at Tyler. His other specialties include allergy, pulmonology, and immunology. Dr. Klein also consults on childhood tuberculosis and asthma in Croatia for the U.S. State Department.

ROBERT KOTLER, MD, FACS
practices facial plastic and reconstructive surgery in Beverly Hills, California. Dr. Kotler is commissioner and regional consultant to the Medical Board of California. He also teaches at UCLA Center for the Health Sciences.

JESSE M. KRAMER, MD
is a dermatologist practicing in Santa Rosa, California. He teaches family medicine physicians through the University of California in San Francisco.

DAVID B. LARSON, MD, MSPH
is a psychiatrist certified in marriage and family therapy; his particular interest is the influence of religious commitment on physical and mental health. Dr. Larson has worked for the National Institutes of Health and the U.S. Department of Health and Human Services. He currently serves as an adjunct faculty member for several universities.

DANA J. LAWRENCE, DC, FICC
has been a faculty member at the National College of Chiropractic in Lombard, Illinois, for more than 15 years. He is also editor of the school's Journal of Manipulative and Physiological Therapeutics.

NORMAN S. LEVY, MD, PhD, FAAO, FACS
practices medicine in Gainesville, Florida, and teaches at the University of Florida. Dr. Levy is former chief of ophthalmology at the Veterans Administration hospitals in Gainesville and Lake City, Florida.

PHILIP LEVY, MD, FACE
practices at the Phoenix Endocrinology Clinic, Ltd., and teaches at the University of Arizona School of Medicine in Tucson. He is an active member of both the American Diabetes Association and the Endocrine Society.

JOHN E. LONSTEIN, MD
is a board-certified orthopedic surgeon and past president of the Scoliosis Research Society. Dr. Lonstein teaches at the University of Minnesota and practices with Twin Cities Spine Surgeons, Ltd. He is also chief of Spine Service and Cerebral Palsy Spine Service at Gillette Children's Hospital in Minnesota.

DAVE MANNINO, MD, FACCP
works at the Centers for Disease Control and Prevention at the National Center for Environmental Health in Atlanta. He teaches at the Emory School of Public Health.

ROY J. MATHEW, MD
teaches at Duke University Medical Center in Durham, North Carolina. He is also director of the Alcoholism and Addictions program, which provides treatment for people with alcoholism and drug addiction and offers consultation services for other medical specialists regarding addictions. Dr. Mathew's research focuses largely on the effects of alcohol and drugs on the brain and behavior.

ALEXANDER MAUSKOP, MD, FAAN
is director of the New York Headache Center and the not-for-profit New York Headache Foundation. He also teaches clinical neurology at the State University of New York, where he conducts research on the role of magnesium in headaches.

JEFFREY MIGDOW, MD
directs yoga-teacher training at Kripalu Center in Lenox, Massachusetts. He began his yoga training more than 20 years ago and has been teaching Kripalu yoga for 7 years. In his medical practice, Dr. Migdow counsels patients on lifestyle and recommends a wide variety of homeopathic, nutritional, and other therapies.

JOHN R. MOFFETT, PhD
is a research scientist in the Biology Department at Georgetown University in Washington, D.C. His specific areas of research are neurotransmitters in the visual system and toxins released by immune cells.

ANNE MOORE, MD
teaches clinical medicine at Cornell University Medical College and chairs the New York Hospital breast cancer tumor board. Board certified in internal medicine with subspecialties in hematology and oncology, Dr. Moore is also on the staff of the New York Hospital-Cornell Medical Center.

LEN OCHS, PhD
is a social psychologist who has spent 15 years developing computerized biofeedback instrumentation. Dr. Ochs is past president of the Biofeedback Society of New York.

STEPHEN OLMSTEAD, MD
practices internal medicine and cardiology in Seattle, where he also teaches at the University of Washington.

ELSA RAMSDEN, EdD, PT
is a licensed physical therapist and certified medical psychologist who is on the faculty of the University of Pennsylvania, Widener University, Temple University, and Beaver College. She has also taught overseas at the University of Queensland in Brisbane, Australia, and the University of Uppsala, Sweden, and was a Fulbright senior scholar to Australia.

JOHN C. REED, MD, MD(H)
is a board-certified family physician who practices with the Arizona Center for Health and Medicine in Phoenix. After medical school, he served as an Indian Health Service officer in southern Arizona. Dr. Reed has integrated acupuncture, homeopathy, and osteopathic medicine into his medical practice. He has consulted for the Office of Alternative Medicine at the National Institutes of Health and was coeditor of that office's report, Alternative Medicine: Expanding Medical Horizons.

NORMAN E. ROSENTHAL, MD
serves as chief of the Section on Environmental Psychiatry at the National Institutes of Health, where he has worked since 1979. Dr. Rosenthal is a former president of the Society for Light Therapy and Biological Rhythms.

BEVERLY RUBIK, PhD
is founding director of the Center for Frontier Sciences at Temple University in Philadelphia. Her particular interests in the field of alternative medicine include spiritual healing, acupuncture, and homeopathy.

MILDRED SEELIG, MD, MPH
teaches nutrition at the University of North Carolina, Chapel Hill, and preventive medicine at Emory University in Atlanta. Dr. Seelig is editor emeritus of the Journal of the American College of Nutrition.

WINIFRED SEWELL, MS, DSc
is a fellow of the Medical Library Association. She has taught at the University of Maryland School of Pharmacy as well as the College of Library and Information Services.

J. JAMISON STARBUCK, JD, ND
practices family medicine in Missoula, Montana. A former practicing attorney, she is past president of the American Association of Naturopathic Physicians and a member of the Homeopathic Academy of Naturopathic Physicians.

JAMES P. SWYERS, MA
is a science writer and editor who formerly served as managing editor of Alternative Medicine: Expanding Medical Horizons, a report published by the Office of Alternative Medicine at the National Institutes of Health. Before turning to journalism, he worked as a research biochemist and molecular biologist.

MICHAEL A. TANSEY, PhD
is an EEG neurofeedback clinician and researcher. He was a founding member of the Executive Council of the National Registry of Neurofeedback Providers.

DICK W. THOM, DDS, ND
teaches clinical and physical diagnosis at the National College of Naturopathic Medicine in Portland, Oregon. He is also a clinic supervisor at the Portland Naturopathic Clinic and maintains a general family practice at the Beaverton Center for the Healing Arts in Beaverton, Oregon.

ALEX A. TIBERI, OMD, LAc
is chairman of the Department of Oriental Medicine at the Pacific College of Oriental Medicine in San Diego. At his private practice at the Pacific Center of Health, he specializes in acupuncture for sports medicine. Dr. Tiberi has also served as a national examiner for the National Commission for the Certification of Acupuncturists.

ANDREW J. VICKERS
directs the information service at the Research Council for Complementary Medicine in the United Kingdom. He also teaches research methodology at the University of Westminster and the London School of Acupuncture.

ROBERT C. WARD, DO, FAAO
teaches biomechanics and family medicine at Michigan State University's College of Osteopathic Medicine. He was in private family practice for 12 years prior to teaching.

CAROLINE WELLBERY, MD, PhD
teaches family medicine at Georgetown University in Washington, D.C., and practices at the university's Ft. Lincoln clinic.

PICTURE CREDITS

All illustrations in this book were created by **Totally Incorporated.** Individual artists are listed below in alphabetical order.

Roxanna Drake
Carol Hilliard
Leslie Lien
Peter Malamas
Tipy Taylor
Patrick Wilson

A-Z Guide to Alternative Therapies Section Book 2:
The sources for the illustrations are listed below. Page numbers are in boldface.

All rights reserved. Corel Stock Photo Library 2, CD ROM: *The Alps in Spring* #207008: **4** (5th image in column on left), **5** (2d, 4th images in column on right), **12, 141**; *Barbecue and Salads* #294000: **157**; #294002, #294055: **9** (top right), **147** (3d and 4th images in column); *Colors and Textures* #403069: **119**; #403096: **5** (5th image in column on left), **64**; *Cuisine* #333056, #333022: **9** (top right), **147** (2d and 6th images in column); *Desserts* #297003: **9** (top right), **147** (1st image in column); *Everyday Objects* #373090: **5** (1st image in column on right), **38**; *Fabulous Fruit* #332095: **9** (top right), **147** (5th image in column), **152**; *Fruits and Nuts* #322069: **9** (top left image), **144**; *Japanese Gardens* #334081: **4** (1st image in column on right), **5** (4th image in column on left; 3d image in column on right), **14, 130**; *Light Pattern* #403069: **117**; *Masters IV* #402076: **4** (6th image in column on left), **170**; *Nepal* #187096: **5** (6th image in column on right), **42**; *People II* #376005: **5** (3d image in column on left), **165**; *Spices and Herb Textures* #362069, #362003, #362002, #362043, #362060, #362037, #362009: **71**. Richard Crist: **68-69**. Chinese symbol traced by John Drummond: **4** (1st image in column on left), **57**. Mark Ledzian: **172-181**. Art by Brian Leister: **7** (bottom image), **47**. Jerry Pavia, *The Virtual Garden* © 1997, Time-Life Inc.: **4** (2d image in column on right), **7** (top image), **8** (bottom right 2), **11** (2d image in column), **66, 70, 74-102**. Robin Reid: **4** (3d image in column on right), **121, 124-129**. Totally Incorporated: **4** (2d, 3d, 4th images in column on left; 4th, 5th images in column on right), **5** (1st, 2d images in column on left; 5th image in column on right), **8** (top left 2), **9** (top right; bottom 2), **10, 11** (1st, 3d, 4th images in column), **16-36, 61, 104, 147** (Pyramid), **163, 164, 167, 169, 182-193.**

ACKNOWLEDGMENTS

The editors wish to thank the following individuals and institutions for their valuable assistance in the preparation of this volume:

American Chiropractic Association, Arlington, Va.; Lucille Arcouet, National Education Coordinator, Nelson Bach USA, Wilmington, Mass.; Denise Bowles-Johnson, LMT, Creative Body Therapies, New Haven, Conn.; Al Bumanis, National Association for Music Therapy, Silver Spring, Md.; Patricia Kaminski, Flower Essence Society, Nevada City, Calif.; William J. Lauretti, DC, Bethesda, Md.; Barbara Mitchell, National Acupuncture and Oriental Medicine Alliance, Olalla, Wash.; Joyce Morris, Reiki Center of Los Angeles, Encino, Calif.; Perelandra, Jeffersonton, Va.; Holly H. Shimizu, Lewis Ginter Botanical Garden, Richmond, Va.; James P. Swyers, MA, Takoma Park, Md.Marian Abousief, Terese Murphy Austin, Univ. of Michigan, Ann Arbor; Kathryn Bryan, Bethesda, Md.; James A. Bryant, Office of Alternative Medicine, NIH, Rock-ville, Md.; Karen Childs, Washington, D.C.; Jim Cirigliano, Torrance, Calif.; Anne DeBevoise, Glendale, Calif.; Alice D. Domar, PhD, Harvard Medical School, Cambridge; Kathleen Enberenz, RENFREW, Philadelphia; Mary Lee Esty, Washington, D.C.; Julia Euling, Sydbury, Mass.; Carol Fedora, Univ. of Michigan; Mitchell Fleisher, MD, Arrington, Va.; Richard Friedman, PhD, State Univ. of New York-Stony Brook, Department of Psychiatry and Behavioral Science, N.Y.; Jim Gray, PhD, The American Univ., Washington, D.C.; Judith Graykowski, Univ. of Michigan; Kate Griffie, Kline and Company, Fairfield, N.J.; Tracy Harnish, Univ. of Michigan; Lucy Henderson, Orinda, Calif.; Roger Jahnke, OMD, Goleta, Calif.; Wayne B. Jonas, MD, Alexandria, Va.; Joan Klyhn, New Age Health Spa, Neversink, N.Y.; Diane Lawther, Julie J. Lea, Univ. of Michigan; Lisa Lefferts, Mothers and Others for a Livable Planet, Hyattsville, Md.; Ginger Lepre, Gary Litovitz, MD, Dominion Hospital, Falls Church, Va.; Robert McCaleb, Herb Research Foundation, Boulder, Colo.; Sarah Neises, Univ. of Michigan; G.R. Oberg, MD, The Crystal Lake Center for Allergy and Environmental Medicine, Crystal Lake, Ill.; Mary T. Panek, Josie Barnes Parker, Tammy M. Pearson, Linda P. Powers, Univ. of Michigan; Jon L. Richter, DMD, PhD, Richter Center for Treatment of Breath Disorders, Philadelphia; Jolie Martin Root, Boca Raton, Fla.; Barbara S. Schneidman, MD, MPH, American Board of Medical Specialties, Evanston, Ill.; Elaine Wu Stephenson, Univ. of Michigan; Colin M. Thomas, Washington, D.C.; Devon Thomas, Univ. of Michigan; Michael Tims, Cash Grocer, Alexandria, Va.; Jeremy Waletsky, MD, George Washington Univ., Washington, D.C.; Thomas A. Wehr, MD, NIMH, Rockville, Md.; Rita Lynn Wilson, Univ. of Michigan; William Wittman, MD, Falmouth, Mass.; Karen Beth Zamanick, MD, Northwestern Memorial Hospital, Chicago; Laura Zylstra-Garth, Washington, D.C.

CONTENTS ▶

10

INTRODUCTION ▶

When you or someone you love is ill or suffering even a minor ailment, you want to know you are making the best choices about treatment. On the eve of the 21st century, those choices are more plentiful than ever. Even as healthcare practitioners embrace the technological advances and the research breakthroughs occurring in modern medicine, they are turning with new interest to the alternative, or natural, therapies from medicine's foundations. Venerable healing practices, from acupressure and herbal remedies to yoga and meditation, are increasingly taking their place alongside modern forms of treatment such as immunotherapy and laser surgery.

In the context of the many options available, these pages offer clear, concise information on hundreds of health problems, ranging from relatively benign conditions to the most serious diseases. For any given ailment, conventional therapeutic approaches represent the best of modern medical science and mainstream medical practices. Alternative therapies also stand on extensive evidence of their benefits—even if those benefits sometimes defy scientific understanding.

In the end, the best decision will be the one you make in conjunction with your healthcare practitioner. The goal of this volume is to provide a solid base of knowledge to help in that process, so you can make informed—and thus more confident—choices about healthcare.

HOW TO USE THIS BOOK ▶

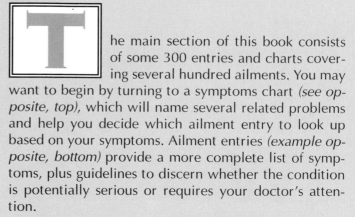

The main section of this book consists of some 300 entries and charts covering several hundred ailments. You may want to begin by turning to a symptoms chart *(see opposite, top)*, which will name several related problems and help you decide which ailment entry to look up based on your symptoms. Ailment entries *(example opposite, bottom)* provide a more complete list of symptoms, plus guidelines to discern whether the condition is potentially serious or requires your doctor's attention.

After explaining what causes the ailment, each entry describes conventional and alternative treatment options; for more information about types of therapies, turn to the **Dictionary of Conventional Medicine and Alternative Therapies,** beginning on page 18.

While reading an ailment entry, you may be referred to other entries or to the **Emergencies/First Aid** section. Plain bold type is used to emphasize a concept, or to indicate a therapeutic technique or a subcategory of the main ailment.

Other sections are useful as references or to supplement information in the ailment entries. For an overview of health concerns specific to women, men, children, and the elderly, consult the **General Guidelines to Health** starting on page 30. **Your Medicine Chest** on page 78 describes the various herbs, homeopathic remedies, and over-the-counter drugs you should have at hand in your home. Finally, the **A - Z Guide to Alternative Therapies,** offers an in-depth look at the wide variety of healing approaches—some dating to the dawn of civilization—that are used to treat ailments ranging in severity from the common cold to skin cancer. This section follows page 895, and has its own pagination. If you can't find the ailment you're looking for, check the general index starting on page 882, to see if it's listed by an alternate name. For example, "pinkeye" is not in the ailments section, but you will find it in the index with page numbers for the ailment entry "conjunctivitis," another name for this eye infection.

If you want more information about one of the ailments or treatment options presented in the book, contact any of the groups listed in the appendix under **Health Associations and Organizations.**

SYMPTOMS CHARTS

Some symptoms, such as abdominal pains, can be caused by any of several different ailments. Charts are a convenient way to identify an ailment by your symptoms and to locate the appropriate ailment entry. To use these charts, start in the far left column and read down until you find the set of symptoms that corresponds most nearly to your own. Read across to find the name of an ailment you can look up for a description and information about causes, treatment, and prevention. Symptoms charts are listed alphabetically with ailment entries.

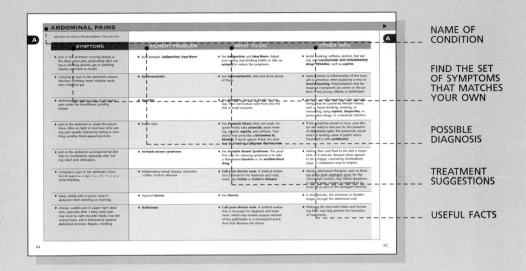

NAME OF CONDITION

FIND THE SET OF SYMPTOMS THAT MATCHES YOUR OWN

POSSIBLE DIAGNOSIS

TREATMENT SUGGESTIONS

USEFUL FACTS

AILMENT ENTRIES

Each of the nearly 300 ailment entries in this book follows a consistent format. Symptoms and information about when you need to call your doctor are listed first. Each entry describes the ailment and how it affects your body. Next, the entry outlines the underlying causes of the ailment and the tests and procedures your doctor may use to confirm a diagnosis. The treatment segment presents conventional and alternative recommendations for curing the problem or alleviating the symptoms. Most ailment entries conclude with advice on preventive measures you can use to stay healthy.

WHAT TO EXPECT AT THE DOCTOR'S OFFICE

ILLUSTRATION AND QUICK EXPLANATION OF AILMENT

CONVENTIONAL AND ALTERNATIVE TREATMENTS

ADVICE ON WHEN TO CALL YOUR DOCTOR

POSSIBLE CAUSES

WHAT YOU CAN DO AT HOME

VISUAL GUIDE TO TREATMENT

ADVICE ON STAYING HEALTHY

DICTIONARY OF CONVENTIONAL MEDICINE AND ALTERNATIVE THERAPIES ▶

The world of medicine can seem bafflingly complex, with numerous fields of specialization apportioned between two broad sectors, generally called conventional and alternative. The definitions and explanations on the following pages offer a map of the terrain, one that covers all of the medical disciplines and therapeutic options cited in this book.

The distinction between conventional and alternative approaches to medicine is best understood in terms of basic perceptions of health. Conventional medicine, also called biomedicine, typically views health as an absence of disease. The main causes of illness are considered to be pathogens—bacteria or viruses—or biochemical imbalances. Scientific tests are often used in diagnosis, and drugs, surgery, and radiation are among the key tools for dealing with the problems. Alternative medicine, by contrast, tends to view health as a balance of body systems—mental, emotional, and spiritual, as well as physical. All aspects of a person are seen as interrelated—a principle called holism, meaning "state of wholeness." Any disharmony is thought to stress the body and perhaps lead to sickness. To fight disease, alternative medicine uses a wide range of therapies to bolster the body's own defenses and restore balance.

For suggestions on finding and working with a doctor or an alternative practitioner, see page 29.

CONVENTIONAL MEDICINE: MEDICAL SPECIALTIES

ALLERGY AND IMMUNOLOGY

Allergy is a subspecialty of immunology, the study of the workings of the immune system. Allergists treat such conditions as asthma, eczema, and hay fever—immune responses brought on by artificial or naturally occurring allergens in water, food, or the air.

ANESTHESIOLOGY

Anesthesiologists chemically induce unconsciousness in patients undergoing surgery, and they treat any heart or respiratory complications that may arise at that time. They may also provide and monitor various types of pain relief during other types of medical procedures, such as childbirth.

DENTISTRY

This field includes numerous specialties relating to the care of the teeth, gums, and jaws. **Dental surgeons** hold four-year dental degrees and emphasize family practice. **Orthodontists** have two additional years of specialized training in positioning teeth. **Oral surgeons,** with three years of added training, perform surgery for such conditions as temporomandibular joint syndrome and jaw reconstruction.

DERMATOLOGY

Dermatologists treat problems of the skin, mouth, hair, and nails—conditions such as acne, psoriasis, allergies, and skin cancer.

EPIDEMIOLOGY

Epidemiology is the statistical study of disease among populations or groups of people. Once dedicated to infectious diseases and epidemics, this specialty has expanded to cover noninfectious diseases such as cancer and heart disease.

FAMILY PRACTICE

Family practice physicians are generalists. Most of them provide a wide range of care, and they usually place special emphasis on looking after the medical, psychological, and social needs of families on a continuing basis. They will refer complicated problems to specialists.

INTERNAL MEDICINE

Internists focus on adult care and are experts on the workings of the internal organs and body systems. They treat a broad spectrum of problems, ranging from common complaints to severe diseases. Subspecialties of internal medicine include **cardiology,** which addresses disorders of the heart, lungs, and blood vessels (angina or atherosclerosis, for example); **endocrinology,** which covers disorders of the endocrine glands (diabetes or thyroid problems, for example); **gastroenterology,** targeting diseases of the digestive system, including stomach ulcers or colitis; **hematology,** which treats diseases of the blood, spleen, and lymph nodes (anemia or leukemia, for example); **infectious diseases,** focused on bacterial and viral diseases such as AIDS or meningitis; **nephrology,** dealing with problems of the kidneys; **oncology,** which is concerned with all forms of cancer; **pulmonology,** which treats the lungs and airways in conditions such as pneumonia, pleurisy, or emphysema; and **rheumatology,** which addresses diseases of the joints, muscles, bones, and tendons (arthritis, for example).

MEDICAL GENETICS

Medical geneticists counsel potential parents on the risks of passing on hereditary disorders, and diagnose such disorders in children after they're born.

NEUROLOGY

Neurologists focus on dysfunctions of the brain, spinal cord, peripheral nerves, and other parts of the nervous system. They frequently act as consultants to other physicians in determining the cause of such symptoms as dizziness or headaches, and they treat disorders ranging from Alzheimer's disease to multiple sclerosis.

NUCLEAR MEDICINE

Specialists in nuclear medicine administer radioactive materials internally to identify and treat disorders in body tissues and organs. Thyroid cancer, for example, can be detected and attacked with radioactive iodine, which is absorbed by thyroid cells.

OBSTETRICS AND GYNECOLOGY (OB-GYN)

Obstetrician-gynecologists care for women during pregnancy and childbirth. They also deal with female reproductive tract disorders, such as endometriosis, as well as conditions caused by imbalances in hormone production. They perform surgery, including Cesarean sections, tubal ligations, and hysterectomies.

OPHTHALMOLOGY

Ophthalmologists treat eye and vision problems, such as glaucoma or cataracts, often with drugs or surgery. They have medical degrees, unlike optometrists, who are licensed only to diagnose vision problems and prescribe glasses and contact lenses.

OTOLARYNGOLOGY (EAR, NOSE, AND THROAT)
Otolaryngologists deal with disorders of the ear, the nose, the throat, and related areas of the head and the neck. They are experts in assessing and treating hearing problems and sinus conditions as well as many other problems, and all are surgeons, trained to perform operations for such conditions as tonsillitis and deviated septum.

PATHOLOGY
Pathologists are trained to recognize the causes, the effects, and the characteristics of disease. They conduct their work primarily through laboratory analysis of tissue samples and

body fluids. They perform autopsies, and they also examine biopsies, often in order to determine the presence of cancer; they routinely serve as consultants to other physicians.

PEDIATRICS
Pediatricians specialize in the medical problems of children, from birth through adolescence, treating such ailments as asthma, diaper rash, chickenpox, abnormal growth and development, and sports-related injuries.

PHYSICAL MEDICINE AND REHABILITATION
Physiatrists work with patients who are injured or physically disabled, especially if the problem is musculoskeletal, neurological, or cardiovascular. They provide pain relief and help the patient regain or achieve a higher level of psychological and physical functioning.

HOW SPECIALISTS ARE CERTIFIED

Medical doctors in every state are required by law to have a license to practice; it is issued by a state licensing board upon their graduation from an accredited medical school and upon passage of a licensure exam. Many then continue their training in order to become specialists, and at the end of the process, they typically seek certification by a board of experts. In most cases, the board will be one that operates under the authority of a national oversight group, the American Board of Medical Specialties (ABMS).

To be certified by an ABMS-recognized board, doctors must complete a residency program lasting from three to seven years, depending upon the specialty, and pass an examination prepared and scored by the board's members. Some specialty boards allow doctors to apply for certification upon completing their residency; others—mostly surgical boards—require doctors to practice for a certain number of years and complete a set number of medical procedures before they can take the exam.

Specialists may go on to become subspecialists, which usually involves additional training and perhaps several years of practice, then passing an additional subspecialty exam admin-

istered by their primary specialty board. These boards sometimes require doctors to pass exams every 7 to 10 years in order to keep their certification.

The American Board of Medical Specialties, by far the best-known and most widely accepted certification authority, oversees 37 areas of specialization and 75 subspecialties. It does not have the certification field to itself, however. Certificates are also issued by self-designated boards—some entirely reputable, some not. These self-designated boards may not require that a specialist get extra training or pass an exam; in the most dubious cases, they may offer an impressive-looking diploma after a doctor merely attends a weekend course—or for no more than the payment of a fee.

With the growth of managed care programs, board certification has become a benchmark for doctors' qualifications, and most hospitals insist that a doctor be certified by one of the 24 member boards of the ABMS to have admitting privileges. Nonetheless, many doctors who are not board certified provide quality care—and it should be remembered that a certificate is never a measure of a doctor's personality or compassion. ■

PREVENTIVE MEDICINE

Preventive medicine specialists develop regimens to help at-risk groups learn healthful habits and avoid disease and injury. Their recommendations may address diet, behavior, occupational or environmental factors, and public awareness about healthcare.

PSYCHIATRY

Psychiatrists are physicians specializing in the treatment of mental, emotional, or addictive illnesses—among them, depression and anorexia nervosa. Like psychologists and clinical social workers, they use psychotherapy, but only psychiatrists have medical degrees and can prescribe drugs.

RADIOLOGY

Radiologists use external radiant energy in many forms to diagnose and treat diseases. Among their procedures are x-rays (including mammography), computed tomography (CT), positron emission tomography (PET), magnetic resonance imaging (MRI), and angiography.

SURGERY

General surgeons perform a wide range of operations involving many parts of the body. In addition, they are trained to recognize problems that should be referred to more highly specialized surgeons who must go through additional training and certification by their own surgical boards. These specialized categories include **colorectal,** to treat the lower digestive tract; **neurosurgery,** which deals with peripheral nerves as well as the brain and spinal cord; **orthopedic,** for problems in the musculoskeletal system; **otolaryngologic,** dealing with the head and neck; **plastic surgery,** to reconstruct, repair, or improve the appearance and function of any part of the body; and **cardio/thoracic,** focusing on the chest, especially the heart and lungs.

UROLOGY

Urologists specialize in genital and urinary tract disorders. Among the conditions they treat—by surgery, if necessary—are kidney stones, chronic bladder infections, and prostate problems. ■

ALTERNATIVE THERAPIES

ACUPRESSURE

This therapy involves pressing points on the body with fingers or hands to alter the internal flow of a supposed vital force or energy called chi (pronounced "chee"), strengthening it, calming it, or removing a blockage of the flow. Acupressure is one of a number of treatment methods regularly used in traditional Chinese medicine, or TCM, a system of healthcare that originated in China thousands of years ago and is still widely practiced in Asian countries today.

According to TCM, acupressure points are aligned along 14 bodily meridians, or pathways *(illustration, pages 22-23).* Twelve of the meridians are bilateral; that is, identical versions of them (with the same sets of points) exist on both sides of the body. The other two are unilateral, running along the midline of the body. The 14 meridians do not correspond to any known physiological processes or anatomical structures in the body, such as nerves or blood vessels. Nevertheless, some well-controlled studies suggest that acupressure can be effective for a number of health problems, including nausea, pain, and stroke-related weakness. A single point may be pressed for relief from a particular symptom or condition; or to promote overall well-being of the body, a series of points can be worked on in a specific order.

Acupressure can be administered by someone trained in the technique or it may be practiced at home. The force used on different points varies, but in general, most points call for a steady, downward pressure lasting one to two minutes. If you are applying pressure to a point several times in succession, complete this process on one side of the body before switching to the other side.

The risks of acupressure are minimal, provided certain cautions are observed. During pregnancy, the points designated Spleen 6 and Large Intestine 4 should never be used; avoid the abdominal area entirely, if possible. Never apply pressure to open wounds, varicose veins, tumors, inflamed or infected skin, sites of recent surgery, or areas where a broken bone is suspected.

ACUPUNCTURE

Acupuncture, like acupressure, is based on the traditional Chinese theory of meridians—energy pathways that are believed to run through the body, carrying the vital force or energy called chi. In this therapy, the flow of chi is controlled by the insertion of hair-thin needles at specific points—the same meridian-aligned ones used in acupressure *(illustration, pages 22-23).* Unlike acupressure, acupuncture must be performed by a trained practitioner.

An average treatment involves the insertion of 5 to 15 fine needles. They may penetrate as little as a fraction of an inch (on the fingertips, for example) or as much as three or four inches (where a thick layer of fat or muscle exists). The procedure usually causes little pain, although often there may be a tingling or heavy sensation. In addition to (or sometimes instead of) inserting needles, acupuncturists may opt for a treatment called moxibustion. This consists of applying heat directly above acupuncture points by means of small bundles of smoldering herbs, usually mugwort leaf.

The ability of acupuncture to relieve pain in many patients is well documented, and the physical basis of the pain relief has been demonstrated through laboratory tests on animals; acupuncture releases endorphins and other forms of neurotransmitters that serve as the body's natural painkillers. However, researchers remain unclear as to how acupuncture is able to provide long-lasting pain relief. Along with its pain-controlling benefits, acupuncture has been found effective in stroke rehabilitation and in providing relief from nausea. It has also been recommended as a treatment for drug addiction. The practice of acupuncture is licensed in 26 states and the District of Columbia.

AROMATHERAPY

In aromatherapy, the essential oils of plants are used to promote relaxation and help relieve the symptoms of certain ailments. Essential oils are extremely concentrated fragrant extracts, cold-pressed or steam-distilled from blossoms, leaves, or roots. The oils are diluted with so-called carrier oils, such as almond or soy, and can be applied through massage, mixed with water and used as compresses on the skin, added to a bath, or diffused into the air and inhaled. Essential oils should never be ingested; one drop of oil can be equivalent to an ounce or more of a whole plant. Taken internally, the oils of such plants as thuja, wormwood, mugwort leaf, tansy, hyssop, and sage are toxic, and they can even be lethal.

Aromatherapists believe that the fragrance of the oils has a soothing effect on the brain's limbic system, which is involved in memory, emotion, and hormone control. Some practitioners also theorize that the oils are absorbed through the skin and work directly in the body. However, critics of aromatherapy suggest that the relaxation attributed to the oils may actually be due to their application by massage, hot baths, and other pleasant methods.

AYURVEDIC MEDICINE

Ayurvedic medicine is a system of diagnosis and treatment that has been practiced in India for more than 5,000 years. The term Ayurveda comes from the Sanskrit roots *āyur,* which means "life," and *veda,* meaning "knowledge." Ayurvedic theory holds that all diseases of the body arise from stresses in the awareness, or consciousness, of the individual; the stresses lead to unhealthy lifestyles, producing a cycle of ill health. Physical manifestations of disease are attributed to the imbalance of three basic physiological principles, called *doshas.* The *vata* dosha represents the kinetic energy of the body; vata makes the heart beat, causes blood to flow, and stimulates brain and nerve functions. The *kapha* dosha is potential energy, responsible for physical strength and the lubrication of tissues. The *pitta* dosha, considered a mediator between vata and kapha, governs the metabolic processes of the body, from digestion to cell operation. If these three principles cease to operate in harmony, sickness ensues. Evaluation of the doshas is performed by a technique called *nadi vigyan,* which involves taking the pulse at the wrist; this assessment determines the precise form treatment will take.

Ayurvedic practitioners prescribe a variety of precise body postures, all derived from the age-old discipline of yoga, along with breathing exercises and meditative techniques *(see Mind/Body Medicine: Yoga, page 27).* In addition, practitioners use herbs, emetics and enemas, oil massage, and dosha-specific diets toward a goal of helping detoxify the system and bring it back into balance.

Some Ayurvedic herbal mixtures have been found to contain high levels of lead and can be toxic. Be sure to thoroughly investigate the ingredients of any remedy before using it; don't hesitate to ask the practitioner about this.

BODY WORK

Body work is an umbrella term for the many techniques, both ancient and modern, that promote relaxation and treat ailments (especially those of the musculoskeletal system) through lessons in proper movement, postural reeducation, exercise, massage, and various other forms of bodily manipulation. Some types of body work—including massage, qigong, reflexology, shiatsu, and t'ai chi—can be practiced at home. Others may require the guidance of a trained professional. Forms of body work include the following:

- ◆ **The Alexander technique** focuses on correcting habitual posture and movement patterns that are believed to damage or impair the body's functioning.
- ◆ **Aston-Patterning** is a technique that tailors guided movement and postural retraining to the particular characteristics of each client's body.
- ◆ **The Feldenkrais method** features individual sessions performed by a trained practitioner, during which verbally directed exercises, touch, and movement are used to teach new patterns in order to improve posture, movement, and breathing.
- ◆ **Hellerwork,** an offshoot of **Rolfing** (Structural Integra-

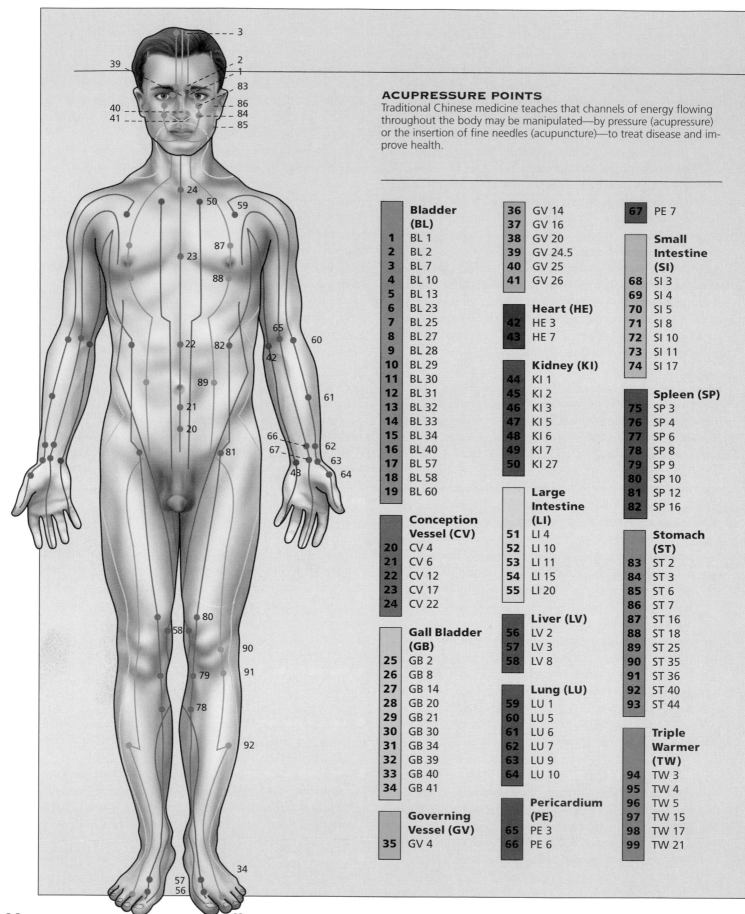

ACUPRESSURE POINTS

Traditional Chinese medicine teaches that channels of energy flowing throughout the body may be manipulated—by pressure (acupressure) or the insertion of fine needles (acupuncture)—to treat disease and improve health.

Bladder (BL)
1 BL 1
2 BL 2
3 BL 7
4 BL 10
5 BL 13
6 BL 23
7 BL 25
8 BL 27
9 BL 28
10 BL 29
11 BL 30
12 BL 31
13 BL 32
14 BL 33
15 BL 34
16 BL 40
17 BL 57
18 BL 58
19 BL 60

Conception Vessel (CV)
20 CV 4
21 CV 6
22 CV 12
23 CV 17
24 CV 22

Gall Bladder (GB)
25 GB 2
26 GB 8
27 GB 14
28 GB 20
29 GB 21
30 GB 30
31 GB 34
32 GB 39
33 GB 40
34 GB 41

Governing Vessel (GV)
35 GV 4

36 GV 14
37 GV 16
38 GV 20
39 GV 24.5
40 GV 25
41 GV 26

Heart (HE)
42 HE 3
43 HE 7

Kidney (KI)
44 KI 1
45 KI 2
46 KI 3
47 KI 5
48 KI 6
49 KI 7
50 KI 27

Large Intestine (LI)
51 LI 4
52 LI 10
53 LI 11
54 LI 15
55 LI 20

Liver (LV)
56 LV 2
57 LV 3
58 LV 8

Lung (LU)
59 LU 1
60 LU 5
61 LU 6
62 LU 7
63 LU 9
64 LU 10

Pericardium (PE)
65 PE 3
66 PE 6

67 PE 7

Small Intestine (SI)
68 SI 3
69 SI 4
70 SI 5
71 SI 8
72 SI 10
73 SI 11
74 SI 17

Spleen (SP)
75 SP 3
76 SP 4
77 SP 6
78 SP 8
79 SP 9
80 SP 10
81 SP 12
82 SP 16

Stomach (ST)
83 ST 2
84 ST 3
85 ST 6
86 ST 7
87 ST 16
88 ST 18
89 ST 25
90 ST 35
91 ST 36
92 ST 40
93 ST 44

Triple Warmer (TW)
94 TW 3
95 TW 4
96 TW 5
97 TW 15
98 TW 17
99 TW 21

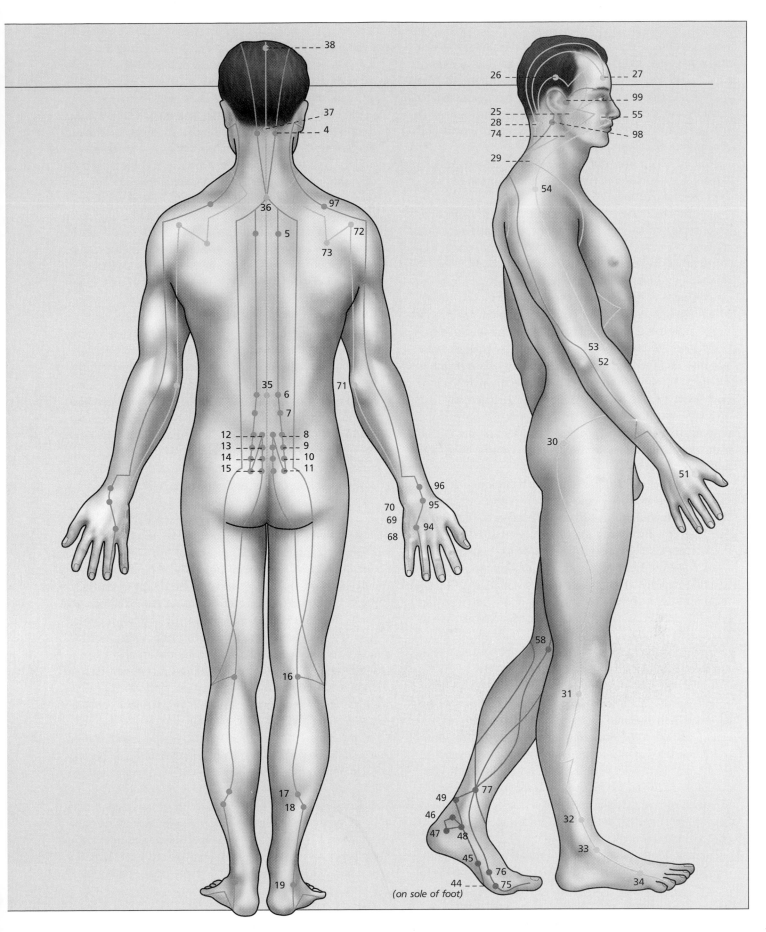

(on sole of foot)

tion), combines touch and movement retraining to teach stress-free methods for performing everyday activities.

◆ **Massage** includes an assortment of manual therapies that manipulate the soft tissues of the body in order to reduce tension and stress, increase circulation, aid the healing of muscle and other soft-tissue injuries, control pain, and promote overall well-being.

◆ **Myotherapy** is a form of deep massage used to reduce tension and pain originating in specific points in the muscle layers of the body.

◆ **Qigong** ("chee-goong"), an ancient Chinese discipline, emphasizes breathing, meditation, and stationary and moving exercises to enhance the flow of energy or chi (sometimes also spelled "qi") through the body.

◆ **Reflexology** involves the manipulation of specific areas on the feet—and sometimes the hands—with the goal of bringing the body into homeostasis, or balance. According to reflexologists, distinct regions of the feet (*illustration, page 25*) correspond to particular organs or body systems, and the stimulation of the appropriate region is intended to eliminate energy blockages thought to produce pain or disease in the associated structures. The arrangement of reflexology areas on the feet mirrors the organization of the body to the extent that organs on the right side of the body are represented on the right foot, and so with the left.

Reflexology features a few basic techniques that can be performed either by yourself or by a partner. The basic thumb technique uses the inside edge of the thumb pad (the side away from the fingers) to "walk" along reflex areas; walking consists of a forward, creeping movement, with the first joint of the thumb bending and unbending slightly as the digit inches ahead. The finger technique uses the same walking motion but with the edge of the index finger closest to the thumb. When working a specific area, one hand should work and the other should hold the foot in a comfortable position with the sole flat and toes straight.

Practitioners of reflexology claim that it can relieve a wide variety of ailments. Critics say that treatments are no more than glorified foot massages.

◆ **Rolfing,** also called Structural Integration, is based on the belief that proper alignment of the various parts of the body is necessary for physical and emotional health. The method uses deep massage and movement exercises to loosen or release adhesions in the fascia—the connective tissue covering muscles—in an effort to bring the body back into correct alignment.

◆ **Shiatsu,** a Japanese technique similar to acupressure, uses finger and thumb pressure on precise body points to encourage the proper flow of chi—or ki, as the Japanese call it—a vital force or energy believed to circulate through the body.

◆ **T'ai chi,** one style of qigong, is a martial art involving meditation and slow, flowing self-guided movements that follow set forms. It is intended to affect the flow of chi (energy) and bring about physical self-awareness.

◆ **Therapeutic Touch** does not involve actual physical contact, despite its name. The practitioner's hands move in slow, rhythmic motions two to six inches above the patient in an effort to detect what are said to be blockages in the body's energy field that may cause or contribute to illness. The technique was devised a few decades ago as a contemporary version of various ancient practices in which a healer consciously strives to direct and focus energy to the receiver to balance and unblock energy flows. Sessions typically last about 20 minutes and are said to produce a sense of relaxed well-being as well as relief from pain and other symptoms.

◆ **Trager Psychophysical Integration** (Trager approach) features gentle touch and rhythmic rocking and shaking movement, along with a series of directed body exercises intended to help identify and correct chronic tension patterns that affect posture and movement. Research suggests that it is beneficial for people with severe neuromuscular problems produced by injury or such diseases as multiple sclerosis or muscular dystrophy.

CHINESE HERBS

The use of herbs, along with acupuncture and acupressure, is a major component of the system of traditional Chinese medicine, or TCM. Doctors of traditional Chinese medicine usually practice under the title "licensed," or "certified," acupuncturist, and they prescribe herbal combinations according to complex rules of diagnosis, which are intended to help the body correct imbalances of energies. In TCM, ailments are believed to be caused by disturbances in the bodily flow of a type of energy called chi, or by a lack of balance in the complementary states of yin (which is characterized by darkness and quiet) and yang (which is characterized by light and activity).

Chinese herbs, like other TCM remedies (such as minerals and animal products, like hide and bone), can be prepared in numerous ways: steeped in hot water to make a tea or infusion; boiled to produce a stronger solution called a decoction; used to make powders, pills, or syrups that may all be taken internally; and fashioned into plasters or poultices that are applied to the skin. Treatments should be prescribed and monitored by a trained practitioner, because some Chinese herbs can be toxic in large doses; others, such

REFLEXOLOGY AREAS

Manually working specific areas on the feet is thought by proponents of reflexology to improve the function of corresponding organs and body parts. For more information, see page 24.

RIGHT BOTTOM

BRAIN

LEFT BOTTOM

SINUS / HEAD / BRAIN

SIDE / NECK

PITUITARY / PINEAL

SINUS / HEAD / BRAIN

THROAT / NECK / THYROID

EYES / EARS

ESOPHAGUS

EYES / EARS

LUNG / BREAST

THYMUS

HEART

ARM

THYROID / BRONCHI

LUNG / BREAST

SHOULDER

SOLAR PLEXUS

ARM

DIAPHRAGM

SHOULDER

GALL BLADDER

ADRENAL GLANDS

DIAPHRAGM

LIVER

KIDNEYS

STOMACH

WAISTLINE

DUODENUM

SPLEEN

ASCENDING COLON

TRANSVERSE COLON

PANCREAS

ILEOCECAL VALVE AND APPENDIX

URETER TUBES

WAISTLINE

SMALL INTESTINE

BLADDER

DESCENDING COLON

SCIATIC

SACRUM / COCCYX

SIGMOID COLON

SCIATIC

RIGHT OUTSIDE

SCIATIC
PELVIC AREA
HIP / BACK / SCIATIC
OVARY / TESTICLE
PROSTATE / UTERUS / RECTUM / SCIATIC
LYMPH / GROIN / FALLOPIAN TUBE
UTERUS / PROSTATE
BLADDER
BREAST / LUNG
SINUS / HEAD / BRAIN
ARM / SHOULDER
LOWER BACK

RIGHT INSIDE

CERVICAL THORACIC LUMBAR SACRUM / COCCYX

SPINAL COLUMN

LYMPH / GROIN / FALLOPIAN TUBE

KNEE / LEG / HIP / LOWER BACK

CHEST / LUNG / BREAST / BACK

TOP RIGHT

as safflower flowers, should be used with caution during pregnancy. Complex mixtures should be formulated only by a trained practitioner.

In recent years, Chinese herbal medicine has been subjected to increasingly rigorous study in China, the United States, and elsewhere. The evidence indicates that although some remedies do not perform as claimed, others are effective. In China today, herbal remedies are often prescribed along with modern biomedical treatments.

CHIROPRACTIC

Chiropractic, a system of healing taught in its own five-year medical colleges and licensed in all 50 states according to standards set by the Council of Chiropractic Education and the Federation of Chiropractic Licensing Boards, is based on the idea that the human body has an innate self-healing ability and seeks homeostasis, or balance. According to chiropractic theory, the nervous system plays a significant role in maintaining homeostasis—and hence health. But problems in the joints, called subluxations, are believed to interfere with proper functioning of the nervous system, and as a result, the body's ability to maintain optimal health is diminished. Chiropractors seek to bring the body back into balance through manual manipulation of the spine and other joints and muscles, allowing the neuromusculoskeletal system to function smoothly.

Today, chiropractors are divided into two major camps. One, traditionalist in stance, sees subluxations as the cause of most ailments. The other, considered progressive, aims at establishing chiropractors as providers of primary care, emphasizing the treatment of back pain and musculoskeletal problems, along with manipulation.

Although chiropractic is categorized as alternative medicine, it has gained a degree of acceptance, in part because of a number of recent studies that have shown it to be quite effective in treating problems such as acute lower-back pain. The services of chiropractors are covered by Medicare and, in many states, by Medicaid and most major private plans.

HERBAL THERAPIES

Herbal medicines are prepared from a variety of plant materials—leaves, stems, roots, bark, and so on. They usually contain many biologically active ingredients and are used primarily for treating mild or chronic ailments. (At least a quarter of all conventional pharmaceuticals include some of the same ingredients, although generally in purified form.) Herbs can be prepared at home in many ways, using either fresh or dried ingredients. Herbal teas and infusions can be steeped to varying strengths. Roots, bark, or other plant parts can be boiled into strong solutions called decoctions. Honey or sugar can be added to infusions and decoctions to make syrups. In stores, herbal remedies can also be purchased in the form of pills, capsules, or powders, or in more concentrated liquid forms called extracts and tinctures. They can be applied topically in creams or ointments, soaked into cloths and used as compresses, or applied directly to the skin as poultices.

In the United States today, herbal remedies are not regulated and come in unpredictable strengths; the amount of the active ingredients varies greatly, depending on whether more than one species of the herb is used and how and when the herb is gathered and prepared. Because some herbs can be toxic or carcinogenic, all herbs should be used under the guidance of a healthcare practitioner familiar with herbal medicine.

Across the spectrum of alternative medicine, the use of herbs is varied: Naturopathic medicine, traditional Chinese medicine, and Ayurvedic medicine all differ in how diseases are diagnosed and what herbal remedies are prescribed. For more information on herbal medicines, see About Herbal Preparations (pages 911–912).

HOMEOPATHY

Homeopathy, founded by a German physician named Samuel Hahnemann in the 1790s, is based on the idea that "like cures like"; that is, substances that cause certain symptoms in a healthy person can also cure those same symptoms in someone who is sick. This so-called law of similars gives homeopathy its name: "homeo" for similar, "pathy" designating disease. In his experiments, Hahnemann developed a method of "potentizing" homeopathic remedies by diluting them in a water-alcohol solution and then vigorously shaking (or succussing) the mixtures. The results convinced him that a high degree of dilution not only minimizes the side effects of the remedies but also simultaneously enhances their medical efficacy.

Modern homeopaths usually prescribe doses at dilution ratios ranging from 1x (1 part substance to 9 parts dilution medium) to 200c (200 repetitions of diluting 1 part substance with 99 parts dilution medium); higher ratios are indicated with an "m," for a 1 to 999 ratio. (See also About Homeopathic Remedies, page 913.) Critics of homeopathy argue that, in the more extreme dilution ratios (which are considered higher potencies), the remedies may not contain even a single molecule of the original healing substance. Nonetheless, studies have shown that homeopathic remedies may be effective for certain disorders, such as childhood diarrhea, hay fever, asthma, and the flu. Further research is now being conducted under the auspices of the National Institutes of Health.

Most homeopathic remedies have undergone "provings," or medical observations in which healthy individuals are given doses of undiluted homeopathic substances. Mental, emotional, and physical changes brought on during these tests help provide homeopathic physicians with a better understanding of which remedy will best suit a particular set of symptoms. Over the past 200 years, provings for almost 2,000 substances have been conducted.

The majority of homeopaths practice "constitutional" homeopathy, based on the idea that each person's constitution—or mental, physical, and emotional makeup—may need to be treated along with any specific ailments. Classically, only one homeopathic medicine is used at a time. An extensive patient history is taken and the patient's physical and psychological symptoms are observed, then an initial prescription is made. If the medication does not have the desired effect or if the symptoms persist, a second analysis is done and a second prescription is given. This process continues until the correct medication for the underlying ailment is found. Constitutional treatment is generally used for chronic problems; acute, or short-term, ailments are usually treated with remedies specific to the illness.

Recently, over-the-counter combination homeopathic remedies have become available for a wide variety of common ailments. These products contain several of the most common remedies for a particular problem and can be useful for self-treatment of minor conditions. For prolonged or serious illness, a professional homeopath can prescribe specific single remedies.

Homeopathic practitioners usually have prior medical training, such as a degree in medicine, osteopathy, or naturopathic medicine. The pharmaceuticals they prescribe are recognized and regulated by the FDA, and may be purchased over the counter at specialty drugstores.

HYDROTHERAPY

Hydrotherapy, literally meaning water therapy, uses ice, liquid, and steam to relieve the symptoms of numerous types of infections, acute and chronic pain, circulatory problems, and more. Treatments include wraps, sprays, and douches, as well as steam rooms and saunas, and both hot and cold baths—among them, whirlpool baths, hand or foot baths, and sitz baths, which involve immersion of only the pelvic area. The aim is to stimulate an immune response or to detoxify the body by changing body temperature. Hydrotherapy is often used by naturopaths.

MIND/BODY MEDICINE

This umbrella term covers activities and therapies that focus on the interrelationship of mind and body; the goal in all forms of mind/body medicine is to address particular disorders and promote overall health by combining both mental and physical approaches. Yoga, for example, involves both physical movement and a meditative state of mind, and may serve the dual purpose of improving a person's physical condition and combating emotional problems such as depression and anxiety. As noted below, the two-way connection between mind and body is exploited in many ways to influence the hormonal, nervous, and immune systems.

◆ **Biofeedback** uses computerized machines to measure and display body functions and states such as heart rate, skin temperature, muscle tension, and brain activity. By monitoring these functions through stages of rest and activity, patients are able to see how and why they change, and eventually can learn to control them.

◆ **Guided imagery** teaches patients to imagine scenarios that may help influence certain physiological conditions. A cancer patient, for example, may imagine a tumor dissolving under an attack by immune system "bullets." While there are no conclusive studies on imagery, patients often report physical and psychological benefits.

◆ **Hypnotherapy,** administered by a professional, uses a relaxed, focused state of awareness to help change physiological and psychological reactions to pain, illness, or anxiety. Self-hypnosis may be learned and applied to certain conditions as well.

◆ **Meditation** includes a number of different Asian and Western practices. All share the basic characteristics of sitting or resting quietly, often with the eyes closed, and performing mental exercises designed to relax the body and focus concentration.

◆ The **relaxation response** is a state of psychological and physiological rest characterized by lowered oxygen consumption and reduced heart rate. It can be induced by many different techniques, including **meditation, yoga, t'ai chi, qigong,** and **hypnotherapy.** This deep relaxation can relieve stress and its many symptoms.

◆ **Spirituality** is a source of relaxation and comfort for many people, whether it involves practicing a particular religion or contemplating spiritual values outside of a religious context.

◆ **Support groups** bring together people who are suffering from the same disease or similar types of trauma. Within the group, they can share experiences and feelings, which may yield great psychological benefits and perhaps improve the functioning of their natural bodily defenses as well.

◆ **Yoga** is a series of body positions and movements developed over thousands of years to calm the mind, relax the body, and ease the spirit (see also Ayurvedic Medicine, *page 21).* Meditation and breathing exercises lead into cycles of stretches and poses that may vary from session to session. Yoga can be learned and practiced at home; however, modified movements may be required during pregnancy or if a person has a condition such as heart disease. A yoga specialist can recommend the appropriate adjustments.

NATUROPATHIC MEDICINE

Naturopathic medicine provides holistic, or whole body, healthcare by taking advantage of resources drawn from numerous traditional healing systems. Dating back to the early part of the 20th century, naturopathy is organized around three fundamental principles: The physician should strive to aid the body's natural healing abilities; the root cause of an illness should be addressed rather than its symptoms; and above all, only therapies that cause no harm should be used (which means that toxic drugs and surgery are avoided whenever possible).

A naturopathic doctor, or ND, may pay considerable attention to a patient's lifestyle, since naturopathic theory holds that physical, psychological, and even spiritual elements can all contribute to disease. In treating patients, the naturopathic practitioner may use a number of alternative therapies, including homeopathy, herbal remedies, traditional Chinese medicine, spinal manipulation, nutrition, hydrotherapy, massage, and exercise.

Doctors of naturopathy train at accredited four-year naturopathic medical schools. The first two years include many of the same core science classes as regular medical schools, while the final two years focus on training in natural healing techniques. At present, naturopathic doctors are licensed to practice in nine states; most other states allow them to practice in limited ways. Many private insurance plans cover naturopathic care.

NUTRITION AND DIET

Conventional and alternative practitioners alike acknowledge the importance of a healthful diet. Alternative practitioners, however, place more emphasis on dietary intervention in some conditions where conventional medicine would resort first to drugs or even surgery. Treatment of atherosclerosis, for example, may take the form of an extremely low-fat diet along with a program of meditation, exercise, and support-group therapy.

Some diets, such as traditional Japanese and Mediterranean ones, contain small amounts of animal fat. Because they are low in saturated fats, these diets appear to protect against heart disease and some forms of cancer. Vegetarian diets have been shown to lower blood pressure and reduce the risk of cardiovascular disease and some cancers. Particular foods may be beneficial: Garlic, for example, is said to reduce the levels of cholesterol in the bloodstream and protect against some forms of cancer.

Vitamins and mineral supplements figure in the dietary recommendations of many therapies. Although some vitamins, such as A and D, are fat-soluble and can reach toxic levels in the body if not carefully monitored, others, like vitamin C, are water-soluble and are not stored; any bodily excess is usually excreted. Generally, vitamins and minerals are recommended for daily use as a preventive measure. They often come in tablet form, and doses are measured by weight in milligrams (mg), or thousandths of a gram; in micrograms (mcg), or millionths of a gram; or in a universal standard known as international units (IU). Orthomolecular medicine, a form of nutrient therapy, uses combinations of vitamins, minerals, and amino acids normally found in the body to treat specific conditions, such as asthma, heart disease, depression, and schizophrenia. Such therapy can also be used to maintain general good health.

OSTEOPATHY

Osteopathy focuses on correcting structural problems in the musculoskeletal system to improve overall bodily functioning. To restore structural balance and thus help a patient regain health, an osteopathic physician will combine manipulation of the joints, physical therapy, and instruction in proper posture. Because osteopathic care is holistic, or targeted at the whole body, the doctor also considers psychological factors, lifestyle, and diet in addressing an illness and maintaining health.

Ever since it was founded by an American doctor named Andrew Taylor Still in the late 19th century, osteopathy has blended all aspects of conventional medicine with its central tenets of the importance of the body's structure and its predisposition toward health over illness. Doctors of osteopathy, or DOs, train at their own four-year medical colleges and can enter either MD or DO residency programs. They are licensed to practice in all 50 states, and can prescribe drugs, perform surgery, and further specialize in any of the medical subspecialties, such as cardiology, neurology, or obstetrics and gynecology.

Apart from the emphasis they place on musculoskeletal function and alignment (an emphasis that can vary from doctor to doctor), most osteopathic physicians practice much like conventional medical doctors. ∎

HOW TO CHOOSE A HEALTHCARE PRACTITIONER

Becoming a patient means becoming a consumer, with the same options and rights as a purchaser of any other service or product. To ensure satisfaction in the medical marketplace, you need to know how to find or change doctors, what sort of relationship to expect, and when to seek a second opinion.

CONVENTIONAL MEDICINE

For a doctor who will oversee your general health (and also suggest specialists when necessary), a good choice within conventional medicine is a family physician with an emphasis on long-term primary care. When looking for candidates, ask for names and recommendations from a regional hospital or medical school, or try a local pharmacist. You may find that family and friends can provide valuable opinions based on their experience with particular doctors. In your search, don't hesitate to act on personal considerations such as a preference for a male or female doctor, or an older or younger one. If you have beliefs or philosophies that play a major role in your healthcare, be sure that you choose a doctor who will respect your views. If board certification is important to you, medical directories—such as the *Directory of Medical Specialists,* published for the American Board of Medical Specialties—can provide the necessary information; these directories can usually be found at a local library. *(For more information on board certification, see page 19.)*

The doctor-patient relationship is built on mutual respect, trust, and communication; you should keep this in mind as you evaluate someone you are considering as your regular physician. Your doctor should take time to explain procedures to you and discuss optional treatment plans—all the while avoiding confusing medical jargon and allowing you to ask questions and add observations of your own. Although bedside manner is not a gauge of skill, a physician should be friendly and approachable. But keep up your end of the doctor-patient commitment by being on time for your appointments, following through on all treatment plans, and reporting any new symptoms or adverse drug responses immediately.

If you are ever given a diagnosis that requires surgery, involves a debilitating or fatal disease, or calls for very complex or costly treatment, you should seek a second opinion. You have an absolute right to one; moreover, some insurance plans actually require a second opinion before approving certain medical procedures. Your doctor should readily provide you with a referral upon request and also should be prepared to share your medical records with other physicians. If you are reluctant to ask for a referral, call a local hospital or medical school to get one, or consult medical directories in your local library.

ALTERNATIVE MEDICINE

When searching for an alternative practitioner, you may want to begin with a recommendation from a conventional doctor. Illness-related self-help groups and books on alternative healing can also be good sources for names. You should fully investigate any alternative practitioner's background and experience and be aware of any licensing requirements in your state or district. Be extremely suspicious of anyone who expresses hostility or derision toward mainstream medicine or makes grandiose claims for a cure. Get explicit information about the treatment you will receive, and remember that *you* are in charge of the entire treatment process. Above all, trust your own instincts and judgment. ■

GENERAL GUIDELINES TO HEALTH ▶

This section is a brief summary of basic health issues related to different stages of life—beginning with infancy, moving into childhood and adolescence, and continuing through maturity and old age. Understanding normal human development and the potential problems males and females face throughout life is one of the keys to establishing a personal plan for healthful living. By adopting good habits and making sensible lifestyle choices at an early age, you can help ensure full, healthy lives for yourself and other family members.

CONTENTS

CHILDREN'S HEALTH

A new baby is probably the most exciting and challenging event a family experiences. A good prenatal program will see that you and your partner are well prepared to care for the new family member. Most babies are born with everything they need to grow into healthy adults, but it's never too early to start preventive healthcare practices to ensure your child's long-term health and well-being.

Every child should have regular medical checkups, learn to practice good hygiene and nutrition, and get plenty of rest and exercise. For the first several years, a family doctor or pediatrician should monitor your baby's development and be on call when the inevitable childhood ailments come along. A baby gets a hepatitis shot shortly after birth and should have a complete course of inoculations before the age of two. Your state or locality will require inoculations against certain infectious childhood diseases, and no child should start school without them. *(See the Immunization Schedule, opposite.)*

Most children develop in size, stature, and motor skills at roughly the same age, but don't be overly concerned if your child's milestones are slightly different from those of other children in the family or the neighborhood. If your child's development differs significantly or consistently from that of peers, you may want to consult your pediatrician. In addition to your child's physical health, mental and emotional well-being needs to be developed and nurtured. Affection and support from family and friends help encourage self-confidence, and interacting with children of a similar age cultivates important socialization skills.

INFANCY (BIRTH TO 1 YEAR)

Even though an infant seems helpless, the first year of life is a period of remarkable growth and development. Care for your child's health during this period begins with a complete physical examination at birth, during which your baby's heart rate, breathing, and reflexes will be checked. The remains of the umbilical cord usually fall off within the first two weeks. Until then, clean the stump every day with alcohol and keep it dry. If your baby boy has been circumcised, keep his penis dry and cover it at each diaper change with a gauze pad moistened with petroleum jelly until healing is complete.

A newborn's head has two soft spots, or fontanels, where the skull plates have not yet fused together. The smaller spot on the back of the head usually closes 8 to 12 weeks after birth; the larger spot in the front generally closes between 6 and 18 months. Even though the brain is covered by a tough membrane, these soft spots should be safeguarded from injury. The fontanels will rise and fall as the baby breathes or cries. If you notice an unusually bulging or sunken soft spot, however, notify your doctor.

Usually for the first six months, a baby's nutritional needs are satisfied by either breast milk or infant formula; breast-feeding is also often supplemented by the occasional bottle. A big advantage of breast-feeding is that breast milk helps the baby's immune system fight off infections and may help protect against allergies in the future. At about six months your infant may be ready to start eating soft foods; drinking from a cup typically comes a few months later. Your pediatrician can advise you about weaning your child completely from the breast or the bottle. Most children triple their birthweight during this first year. *(See Growth Charts, pages 34-35.)*

Spitting up a small amount of milk or food soon after eating is normal for an infant, as he gets rid of swallowed air and gas. If he vomits frequently and has a fever or diarrhea, or if you see blood or green bile in the vomit, however, call your pediatrician. In newborns, stools are greenish black or mustard-colored and may be very watery; breast-fed babies usually have more bowel movements than those fed on formula. To prevent diaper rash, change diapers before or after each feeding, after each bowel movement, and every time the baby wakes from a sleep. Wash and dry the diaper area at each change; if you see signs of irritation, apply a mild skin ointment or barrier cream.

The baby's first vocal response is crying, which usually stops when he is held or fed. *(See Colic.)* At one to two weeks your baby will start following your eyes with his own, and at four to six weeks he may smile at a nearby face; what looks like a smile before this age is probably just a reaction to intestinal gas. By about 12 weeks you can expect to hear his first laugh. Sometime between 5 and 10 months, most babies get their first teeth, and some babies have as many as eight teeth by their first birthday.

At the age of about three to four months, many babies are able to raise their head and shoulders when lying on their stomach. By six months, an infant may be able to sit up with some help. Most children learn to crawl at about eight months, and about the time of their first birthday they take their first independent steps. Children of this age may also point with their fingers and speak a few intelligible words, including "mama" and "dada."

Some babies have patches of discolored skin, or birthmarks, on their face or body. Most birthmarks are harmless and fade away as the child ages, although tan, brown, or purplish red birthmarks may be permanent. Because some skin marks are disfiguring, and in rare cases carry a risk of cancer, ask your doctor about treatment options.

Children are naturally inquisitive and need to be protected from accidentally hurting themselves. Before your child starts to crawl, take steps to childproof your home. You can, for example, install safety gates at the top and bottom of stairs and put childproof latches on doors and cabinets; you may also want to put protective covers over electrical outlets. If your child injures himself, refer to the Emergencies/First Aid section for appropriate care. Infants may also have minor health problems, including anal fissures, croup, diarrhea, constipation, eczema, gastroenteritis, and jaundice.

A baby should sleep on a firm mattress. Some experts recommend that to prevent your baby from being smoth-ered in bed, you should not cover him with a fluffy comforter or blanket, and should keep all pillows or stuffed animals out of the crib during the first year. Sudden infant death syndrome (SIDS), or crib death, happens to some babies in their sleep without apparent cause. SIDS strikes about 1 out of 2,000 babies in the first year, affects more boys than girls, and occurs more frequently in colder months. Placing the baby on his back or side to sleep is believed to reduce the risk of SIDS.

YOUR PRESCHOOL CHILD (AGES 1 TO 5)

The next few years are a period of rapid development. Your child's individuality becomes more apparent, especially as language skills improve. At 18 months she can stack blocks, throw a ball, and push toys around the room. She will soon be able to run, walk up and down stairs without help, and feed herself with a spoon.

IMMUNIZATION SCHEDULE

DISEASE	Birth	2 Months	4 Months	6 Months	6-18 Months	12-15 Months	12-18 Months	4-6 Years	11-12 Years	14-16 Years
Hepatitis B			△							▲
Diphtheria										■
Tetanus										■
Pertussis (whooping cough)										
Hemophilus influenzae B				●						
Polio										
Measles									□	
Mumps									□	
Rubella (German measles)									□	
Chickenpox							O			

Immunization against contagious diseases is one of the most important aspects of preventive healthcare, protecting not only individuals but the general public. Because certain types of immunization are effective only for limited periods, booster shots are required to maintain immunity. The inoculations listed above are recommended for all children by the Advisory Committee on Immunization Practices. State and local health authorities may recommend or require specific inoculations before a child can attend public school. From time to time, other inoculations may be recommended or required to prevent or control the spread of communicable diseases.

Key

△ If not given at birth.

□ If not given at 4-6 years.

O If your child is older and has not yet had chickenpox, this vaccine may be given at any time.

▲ If your child was not inoculated as an infant, this shot should be given before leaving high school.

■ Booster needed every 10 years.

● Depending on the vaccine used, may not be required.

Some children use simple words at about one year, but long before they start putting words together as statements, they understand and respond with actions to much of what you say. During the second year a child may be easily frustrated and throw temper tantrums. Learning to disregard such outbursts, while praising your child's positive behavior, is a parent's best course of action.

Two-year-olds are able to run well and are beginning to dress and undress themselves. Most children are toilet-trained by this age and stay dry all day, although some, particularly boys, may not stay dry all night until age five or six. Their vocabularies expand dramatically, and by her third birthday, your child will probably be speaking short sentences. She will crave your affection and approval, and will understand your disapproval. Between 18 months and three years, a child becomes more responsive—and sometimes deliberately unresponsive—to parental guidance. During this period, sometimes called the terrible twos, children are developing a sense

of independence as well as responsibility. As much as children enjoy praise for things they do well, don't be surprised when they occasionally answer "no" to your requests.

Three-year-olds learn to use simple sentences, get dressed and undressed with help, and use the toilet on their own. They will play with more complicated toys, such as swings, slides, and tricycles. They are now more interested in interacting with playmates, rather than just playing alongside them as one- and two-year-olds do. At this age, signs of sibling rivalry and jealousy are not unusual. If your child hasn't done so already, he is likely to stop sucking his thumb or finger during this year.

By the age of four, children are using more complex sentences. A sense of imagination may make your child fear the dark or imaginary monsters; such fears are normal and usually disappear in a year or two. Five-year-olds have the motor skills to hop on one foot and skip. Physical independence and curiosity make young children particularly acci-

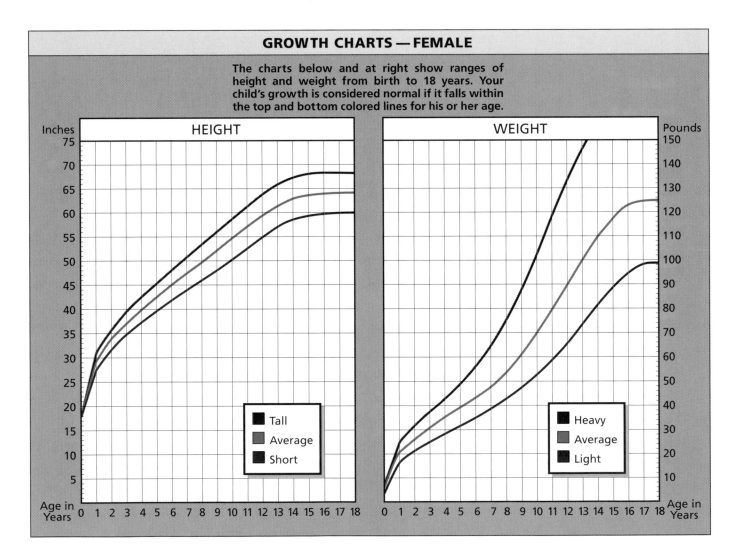

GROWTH CHARTS — FEMALE

The charts below and at right show ranges of height and weight from birth to 18 years. Your child's growth is considered normal if it falls within the top and bottom colored lines for his or her age.

dent prone. Most scrapes and bruises heal quickly, but some injuries may require medical attention. You and your family should be alert for hazards to children—such as fires or unfenced pools—that could cause severe injuries.

The preschool child may contract such illnesses as the common cold, flu, or strep throat, especially when exposed to other children in group activities. Many childhood illnesses are accompanied by fever. Unlike an adult, a child under the age of eight may suffer no ill effects from a temperature as high as 106°F (41.1°C), although a child between one and three years with a fever over 101°F (38.3°C) may suffer febrile seizures. Such seizures are frightening to a parent but are rarely life-threatening to the child. *(See Emergencies/First Aid: Seizures.)*

YOUR SCHOOL-AGE CHILD (AGES 6 TO 12)
By age six, most children enter elementary school, where the relaxed atmosphere of preschool and kindergarten is re-placed with more structure and regimentation. In the classroom and in organized sports, the school-age child is presented with opportunities for intellectual, physical, and psychological growth. Many children develop close friendships, usually with children of the same sex. Your child will begin learning to read and write; those who experience unusual difficulty with schoolwork can be tested for developmental problems, such as attention deficit disorder, or specific learning disabilities, such as dyslexia.

Once a child starts school, she is likely to be exposed to chickenpox and other infectious illnesses. Baby teeth begin to fall out, usually painlessly. Except for wisdom teeth, the permanent teeth are usually in place by the early teens. Your child should have dental examinations every six months, and if the teeth do not come in straight, you may want to consult an orthodontist about corrective work.

Some children between the ages of three and nine experience severe, recurring "growing pains" in the arms and

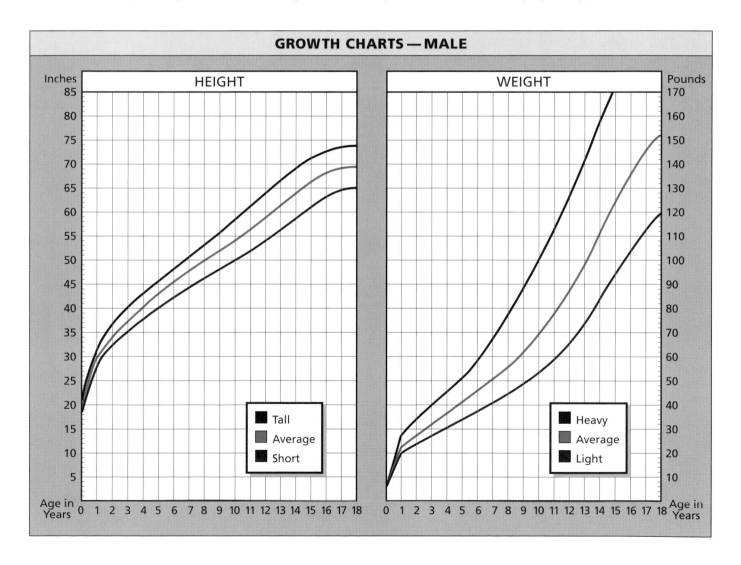

legs. In most cases these pains occur in the evening and last a few hours but are not a serious health problem. Children may also complain about recurring headaches or stomachaches. As your child becomes more independent and adventurous, the likelihood of accidental injury also increases. To minimize the risks, teach your child how to cross streets and ride a bicycle safely, how to swim, and how to use a seat belt when riding in a car. Instruct your child that knives, guns, and tools are not toys and are not to be used without parental guidance.

You should also explain to your child the hazards of contact with strangers, the difference between "good" and "uncomfortable" touching, when to say "no," and other precautions against potential child abuse.

For most girls, puberty begins sometime after the 10th birthday, for boys sometime after the 11th. Early signs of puberty in girls include growth of pubic hair, breast development, and a noticeable increase in physical size. Early signs of puberty in boys include enlargement of the testicles and penis and the emergence of pubic hair. A year or two later, boys begin to grow rapidly in weight and stature. If your child shows signs of puberty before the age of eight, you should speak with your doctor. Although the underlying cause of premature, or precocious, puberty may simply be an early-maturing endocrine system, it is wise to check for other potential disorders. In any case, remember that preadolescent children who are beginning to mature physically are still children mentally and emotionally and need to be treated as such.

ADOLESCENCE (AGES 13 TO 18)

During the teenage years, or adolescence, your child becomes more independent and socially mature, and takes on many adult physical attributes. In girls, menstruation typically begins between 11 and 14. Pubic hair, breasts, and all sweat glands are usually developed by age 14. The growth spurt that began at 10 or 11 usually slows down after the first menstrual period. It is not unusual for adolescent girls to suffer from painful menstruation; they may not establish regular menstrual patterns until about 17. If your daughter is 15 and has had no significant physical growth, or by 17 has not begun to menstruate, discuss delayed puberty with your doctor. If she has severe menstrual problems, she may need a pelvic exam by a pediatrician-gynecologist; in any case, girls should have a pelvic exam by their 18th birthday, and earlier if they are sexually active.

At 13 or 14 your son's voice box begins to grow and his voice begins to change. Underarm and facial hair, as well as sweat glands, begin to develop between 13 and 15, and most boys are able to ejaculate seminal fluid by this age. The growth spurt that began between 13 and 15 usually ends at around 17 or 18. If your son is 15 and has had no significant physical growth, or if his voice has not begun to change by 16, discuss delayed puberty with your doctor.

It is natural for adolescents to explore and experiment with their own sexuality, often through masturbation. They start to develop relationships with members of the opposite sex, and some may experiment with homosexual relationships, although few will ultimately become gay or lesbian. As your child enters puberty, you should explain the changes your child is experiencing, the differences between sex and love, homosexuality, and the potential consequences of unprotected sex—including pregnancy and sexually transmitted diseases.

Rapid physical and hormonal growth may cause other changes, such as vision problems, iron deficiency anemia, and acne. A common infectious disease that affects children of all ages, but especially adolescents, is mononucleosis. Eating disorders, including anorexia nervosa and bulimia, sometimes affect teenage girls and young women; the warning signs are extreme weight loss, fluctuating weight, or binge-and-purge eating. Some adolescents, especially girls, are susceptible to migraine headaches. More girls than boys are subject to scoliosis, a sideways curvature of the spine; many schools routinely screen children for this condition.

The physical, intellectual, and psychological development that occurs during adolescence may be associated with emotional or behavioral instability: It is not uncommon for teenagers to suffer depression, anxiety, and panic attacks. Out of curiosity, in response to depression or other trauma, or as a result of peer pressure, many adolescents experiment with drugs, alcohol, and tobacco. You should discuss with your child the potential health hazards, as well as the social and legal repercussions, of smoking, drinking, and drug abuse. ∎

THE HEALTHY ADULT

Early adulthood is, for most people, a period of good health. A young adult is more likely to have an accidental injury than a systemic disorder, but a few ailments, such as testicular cancer and multiple sclerosis, tend to strike young and middle-aged people rather than the elderly.

GOOD HEALTH HABITS

To keep your body in top shape, you should exercise regularly, eat a balanced diet, keep your weight within sensible limits, drink alcoholic beverages only in moderation, avoid abuse of legal or illegal drugs, and not smoke.

If you have a chronic ailment or condition, or if you think you have a hereditary predisposition to a certain disorder, advise your family doctor and educate yourself to recognize the likely symptoms. For example, if you are overweight or have a family history of diabetes, you are at some risk of developing Type 2 (noninsulin-dependent) diabetes as you approach middle age. Early detection of the disease is critical; even though there is no cure, it can be effectively controlled.

HEALTHCARE OPTIONS

Choosing a family doctor or other healthcare provider and carrying adequate health insurance give you protection against unexpected disease or injury. Most employers offer basic health programs to ensure productivity in the workplace. At the very minimum, look into a low-cost major medical policy that covers the potentially devastating expense of a catastrophic medical situation.

Periodic checkups may help detect health problems in their early stages, when treatment is likely to be most effective. Even if you received childhood inoculations against tetanus and diphtheria, your immunizations should be renewed every 10 years. A dental examination every six months will help detect tooth and gum problems, and if necessary an annual checkup by an ophthalmologist will monitor any vision problems. (See Women's Health and Men's Health, on the following pages.)

EMOTIONAL WELL-BEING

In addition to maintaining physical health, it is important to keep your mental and emotional health under control. Learning to cope with the changes and personal crises of life can have a direct effect on your physical well-being, while stress and anxiety place you at greater risk for a variety of health problems. Sometime after the age of 40, some people experience a so-called midlife crisis, as they reflect on their own aging and accomplishments. If you find yourself overwhelmed by self-examination or depression at any stage of your life, you should seek professional counseling. ■

HEIGHT AND WEIGHT GOALS

WOMEN			
Height	Small Frame	Medium Frame	Large Frame
4'10"	102-111 lbs.	109-121 lbs.	118-131 lbs.
4'11"	103-113	111-123	120-134
5'0"	104-115	113-126	122-137
5'1"	106-118	115-129	125-140
5'2"	108-121	118-132	128-143
5'3"	111-124	121-135	131-147
5'4"	114-127	124-138	134-151
5'5"	117-130	127-141	137-155
5'6"	120-133	130-144	140-159
5'7"	123-136	133-147	143-163
5'8"	126-139	136-150	146-167
5'9"	129-142	139-153	149-170
5'10"	132-145	142-156	152-173
5'11"	135-148	145-159	155-176
6'0"	138-151	148-162	158-179
MEN			
5'2"	128-134 lbs.	131-141 lbs.	138-150 lbs.
5'3"	130-136	133-143	140-153
5'4"	132-138	135-145	142-156
5'5"	134-140	137-148	144-160
5'6"	136-142	139-151	146-164
5'7"	138-145	142-154	149-168
5'8"	140-148	145-157	152-172
5'9"	142-151	148-160	155-176
5'10"	144-154	151-163	158-180
5'11"	146-157	154-166	161-184
6'0"	149-160	157-170	164-188
6'1"	152-164	160-174	168-192
6'2"	155-168	164-178	172-197
6'3"	158-172	167-182	176-202
6'4"	162-176	171-187	181-207

By keeping your weight within these ranges, you join those people identified by the Metropolitan Life Insurance Company as having fewer illnesses and longer lives than the general population.

WOMEN'S HEALTH

All women should have a periodic checkup by a family doctor, a women's health specialist, or another licensed healthcare provider. The checkup should include appropriate blood, urine, and stool tests; a pelvic examination to check the health of the reproductive organs; and a Pap smear and breast examination to detect early signs of cervical cancer and breast cancer. If you are over 50 or have entered menopause, you should have an annual breast x-ray, or mammogram, which can detect tumors before they can be felt. (When to begin annual mammograms is a controversial issue, with some doctors suggesting that they begin as early as the age of 35.) If a lump appears—or if you detect a lump through your own breast self-examination—your doctor will follow up with appropriate tests, even though most breast lumps are benign. (See Breast Cancer, Breast Problems, Cervical Problems, Ovary Problems, Uterine Problems, Vaginal Problems.)

THE REPRODUCTIVE PROCESS

During fetal development of a female baby, millions of egg cells are created and stored in her two ovaries. When puberty begins, the ovaries start releasing eggs in the process called ovulation. Normally, ovulation alternates between the two ovaries, with one egg being released about every 28 days. The egg then travels toward the uterus through the fallopian tube. If sexual intercourse has occurred within 72 hours before or 24 hours after ovulation, millions of male sperm cells are swimming toward the egg. If a single sperm penetrates the egg, fertilization occurs. Normally, the fertilized egg implants itself in the lining of the uterus, or endometrium, where it will develop into an embryo. If the egg is not fertilized, it and the blood-filled endometrium are expelled from the uterus during menstruation.

If two eggs are released by the ovaries and fertilized by separate sperm cells, the eggs develop into fraternal twins. If the fertilized egg splits in two early in its development, identical twins occur. In rare cases, three or more fertilized eggs develop; such multiple conceptions can be either identical or fraternal, or a combination of the two.

MENSTRUATION

The menstrual cycle varies from individual to individual. On average, a menstrual period begins every 28 days and lasts 4 days, although periods from 23 to 35 days apart and lasting from 2 to 7 days are still considered normal. Most women use either vaginal tampons or sanitary pads to absorb the flow of blood. A tampon should not be left in the vagina for longer than eight hours, because extended use of a single tampon has been linked to toxic shock syndrome, especially in women under the age of 30.

Unusual stress or long-distance travel may upset your regular menstrual cycle. Irregular periods are also common in young women who have just begun to menstruate and in older women nearing menopause. Absence of a period typically indicates pregnancy but may be due to stress, excessive exercise or athletic activity, obesity, anorexia nervosa, or other illnesses. During their menstrual periods some women experience abdominal pain, cramps, or low-back pain. Hormonal changes can cause unusually heavy periods—those that last more than seven days—and irregular menstrual cycles. If, after years of relatively pain-free periods, you start having menstrual pain or heavier-than-usual menstrual flow, you should notify your doctor. The unusual pain or the heavy flow may be caused by a tumor in the uterus, endometriosis, or pelvic inflammatory disease.

Premenstrual syndrome (PMS) strikes some women with varying degrees of severity about a week before a period begins. Hormonal imbalances may cause temporary breast tenderness, swelling, water retention, weight gain, food cravings, or mood swings. If menstruation has not begun by the time a young woman turns 17, she should see her doctor to determine if she has a disorder in her reproductive or endocrine system.

PREGNANCY

One of the first indications of pregnancy is the absence of a menstrual period. Other early signs are tender or swollen breasts, frequent urination, and perhaps nausea or vomiting. Pregnancy test kits available at most drugstores test your urine for a hormone that is present only when you are pregnant, but at-home tests are not always accurate, especially in the early days of a pregnancy. As soon as you think you might be pregnant, you should see a doctor or visit a healthcare center for more accurate testing.

On average, babies are born 266 days—or 38 weeks—after fertilization. Even if you can't tell exactly when fertilization occurred, you can estimate the baby's due date with reasonable accuracy, especially if your periods are regular: From the first day of your previous menstrual period, add 40 weeks, or 280 days. As a convenient benchmark, doctors commonly divide pregnancy into three trimesters of 13 weeks. In terms of the baby's development, the first trimester is perhaps the most important; the microscopic embryo grows to a fetus about three inches long, and all its major organs are formed. The baby is enclosed in amniotic fluid and is connected to the mother's circulatory system by the umbilical cord. During the second and third trimesters, the baby's organs and limbs continue to develop. Although birth size and weight can vary considerably, a typical full-term baby is about 20 inches long and weighs about 7½ pounds.

Babies born between the 20th and 35th week of pregnancy are considered premature; some do not survive the birthing process and are stillborn. In general, a baby's chance of survival increases the longer it stays in the womb.

Even though 1 in 4 pregnancies ends in miscarriage before the 13th week of pregnancy, the majority of these happen early—often before a woman even knows she is pregnant. Such spontaneous abortions occur because of genetic abnormalities or developmental defects in the baby. Miscarriages due to falls, injury, or stress are very rare. *(See Pregnancy Problems.)*

PRENATAL CARE

Proper prenatal care should begin as soon as you know you are pregnant. Your doctor will warn you that using tobacco, alcohol, and drugs—whether they are prescription or over-the-counter, legal or illegal—is potentially hazardous to your baby's development. Proper nutrition is very important, and the quality of the food you eat is more important than quantity. A good diet during pregnancy will be high in fresh fruits and vegetables but low in sugar and salt, with a sensible balance of vitamins, minerals, proteins, and fats. Most pregnant women gain between 20 and 30 pounds before delivery. Of this weight, 6 to 9 pounds will be the baby; the rest is due to breast and uterus enlargement, increased blood supply, amniotic fluid, and the placenta.

During pregnancy you may develop varicose veins, hemorrhoids, backaches, anemia, constipation, or heartburn; if you are over 35 you are at a slightly greater risk of developing diabetes or high blood pressure. These problems usually subside or disappear soon after the baby is born. If your nipples are inverted, you can place plastic or rubber inserts inside your bra after the 15th week of pregnancy; the suction of these inserts will draw out the nipples by the time your baby is born so you can breast-feed successfully.

Children born to women over the age of 35 are at slightly greater risk of having chromosomal abnormalities, such as Down syndrome. If one or both sides of the family have a history of any chromosomal disorders, you may want to have genetic counseling to determine the likelihood of your child's inheriting a given problem. Prenatal tests such as amniocentesis and ultrasound imaging may help detect such disorders early in the pregnancy.

If you should contract either toxoplasmosis or German measles (rubella) during your pregnancy—especially in the first trimester—your baby is at risk of a major congenital defect. Blood tests before you get pregnant can determine whether you are immune to either disease. Rubella is entirely preventable by vaccination, and all women should be protected against it. If you are not already immune, you should be vaccinated against it and then wait three months before you start trying to get pregnant. The parasite that causes toxoplasmosis is carried by raw meat and cat feces. If you are not immune to toxoplasmosis, your doctor can suggest ways to guard against infection.

A relatively rare, though preventable, disease occurs when the mother's blood is incompatible with the baby's blood because of the so-called Rh factor. Although the mother is unaffected, the incompatibility can cause the baby serious blood disorders that could result in anemia or even death. Your doctor can determine if your child is at risk of developing Rh disease and can recommend preventive treatment—usually inoculation with the drug Rh immunoglobulin early in the third trimester and again after the birth to protect the next child. For other potential complications, see Pregnancy Problems.

LABOR AND DELIVERY

Before the baby is due, you should consider your birthing options. Your doctor or prenatal clinic can provide information about various natural-childbirth approaches, as well as the pros and cons of using drugs or anesthetics to relieve pain during delivery. An injected epidural anesthetic alleviates the pain while still allowing you to remain awake and aware of the birth, and it tends to have fewer potential side effects than a general anesthetic.

The need for surgical procedures depends on a number of circumstances, and you may want to discuss the various options with your obstetrician. During normal delivery, the vaginal opening can be surgically enlarged in a procedure called episiotomy. In a Cesarean section, the baby is surgically removed from the womb. A C-section delivery may be elective or may be used in an emergency when the life of the mother or child is at risk.

The first signs of labor may be difficult to detect. Some women have so-called Braxton Hicks contractions for a few weeks before the due date; they occur irregularly, will not increase in intensity, and do not indicate the beginning of labor. For most women, the start of active labor is indicated when "the water breaks." This release of the amniotic fluid that protects the baby can be anything from a trickle to a gush of fluid from the vagina. Other signs can include a light discharge of blood-tinged mucus or uterine contractions at regular intervals.

Labor is divided into three stages. During the first and longest stage, uterine contractions cause the cervix to open so the baby can leave the uterus; this may take 12 hours or more for first-time mothers. During the second stage, uterine contractions actually push the baby out of the uterus; for first-time mothers, this may last several hours, although a child is sometimes delivered after only a few minutes. The final stage of labor consists of expelling the placenta, a quick and relatively painless process. After a woman's first delivery, labor is usually shorter, on average between 4 and 8 hours, because the uterus and vaginal muscles are more flexible. If you should go into delivery sooner than expected and you are not with your obstetrician, midwife, or family doctor, follow the guidelines in Emergencies/First Aid: Emergency Childbirth.

BREAST-FEEDING AND AFTER

Although breast-feeding is an entirely natural process, both you and your new baby not only must learn how to do it but also must establish a comfortable routine. This may take several days, so don't be frustrated if you have difficulty at first; your doctor, nurse, or midwife will offer advice as needed. For the first two to three days of nursing, the baby receives colostrum, a thin, sticky fluid rich in protective antibodies; but colostrum is soon replaced by actual milk. Some women may wean their baby to a bottle (and formula) after only a few weeks. In any event, after several months you can introduce your baby to bottled water and juice, and later to solid foods. You and your baby will know when she is ready to be weaned from the breast or bottle.

Some women who breast-feed their babies develop engorged breasts or cracked nipples; if this happens, ask your healthcare practitioner for appropriate treatment. A new mother may feel varying degrees of postpartum depression for a few weeks after the baby is born, a condition generally attributable to fatigue, hormonal recovery, and emotional changes. If you feel overwhelmed by these "baby blues," you should discuss the situation with your doctor.

INFERTILITY

If you have been trying to get pregnant for a year or more without success, you and your partner should investigate possible causes of infertility. In women, causes may include the failure of an ovary to release an egg, a blockage or other abnormality in the fallopian tubes, a disorder of the uterus or cervix, or a sexually transmitted disease (STD). While many cases of infertility can be resolved successfully, the alternatives include artificial insemination, surrogate fertilization, and adoption. *(For information about male infertility, see Men's Health, pages 42-43.)*

Fertility is definitely affected by age. In both men and women, fertility peaks sometime in the twenties. After the age of 37, a woman's fertility begins to decline significantly. Whereas men produce sperm most of their lives, a woman cannot conceive a child after menopause.

FAMILY PLANNING

Every woman should consider the consequences of becoming sexually active: It takes only one act of sexual intercourse to become pregnant. There are a number of ways to be sexually active and prevent conception.

Natural family planning is the practice of determining the fertile and infertile days of a woman's menstrual cycle to predict when she is likely to ovulate and therefore likely to conceive. Coordinating intercourse with ovulation can be helpful in becoming pregnant; conversely, abstaining from sexual intercourse during the time near ovulation can serve as a form of contraception.

Modern natural family planning originates from the rhythm method, first introduced in the 1930s, in which a woman predicts ovulation based on the timing of her previous menstrual cycle. This method is not particularly effective and is no longer recommended. Modern forms of natural family planning include a method that relies both on observations of cervical mucus and on basal—or resting—temperature readings to determine a two- to three-day window during which ovulation will occur. Advocates of modern forms of natural family planning suggest that preventing pregnancy usually involves 10 to 14 days of abstinence from intercourse each month.

Preventing sperm from reaching an unfertilized egg is called barrier contraception. Methods include a man's use of a condom and a woman's use of a diaphragm, female condom, or cervical cap. All barrier methods are more effective in combination with spermicidal cream or gel that destroys sperm on contact. An intrauterine device (IUD) inserted in the uterus prevents a fertilized egg from becoming implanted in the uterine wall; although IUDs can be highly effective, some women who use them experience uncomfortable and occasionally serious side effects. Women under the age of 30 who use internal contraception devices are also at somewhat elevated risk of developing toxic shock syndrome.

Hormone-based birth control—using either oral pills or timed-release capsules implanted under the skin—is among the most effective means of contraception. The synthetic hormones temporarily suppress the release of eggs from the ovaries while allowing menstruation to continue. Contraceptive pills or capsules must be prescribed by a physician, who will advise about the most appropriate type, their potential side effects, and other complications, which these days are rare. After discontinuing birth-control pills, most women resume normal ovarian function and can conceive successfully.

Sterilization is a permanent form of contraception. Treatment for some diseases, such as cervical or uterine cancer, requires a hysterectomy—the surgical removal of the uterus and often the ovaries, fallopian tubes, and cervix. After bearing one or more children, some women elect to have their tubes surgically severed or tied, effectively preventing contact between eggs and sperm.

On rare occasions, an egg will be fertilized and implanted outside the uterus in the fallopian tube. This is called an ectopic pregnancy—a painful and potentially life-threatening condition for the mother, requiring the fetus to be surgically aborted. Elective abortions are generally performed during the first trimester of pregnancy, typically by a method known as dilation and curettage (D and C) of the uterus.

OTHER SEXUAL CONCERNS

An active sex life that includes multiple partners raises concerns about sexually transmitted disease (STD), or venereal disease (VD). Direct body contact and exchange of fluids during intercourse and oral sex leave partners open to such highly contagious diseases as syphilis, gonorrhea, genital herpes, and genital warts, as well as to transmission of the human immunodeficiency virus (HIV), the cause of AIDS (acquired immune deficiency syndrome). While bacterial STDs can usually be cured, viral STDs generally cannot, which can mean lifelong consequences for affected people; AIDS is eventually fatal.

Male condoms, properly used, can prevent some STDs but should not be considered 100 percent effective. If any symptoms of an STD appear, both partners should be checked by a doctor immediately, and any person with a known STD should avoid sexual contact entirely. Every woman has the right to know whether her partner has ever had an STD, and should not be afraid to ask.

SEXUAL DYSFUNCTION

A woman's sexual desire, or libido, naturally fluctuates; there may be times when she is not interested in having sex at all. This may be due to illness, the side effects of certain medications, stress, depression, or problems in the relationship. If your sexual desires are diminished for an extended period of time, if sexual intercourse is consistently uncomfortable, or if you are unable to have an orgasm, you may wish to discuss the problem with your doctor. (See Sexual Dysfunction.)

MENOPAUSE

Sometime between the ages of 40 and 55, most women's supply of eggs becomes depleted, and the ovaries no longer produce the quantities of estrogen—the primary female hormone—needed for the menstrual cycle to continue. For a period of several years the interval between menstrual periods becomes longer. Eventually, ovulation ceases, menstruation stops altogether, and pregnancy is no longer possible. This is menopause, the natural endpoint of a woman's reproductive years.

Other symptoms of menopause may include hot flashes, felt predominantly in the upper body; drying and thinning of the vaginal walls, which may cause painful intercourse; and various emotional complications. Elderly women and women who have had many children may lose strength in the pelvic muscles that hold the uterus or cervix in place. These conditions are usually minor, but treatment may be necessary if the symptoms cause undue discomfort. (See Uterine Problems, Cervical Problems.) The threat of osteoporosis is a serious concern for postmenopausal women, as decreasing amounts of estrogen just after menopause speed up depletion of calcium in the bones. To help counter some of the effects of menopause, ask your doctor about the pros and cons of hormone replacement therapy (HRT). (See Menopausal Problems.)

OTHER HEALTH CONCERNS

Among treatable ailments that tend to afflict women are urinary tract infections (including bladder infections), irritable bowel syndrome, and yeast infections. Some women are predisposed to chronic ailments such as arthritis, diabetes, obesity, and the eating disorders bulimia and anorexia nervosa.

Of all the health issues that concern women, probably the most significant is cancer. While the disease strikes a relatively small percentage of women, the incidence of various types of cancer is rising as other ailments are brought under control. Every woman should be alert to the warning signs of cancer in any part of the body and should see a doctor at once if a suspected symptom appears. If symptoms persist, or if you feel unsure, get a second opinion. If a tumor is discovered, whether it is benign or malignant, discuss treatment options with a specialist to be sure that you get the most appropriate treatment possible. (See Cancer.) ∎

MEN'S HEALTH

Every man should establish basic habits that will help ensure decades of continuing good health. First and foremost is a balanced diet that provides proper nutrition and keeps your body weight within recommended limits for your height and build. It is a good idea to start exercising at an early age, through either active sports or a regular fitness program. The importance of physical fitness continues into a man's middle years and beyond. An active lifestyle that includes regular exercise can help prevent obesity and can also be an important aspect of your mental and emotional well-being, especially as a means of relieving stress.

A regular physical checkup by a family physician or health service monitors your heart, lungs, and circulation, and includes analysis of your blood, urine, and stool for such things as blood sugar, cholesterol, and signs of systemic diseases. After the age of 50, your physical is likely to include a digital check of your prostate gland. Depending on your overall health and family history of specific ailments, you may need other tests, such as an electrocardiogram (ECG) to check heart function, a sigmoidoscopy to check for colorectal cancer, or a stress test to check your cardiovascular system.

It is always important to report any apparent symptoms of disease or physical disorders to your doctor without delay, and to ask about any unusual conditions, changes in your body, or reduced physical ability. The essential keys to keeping diseases and disorders at bay are prevention, early detection, and prompt, professional treatment.

THE REPRODUCTIVE SYSTEM
After puberty, a man's testicles manufacture sperm cells and the male sex hormone testosterone continuously into old age. Sperm and fluids from the seminal vesicles and the prostate gland combine to create semen, which is ejaculated through the urethra during orgasm. If semen is not ejaculated in a few days, the sperm cells are reabsorbed and replaced. In a typical ejaculation about 500 million sperm cells are expelled, even though only one is needed to fertilize an egg cell. Since sperm can live in a woman's reproductive tract for up to 72 hours, fertilization can occur up to three days after sexual intercourse.

SEXUAL DYSFUNCTION
Impotence—not being able to have an erection or to maintain it long enough to reach orgasm—afflicts most men at some time or other. Temporary impotence can occur if you drink too much alcohol, when you are overly excited, or during an emotional crisis. Premature ejaculation occurs under some of the same circumstances and can be frustrating to both you and your partner. Both problems tend to disappear when the underlying cause goes away. If either problem occurs regularly or persists in spite of your best efforts, you should see a doctor or a sex therapist to discuss treatment options. (See Sexual Dysfunction.)

Various disorders of the sexual organs can complicate or prevent normal sexual activity. You should visually examine your penis and testicles on a regular basis, and report any abnormalities to your doctor. (See Penile Pain, Testicle Problems, Testicular Cancer.)

INFERTILITY
Most men have no problem fathering children, but there is perhaps nothing more upsetting to a couple than finding out that one person is infertile. Two of the most common causes of infertility in men are low sperm count and poor sperm motility. Other men have difficulty controlling the timing of their ejaculations, or they may ejaculate little or no semen. Various other genital disorders can cause infertility, among them varicocele, or enlarged veins in the scrotum, and inflammation of the testicles, sometimes caused by mumps. Fortunately most such conditions can be remedied with proper treatment.

SEXUAL RESPONSIBILITY
A man has an obligation to father children in a responsible fashion and to share with a woman the decision to let pregnancy begin. Withdrawing the penis during intercourse prior to ejaculation is not an effective way to prevent fertilization. A more reliable preventive method is to use a condom, which physically blocks sperm from entering the vagina; condoms are even more effective if the woman also uses a spermicidal cream.

Sterilization is a reliable, but usually permanent, form of male contraception, which some men choose after having children. In a surgical procedure called vasectomy the vas deferens is severed and tied off, preventing sperm from reaching the urethra and being ejaculated. A vasectomy does not affect a man's ability to have erections and orgasms. In theory, vasectomies can be surgically reversed, but in practice, reversal is fully successful in only about 30 percent of cases. (See Women's Health, pages 38-41, for more information about fertilization and contraception.)

Condoms are also an effective means of preventing sexually transmitted diseases (STDs), which can result from either heterosexual or homosexual contact. STDs are by definition highly contagious, and men with active sex lives and multiple partners should be alert to the possibility of being infected and of transmitting disease. At the first symptom of an apparent STD, see a doctor and have a thorough physical checkup. If you know or suspect you are carrying an STD, avoid any sexual contact until you get a complete diagnosis and medical treatment if necessary.

SYSTEMIC DISORDERS

Numerous ailments can strike men at any time in their adult lives. Men are somewhat more likely than women to suffer cardiovascular ailments, such as atherosclerosis and heart attacks. They are also at somewhat greater risk for lung cancer and gastrointestinal problems, although those tendencies may be changing as people become more conscious of the importance of good diet and the hazards of smoking.

You should discuss with your doctor any sores, lumps, or discoloration that appears anywhere on your body. The same is true for difficulties with urination, sexual dysfunction, or any other apparent physical symptoms. It is important to understand any disorders that may have been passed on from one generation of your family to another, whether they are benign conditions like hair loss or potentially fatal diseases like diabetes or cancer. Being conscious of such inherited tendencies and alert to their warning signs can make the difference between a healthy life and early disability. If you have a family history of a systemic ailment, or recognize the potential symptoms of some other disorder, consult a doctor and discuss preventive measures. A change in lifestyle at an early age may be the key to long-term health.

OTHER MALE CONCERNS

Poor hygiene is associated with urinary tract infections and cancer of the penis, and more uncircumcised than circumcised men develop these problems. Uncircumcised men should wash under the foreskin daily. *(See Penile Pain.)* You should also carefully self-examine your testicles for lumps or enlargement once a month. Testicular cancer, although rare, is most likely to strike men under the age of 40. If you experience any pain or swelling in the testicles or scrotum that is not readily explained, see your physician. *(See Testicle Problems.)*

Bladder and prostate problems develop gradually over a period of years, which is why many men accept difficulty in urination and ejaculation as normal consequences of aging. The prostate is a walnut-sized gland that partially surrounds the urethra—the tube that takes urine out of the bladder. Over time the prostate can swell, constricting the urethra and causing frequent, painful urination. *(See Blad-der Infections, Prostate Problems, Urinary Problems.)*

An unrelated disorder, prostate cancer is the most common type of cancer in men, especially those over 50. As with all cancers, early detection is critical for successful treatment; therefore it is important to have regular physical checkups and to be examined if symptoms appear. Although medical intervention remains somewhat controversial, you should discuss any apparent difficulties with your doctor, who can inform you about the latest research findings and recommend appropriate treatment.

MENTAL HEALTH

Men and women alike can be challenged by emotional and psychological difficulties, often in times of personal crisis but sometimes as a recurring or lifelong problem. If you tend to react to stress in your life with anger or depression, or if you have difficulty coping with enforced or accidental changes—such as the breakup of a relationship, the loss of a job, or the death of a family member or friend—you may benefit from professional counseling or therapy, with or without medication.

Some people are considered Type A personalities, given to aggressive attitudes and stressful patterns of behavior. Although women can have such traits too, men seem to be particularly disposed. Some studies associate aggressive behavior and a stressful lifestyle with such ailments as high blood pressure, gastrointestinal problems, and some forms of cancer. Authorities believe that learning to control such tendencies can have a beneficial effect on overall health.

Emotional well-being is as important as physical fitness, and your emotional and mental state can have a profound effect on your physical health. This is particularly true when disease strikes. A positive, realistic attitude—as well as a clear understanding of the ailment—can be an important contribution to a successful recovery. ■

GROWING OLDER

Thanks to monumental advances in medical science and the healing arts, most people today can look forward to longer, more productive lives than their grandparents might have imagined. Men born in the second half of the 20th century can expect to live an average of more than 70 years; for women the average life span is more than 75 years.

Adequate exercise, proper nutrition, and appropriate medical care when needed can help keep you in good physical and mental health through your middle years—between 40 and 65—and well into old age. On the other hand, poor nutrition, obesity, systemic diseases, and excessive use of tobacco, alcohol, and drugs tend to accelerate the inevitable process of aging.

THE AGING PROCESS

Physical fitness and mental productivity generally peak in the mid-twenties and stay stable for many years. Eventually, however, all body systems begin to become less efficient. You may not start to notice changes until you are in your forties or fifties, but sometimes the effects of aging come on without warning. For many people, the first sign of aging is loss or graying of hair. Hair loss that begins while you are still in your twenties is usually hereditary, but whenever it occurs, it is nearly impossible to prevent.

Accumulation and redistribution of body fat may also contribute to a changing appearance. In middle age, a man's excess fat tends to settle at the abdomen; in women, fat gravitates to the breasts, abdomen, and hips. Bones reach their maximum density between the ages of 25 and 35, and their slow erosion to osteoporosis may result in losing several inches of height by the late seventies, while also contributing to lower body weight. Bones may also develop calcification and lose protective cartilage at the joints, or may develop other symptoms of arthritis.

Over the years your skin slowly thins, loses elasticity, and begins to wrinkle, especially on the face and hands. Age spots or patches that appear on the backs of the hands and elsewhere are usually harmless and may actually disappear over time. The best thing you can do for your skin is to avoid overexposing it to the sun. What was once considered a healthy tan—or even one severe sunburn at an early age—is now considered a potential risk factor for skin cancer. Itchy, reddened skin and other forms of dermatitis may also be associated with aging. Cosmetic surgery may tighten areas of loose skin and eliminate existing wrinkles for a time, but the skin and underlying fat layers will continue to grow thinner and new wrinkles will eventually appear.

Disorders of the joints and the skeletal system may become apparent as people get older, making arthritic conditions some of the more widespread ailments of the elderly. *(See Arthritis, Joint Pain.)* The combination of slower reflexes and a deterioration in the sense of balance makes older people prone to falls and other accidents. Brittle bones, weaker muscles, and thinner skin mean that such accidents may also have more serious consequences. The healing process is much slower in older adults than in younger people, so relatively minor injuries can become serious, even life-threatening.

Exercise and good nutrition can help keep your body limber and strong, although muscles, too, will atrophy naturally over time. Shrinking gum tissue can cause teeth to become loose and susceptible to decay, so regular dental checkups and corrective dental work are important for good oral health. If tooth and gum deterioration interferes with eating, or if you begin to lose your teeth, you should speak with your dentist about being fitted for dentures. *(See Gum Problems, Toothache.)*

SENSORY CHANGES

Each of the physical senses tends to degenerate as you age, at varying rates for different people. When you first detect changes in your vision, see an ophthalmologist about glasses or contact lenses to correct near- or farsightedness. Adults over 60 may be susceptible to glaucoma, cataracts, and macular degeneration; these conditions, if left untreated, can eventually lead to partial or total blindness. Because eyesight tends to deteriorate slowly, you may not be aware of progressive vision loss, so you should schedule an annual vision exam to check your eyes for these disorders. *(See Vision Problems.)*

Hearing loss is usually a gradual process that may be noticeable after age 40; some people may notice significant loss over time while others may notice little change. *(See Hearing Problems, Tinnitus.)* Your senses of smell and taste will also become less acute, but the gradual loss is usually a problem only if it adversely affects your appetite. Older people are more susceptible to **hypothermia, heatstroke,** and **heat exhaustion** than are younger people *(see these entries in* Emergencies/First Aid*)*. Temperature sensitivity may be affected by circulatory problems or a thyroid problem.

SYSTEMIC CHANGES

All your internal systems become less efficient as you age. The muscles of your heart and blood vessels lose some of their elasticity, making it harder for blood to circulate through your body. Cardiovascular deterioration eventually makes physical exertion very tiring. Because your heart has to work harder to do its job, a slight increase in blood pressure is normal; a significant increase may mean you are at risk for having a heart attack or stroke; adults who smoke are at markedly greater risk of stroke. Regular physical exercise—walking, swimming, golf, or tennis—will help keep your cardiovascular system healthy, but consult your doctor before you start any new exercise programs.

Urinary tract infections such as kidney and bladder infections become more common with increasing age and can lead to more serious repercussions. Older adults are also susceptible to gastrointestinal problems, such as irritable bowel syndrome and diverticulitis. Poor diet may cause anemia to develop in older adults. Elderly adults are also prone to suffer from incontinence and constipation.

Your body's immune system is also likely to become less effective with age. You may find yourself more susceptible to common illnesses, and whenever you get them you may take longer to recover than you did in the past. Many doctors recommend that adults over 65 get an annual flu shot to protect against active strains of the influenza virus. Some older people may need a pneumococcal shot to prevent pneumonia.

For various reasons, your risk of developing cancer becomes more likely after the age of 50. You should advise your doctor of any family history of a particular form of cancer and educate yourself about its possible warning signs. Women should be particularly alert to signs of breast cancer, uterine cancer, cervical cancer, and ovarian cancer. Men should be aware of the warning signs of prostate and testicular cancer, and should understand that they are statistically at somewhat higher risk than women for lung and colorectal cancer.

Aging also affects the brain and the nervous system. Mild tremors in the hand or head are common in older adults; for many people this is harmless, but it may be a symptom of Parkinson's disease. Forgetfulness, partial memory loss, and progressively increasing confusion have many causes, ranging from minor infections or sleep deprivation to stroke or Alzheimer's disease. If you notice such symptoms in yourself or in another adult family member, arrange a medical examination to determine the cause.

MAKING ADJUSTMENTS

Physical changes related to aging will be accompanied by changes in your personal life. Retirement and adopting a slower-paced lifestyle may have a substantial psychological effect that some people find difficult to accept. Finding new outlets—travel, volunteer work, or pursuing a lifelong interest—can ease the adjustment to a different role in your family and community.

Around the house, a modest investment in safety—grab rails in the bathtub or shower, reinforced stair banisters, and securely fastened floor coverings, for example—can help prevent accidents. If balance or mobility becomes a problem, using a cane or a walker may be a wise decision. At some point, because of declining vision and physical reflexes, most older adults find it prudent to stop driving a car.

Retirement communities offer many benefits for older adults, but the decision to change one's lifestyle in a major way should be made with a clear understanding of the financial and social consequences, and the possibility of some initial emotional trauma. The death of friends or a spouse will inevitably cause grief and perhaps anxiety about changes in your own life. If you feel overwhelmed by your feelings, or if you or others around you sense you are suffering from depression, you should seek help from your healthcare practitioner or a counselor.

CARING FOR THE ELDERLY

The time-honored concept of younger family members caring for an older generation is still valid, but for many people today it is unrealistic or impossible. If you choose to be a primary caregiver, you may find that enrolling an older person in a day-care program eases the mental and physical strain associated with such care over the long term. If caring for a chronically ill or bedridden person at home yourself is not feasible or acceptable, you can consider home care by a trained nurse or other provider, on either a part- or full-time basis.

The time may come when you need to place an elderly spouse or parent in a nursing home or similar facility. This is not an easy decision, but it may be the best solution, especially when the person is ill, family members are far away, or at-home facilities are inadequate or unsuitable. With careful research and planning, a suitable and caring environment for any elderly person can be found. ■

EMERGENCIES/ FIRST AID ▶

CONTENTS

What to Do in an Emergency

1 Call 911 or your emergency number, or tell someone nearby to do so.

2 Check the victim's ABCs *(right)*.

3 Stop any severe bleeding *(page 48)*.

4 Prevent shock *(page 75)*.

5 Try to determine what happened. Look around the scene for any clues, such as a Medic Alert tag on the victim or an open container of a poisonous chemical.

The Recovery Position

Placing an unconscious victim who is breathing in the recovery position will keep the airway open. CAUTION: Do not place the victim in this position if you suspect a neck or back injury.

Support the victim's head and roll him onto his stomach. Bend the victim's arm and knee that are closest to you. Carefully tilt back the head so the airway remains open.

Checking the ABCs:
AIRWAY, BREATHING, CIRCULATION

A

OPENING THE VICTIM'S AIRWAY.
Gently tilt back the victim's head and lift the chin. CAUTION: If you suspect a head, neck, or back injury, just lift the chin.

B

LOOKING, LISTENING, AND FEELING FOR BREATHING.
Look for the victim's chest to rise. Put your ear to the victim's mouth, and listen and feel for exhaled air; chest movement alone might not mean breathing.

C

CHECKING FOR A PULSE.
Gently press two fingers, not your thumb, in the depression on the side of the victim's neck, next to the Adam's apple, and feel for a pulse.

CHECKING FOR AN INFANT'S PULSE (UP TO 1 YEAR OLD).
Gently press two fingers, not your thumb, on the inside of the infant's arm between the elbow and shoulder, and feel for a pulse. If you do not feel a pulse, listen for a heartbeat.

BLEEDING

CAUTION: If you suspect a head, neck, or back injury, see page 66.

1 **Lay the victim flat on his back**. Raise the victim's feet several inches. If possible, elevate the wound above heart level.

2 **Check the victim's ABCs** *(page 47)*. **If the victim is not breathing or does not have a pulse or heartbeat, begin CPR** *(pages 50-53)*.

3 **Remove any visible objects from the wound.** CAUTION: Do not remove any object or pull on any clothing that is stuck in the wound. Do not probe the wound or disturb it in any way.

4 **Apply direct pressure to the wound with a clean cloth or your hand.** If blood seeps through the cloth, do not remove it; put another cloth on top and keep pressing. You may need to apply firmer pressure if blood continues to seep through. For an embedded object, put pressure around the wound, not on the object.

5 **If the bleeding does not stop, apply pressure to an arterial pressure point.** Keep direct pressure on the wound as you press the arterial point. Do not apply pressure to arteries leading to the head or neck unless bright red blood is spurting from an injured neck artery.

6 **When the bleeding stops, apply a bandage.** Do not remove any cloths placed on the wound to help stop the bleeding; place a clean cloth over the wound. If there is an object embedded in the wound, bandage around it to support it.

7 **Keep the victim calm and still.**

Applying direct pressure. Use a clean cloth, or your hand alone if necessary, to put pressure directly on the wound. Hold the edges of flesh together.

Applying pressure to an arterial pressure point. Apply pressure with your fingers held flat against the arterial pressure point that is closest to the wound, between it and the heart.

Bandaging a wound. Wrap a bandage or a clean cloth around the wound; tie it in place.

BURNS

CAUTION: If you suspect a head, neck, or back injury, see page 66.

1 Remove the victim from the cause of the burns.

2 Remove any clothing or jewelry from the burned area. CAUTION: Do not remove any hot or smoldering clothing that is dry or is stuck to the burned skin. Do not breathe or cough on the burned skin.

3 Cover small burns with wet cloths. If the burned area is smaller than the size of the victim's chest, loosely cover it with a sheet or towel that has been soaked in cold water, or hold the burned skin under cold running water. CAUTION: Do not place ice on the burned skin. Do not break any blisters. If the burned area is larger than the size of the victim's chest, do not apply water or cover the burn.

4 Separate burned fingers or toes. If fingers or toes have been burned, gently place dry cloth dressings between them. CAUTION: Do not use cotton or any adhesive bandages.

5 Loosely cover the burned skin with a clean, dry cloth. If fluid oozes through the cloth, place another cloth over it. CAUTION: Do not spread any ointments, lotions, butter, baking soda, or ice on the burn.

6 Elevate a burned arm or leg above the level of the victim's heart.

IMPORTANT!

◆ Call 911 or your emergency number if the burns involve more than one body part or the face, neck, hands, feet, or genitals, or if the victim has trouble breathing. Call if the victim is a child or is elderly.

◆ Call 911 or your emergency number if the burns are caused by chemicals. See the box below.

◆ If you suspect that the victim has been electrocuted, see Electric Shock *(page 59)*.

◆ If the victim has a chemical burn in the eye, see Eye Emergencies *(page 62)*.

◆ If the victim spilled a chemical that caused the skin to freeze, give first aid for chemical burns, then give first aid for frostbite *(page 69)*.

◆ If the victim spilled a chemical that was absorbed through the skin without burning it, see Poisoning *(page 73)*.

DEEP BURNS

For deep burns (indicated by charred or white skin), you should also check the victim's ABCs *(page 47)*.

CLOTHING ON FIRE

1 Lay the person on the ground so the burning clothing is on top.
2 Smother the flames with a blanket, coat, or any other cloth that is nearby and handy. Direct the flames away from the person's face, or **tell the victim to roll over slowly.**

CHEMICAL BURNS

SYMPTOMS

◆ Burn marks   ◆ Blisters
◆ Headache   ◆ Dizziness
◆ Breathing problems ◆ Abdominal pain
◆ Seizures   ◆ Unconsciousness

1 Remove the victim from the chemical.
2 Flush the burn with water and remove contaminated clothing. Place the burned area under running water for at least 15 minutes to dilute the chemical. As you flush the burn, remove any jewelry or clothing that may have come in contact with the chemical. CAUTION: For a dry chemical, such as lime, brush off any particles before flushing with water.
3 Check the victim's ABCs *(page 47)*.
4 If the victim is not breathing or does not have a pulse or heartbeat, begin CPR *(pages 50-53)*.
5 Cover the burn with a clean, dry cloth.

CARDIAC AND RESPIRATORY ARREST

CPR

Treatment for cardiac or respiratory arrest is called cardiopulmonary resuscitation (CPR). The goals of CPR are to open the airway, reestablish breathing, and reestablish circulation. It is best to give CPR only if you have been trained in the procedure.

CAUTION: If you suspect a head, neck, or back injury, see page 66.

1 Lay the victim flat on his back.

2 Sweep the victim's mouth. CAUTION: If you see an object lodged in the victim's throat, do not try to retrieve it, as this might force the object farther down the airway; give first aid for choking (page 54).

3 Open the victim's airway. Gently tilt back the victim's head and lift the chin.

4 Look, listen, and feel for breathing. Be sure to put your ear to the victim's mouth; chest movement alone might not mean breathing.

5 If the victim is not breathing, give breaths. Watch for the chest to rise with each breath; let the chest fall before you give the second breath. If the victim's chest does not rise, gently tilt his head farther back and try again to give two slow breaths. If the chest still does not rise, give first aid for choking (page 54). CAUTION: If the head is tilted too far or not far enough, you may not successfully open the airway.

6 Check for a pulse.

IMPORTANT!

◆ If the victim is not breathing and does not appear to be choking, call 911 or your emergency number, or tell someone nearby to do so; then begin CPR (below). But if you suspect choking, see page 54.

◆ If the victim is having trouble breathing, treat for breathing problems (page 212).

◆ If you suspect that the victim is having a heart attack, see page 67.

SYMPTOMS

◆ Pale or bluish face
◆ Chest does not rise or fall
◆ No heartbeat or pulse
◆ Unconsciousness
◆ No exhaled breath

Finger sweep, adult. Hold the victim's tongue and lift the chin. Slide your index finger down the inside of the cheek and sweep out any loose objects.

Giving breaths, adult. Pinch the nose shut and seal your lips tightly around the mouth. Give two slow breaths; remove your mouth between breaths.

Checking the pulse, adult. Gently press two fingers, not your thumb, in the depression on the side of the victim's neck, next to the Adam's apple; feel for a pulse.

7 **If you feel no pulse, give chest compressions.** See the illustrations at right.

8 **Repeat steps 3, 4, and 5.** If the victim is an infant or a child younger than eight years old, give only one breath.

9 **Give chest compressions, breaths, and recheck for a pulse.** For an adult or child over eight years old, repeat a series of 15 chest compressions, followed by two breaths, 4 times; then recheck for a pulse. For an infant or a child younger than eight years old, repeat a series of 5 chest compressions, followed by one breath, 10 times; then recheck for a pulse. Repeat the series of chest compressions, breaths, and pulse checking until the victim has a pulse or begins to breathe on his own, or until medical help arrives.

10 **If the victim is not breathing but has a pulse, give breaths.** For an adult or child over eight years old, give 1 breath every five seconds. Check the pulse every 12 breaths. For a child between one and eight years old, give 1 breath every four seconds; check the pulse every 15 breaths. For an infant, give 1 breath every three seconds; check for a pulse or heartbeat every 20 breaths. Continue until help arrives.

Placing your hands, adult. Place your middle finger in the notch where the ribs meet the bottom of the breastbone. Put your index finger next to and above your middle finger. Place the heel of your other hand next to and above your index finger. Remove your fingers and place that hand over your other hand; interlace your fingers and keep them up, off the chest.

Giving chest compressions, adult. Position yourself so that your shoulders are directly over your hands; keep your arms straight. Press down forcefully to depress the victim's breastbone 1 1/2 to 2 inches. Release the pressure, but don't lift your hands off the chest. Give 15 chest compressions, at the count of "one and two and three and...." CAUTION: Do not rock back and forth.

CONTINUED ▶

INFANT (UP TO 1 YEAR OLD)

SWEEP, BREATHS, PULSE

Finger sweep. Hold the tongue and lift the chin. Look in the mouth; if you can see an object and think you can easily remove it, slide your little finger down the inside of the cheek and sweep out the object.

Giving breaths. Keep the chin lifted with one hand and seal your lips over the nose and mouth. First give two breaths, then one thereafter. Remove your mouth between breaths. Breathe forcefully but not so hard that air goes into the stomach.

Checking the pulse. Gently press two fingers, not your thumb, on the inside of the infant's arm between the elbow and shoulder. If you do not feel a pulse, listen for a heartbeat.

CHEST COMPRESSIONS

Placing your hands. Place your index finger just below an imaginary line between the nipples, in the center of the chest, on the breastbone. Place your two middle fingers next to and below your index finger, then lift your index finger. Use your free hand to help keep the infant's head tilted back.

Giving chest compressions. Bend your elbow slightly and press straight down on your fingers, depressing the infant's breastbone $1/2$ to 1 inch. Release the pressure, but don't lift your fingers. Give five chest compressions, at the count of "one two three...." CAUTION: Do not rock back and forth.

See pages 50-51 for complete instructions.

CHILD (BETWEEN 1 AND 8 YEARS OLD)

SWEEP, BREATHS, PULSE

Finger sweep. Hold the victim's tongue and lift the chin. Slide your index finger down the inside of the cheek and sweep out any loose objects.

Giving breaths. Pinch the nose shut and seal your lips tightly around the mouth. Give two slow breaths initially; give one breath thereafter. Remove your mouth between breaths.

Checking the pulse. Gently press two fingers, not your thumb, in the depression on the side of the victim's neck, next to the Adam's apple, and feel for a pulse.

CHEST COMPRESSIONS

Placing your hands. Place two fingers of your right hand in the notch where the ribs meet the bottom of the breastbone. Place the heel of your left hand next to your right index finger, keeping your fingers off the child's chest. Now remove your left hand and put the heel of your right hand where the left hand was. Use your left hand to keep the child's head tilted back *(below)*.

Giving chest compressions. Position yourself so that your shoulders are directly over the child's chest; keep your arm straight. Press down forcefully on your hand to depress the child's breastbone 1 to 1½ inches. Release the pressure, but don't lift your hand. Give five chest compressions, at the count of "one and two and three and...." CAUTION: Do not rock back and forth.

See pages 50-51 for complete instructions.

CHOKING

IMPORTANT!

◆ If you suspect that an object is caught in a victim's throat and he cannot cough, breathe, speak, or cry, call 911 or tell someone nearby to do so. Begin first-aid treatment for choking *(below)*. If you are the victim, see the box below, right. If the victim is an infant (up to one year old), see the box on page 56.

◆ If you suspect that an object is caught in a victim's throat but he is able to cough, breathe, talk, or cry, do not intervene. But be prepared to act if the situation worsens.

CAUTION: If you suspect a head, neck, or back injury, see page 66.

1 **Do not try to retrieve an object lodged in the victim's throat.** This might force the object farther down the airway.

2 **Give abdominal thrusts (the Heimlich maneuver).** Continue giving abdominal thrusts until the object is dislodged or until the victim loses consciousness. CAUTION: If the victim is pregnant or obese, place your fist on the middle of the victim's breastbone; do not place your hands on the ribs or on the lower edge of the breastbone.

3 **If the victim loses consciousness, lay him flat on his back.**

4 **Sweep the victim's mouth.** CAUTION: Remember, do not try to retrieve an object lodged in the victim's throat.

5 **Open the victim's airway.** Gently tilt back the victim's head and lift the chin.

6 **Look, listen, and feel for breathing.** Be sure to put your ear to the victim's mouth; chest movement alone might not mean breathing. If the victim is breathing, give first aid for unconsciousness *(page 71)*.

7 **Breathe twice into the victim's mouth.** Watch for the victim's chest to rise with each breath; let the chest fall before you give the next breath. If the victim's chest does not rise with each breath, gently tilt the head farther back and try again to give two slow breaths.

Abdominal thrust. Place your arms around the victim's waist. Make a fist with one hand and place it in the middle of the victim's abdomen, just above the navel and below the ribs. Hold your fist with your other hand. Give quick, repeated thrusts, pushing inward and upward.

Finger sweep. Hold the victim's tongue and lift the chin. Slide your index finger down the inside of the cheek and sweep out any loose objects.

Breathe into the victim's mouth. Pinch the victim's nose shut and seal your lips tightly around the mouth. Give two slow breaths; remove your mouth between breaths.

8 **If the victim's chest still does not rise, give five abdominal thrusts.** CAUTION: Do not press to either side as you thrust.

9 **Sweep the victim's mouth, make sure the airway is open, and breathe twice again into the victim's mouth.**

10 **If the victim's chest still does not rise, give abdominal thrusts, sweep the mouth, and give breaths.** Give five abdominal thrusts. Sweep the victim's mouth, and give two slow breaths. Repeat this sequence of abdominal thrusts, sweeps of the mouth, and slow breaths until the object is dislodged or until medical help arrives.

11 **If the object is dislodged but the victim is not breathing, begin CPR** *(pages 50-53).*

Abdominal thrust. Position the heel of one of your hands against the middle of the victim's abdomen, just above the navel and below the ribs. Place your other hand on top of the first. Give quick thrusts, pressing your hands inward and upward.

SELF

Give yourself abdominal thrusts until the object is dislodged. Get medical help to check for complications arising from either the choking episode or the first aid. CAUTION: If you feel or see an object lodged in your throat, do not try to retrieve it, as this might force the object farther down your airway.

Abdominal thrust. Make a fist with one hand and place it in the middle of your abdomen, just above the navel and below the ribs. Hold your fist with your other hand. Keeping your elbows out, press your fist with a quick, upward thrust into your abdomen.

Abdominal thrust with the help of an object. Make a fist with one hand and place it in the middle of your abdomen, just above the navel and below the ribs. Bend over the back of a chair, a countertop, or some other firm, hard object and forcefully press it against your fist.

CONTINUED ▶

INFANT (UP TO 1 YEAR OLD)

1 **Give back blows and chest thrusts.** Give four back blows. If the object is not dislodged, give four chest thrusts. Repeat sets of four back blows and four chest thrusts until the object is dislodged or the infant loses consciousness.

2 **If the infant loses consciousness, sweep the infant's mouth with your little finger.** CAUTION: Do not try to retrieve an object lodged in the infant's throat.

3 **Give breaths.** If the infant isn't breathing, give two breaths into the mouth and nose. If the infant's chest does not rise with each breath, gently tilt the head farther back and try again to give two breaths.

4 **If the infant's chest does not rise with breaths, continue giving breaths, back blows, and chest thrusts and sweeps of the mouth.** Repeat a sequence of two breaths, four back blows, four chest thrusts, and a sweep of the mouth until the object is dislodged or until medical help arrives.

Back blow. Lay the infant facedown on your lower arm, supporting the head with your hand. Hold the chin between your index finger and thumb. Strike the back between the shoulder blades with the heel of your other hand.

Chest thrust. Turn the infant onto his back, with his head lower than the rest of his body. Place your index and middle fingers on the breastbone just below the nipples. Give quick thrusts.

Finger sweep. Hold the infant's tongue and lift the chin. If you see an object and believe that you can easily remove it, slide your little finger down the inside of the cheek and sweep the object out.

Breathe into the infant's mouth. Keep the head tilted with one hand and the chin lifted with your other. Tightly seal your lips around the mouth and nose. Give two breaths; remove your mouth between breaths. Breathe forcefully but not so hard that air goes into the infant's stomach.

DROWNING OR NEAR-DROWNING

◆ If a victim is floating facedown in the water or is having difficulty swimming, call 911 or your emergency number, or tell someone nearby to do so; begin the first-aid steps described here.

SYMPTOMS

◆ Cold, pale skin   ◆ Blue face
◆ Unconsciousness   ◆ No exhaled breath

CAUTION: If you suspect a head, neck, or back injury, see page 66.

1 **Pull the victim to safety.** CAUTION: Be careful if you stretch out your arm or leg to the victim; the victim may inadvertently pull you into the water. Try to keep the victim's head, neck, and back aligned as you pull him to shore; if possible, slip a board under his back to tow him or to carry him out of the water.

2 **Check the victim's ABCs** *(page 47).* **If the victim is not breathing or does not have a pulse or heartbeat, begin CPR** *(pages 50-53).*

3 **Place the victim in the recovery position** *(page 47).* CAUTION: Do not place the victim in the recovery position if you suspect a neck or back injury, perhaps caused by a diving accident.

4 **Remove any wet clothing and cover the victim with a coat, blanket, or dry clothing.**

5 **Keep the victim still and quiet while you wait for medical help to arrive.**

WATER RESCUE

Unconscious victim. If possible, wade out and tow the victim faceup to shore; be careful of strong currents. If the water is too deep for wading, look for a boat to use to get to the victim. If there is no boat nearby and you are a strong swimmer, swim out to the victim and tow him faceup to shore. Otherwise, get help.

Conscious victim. Pull the drowning victim to safety with the help of a stick, oar, rope and life ring, towel, or nearby boat. If necessary, wade toward the victim, but be careful of strong currents. CAUTION: Do not swim out to the victim, unless you have been trained in water rescues.

ICE RESCUE

Unconscious victim. If you can't reach the victim, tie a rope to a tree and then around your waist; slide on your belly to the victim. Otherwise, form a human chain with rescuers lying flat on the ice, and pull the victim to shore. CAUTION: Stay as far away as possible from the break in the ice.

Conscious victim. Tell the victim not to climb out but to hang on to the edge of the ice. Pull the victim out with the help of a big stick, rope, or ladder. Or form a human chain with rescuers lying flat on the ice.

EAR EMERGENCIES

Foreign Objects

1 Shake the object out. Tilt the victim's head so that the affected ear is near the ground. Ask the victim to shake his head, or shake it for him. CAUTION: Do not hit the victim's head to try to free the object.

2 Pick the object out. If the object does not fall out, look into the ear. If you can see the object and it is pliable but is not a live insect, try to remove it with tweezers. CAUTION: Never poke at an object. Do not try to pick out a hard object such as a bean or a bead.

3 If there is a live insect inside the ear, kill the insect by pouring a small amount of oil, vinegar, or alcohol onto it. This will help alleviate pain. Then float the insect out with warm, not hot, oil.

4 If the object is securely lodged in the ear, take the victim to the nearest hospital.

3

Floating an insect out of the ear. Tilt the victim's head so that the affected ear is toward the sky. Gently pull the victim's earlobe backward and upward, and pour a little warm mineral, olive, or baby oil into the ear. This should float the insect out of the ear.

Blood or Other Fluids from inside the Ear

1 Loosely cover the ear with a clean cloth and tape the cloth in place. CAUTION: Do not try to stop the drainage. Do not try to clean the ear.

2 Lay the victim flat on his back. CAUTION: If you suspect a head, neck, or back injury, see page 66.

ELECTRIC SHOCK

CAUTION: If you suspect a head, neck, or back injury, see page 66.

1 **Stop the flow of electricity.** Unplug the electrical appliance or turn off the house's main power switch. If you are not able to do this, separate the victim from the live current. CAUTION: Do not touch the victim's skin while he is still touching the live current. Do not touch the electrical wire.

2 **Check the victim's ABCs** *(page 47)*. **If the victim is not breathing or does not have a pulse or heartbeat, begin CPR** *(pages 50-53)*.

3 **Check for and treat any other serious injury.** Treat any entry and exit burns *(page 49)*.

4 **Make the victim comfortable.** Cover the victim with a coat or blanket. Do not place a pillow under the head; this might cause the airway to become blocked.

Separating the victim from the current. Stand on a pile of clothes, a book, or a piece of wood; make sure you are not standing in a pool of water. Use a dry, nonconductive material such as a wooden broom handle or a chair to separate the victim from the live current.

EMERGENCY CHILDBIRTH

Preparing the Mother

1 Make the mother comfortable. Place her on a large, flat area with pillows or other comfortable, supportive materials. Put a clean sheet or newspapers under her. Make sure she is warm. Help her remove any clothing below her belly.

2 Keep the mother calm. The mother may be in great pain; tell her to take deep, slow breaths.

3 Wash your hands with soap and water. Scrub under your fingernails with soap and water, and remove all of your jewelry.

The Delivery

1 Bloodstained fluid will appear. It is normal for there to be some bloodstained fluid; do not be alarmed. CAUTION: Get immediate medical help if the mother bleeds more than 1 to 2 cups of blood before, during, or after delivery.

2 Support the baby as he emerges. The baby will be slippery; you may want to use a clean, dry towel to hold him. CAUTION: Do not pull on the baby.

3 Make sure the umbilical cord is not around the baby's neck. If the umbilical cord is wrapped around the baby's neck, hook your finger underneath it and gently slip it over the baby's head.

Support the baby. Most babies emerge headfirst. Support his head, and the rest of his body, as he emerges. He will naturally turn to one side and the rest of his body will follow.

4 **The baby's shoulder may get stuck.** If a shoulder seems stuck, gently press just above the mother's pubic hair or raise her legs up; tell her to push hard.

5 **The baby may still be in the amniotic sac.** If this is the case, tear the sac open.

6 **The baby's head may not emerge first.** If this happens, gently press just above the mother's pubic hair. Note the time. Support the baby's body as he emerges. If the head is not delivered within three minutes, lift the baby's body to expose his face so he can breathe. Tell the mother to keep pushing. CAUTION: Do not pull the baby out of the vagina.

Let a breech baby breathe. Lift the baby's body upward until you can see his face. Clean the baby's mouth and nose with a clean, dry towel.

After the Birth

1 **Help the baby begin to breathe.** Hold the baby so fluids drain from his mouth and nose. Clean his mouth and nose with a clean, dry towel. If he is not breathing, hold him so his head is lower than his feet and tap his soles. Immediately rub his back. If this doesn't work, begin CPR (pages 50-53).

2 **Dry and wrap the baby.** Use a clean, dry towel; do not wash off any white material on his body. Wrap him in a clean, dry towel.

3 **Tie a string around the umbilical cord.**

4 **Save the placenta.** The mother will usually expel the placenta within 30 minutes. Place it in a container to give to medical personnel. If it is not entirely expelled within 30 minutes, get immediate medical help. Do not pull on the umbilical cord or try to get the placenta out.

5 **Massage the mother's lower abdomen.** After the placenta is expelled, rub the mother's lower abdomen to help control any bleeding.

6 **Keep the mother and baby warm until medical help arrives.**

Drain the baby's fluids. Hold the baby so his head is lower than his feet and turn his head sideways.

Tie off the umbilical cord. Use a string or shoelace and tie it tightly around the umbilical cord at least four inches from the baby's navel. CAUTION: Do not use thread to tie the umbilical cord.

EYE EMERGENCIES

Foreign Objects

CAUTION: Do not touch or attempt to remove anything embedded in the eye. If the object is large, such as a pen, place a paper cup over the eye so that it supports the object; you may need to punch a hole in the cup. Tape the cup in place. Cover the victim's other eye with a clean cloth to help keep the injured eye from moving. If the object is small, cover both eyes with a clean cloth and loosely tie it in place.

1 **Wash your hands with soap and water.**

2 **Look for the object.** Ask the victim to slowly roll his eyes as you look for the object. CAUTION: Do not let the victim rub his eye.

3 **Cause tears to form in the eye.** If you see the object, gently pull the upper eyelid down over the lower eyelid. This will cause tears, which may wash the object out.

4 **Remove a visible object.** If the object does not wash out with tears, flush it out with running water or lift it off with a clean, damp cloth. Alternatively, the victim can open his eyes underwater in a bowl of fresh tap water. Once the object is out, the victim should take out any contact lenses. CAUTION: Do not use tissue or cotton to lift off the object. Do not lift off an object that is on the victim's iris or pupil.

5 **Remove an object from the lower eyelid.** If you see the object on the lower eyelid, flush it out with water or lift it off with a clean, damp cloth. Once the object is out, the victim should take out any contact lenses.

Lifting an object off the lower eyelid. Tell the victim to look up, and gently pull down the lower eyelid. Lift the object off the eye with a clean, damp cloth. CAUTION: Do not use tissue or cotton to lift off the object.

6 **Remove an object off the upper eyelid.** If you do not see the object on the eye or inside the lower eyelid, lift the victim's upper eyelid. If you see the object on the upper eyelid, flush it out with water or lift it off with a clean, damp cloth. Once the object is out of the eye, flip the upper eyelid back into place. The victim should now take out any contact lenses. CAUTION: Do not use tissue or cotton to lift off the object.

Raising the upper eyelid. Tell the victim to look down. Place a cotton swab, matchstick, or coffee stirrer across the upper eyelid. Hold the victim's upper eyelashes and eyelid, and fold the upper eyelid over the matchstick.

7 **If necessary, cover both eyes and get medical help.** If you cannot find or remove the object, or if the victim is in pain or has difficulty seeing after you've removed the object, cover both eyes with a clean cloth and tie it in place. Take the victim to the nearest hospital.

Covering both eyes. Place a clean cloth over the injured eye. Wrap another clean cloth around the victim's head so that it covers both eyes; tie it in place.

Chemical in the Eye

CAUTION: Do not waste any time to begin flushing the eye, and make sure that water is getting underneath both eyelids. Do not put anything other than water in the eye. Do not let the victim rub his eye.

1 **Flush the eye with water.** See the illustration at right. If you cannot get the victim to a faucet, keep flushing the eye with glasses of water for 15 minutes, making sure that the water flows across the eye away from the inner corner.

Flushing the eye. Hold the person's open eye under running water from a faucet for at least 15 minutes. The water should run from the inside of the eye to the outside. If both eyes are affected, let the water run over both eyes.

2 **Ask the victim to remove his contact lenses, if he is wearing any.**

3 **Cover the eye.** After flushing the eye, cover it with a clean cotton cloth. Then tie a bandage over both eyes; this will help inhibit movement of the affected eye.

4 **Identify, if you can, the chemical that caused the burn.** At a minimum, be prepared to tell emergency medical personnel whether the chemical was wet or dry.

FRACTURES AND DISLOCATIONS

CAUTION: If you suspect a head, neck, or back injury, see page 66.

1 **Check the victim's ABCs** *(page 47)*. **If the victim is not breathing or does not have a pulse or heartbeat, begin CPR** *(pages 50-53)*.

2 **Do not move the victim.** CAUTION: Do not move someone with an injured hip, pelvis, or upper leg unless it is absolutely necessary. If you must move him to safety, immobilize the victim's head between your arms, grab his clothes at his shoulders, and drag him.

3 **Check for and treat any other serious injuries.** CAUTION: If the victim is bleeding around or near a broken bone, do not wash or probe the wound. Place a clean cloth over the wound and tie a bandage over it.

4 **Immobilize the injured bone or joint.** If a finger or toe is broken, apply a cold compress to it and elevate it above the level of the victim's heart. Place a small cloth or piece of cotton between the injured digit and an uninjured one, and then tape them together. See the illustrations opposite for instructions on how to immobilize an injured leg or arm. CAUTION: Do not attempt to straighten or change the position of any misshapen bone or joint. When applying a sling or splint, do not cut off blood circulation to the injured limb. Do not tie the splint in place over the break.

IMMOBILIZING AN INJURED ARM

LOWER ARM, WRIST, OR HAND

STABILIZE THE INJURED ARM

Stabilizing the arm. Support the injured bone or wrist with your hands, and place the lower arm at a right angle over the victim's chest. The victim's thumb should be pointing upward. Place the arm and wrist on a magazine or newspaper padded with a towel or pillow, and tie the magazine in place.

PLACE THE ARM IN A SLING

1 Position a cloth to be used as a sling. Locate a large piece of cloth or a long-sleeved shirt or sweater; fold the cloth in half, so it forms a triangle. Slide the cloth or shirt between the victim's arm and body, so the long side of the cloth or the shirt's top is closest to the uninjured arm.

2 Tie the cloth in place. Pull one end of the cloth behind the victim's neck; place the other half over the injured arm. Tie the sling over the shoulder of the uninjured side; fold over any extra material that is behind the elbow and pin it in place. Make sure the sling is snug but not tight.

UPPER ARM, SHOULDER, OR COLLARBONE

STABILIZE THE INJURED SHOULDER OR COLLARBONE

1 Support the injured bone or joint with your hands. Position the injured arm across the chest, thumb pointing up, and place it in a sling (above).

2 Secure the sling in place. Tie a piece of cloth around the sling and the victim's chest and arm.

IMMOBILIZING AN INJURED LEG

LOWER LEG

SPLINT THE LOWER LEG

Using boards as a splint. Locate two long boards; one should extend from the victim's hip to the heel, and the second should stretch from the groin to the heel. Pad the boards with blankets or pillows, then place the boards so the padded side touches the injured leg. Tie the boards in place at the groin, thigh, knee, and ankle.

Using a blanket as a splint. If boards are unavailable, roll up a blanket, place it between the victim's legs, and tie the victim's legs together at the groin, thighs, knees, and ankles.

UPPER LEG OR HIP

SPLINT THE UPPER LEG OR HIP

CAUTION: Do not splint an injured upper leg or hip unless you have to move the victim. Do not tie the splint in place over the break.

Using boards as a splint. Locate two long boards: one to extend from the victim's armpit to the heel, and the other from the groin to the heel. Pad the boards with blankets or pillows, then place the boards padded side in. Tie the boards in place at the chest, waist, groin, thigh, knee, and ankle.

HEAD, NECK, AND BACK INJURIES

CAUTION: Do not move the injured person unless it is absolutely necessary.

1 Keep the victim calm and completely still.

2 Check the victim's ABCs *(page 47)*. **If the victim is not breathing or does not have a pulse or heartbeat, begin CPR** *(pages 50-53)*. CAUTION: When opening the victim's airway, just lift the chin. If you need to place the victim on his back, support his head, neck, and back together and carefully roll him onto his back; make sure you keep the head, neck, and back aligned as you roll him. It is best to have at least one other person help you do this.

3 Treat obvious injuries.

4 Make the victim comfortable. Keep the victim warm, with a blanket or coat, until medical help arrives. CAUTION: Do not put a pillow under the head, as this might cause the airway to become blocked. Do not give him anything to eat or drink.

5 Keep the airway open. If the victim begins to choke or vomit or becomes unconscious, support his head, neck, and back together and carefully roll him onto his side. It is best to have someone else help you do this. CAUTION: Make sure that the victim's head and neck move with his body.

IMPORTANT!

◆ Call 911 or your emergency number.

◆ If you suspect the victim has suffered a head injury and he is bleeding from his ear, eye, or nose, give first aid as described below and then give first aid for ear emergencies *(page 58)*, eye emergencies *(page 62)*, or nose emergencies *(page 72)*.

◆ If you can, find out how the victim was injured. A head, neck, or back injury is particularly likely if the victim was in an accident involving sudden acceleration or deceleration (as in car accidents) or from jumping or diving, or if there are gunshot wounds to the head or chest. Multiple wounds and unconsciousness after physical trauma are other possible indicators.

SYMPTOMS

Head Injuries

◆ Head wound
◆ Bruise or lump on scalp
◆ Bleeding from ear, nose, or mouth that is not due to injury to those areas
◆ Fluid draining from ear or nose
◆ Black eyes
◆ Bruise behind ear
◆ Headache, nausea, or vomiting
◆ Altered mental state
◆ Vision changes
◆ Slurred speech
◆ Irregular pulse
◆ Unconsciousness

Neck or Back Injuries

◆ Pain in back or neck
◆ Tingling sensation in arms or legs
◆ Loss of movement in arms or legs
◆ Loss of bladder or bowel control
◆ Odd position of head, neck, or back
◆ Unconsciousness

HEART ATTACK

CAUTION: If you suspect a head, neck, or back injury, see page 66.

1 **Check the victim's ABCs** *(page 47).* **If the victim is not breathing or does not have a pulse or heartbeat, begin CPR** *(pages 50-53).*

2 **Make the victim comfortable and keep him calm.** Loosen any tight clothing, especially around the victim's neck, chest, and waist. If the victim is unconscious, place him in the recovery position *(page 47).* Keep the victim warm; if necessary, cover him with a blanket or additional clothing. Stroke the victim's forehead with a cool, wet cloth. CAUTION: Do not try to revive an unconscious victim by slapping or shaking him or throwing cold water on him. Do not give the victim anything to eat or drink.

3 **Continue to monitor the victim's breathing and pulse, and if necessary, begin CPR.**

HEATSTROKE AND HEAT EXHAUSTION

SYMPTOMS

Heatstroke

◆ Body temperature above 102°F
◆ Flushed, dry, hot skin
◆ Constricted pupils
◆ Confusion
◆ Rapid pulse
◆ Seizures
◆ Unconsciousness

Heat Exhaustion

◆ Cool, clammy skin
◆ Excessive perspiration
◆ Dilated pupils
◆ Rapid pulse
◆ Headache
◆ Nausea or vomiting
◆ Abdominal or limb cramps
◆ Dizziness
◆ Unconsciousness

Heatstroke

Cool the victim. Quickly move the victim to a cooler site. Place cool, wet cloths on the forehead and torso, or wrap the victim in wet towels or sheets. Fan him with an electric fan, a hair dryer set on cold, or your hand. CAUTION: Do not use an alcohol rub to cool the victim; do not give him anything to eat or drink.

Heat Exhaustion

1 Move the victim to a cooler site.

2 Have the victim lie or sit down, and elevate his feet.

3 Cool the victim. Place cool, wet cloths on the forehead and torso, or wrap the victim in wet towels or sheets. Fan the victim with an electric fan, a hair dryer set on cold, or your hand. CAUTION: Do not use an alcohol rub to cool the victim.

4 Give the conscious victim a cool drink. If the victim is conscious and is able to swallow and breathe without difficulty, give him salt water (1 tsp salt mixed with 1 qt water) to sip. CAUTION: Do not force the victim to drink; do not give him anything that is alcoholic or caffeinated.

5 If the victim's condition does not improve, call 911 or your emergency number.

HYPOTHERMIA AND FROSTBITE

Hypothermia

CAUTION: If you suspect a head, neck, or back injury, see page 66.

1 Check the victim's ABCs *(page 47).* If the victim is not breathing or does not have a pulse or heartbeat, begin CPR *(pages 50-53).* CAUTION: Hypothermic victims often have very slow and weak pulses; therefore, take a little extra time and care to check for the pulse.

2 Gently take or lead the victim to shelter. Change the victim into dry clothing.

3 If medical help is unavailable, slowly rewarm the victim. Cover the head and neck. Use your own body heat, blankets, or aluminum foil to slowly warm the victim. Place warm compresses to the neck, chest, and groin. If the victim is conscious and can swallow, give warm, sweetened, nonalcoholic beverages to sip. CAUTION: Do not use any form of direct heat, such as an electric blanket, to warm the victim.

Frostbite

CAUTION: If there is any chance of the skin refreezing, do not thaw it. Move the victim out of the cold and wait for emergency help.

1 Move the victim to a nearby shelter. Remove any tight clothing or jewelry.

2 If you can keep the frostbitten skin warm and help will not arrive soon, slowly thaw the skin. Place frostbitten hands or feet in a bowl of warm, not hot, water for at least 30 minutes. Gently stir the water, and add warm water as it cools. Or soak a cotton cloth in warm water; resoak the cloth to keep it warm. If water is not available, use your own skin, blankets, or newspaper to warm the skin. CAUTION: Frostbitten skin may be permanently damaged if warmed too quickly; do not use direct heat, such as an electric blanket. Do not massage the skin.

3 Dry the thawed skin and keep it warm. Once the damaged skin is soft and sensation returns, place a clean, dry cloth over the skin; place clean, dry cloths between frostbitten toes and fingers. Wrap the skin with dry cloths in order to keep it warm.

4 Do not let the victim smoke or drink alcohol while you wait for medical help.

INTERNAL BLEEDING

SYMPTOMS

◆ Bruises
◆ Coughing or vomiting blood
◆ Rectal bleeding
◆ Vaginal (but not menstrual) bleeding
◆ Blood in urine
◆ Bleeding from the nose or ear
◆ Skull, chest, or abdominal wounds
◆ Dizziness
◆ Fainting
◆ Weak pulse
◆ Shortness of breath
◆ Shallow breathing
◆ Dilated pupils
◆ Pale, clammy skin

CAUTION: If you suspect a head, neck, or back injury, see page 66.

1 Check the victim's ABCs *(page 47)*. **If the victim is not breathing or does not have a pulse or heartbeat, begin CPR** *(pages 50-53)*. While you wait for medical help, periodically recheck the victim's ABCs.

2 Keep the victim calm and still. Do not give him anything to eat or drink.

3 If the victim's arm or leg is swollen or misshapen, immobilize it *(page 65)*.

4 Begin treatment for shock *(page 75)* while you wait for medical help.

LOSS OF CONSCIOUSNESS

CAUTION: If you suspect a head, neck, or back injury, see page 66.

1 **Check the victim's ABCs** *(page 47).* **If the victim is not breathing or does not have a pulse or heartbeat, begin CPR** *(pages 50-53).*

2 **Remove the victim from an injurious site.**

3 **Loosen any tight clothing, especially around the victim's neck.**

4 **Place the victim in the recovery position** *(page 47).*

5 **Keep the victim warm, with a blanket or coat, until medical help arrives.** Stroke the victim's forehead with a cool, wet cloth. CAUTION: Do not try to revive the victim by slapping or shaking him or throwing cold water on him. Do not place a pillow under the head, as this might cause the airway to become blocked.

NOSE EMERGENCIES

SYMPTOMS

Foreign Objects

◆ Irritation
◆ Difficulty breathing through nostril
◆ Foul-smelling discharge from nostril
◆ Bleeding from nostril

Nosebleed

◆ Bleeding from nostril
◆ Bleeding in the back of the throat
◆ Gagging
◆ Choking

Foreign Objects

CAUTION: Do not use tweezers or other tools to try to remove the object. Do not ask the victim to inhale sharply.

1 Ask the victim to try to blow out the object. Press the unaffected nostril with one finger; ask the victim to blow his nose. If the object is not dislodged, ask the victim to sniff some pepper to help him sneeze and blow the object out.

2 If the object is still not dislodged, take the victim to the nearest hospital.

Nosebleed

CAUTION: If your nose is misshapen or misaligned, or you have swelling, pain, or bruises around your eyes, your nose may be broken. Sit down and press a cold cloth against your nose. Ask someone to take you to the nearest hospital.

1 Sit down.

2 If there are clots of blood in your nose, try to blow them out, once.

3 Pinch your nose shut. Hold both nostrils, below the bridge, between your thumb and index finger for 10 minutes. Breathe through your mouth.

4 If the bleeding does not stop, place a cloth packing in the bleeding nostril. Roll a small, clean cloth and place it in the bleeding nostril; hold both nostrils between your thumb and index finger. CAUTION: Do not push the cloth too far into the nose; make sure that you will be able to pull it out.

5 Once the bleeding stops, place a cold cloth over your nose and face.

6 Remove the cloth packing in your nostril after 30 to 60 minutes. It is best to dampen the cloth before removing it. Do not blow or pick your nose, strain yourself, or bend over for 24 hours. Rub petroleum jelly inside the nostril to help prevent further bleeding or drying.

POISONING

CAUTION: If you suspect a head, neck, or back injury, see page 66.

1 **Check the victim's ABCs** *(page 47)*. **If the victim is not breathing or does not have a pulse or heartbeat, begin CPR** *(pages 50-53)*.

2 **Try to identify the poison.** If possible, ask the victim what he swallowed or inhaled. Otherwise, look around for any open or nearby containers of chemicals or for any plants or household items that the victim may have swallowed; sniff the air for unusual odors.

3 **Call your local poison control center or 911.** Tell emergency personnel what chemical, plant, or household item the victim swallowed. Wait for instructions as to how to proceed.

4 **Follow the instructions given by the poison control center or by 911 personnel.** Depending on the poison, you may be instructed to induce vomiting by giving the victim syrup of ipecac, to give milk or water to drink, or to give activated charcoal. CAUTION: Do not try to induce vomiting unless told to do so; do not induce vomiting if it has been more than one hour since the victim ingested the poison. Do not give the victim anything to eat or drink unless told to do so. Do not rely on poisoning instructions given on container labels.

5 **Place the victim in the recovery position** *(page 47)*.

6 **Save any vomit for medical personnel.**

IMPORTANT!

◆ If chemicals have splashed or spilled into the victim's eyes, see Eye Emergencies *(page 62)*.

◆ If chemicals have splashed or spilled onto the victim's skin, see Burns *(page 49)*.

◆ If the victim inhaled poisonous gas, take him to fresh air and then begin the first-aid steps for poisoning described here.

◆ Since a poisoning victim may exhibit few symptoms or symptoms that are not listed below, it is very important to examine the scene for clues.

SYMPTOMS

◆ Headache	◆ Chills
◆ Dizziness	◆ Drowsiness
◆ Fever	◆ Burns on skin
◆ Abdominal pain	◆ Nausea or vomiting
◆ Vision problems	◆ Breathing problems
◆ Seizures	◆ Unconsciousness
◆ Unusual breath odor	

POISONOUS HOUSEHOLD ITEMS

In addition to this list of poisonous household items, many cleansers, detergents, deodorizers, and disinfectants are poisonous. Drugs, medications, herbal remedies, and vitamins, whether prescription or over the counter, may be poisonous if mixed together, mixed with alcohol, or taken in large quantities. Call your local poison control center about specific items.

◆ Alcohol	◆ Iron pills	◆ Polishes
◆ Antifreeze	◆ Lye	◆ Solvents
◆ Fuels	◆ Mothballs	◆ Tobacco products
◆ Herbicides	◆ Paint	◆ Turpentine
◆ Insecticides	◆ Pesticides	◆ Windshield fluid

POISONOUS PLANTS

There are hundreds of potentially poisonous plants in the U.S. Many plant parts, including seeds, berries, nuts, and bulbs, are potentially poisonous. If you have a question about a plant, call your local poison control center. Some of the most poisonous plants are:

◆ Castor bean	◆ Oleander	◆ Pothos
◆ Dieffenbachia	◆ Philodendron	◆ Water hemlock
◆ Foxglove	◆ Poison hemlock	
◆ Jimson weed	◆ Pokeweed	

SEIZURES

CAUTION: If you suspect a head, neck, or back injury, see page 66.

1 If the victim suspects that he is going to have a seizure or if he begins to lose his balance, help him to the ground.

2 Lay the victim on his side to prevent any vomit from entering his lungs. CAUTION: Do not put your hands in or near the victim's mouth during the seizure.

3 Loosen any tight clothing on the victim.

4 Prevent the victim from injuring himself. Remove eyeglasses. Push away any objects or furniture that might injure the victim if he collides with it. CAUTION: Do not try to restrict his movements, unless he is going to hurt himself.

5 When the seizure has ended, help the victim into a comfortable position on his side. The victim is likely to be tired and confused; he may fall asleep.

6 Check the victim's ABCs *(page 47)*. If the victim is not breathing or does not have a pulse or heartbeat, begin CPR *(pages 50-53)*.

FEBRILE SEIZURES

Seizures in young children or infants are often caused by sudden high fevers. If the child has such a fever, take off his clothes and sponge his body with lukewarm, not cold, water. Call your doctor for further advice. CAUTION: Do not give the child a bath.

SHOCK

IMPORTANT!

◆ Call 911 or your emergency number.

SYMPTOMS

◆ Restlessness or anxiety
◆ Weak, rapid pulse
◆ Cold, clammy, pale skin
◆ Shaking chills
◆ Chest pain
◆ Rapid, shallow breathing
◆ Dizziness or general weakness
◆ Nausea or vomiting
◆ Unconsciousness

CAUTION: If you suspect a head, neck, or back injury, see page 66.

1 **Check the victim's ABCs** *(page 47)*. **If the victim is not breathing or does not have a pulse or heartbeat, begin CPR** *(pages 50-53)*.

2 **Position the victim so he is comfortable.** Unless the victim is more comfortable sitting up, lay him on his back, with his head lower than the rest of his body. If you do not suspect any broken leg bones, elevate the legs 8 to 12 inches. Recheck the victim's airway.

3 **Try to determine the cause of shock and perform first aid for the appropriate emergency.**

4 **Make the victim warm and comfortable.** Loosen any tight clothing and cover the victim with a blanket or additional clothing. Do not use an electric blanket or any other form of direct heat. If the victim is lying down, do not place a pillow under the head, as this might cause the airway to become blocked.

5 **Keep the airway open.** If the victim begins to choke or vomit, turn his head to one side so that the vomit will not block his airway.

6 **If medical help is more than an hour away, give the conscious victim a clean cloth soaked in water to suck on.**

ANAPHYLACTIC SHOCK

IMPORTANT!

◆ If you suspect a severe allergic reaction, the victim may be in anaphylactic shock.

SYMPTOMS

◆ Itching
◆ Flushed face
◆ Dizziness
◆ Nausea or vomiting
◆ Wheezing
◆ Unconsciousness
◆ Hives
◆ Warm skin
◆ Swollen face or tongue
◆ Abdominal cramps
◆ Difficulty breathing

In addition to treating the victim as you would for shock, perform these steps:

◆ **Try to keep the victim calm.**

◆ **Determine if the victim was stung by an insect.** If so, carefully scrape the stinger off the victim's skin. CAUTION: Do not use tweezers; this may push more venom into the skin.

◆ **Administer medicine, if available.** Some people are prone to anaphylactic shock and may have emergency supplies on hand. If this is the case, help the victim with his medicine. This may include giving the victim a shot of epinephrine; follow the instructions on the medication.

SNAKEBITES

SYMPTOMS

Rattlesnake, Copperhead, and Cottonmouth Bites

◆ Increasing pain at bite site
◆ Rapid swelling and skin discoloration at bite site
◆ Twitching skin
◆ Dizziness
◆ Nausea
◆ Sweating
◆ Numbness around mouth

Coral Snake Bites

◆ Pain at bite site
◆ Drowsiness
◆ Slurred speech
◆ Double vision
◆ Sweating
◆ Nausea
◆ Delirium
◆ Seizures

1 Keep the victim calm and still, and if possible, place the bite below the level of the victim's heart.

2 Identify the snake, if you can. If you have to kill the snake, do not damage its head. CAUTION: Do not endanger yourself by getting too close to the snake.

3 Call 911 or your emergency number and report what kind of snake bit the victim.

4 Check the victim's ABCs (page 47). If the victim is not breathing or does not have a pulse or heartbeat, begin CPR (pages 50-53).

5 If the bite is on the victim's arm or leg, tie a band above it. Loosen the band for a minute or two every 15 to 30 minutes. If swelling extends to the band, move it a few inches higher. CAUTION: Do not apply a band if you suspect that the victim was bitten by a coral snake.

6 If you are sure that the snake was poisonous, the bite occurred within 5 minutes, and it will take more than 30 minutes to get medical help, cut into the bite and suck out the venom. With a sterile razor blade, cut just through the skin and through the bite mark. With a suction cup or your mouth, suck out the venom. CAUTION: Cut along the length of a limb, not across it. Do not make any cuts on the victim's head, neck, or torso. Do not swallow the venom; spit it out. Do not suck the venom if you have open sores in or on your mouth. Do not make any cuts if the victim was bitten by a coral snake.

5

Tie a band above the bite. Use either a belt or scarf to tie a band two to four inches above the bite; the band should be between the bite and the victim's heart. Make sure you can slip your finger between the band and the victim's skin and that you can feel a pulse below the band. If you cannot do this, loosen the band until you can.

7 **Gently wash the bite with soap and water.** Pat, don't rub, it dry.

8 **Remove any constricting jewelry or clothing near the bite.**

9 **Place a clean cloth bandage over the bite.**

10 **Watch for signs of a severe allergic reaction.** See Anaphylactic Shock *(page 75).*

11 **If the victim needs to move, do not let him walk; carry him.**

HEAD SHAPES AND BITE MARKS

NONPOISONOUS SNAKE POISONOUS SNAKE

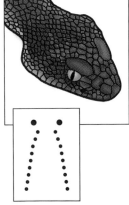

Nonpoisonous snakes tend to leave a bite pattern similar to that shown above, with double rows of bite marks.

Poisonous snakes (except the coral) have a distinctive triangular head; the bite usually includes two fang puncture wounds.

POISONOUS SNAKES IN THE U.S.

There are four types of poisonous snakes in the United States: rattlesnakes, copperheads, cottonmouths (also called water moccasins), and coral snakes (also called harlequin or bead snakes). It is important to be able to recognize the snake that bit the victim so that the proper antivenin can be administered at the hospital.

Rattlesnakes, copperheads, and cottonmouths have triangular heads, slitlike eyes, long fangs, and a similar bite pattern. Rattlesnakes and copperheads shake their tails when disturbed, but only rattlesnakes have rattles on the end of their tails. Cottonmouths can be recognized by the white lining of their mouths.

RATTLESNAKE

COPPERHEAD

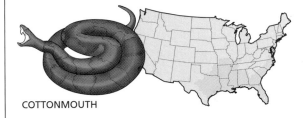

COTTONMOUTH

Coral snakes have red, black, and yellow or white bands and a black snout. They can be distinguished from similarly colored nonpoisonous snakes with the help of this rhyme: "Red next to yellow will kill a fellow; red next to black won't hurt Jack."

CORAL SNAKE

YOUR MEDICINE CHEST

CONVENTIONAL

It is helpful to have some medications for common ailments on hand in your home so that when the occasional cold or flu strikes you'll be prepared. All of the items below are available over the counter (OTC) at most drugstores and supermarkets. When it comes to brand names among OTC classes, most preparations have the same active ingredients and differ only in packaging. Keep in mind that OTC products are still drugs and can have potentially dangerous side effects if misused.

All of these substances should be stored away from light, humidity, and the reach of children. Check expiration dates on all your medications periodically; many of these preparations have a limited shelf life.

Members of your family may have other, specific needs, such as epinephrine for bee allergies. These should also be included in your home medicine chest.

FIRST-AID SUPPLIES

In addition to your home pharmacy, you should also keep a supply of bandages and first-aid materials on hand for emergencies. These items should be stored in clean, airtight containers.

- Adhesive bandages, assorted sizes
- Adhesive tape
- Antiseptic wipes
- Butterfly bandages
- Cold packs (disposable)
- Cotton, both roll and balls
- Cotton-tipped swabs
- Elastic bandage
- First-aid manual
- Gauze bandages, various sizes, in pads and rolls
- Hand wipes (disposable)
- Insect repellent
- Latex gloves
- Safety pins
- Scissors (kept solely for this purpose)
- Sling (triangular bandage)
- Soap
- Sterile nonstick dressings
- Thermometer (if there are children under age five in the household, be sure to include a rectal or ear thermometer)
- Tissues
- Tongue depressors (for finger splints)
- Tweezers

CONVENTIONAL

1 **Antacid** indigestion
2 **Antibiotic cream** cuts, scratches
3 **Antidiarrheal medication**
4 **Antifungal medication** athlete's foot or jock itch
5 **Antihistamine capsules** allergies
6 **Aspirin** or **acetaminophen** pain such as headaches or muscle cramps
7 **Calamine lotion** itching of skin rashes and insect bites
8 **Cough/cold/flu medicine**
9 **Dimenhydrinate tablets** motion sickness
10 **Hydrocortisone cream** skin rashes and insect bites
11 **Hydrogen peroxide** antiseptic for cuts and scratches
12 **Laxative** constipation
13 **Petroleum jelly** chafing
14 **Sunscreen**

ALTERNATIVE

Natural preparations can be used for many common ailments. These herbs, oils, and homeopathic medications can usually be found at health food stores or specialized pharmacies. Oils and homeopathic pharmaceuticals are commonly prepackaged, but herbs may be purchased loose and combined at home to create specific preparations. Don't forget that herbs, like OTC drugs, are powerful substances and should be used with care.

HOMEOPATHIC

1 Aconite colds, croup, fever, shock

2 Apis bites and stings, hives

3 Arnica bruises, dislocated joints, shock

4 Arsenicum album colds, food poisoning, influenza

5 Belladonna earache, fever, headache, infection, heatstroke

6 Bryonia back pain, fever, headaches, influenza

7 Gelsemium fever and influenza

8 Hepar sulphuris abscesses, boils, croup, sore throat

9 Hypericum injury to nerves, insect bites

10 Pulsatilla childhood infections, colds, fever, sinus problems

11 Rhus toxicodendron back pain, chickenpox, influenza, sprains, strains

HERBAL

12 Aloe *(Aloe barbadensis)* apply gel externally for bee stings, sunburn

13 Chamomile *(Matricaria recutita)* tea for indigestion

14 Chickweed *(Stellaria media)* cream for relief of skin irritation

15 Comfrey *(Symphytum officinale)* leaf ointment for cuts but not puncture wounds

16 Dandelion *(Taraxacum officinale)* root decoction as a secretory laxative

17 Elder *(Sambucus nigra)* flower, **peppermint** *(Mentha piperita)*, and **yarrow** *(Achillea millefolium)* hot infusion of equal parts three times daily to relieve sinus pain

18 Flaxseed bulk laxative

19 Gentian *(Gentiana lutea)* hot tea to relieve indigestion

20 Ginger *(Zingiber officinale)* hot infusion of root as needed to relieve nausea

21 Horehound *(Marrubium vulgare)* hot infusion as needed for coughs

22 Marsh mallow *(Althaea officinalis)* hot infusion as needed for coughs

23 Meadowsweet *(Filipendula ulmaria)*, **wild cranesbill** *(Geranium maculatum)*, and **peppermint** *(Mentha piperita)* infusion of equal parts to relieve symptoms of diarrhea

24 Mullein *(Verbascum thapsus)* hot infusion three times daily for coughs; good for children

25 Osha *(Ligusticum porterii)* root for sore throat relief

26 Peppermint *(Mentha piperita)* tea or infusion to relieve indigestion, diarrhea

27 Psyllium *(Plantago psyllium)* bulk laxative

28 Sage *(Salvia officinalis)* gargle infusion for sore throat

29 Sourdock *(Rumex crispus)* decoction three times daily as secretory laxative

30 Tea tree oil *(Melaleuca* spp.) externally for athlete's foot

31 Witch hazel *(Hamamelis virginiana)* distilled, use externally for relief of itching ■

AILMENTS
AND
OPTIONS

Before using any drug or natural medicine mentioned in the following ailment entries, be sure to check with your healthcare practitioner, and check the product packaging or other reliable source of information for any warnings or cautions. You should keep in mind that herbal remedies are not as strictly regulated as drugs.

CONTENTS

CONTENTS CONTINUED

ABDOMINAL PAINS

Read down this column to find your symptoms. Then read across.

SYMPTOMS	AILMENT/PROBLEM
◆ pain in the abdomen; burning feeling in the chest; chest pain, particularly after eating or drinking alcohol; gas or belching; nausea; acid taste in mouth.	◆ Acid stomach; indigestion; heartburn
◆ cramping or pain in the abdomen; nausea; diarrhea; vomiting; fever; malaise; weakness; intestinal gas.	◆ Gastroenteritis
◆ abdominal discomfort, pain, or cramping; pain under the breastbone; possibly, nausea.	◆ Gastritis
◆ pain in the abdomen or under the breastbone, often at night or one hour after eating; pain usually relieved by eating or vomiting; possibly, black-appearing stools.	◆ Peptic ulcer
◆ pain in the abdomen accompanied by diarrhea or constipation, especially after eating; relief with defecation.	◆ Irritable bowel syndrome
◆ cramping or pain in the abdomen; fever; loss of appetite; weight loss; diarrhea; gas; rectal bleeding.	◆ Inflammatory bowel disease; ulcerative colitis; Crohn's disease
◆ sharp, steady pain in groin; lump in abdomen when standing or straining.	◆ Inguinal hernia
◆ intense, sudden pain in upper-right abdomen, especially after a fatty meal; pain may move to right shoulder blade, may last several hours, and is followed by general abdominal soreness. Nausea, vomiting.	◆ Gallstones

WHAT TO DO	OTHER INFO
◆ See Indigestion and Heartburn. Adjust your eating and drinking habits or take an antacid to reduce the symptoms.	◆ Avoid smoking, caffeine, alcohol, fast eating, and nonsteroidal anti-inflammatory drugs (NSAIDs), such as aspirin.
◆ See Gastroenteritis. Rest and drink plenty of fluids.	◆ Gastroenteritis is inflammation of the stomach or intestines often caused by a virus or food poisoning. Hospitalization may be required if symptoms are severe or the patient is very young, elderly, or debilitated.
◆ See Gastritis. Take only liquids for one day; then reintroduce solid food into the diet in small amounts.	◆ Gastritis, an inflammation of the stomach lining, may be caused by lifestyle factors, such as heavy drinking, smoking, or overeating; using aspirin, ibuprofen, or prescription drugs; or a bacterial infection.
◆ See Stomach Ulcers. Rest; eat small, frequent meals; take antacids; avoid smoking, alcohol, aspirin, and caffeine. Your doctor may prescribe a histamine H_2 blocker. If stools appear black, the ulcer may be bleeding. **Call your doctor now.**	◆ If the symptoms persist or recur, your doctor will want to test you for the presence of *Helicobacter pylori,* the bacterium considered the leading cause of peptic ulcers. Treatment is with antibiotics.
◆ See Irritable Bowel Syndrome. The usual first step for reducing symptoms is to take a fiber-based laxative or an antidiarrheal drug.	◆ Adding fiber and fluid to the diet is important, as is exercise. Because stress appears to be a trigger, counseling, biofeedback, yoga, or meditation may be helpful.
◆ **Call your doctor now.** A medical evaluation is necessary for diagnosis and treatment. See Colitis or Crohn's Disease.	◆ Various alternative therapies, such as drinking green leafy vegetable juices for the chlorophyll content, may relieve symptoms. In severe cases, surgery is required to remove all or part of the damaged intestine.
◆ See Hernia.	◆ In this disorder, the intestines or bladder bulges through the abdominal wall.
◆ **Call your doctor now**. A medical evaluation is necessary for diagnosis and treatment, which may involve surgical removal of the gallbladder or a nonsurgical procedure that dissolves the stones.	◆ Reducing fat and meat intake and increasing fiber may help prevent the formation of new stones.

A

SYMPTOMS	AILMENT/PROBLEM
◆ acute, constant abdominal pain radiating to the back and chest; fever; nausea; vomiting; abdominal distention; clammy skin.	◆ Pancreatitis
◆ severe cramping pain that is usually worse on the left side of the abdomen; chills; fever; nausea; history of constipation.	◆ Diverticulitis
◆ sharp pain in the side that moves toward the groin and/or abdomen; frequent urge to urinate; blocked flow of urine; painful urination; cloudy or foul-smelling urine; blood in urine; fever and chills; nausea and vomiting; profuse sweating.	◆ Kidney stones
◆ pain low in the abdomen that is accompanied by painful and frequent urination; constant urge to urinate; possibly, blood in urine.	◆ Urinary tract infection
◆ pain radiating from below the breastbone into the neck and arms; heartburn; vomiting; belching; bloating; difficulty swallowing.	◆ Hiatal hernia
◆ crampy pain in the pelvic area during menstruation.	◆ Menstrual cramps
◆ extremely severe abdominal pain with or without other acute symptoms.	◆ **Emergency conditions:** intestinal obstruction, peritonitis, appendicitis, ileus, pelvic inflammatory disease, heart attack, abdominal aortic aneurysm, ischemic bowel, ruptured ectopic pregnancy, ruptured ovarian cyst, perforated peptic ulcer, anaphylactic shock, chemical burn, diabetic emergency, poisoning.

WHAT TO DO	OTHER INFO
◆ **Call your doctor now** to avoid possible life-threatening complications. See Pancreatic Problems.	◆ The cause is usually heavy drinking or gallbladder disease. To control chronic pancreatitis, avoid alcohol and fatty foods.
◆ **Call your doctor now.** Severe cases may require hospitalization and surgery. Treatment for milder cases usually involves bed rest, stool softeners, a liquid diet, antibiotics, and possibly, antispasmodic drugs.	◆ Although you should eat low-bulk foods during the inflammatory period, a high-fiber diet may be preventive.
◆ **Call your doctor now.** A medical evaluation is necessary for diagnosis and treatment. Commonly, the first step is to drink plenty of water and take a pain reliever until the stone passes.	◆ Infection, blockage, or large stones may make surgery necessary. A new treatment method uses high-energy shock waves to break up the stones without surgery.
◆ If you also have fever, chills, back pain, and possibly, nausea and vomiting, you may have a kidney infection. **Call your doctor now.** See Bladder Infections and Kidney Infections.	◆ Pregnant women, people with diabetes, and nursing-home patients are at greatest risk for serious complications of a urinary tract infection.
◆ See Hiatal Hernia.	◆ Lifestyle changes that may alleviate symptoms include avoiding smoking and alcohol, and eating smaller meals, none within two hours of going to bed.
◆ See Menstrual Problems. Take a pain reliever such as aspirin or ibuprofen.	◆ Chiropractic, acupuncture, or magnesium supplements may help. For severe cramps, your doctor may recommend a prescription anti-inflammatory drug. See also Ovary Problems.
◆ **Call your doctor, 911, or your emergency number now. Follow instructions to obtain immediate medical care.**	

ACHES AND PAINS

SYMPTOMS	AILMENT/PROBLEM
◆ pain and swelling of muscles and joints in an active person; possibly, headache.	◆ Overexertion
◆ achiness with runny nose, sneezing, and cough; possibly, sore throat, headache.	◆ Common cold
◆ achiness with runny nose, sneezing, cough, headache, sore throat, weakness, chills, and fever; possibly, vomiting and/or diarrhea.	◆ Flu
◆ achiness with fever, chills, and chest pain; cough that produces sputum.	◆ Pneumonia
◆ joints painful, red, warm, stiff, and/or swollen; pain worse in the morning.	◆ Inflammatory arthritis
◆ chronic, widespread muscle pain and stiffness, especially in the morning; sleep disturbance and chronic fatigue.	◆ Fibromyalgia
◆ muscle or joint pain with headache, fatigue, malaise, and fever; months before, a circular or oval red rash up to eight inches or more in diameter with a white center may have appeared on the skin, from a tick bite that may or may not have been noticed.	◆ Lyme arthritis, a later stage of Lyme disease

WHAT TO DO	OTHER INFO
◆ Consider anti-inflammatory drugs, heat rubs or massage, a cream containing aspirin, or the homeopathic remedy Arnica. Also, set limits to exercise; pay attention to your body's early signals of overexertion.	◆ The achiness may not be felt until two to three days after the overexertion. People who exercise to maintain a mood uplift need to be especially cautious.
◆ See Common Cold. Rest, drink plenty of fluids, and if needed, take a decongestant.	◆ Vitamin C is widely believed to lessen the severity of colds. The herb echinacea (*Echinacea* spp.) may also help.
◆ See Flu. Rest, drink plenty of fluids, and if needed, take an anti-inflammatory drug to reduce fever and achiness. For prevention, eat a healthful diet to improve your immune defenses.	◆ Flu shots are often recommended for people over 65 and for those with chronic diseases. Children under 18 who may have a viral infection should not take aspirin or aspirin-containing products, which have been linked in young people with the neurological disorder Reye's syndrome. Children under 12 should not take aspirin when ill.
◆ **Call your doctor now.** A medical evaluation is needed for diagnosis and treatment, which may involve antibiotics. If you are elderly, have another serious illness, or fail to improve with treatment, you may need to be hospitalized. See Pneumonia.	◆ Muscle aches are more likely to be caused by an "atypical" pneumonia, which comes on more slowly and is caused by a virus or other microorganism rather than by a bacterium.
◆ See Arthritis. Take an anti-inflammatory drug for pain relief.	◆ The condition may be helped by acupuncture, homeopathy, herbal medicine, and nutritional changes. Aching in joints also may be caused by a noninflammatory arthritis, such as osteoarthritis, in which redness, warmth, and swelling do not occur.
◆ Treatment frequently involves analgesics, a low-dose antidepressant, and/or injection of a local anesthetic, possibly with a corticosteroid, into aching points of the body.	◆ Fibromyalgia was previously believed to be psychogenic but is now recognized as a syndrome with uniform signs and symptoms. Aerobic exercise, stress management, massages, and acupuncture may be helpful.
◆ **Call your doctor now.** The usual treatment is antibiotics. See Lyme Disease.	◆ Lyme arthritis, which is characterized by back and joint pain, can occur months, or even years, after the bite of a deer tick, the cause of Lyme disease.

SYMPTOMS

- persistent, recurrent red spots or swellings on the skin, generally known as pimples; they may become inflamed or pus-filled, and typically appear on the face, chest, shoulders, neck, or upper portion of the back, particularly in adolescents.
- Dark spots with open pores at the center are **blackheads.**
- Spots that bulge under the skin and have no opening are **whiteheads.**
- Red swellings or lumps, sometimes visibly filled with pus, are **pustules,** which develop from blackheads or whiteheads.
- Inflamed, fluid-filled lumps under the skin, which may become as large as an inch across, are **nodules,** or **cysts.**
- Abnormally flushed cheeks and nose are a sign of **rosacea,** an acnelike disorder that affects adults—mostly women—over 30 years of age.

CALL YOUR DOCTOR IF:

- your acne doesn't respond in two to three months to over-the-counter remedies; you may need medical treatment.
- you have severe acne, which may produce cysts under the skin and persistent pimples that may become infected. A dermatologist may recommend prescription drugs to control the condition and prevent permanent scars.
- your skin becomes abnormally flushed around your cheeks and nose. You may have **rosacea,** which can be controlled with appropriate antibiotic medication.

Nearly everyone suffers from outbreaks of pimples at some point in life, making acne one of the most common skin disorders. It starts when tiny hair follicles become plugged with oily secretions from the skin's sebaceous glands. **Blackheads** appear as small, usually flat spots with centers darkened by exposure to air; **whiteheads** are similar lesions without the color. Both types of pimples can develop into swollen, tender inflammations. **Cysts,** or **nodules,** associated with severe cases of acne, are firm swellings below the skin's surface that become inflamed and sometimes infected.

Although acne remains largely a curse of adolescence, about 20 percent of all cases occur in adults. Acne commonly arises during puberty and tends to be worse in people with oily skin. It occurs in both sexes, although teenage boys tend to have the most severe cases. Women are more likely than men to have mild to moderate forms into their thirties and beyond, and are somewhat more susceptible to **rosacea.**

Myths about harmful diets and uncontrolled sex drives causing acne have been replaced by the simple truth that heredity and hormones are behind most forms. Swearing off chocolate or scrubbing your face 10 times a day won't change your predisposition to this unsightly, sometimes painful, and often embarrassing skin disorder.

CAUSES

The cause of acne is not fully understood. While poor hygiene, poor diet, and stress can aggravate acne, they clearly do not cause it. Common **acne vulgaris** in teenagers starts with an increase in hormone production. During puberty, both boys and girls produce high levels of androgens—male sex hormones that include testosterone. Androgens can in turn step up production of sebum, the substance that lubricates the skin and helps it retain moisture, and keratin, a primary constituent of hair. Tiny hair follicles, especially those on the face, neck, chest, and back, can become plugged with sebum and keratin. As the follicles fill up and bacteria multiply, **blackheads** or **whiteheads** form on the skin's surface, a condition called

noninflammatory acne. If the follicle wall ruptures under pressure and sebum leaks into nearby tissue, the result is a **pustule,** or **inflammatory acne.** If pustules become infected, matters are further complicated: The infection can penetrate deep into the skin and create **cysts,** which can rupture and leave temporary or permanent scars.

Various factors appear to make certain people prone to developing acne, such as family history of the condition, stress, and using contraceptives or corticosteroids. Taking oral contraceptives may trigger acne in some women but actually suppress it in others, depending on the type of pill taken. Anabolic steroids taken by some bodybuilders can also lead to severe outbreaks.

Acne has many subtypes. Some forms—**acne neonatorum** and **acne infantum**—occasionally affect newborns and infants, usually boys. A pimply rash appears on the face but usually clears within weeks with no lasting effect. Adults, usually women, who escape their teen years almost pimple free may develop persistent **adult-onset acne** as they get older. In some cases the outbreaks are allergic reactions to cosmetics or foods, while others are linked to menstruation. Both **premenstrual** and **postmenopausal acne** tend to be relatively milder than cosmetic-related flareups.

Despite the normal increase in androgen levels during puberty, some researchers believe that flareups of acne have less to do with an individual's androgen levels than with how that person's skin responds to an increase in the production of sebum. The bacteria *Propionibacterium acnes* and *Staphylococcus epidermidis* occur naturally in healthy hair follicles. If too many of them accumulate in plugged follicles, they may secrete enzymes that break down sebum, promoting localized inflammation. Some people are simply more sensitive than others to this reaction, so that sebum levels that might cause a pimple or two in one person may result in widespread outbreaks, or **acute cystic acne,** in another person.

ROSACEA

W. C. Fields, with his bulbous nose and flushed complexion, may be the best-known victim of rosacea, but fair-skinned women over 30 are actually the most prone to the condition. Rosacea starts with a persistent, abnormal blush on the cheeks and nose, which is made more obvious by consuming spicy foods, hot drinks, or alcohol. The inflammation tends to spread, and a few rosacea patients, usually men, develop a severe form in which the nose becomes red, thickened, and tender.

To control mild cases, your doctor will probably prescribe an oral antibiotic such as metronidazole or a topical corticosteroid. Lotions or gels containing sulfur as an active ingredient may be prescribed or purchased over the counter. Because many rosacea patients also suffer from migraine headaches, some researchers suspect that an intolerance to certain types of food may be a factor. Some cases respond particularly well to large doses of B vitamins, especially vitamin B_2 (riboflavin). In severe cases of rosacea, surgery or laser treatments may reverse the inflammation and swelling.

TREATMENT

The occasional pimple or two need no treatment. Over-the-counter cover-up creams and cosmetics, if used at all, should be water based and hypoallergenic. Even if outbreaks of acne cannot be eliminated, conventional and alternative treatment can provide relief. Conventional medicine favors drug therapies that inhibit sebum and keratin production, limit bacterial growth, or encourage shedding of skin cells to unclog pores. Because many therapies can have potent side effects, any patient with a skin problem should proceed with caution when trying a new treatment.

People with severe, persistent cases need the care of a dermatologist.

CONVENTIONAL MEDICINE

To treat mild acne, your doctor may recommend a topical over-the-counter medication containing benzoyl peroxide or prescribe the antiacne drug tretinoin (retinoic acid), a vitamin A derivative. Before applying the medication, wash the affected area with a mild oil- and scent-free soap. When pus-filled pimples are ready to break, applying a hot towel for a few minutes may encourage the process. Infected pimples should be opened only by a nurse or doctor using surgical instruments and following antiseptic practices. Squeezing pimples yourself may lead to further infection and the possibility of permanent scars.

For moderate to severe cases, a mainstay of treatment is tetracycline, an antibiotic that is usually taken orally, sometimes in combination with topically applied tretinoin. Other useful antibiotics are oral erythromycin and clindamycin.

For chronically inflamed **cysts,** a doctor may prescribe the drug isotretinoin, but because of its potentially severe side effects, the treatment must be monitored carefully, especially in women of childbearing age. A less common treatment option is to inject triamcinolone, a type of corticosteroid, directly into the cysts. This treatment may leave some patients' skin temporarily darkened around the lesion. Because many acne sufferers are relieved by summer sun, a dermatologist may also recommend controlled exposure to ultraviolet light to keep outbreaks in check.

Patients taking antiacne drugs should be alert to possible side effects and interactions. The drugs tretinoin and benzoyl peroxide can leave skin reddened, dry, and sensitive to sunlight. Benzoyl peroxide may inhibit the healing effects of tretinoin, so never apply them at the same time. Taking antibiotics for more than a few weeks may leave women susceptible to yeast infections.

Some adults carry scars or pitted skin from cysts or deep pimples that were scratched or severely infected. Two relatively aggressive surgical procedures can improve the skin's appearance: dermabrasion, in which a dermatologist essen-

ACUPRESSURE

1 Acupressure may help to ease inflammation, hormonal imbalances, and emotional distress associated with acne. Apply firm pressure with your thumb to Large Intestine 11, at the outer end of the elbow crease. Hold for one minute, and repeat on the other arm.

2 To help ease skin irritation, press your right thumb into Large Intestine 4, between the thumb and index finger of your left hand, pushing against the bone above your index finger. Hold for one minute, then repeat on the other hand. Do not use this point if you are pregnant.

tially sandpapers frozen skin, and chemical peeling. Both procedures remove the scarred surface and expose unblemished skin layers. Before considering such treatment, however, discuss the procedures, necessary precautions, and likely results with at least two dermatologists.

ALTERNATIVE CHOICES

Some alternative therapies for acne attempt to reduce inflammation and fight infection. Other approaches use herbal or dietary measures to control factors that may promote acne, such as stress. For mild or moderate acne, these approaches may make sense, but **acne vulgaris** and **rosacea** respond much more slowly than most other ailments to any therapy. Be patient: Many acne treatments take up to a year to produce results.

CHINESE HERBS

Chinese herbal medicine for acne seeks to rid the skin of dampness and heat, which are believed to be causative factors. Preparations commonly used for the purpose include cnidium seed *(Cnidium monnieri)* and honeysuckle flower *(Lonicera japonica).* Consult a practitioner of Chinese medicine for specific formulations and dosages.

HERBAL THERAPIES

Many herbs are used to help heal the skin and soothe inflammation and itching. Among those a trained herbalist may recommend are echinacea *(Echinacea* spp.), calendula *(Calendula officinalis),* tea tree oil *(Melaleuca* spp.), and goldenseal *(Hydrastis canadensis);* tincture of blue flag *(Iris versicolor)* works particularly well with echinacea. Drinking tea made with a combination of nettles *(Urtica dioica)* and cleavers *(Galium* spp.) tincture may be effective. CAUTION: Never use any herbal preparation on newborns without consulting your doctor.

If stress may be contributing to your acne, try relaxing with a cup of tea made from lavender *(Lavandula officinalis)* or chamomile *(Matricaria recutita).* A facial sauna two to three times a week with either of these herbs may also help.

HOMEOPATHY

For minor outbreaks of acne, Hepar sulphuris or Silica, in 6x potency tablets taken three times a day for up to a week, may help speed healing.

NUTRITION AND DIET

Most doctors now believe that acne is not a food-related problem and rarely ask patients to change their diets as a means of reducing outbreaks. Some alternative therapists, however, make a change in diet the basis of treatment. While experts in both camps concede that chocolate, fats, and other suspect foods don't cause acne, debate continues over whether they can aggravate the condition.

Among vitamin and mineral supplements, nutritionists generally suggest zinc, which plays a part in how the body processes hormones. A 30- to 50-mg zinc supplement daily may contribute to reducing inflammation and healing damaged skin. Chromium supplements are said to boost the body's ability to break down glucose. Large amounts of vitamin A may reduce sebum and keratin production, but since large doses can cause

headaches, fatigue, muscle and joint pain, and other side effects, taking megasupplements is not advised unless monitored carefully by your doctor or other healthcare practitioner. Vitamin E, an antioxidant, may also be included in a natural antiacne regimen at doses of 200 to 400 IU a day. Vitamin B_6, which aids in the metabolism of hormones, can be particularly effective for women suffering from premenstrual acne; 50 mg a day is a typical dosage.

AT-HOME REMEDIES

◆ Washing your face gently with unscented, oil-free soap—or even a medicated soap—helps keep your skin clean, but scrubbing already inflamed skin only makes acne worse.

◆ Resist the urge to pop pimples. Let them break when they're ready, then wash gently.

◆ For mild to moderate acne, try over-the-counter treatments that contain benzoyl peroxide.

◆ Expose your acne to sunlight in moderation, but be careful to avoid overexposure.

◆ Men with moderate to severe acne should use a new razor blade every time they shave to lower the risk of infection. Instead of alcohol-based aftershaves, try herbal alternatives that include essential oils of lavender, chamomile, or tea tree.

PREVENTION

Because of acne's association with fluctuating hormone levels and possible genetic influences, many doctors believe there is no way to prevent it. Although the accepted wisdom is that neither good hygiene nor diet can prevent outbreaks, the tips in **Nutrition and Diet** *(left)* may be helpful.

Good general hygiene and sensible skin care are especially important during adolescence. The basics include a daily bath or shower, and washing face and hands with unscented or mildly antibacterial soap. Teenage girls are better off not using cosmetics regularly. And despite claims to the contrary, few if any commercial skin medications have any beneficial effect on acne. ■

SYMPTOMS

Adenoid-related problems produce symptoms in the ears, nose, and throat. Any of the following may be indicative of adenoid problems:

- sleep apnea, in which the sleeping child may interrupt a normal breathing pattern with either short periods of not breathing many times through the night, or longer periods of not breathing—up to 20 seconds—once or twice a night.
- mouth breathing (nasal obstruction).
- snoring (obstructed airway).
- nasal voice.
- secretions from the nose during the day combined with a cough at night, caused by sinus drainage.
- recurring ear infections in association with the above symptoms.

CALL YOUR DOCTOR IF:

- ◆ your child has intervals of not breathing many times each night; this may indicate sleep apnea syndrome, which can cause behavioral problems in children because of sleep disturbances, or in severe cases can put pressure on the cardiac system.
- ◆ you notice your child having difficulty breathing or breathing open-mouthed because of extreme nasal congestion. While these symptoms are not life-threatening, they indicate that your child's adenoids may be obstructing the nasal airway.
- ◆ your child has recurrent ear infections that respond poorly to antibiotic treatment; untreated ear infections can cause hearing loss.

The adenoids, masses of lymph tissue located in the top of the throat behind and above the tonsils *(below, right)*, play a special role during childhood: By making antibodies, they help the young child's body fight respiratory tract infections. From the time your child is three until around the age of seven, the adenoids grow so that they can give extra protection to the lungs and chest. After about the age of eight, they usually begin to shrink, and by the time your child is an adolescent, they have virtually disappeared.

When the adenoids become infected or irritated they swell, often blocking the airway to the nose and the Eustachian tube to the ear, causing mild to severe discomfort and difficulty breathing or hearing. Left untreated, enlarged adenoids can lead to chronic sinusitis, and in severe cases, sleep apnea—in which the child stops breathing for seconds at a time during the night.

You may have grown up in an era when removing the adenoids and tonsils was standard practice and may have undergone one of these procedures yourself. But because doctors now understand more clearly the role of the adenoids in fighting infection, the chances of your child's undergoing an adenoidectomy are much more remote—usually limited to the most severe cases.

CAUSES

The primary reason for chronic adenoid problems is structural: The adenoids grow so large that they block the nasal passages. But infection or irritation, perhaps caused by allergies, can also cause problems by making the adenoids swell.

TREATMENT

Adenoid problems are difficult to diagnose because the symptoms can point to any number of conditions and it is hard to tell even by examination if enlarged adenoids are the cause. Always take your child to a pediatrician or to an alternative practitioner for an examination if he or she has had recurrent ear infections, a blocked nose, or any of the other symptoms listed at left.

CONVENTIONAL MEDICINE

Your child's pediatrician will take a history of your child's ear, nose, and throat problems and probably refer you to either an ear, nose, and throat (ENT) specialist or an allergist for an evaluation of your child's symptoms. The ENT specialist will want to examine your child and may also order x-rays to help determine the size and shape of the adenoids. The allergist will probably test for any sensitivity to airborne allergens (for example, cigarette smoke, dust, pollen, or pet dander).

If allergies are to blame, treatment for the allergies—such as a course of allergy shots to desensitize your child—or elimination of allergens is the appropriate action. If allergies are not the cause, the ENT specialist may recommend surgery to remove the adenoids. Surgery is called for as a first-line defense only in cases of severe sleep apnea, in which the enlarged adenoids can cause chronic pressure on the cardiac system and could possibly lead to heart failure.

THE ADENOIDS

ADENOIDS

TONSILS

Adenoids, like tonsils, are lymph nodes that act as filters against germs. They are small, pink lumps on the back wall of the throat (shown here in yellow), just above the roof of the mouth. When the adenoids become infected, they may swell and hamper breathing.

ALTERNATIVE CHOICES

Alternative therapists usually seek an allergy-related cause first. Always take your child to a professional for evaluation and treatment; at-home care can only alleviate the symptoms.

HERBAL THERAPIES

Echinacea (*Echinacea* spp.) is believed to help fight infection. Cleavers (*Galium aparine*) may help reduce swelling of lymphatic tissue. Consult a medical herbalist for appropriate dosages.

HOMEOPATHY

Because chronic adenoid problems give rise to other problems, you should consult a homeopathic physician for remedies appropriate to the condition as well as to the individual. The practitioner will monitor your child's progress and change remedies if they do not bring relief in a short time.

OSTEOPATHY

Manipulative treatment of the neck, which is thought to drain the lymphatic system, would be the prescribed course of treatment.

AT-HOME REMEDIES

These remedies may alleviate some symptoms, but they will not clear up the underlying condition. Always seek help from a professional when your child has a chronic problem.

◆ For children with allergies, reducing or eliminating environmental irritants can make your child more comfortable. For example, an electrostatic air filter may lower the amount of dust or mold in the house.

◆ A humidifier may help a child who is congested by preventing the mucus from getting too thick. Use a humidifier with a humidistat to ensure the proper amount of moisture in the air, and clean the humidifier thoroughly before and after use.

◆ An over-the-counter decongestant may temporarily alleviate stuffiness.

◆ Chicken soup may also open blocked nasal passages.

SYMPTOMS

The following are among the most common symptoms of AIDS:

- long-term fatigue you can't explain.
- swollen lymph nodes.
- a fever that lasts more than 10 days.
- night sweats.
- unexplained weight loss.
- purplish or discolored lesions on skin or mucous membrane that do not go away.
- persistent, unexplained cough or sore throat.
- shortness of breath.
- persistent colds.
- persistent severe diarrhea.
- yeast infections.
- easy bruising or bleeding that cannot be explained.

CALL YOUR DOCTOR IF:

- you have more than one of the above symptoms; you may not have AIDS, but you do have a condition that requires treatment.

For a person who has contracted the virus that causes AIDS, the long-term outlook is undeniably grim. But a diagnosis of AIDS should not be taken as an immediate death sentence. With proper care the AIDS sufferer can stave off the worst symptoms and live a productive life for many years.

Acquired immune deficiency syndrome (AIDS) is not a single disease in itself. Rather, a severely impaired immune system leaves the AIDS sufferer highly susceptible to a whole host of infections and diseases. AIDS is thought to be caused by the human immunodeficiency virus (HIV), which is spread through infected semen, vaginal fluids, and blood. HIV damages the body's ability to produce adequate numbers of white blood cells called T cells, leaving it unable to fight off invading bacteria or viruses.

Symptoms differ widely from country to country and even from risk group to risk group. In the United States and Europe, AIDS sufferers often develop Kaposi's sarcoma (a rare form of skin cancer), pneumocystis pneumonia, and tuberculosis. In Africa, AIDS usually causes sufferers to waste away from fever, diarrhea, and a persistent cough. Developing any of the 28 or so diseases and sets of symptoms associated with AIDS in the United States and testing positive for antibodies to HIV will almost certainly lead to a diagnosis of AIDS.

In most cases AIDS starts with flulike symptoms that resemble mononucleosis. These may persist for two weeks to a few months after the virus enters the body.

After this first stage, symptoms may disappear for several years. How the AIDS patient takes care of himself or herself during this time is extremely important, because HIV is multiplying in the body, slowly at first and then rapidly. As the virus systematically destroys the cells that fight off infection, the immune system begins to fail and the patient becomes vulnerable to various illnesses and tumors. This stage is sometimes called **ARC,** or **AIDS-related complex.** Full-blown AIDS—the stage in which serious infections begin to develop—may not appear until 5 to 10 years after the onset of HIV infection. Death usually occurs 2 to 3 years later.

Doctors in the United States first recognized AIDS in 1981, but undiagnosed cases had begun showing up in 1979. Before that, AIDS probably existed in Africa and some Caribbean countries.

Although AIDS can strike anyone, it first occurred among homosexual and bisexual men who had many sexual partners. Because many of these men also used recreational drugs such as "poppers" (amyl nitrate), doctors thought at first that the drugs caused the disease. Eventually, research showed that AIDS is transmitted via bodily fluids. That hypothesis was borne out when intravenous-drug users, heterosexuals, and people who got blood transfusions began to contract AIDS.

This most serious health crisis of our time has now reached epidemic levels. Worldwide, more than 14 million people are infected with HIV. In the United States as many as 1.5 million people are thought to have the virus, and the number of AIDS cases doubles every year; in many U.S. cities, AIDS is the leading cause of death for adults 25 to 44 years old.

At greatest risk for AIDS are people who engage in sex without using condoms and infants born to AIDS-infected mothers. Also at great risk are male and female intravenous-drug users who share needles, and people who received blood transfusions or clotting factors between 1977 and 1985, prior to the establishment of standard AIDS screening of donated blood. Currently, as AIDS spreads through the heterosexual population, women make up the fastest-growing group of infected people. In the United States, more than 80,000 women between the ages of 15 and 44 have contracted the virus.

The good news is that AIDS is preventable. Provided you are not at risk because of intravenous drug use, you can avoid HIV infection through a monogamous relationship, or reduce the risk of infection by practicing safe sex—which means, first and foremost, using condoms.

According to recent indicators, more people are taking such precautions. The National Health and Social Life Survey, which was published in 1995, found that nearly 3 in 10 American adults say they have dramatically altered their sexual behavior to lower the risk of contracting AIDS. This landmark study of adult sexual behavior investigated the sex habits and attitudes of about 150 million people. Results of the survey include:

◆ 29 percent reported using condoms more often.
◆ 26 percent said they were likely to be monogamous.
◆ 25 percent said they were choosing their partners more carefully or getting to know them better before being intimate.
◆ 11 percent said they had decided to abstain from sex because they were afraid of contracting AIDS.

CAUSES

Scientists suspect that at least two viruses cause AIDS: **HIV-1** and **HIV-2.** Worldwide, the viruses infect equal numbers of people, but HIV-1 is much more prevalent in North America.

Researchers don't yet know precisely how HIV works, and some are asking whether in fact the virus causes AIDS or merely shows up in conjunction with it. For some reason the immune system can't detect HIV. The virus enters the body through small abrasions or cuts in mucous membranes in the mouth, vagina, or rectum and destroys T cells, so the immune system fails. Patients then develop infections that eventually kill them.

AIDS is not a highly contagious disease. The only way you can get it is to have unprotected vaginal, oral, or anal sex with an infected partner or to share tainted blood, which may occur through IV-drug use or transfusions.

You can't get AIDS from kissing. A protein in human saliva keeps the AIDS virus from infecting white blood cells. The protein attaches itself to white blood cells and protects them from infection. The discovery may lead to new strategies for developing AIDS medicines, such as injecting this protein directly into the bloodstream to keep the virus from attacking blood cells.

You also needn't worry about catching AIDS if you live with someone who has it. HIV cannot be transmitted by toilet seats or objects handled by people who have AIDS. Nor will you get the disease if you share food with someone who is infected, because HIV dies very quickly once it is outside the body.

A

DIAGNOSTIC AND TEST PROCEDURES

Within a few weeks of infection, your body should be producing antibodies to the virus, which your doctor can detect in blood tests. However, your body may take as long as 35 months to produce a detectable level of antibodies, so if you think you've been infected, particularly if you're in a high-risk group, you should be tested for the disease every 6 months.

The first test you'll be given is the ELISA, or enzyme-linked immunosorbent assay. This test is generally reliable, but a positive result (meaning antibodies have been detected) should always be confirmed; the doctor may follow up with the Western blot, a blood test that almost never gives a false-positive reading.

Before deciding to have an AIDS test, make sure you get advice from a counselor. A positive test result for AIDS may cause you profound psychological distress. The counselor can help you deal with the anxiety, grief, and fear you'll probably experience at first.

If you test positive, make sure your doctor gives you a complete workup to detect other sexually transmitted diseases, such as gonorrhea, genital herpes, or syphilis.

It is extremely important that you notify your sexual partners of your diagnosis. They too must be tested and treated.

TREATMENT

Almost everyone who develops full-blown AIDS eventually succumbs to the disease, but antibiotic and antiviral drugs can prolong life for several years. In any event, you should never try to treat yourself for this life-threatening illness: Always seek the advice of a qualified practitioner. And beware of claims made for "miracle" cures. They simply don't exist.

Currently there are several hundred human studies to test drugs for the treatment of AIDS and related conditions. These include antiviral drugs, drugs that modify the immune system, anti-infective drugs, and anticancer drugs.

One study by the National Institute of Allergy and Infectious Diseases (NIAID) has found that a naturally produced protein may rebuild AIDS-damaged immune systems. Called interleukin 2, the protein dramatically increased T cell counts in 6 out of 10 people who took it. However, it did not work for people with advanced AIDS, and it also has severe side effects, including rash, nausea, diarrhea, and depression. Further studies on the protein are being conducted.

Another experimental treatment, now in use in France, is **passive immunotherapy**. The therapy does not increase the life span of AIDS sufferers, but it may keep them from getting as sick as they otherwise might. Patients with advanced AIDS are injected with plasma from healthier HIV-infected donors. Researchers hope the injections will bolster the advanced patients' immune systems and help them fight off diseases associated with AIDS. Initial results have been promising.

Although a number of vaccines to prevent AIDS are under investigation, scientists have had difficulty finding one that works. The theory is that injecting someone with a weakened form of the virus would spur that person's immune system to mount a huge attack against HIV and build up a resistance. Doctors are understandably reluctant to inject anyone with HIV, however, fearing that even a weakened virus might cause AIDS.

In related work, a team of researchers from NIAID has developed a vaccine with a "suicide gene" that allows itself to be killed off once its job is done. The weakened HIV carries an extra gene taken from the herpesvirus. Cells that become infected with HIV then can be selectively destroyed with ganciclovir, a herpes medicine. So far the

---

C A U T I O N !

Seek help immediately if you think you have AIDS, and don't fail to notify your sexual partners if you test positive for HIV. They too will require testing and possibly treatment. In some states the health department will require that sexual partners be notified. Ask your doctor for advice.

vaccine has been examined only in the test tube. Animal and human trials are being planned.

CONVENTIONAL MEDICINE

The current treatment of choice for AIDS patients is the use of powerful antiviral drugs. These include zidovudine, didanosine, and dideoxycytidine. None of these cures AIDS, but they may help stave off the worst symptoms of the disease for several years.

Zidovudine, known better by the trade name AZT, is by far the most widely used and will probably be the first drug your doctor gives you. AZT slows down the virus by interfering with the way it goes about propagating itself. The problem with AZT is that the virus often becomes resistant to it within a few years. AZT also produces side effects such as muscle wasting, extreme nausea, acute headaches, insomnia, hepatitis, dementia, and cancerous lymphomas.

Switching to another drug, such as didanosine, will help temporarily, although this drug produces side effects such as diarrhea, nerve problems, and pancreatitis. Combining drugs is often the most helpful form of treatment.

ALTERNATIVE CHOICES

Combined with medical treatment, many alternative therapies can lengthen and improve the quality of the AIDS patient's life. Studies demonstrate that many AIDS patients respond well to immune-bolstering nutritional programs. Patients also show marked improvement after using stress-reduction techniques. Again, beware of any treatment that claims to be a "miracle" cure.

ACUPRESSURE

Your immune system may function more efficiently if you reduce stress in your life. One acupressure massage that seems to relieve fatigue and tension is known as the Shoulder Well. Press Gall Bladder 21, the highest point of the shoulder muscle midway between the outer tip of the shoulder and the spine. Do this at home several times a day.

ACUPUNCTURE

When combined with Chinese herbs, acupuncture seems to boost immune functions and reduce symptoms of AIDS, including night sweats, fatigue, and digestive problems. Acupuncture may also help your body fight off secondary infections and eliminate lesions. Seek the advice of a qualified practitioner.

AROMATHERAPY

You may also reduce stress by inhaling the aromas of various oils, such as lavender (*Lavandula officinalis*). To heal lesions brought on by AIDS, aromatherapists recommend that you apply the antiviral oils of tea tree (*Melaleuca* spp.) and garlic (*Allium sativum*).

BODY WORK

Several studies indicate that moderate exercise substantially increases immune system activity. In one study, aerobic training boosted immune cells in AIDS patients. Too much aerobic exercise can suppress immunity, however, so ask your doctor to recommend an exercise program for you.

CHINESE HERBS

Many Chinese herbs have been effective in treating symptoms of AIDS such as night sweats, fatigue, neuropathy, and diarrhea. Chinese herbs also may relieve the side effects of some conventional drugs.

Tonic herbs to strengthen the system include astragalus (*Astragalus membranaceus*), ganoderma (*Ganoderma lucidum*), and Asian ginseng (*Panax ginseng*). Licorice (*Glycyrrhiza glabra*) is thought to enhance the immune system and inhibit the herpesvirus.

Trichosanthin, a protein in Chinese cucumber root, has been extracted to form tricosantin, or Compound Q, which seems to purify the blood and ward off a variety of infections.

An extract of shiitake (*Lentinus edodes*) mushrooms has also been successfully used to treat AIDS symptoms.

HERBAL THERAPIES

Herbalists recommend several plant-based medicines for boosting the immune system and

A

strengthening the body. Echinacea (*Echinacea* spp.) increases immune system functions by stimulating T cells, but it may not be as effective in treating AIDS because it stimulates HIV as well. Ask your doctor before trying it.

Garlic (*Allium sativum*) has been used by AIDS patients for its antibacterial and antiviral properties, and some studies have indicated that hyssop (*Hyssopus officinalis*) may be useful in treating Kaposi's sarcoma.

A promising herbal remedy is St.-John's-wort (*Hypericum perforatum*), which contains hypericin, a chemical that has been shown to inhibit the growth of the virus that causes one form of leukemia. Researchers hope that hypericin can be used to reduce AIDS symptoms such as fever and swelling of lymph nodes. Hypericin isn't effective if you just drink St.-John's-wort tea; to get the powerful extract, consult your doctor or a qualified herbal practitioner.

HOMEOPATHY

Besides seeking conventional treatments, you may also wish to consult a homeopathic physician, who will take your complete medical, emotional, and genealogical history and then help you make healthful changes in your lifestyle. In addition, many homeopathic remedies have been helpful in treating the symptoms of AIDS. Hypericum, a homeopathic drug derived from St.-John's-wort, is one remedy a homeopath might prescribe.

HEAT THERAPY

Several studies have shown that HIV is sensitive to heat and becomes increasingly inactive as body temperature is raised above normal for extended periods of time. Raising body temperature stimulates the immune system in general by increasing production of antibodies and interferon, a protein substance produced by virus-invaded cells that prevents reproduction of the virus.

Ask your doctor about the experimental therapy hyperthermia—heat therapy—in which AIDS patients combine hot baths with hot drinks and then wrap themselves in blankets. This should be done only under strict supervision. Heat may elevate your body temperature to dangerous extremes and impair organ functioning.

MIND/BODY MEDICINE

Many doctors and psychologists believe that there is a vital relationship between your emotions and the way your immune system functions. Negative emotions such as guilt, hopelessness, suppressed anger, and fear are common among AIDS patients and may suppress the body's ability to fight off infection. Practitioners of mind/body medicine believe you'll be healthier and live longer if you do everything you can to maintain a positive attitude. Low moments are unavoidable, and you should not chide yourself for having them; but do what you can to avoid dwelling on negative thoughts.

To help, try relaxation techniques such as **biofeedback, yoga,** exercise, and **meditation. Massage** therapy can improve your circulation and give you a greater sense of ease and well-being. The massage should not be too fast or deep, however, or your adrenal system, which releases powerful chemicals in response to real or imagined stress, could become overstimulated and challenge your immune system. Seek the advice of a licensed massage therapist.

Also, try joining a support group to help you deal with the anxiety you may be feeling. Sharing your fears—and also your victories—with others can be of enormous benefit. *(See the Appendix.)*

NUTRITION AND DIET

What you put into your body once you're diagnosed with HIV may have a profound effect on how long you live. With proper nutrition you can strengthen your body's ability to fight the virus.

Avoid foods that impair the immune system. For example, there are some indications that 100 grams of simple sugar—such as honey or refined sugar—can significantly decrease the ability of white blood cells to kill bacteria and viruses for up to five hours. The typical American consumes about 150 grams of sugar a day.

Stay away from alcohol and caffeine, which deplete the body of vitamins and minerals. And smoking heavily tends to increase suppressor T cells and decrease helper T cells (two types of immune cells that, in proper proportion, help keep the immune system in balance).

Eat more foods rich in beta carotene such as

DIET POINTERS

For AIDS patients, nutritionists recommend in particular that you:
- *reduce your consumption of polyunsaturated and saturated fats and oils.*
- *use monounsaturated oils (such as olive oil) and increase your intake of omega-3 fatty acid, which is found in fish but is also effective when obtained through supplements.*
- *eat small portions throughout the day to optimize absorption of nutrients from foods.*
- *eat a balanced meal—65 percent complex carbohydrates, 15 percent protein, and 20 percent fat.*
- *make sure fruits and vegetables are clean and free of parasites and bacteria by steaming them lightly before eating.*
- *eat a wide variety of foods to help avoid becoming sensitized to specific food families.*

---

green, leafy vegetables and orange and yellow vegetables. If you develop candidiasis or other infections common with AIDS, you may want to increase consumption of garlic, which contains the powerful antibiotic allicin.

Take vitamin C supplements to boost your immune system. Some naturopaths and dietitians recommend taking vitamin C until it causes diarrhea, then cutting back to the highest tolerable level; one approach is to take dosages every two hours. CAUTION: You should check with your doctor before trying this approach. Zinc also stimulates the immune system and is antiviral.

AT-HOME REMEDIES
If you have HIV, you may stave off symptoms of AIDS if you:

- eat nutritious, balanced meals to bolster your immune system.
- take vitamin supplements.
- try acupressure exercises to relax.
- take up meditation or yoga to relieve stress.
- try to maintain a positive attitude.
- don't smoke or drink.
- follow a moderate exercise program approved by your doctor.

If you have AIDS:
- eat nutritious, balanced meals to bolster your immune system.
- take vitamin supplements.
- try acupressure exercises to relax.
- take up meditation or yoga to relieve stress.
- try to maintain a positive attitude.
- follow a moderate exercise program approved by your doctor.
- try inhaling or bathing with oils of tea tree and garlic.
- ask a knowledgeable practitioner about herbs such as St.-John's-wort.

PREVENTION

- Condoms reduce the risk of HIV infection. Use a latex condom with the spermicide nonoxynol-9, which has been shown to kill HIV outside the body. Use a condom for all kinds of sex, including oral, anal, and vaginal. This is not necessary if you and your partner are monogamous and not infected.
- Don't use oil-based lubricants, which can eat through condoms.
- Learn the sexual history of a potential partner and ask about HIV test results.
- Don't have sex with prostitutes.
- Don't share a needle if you use intravenous drugs; bleach needles to clean them.
- When in Third World countries, carry a supply of disposable sterile needles in case you require medical injections.
- Get tested every six months if you're in a high-risk group; your sexual partner should be tested as well. ■

SYMPTOMS

The following symptoms are associated with abuse of alcohol:

◆ temporary blackouts or memory loss.

◆ recurrent arguments or fights with family members or friends.

◆ continuing use of alcohol to relax, to cheer up, to sleep, to deal with problems, or to feel "normal."

◆ headache, anxiety, insomnia, nausea, or other unpleasant symptoms when you stop drinking.

◆ flushed skin and broken capillaries on the face; a husky voice; trembling hands; chronic diarrhea; and drinking alone, in the mornings, or in secret. These symptoms are specifically associated with **chronic alcoholism.**

CALL YOUR DOCTOR IF:

◆ you have any of the symptoms above and are unable to stop drinking on your own. You need medical intervention to treat alcoholism. You may also be susceptible to ailments such as cirrhosis, alcoholic hepatitis, and heart disease.

◆ you drink regularly and experience chronic or periodic depression. You may be at risk of suicide.

◆ you have tried to stop drinking and experienced withdrawal symptoms such as headache, anxiety, insomnia, nausea, or delirium tremens. You need medical attention by a physician or a treatment center.

People have been brewing and fermenting alcoholic drinks since the dawn of time. Consumed in moderate amounts, alcoholic beverages are relaxing and in some cases may even have beneficial effects on health (see Atherosclerosis). Consumed in excess, alcohol is poisonous to human systems and is considered a drug. Nearly 100,000 Americans die each year as a result of alcohol abuse, and alcohol is a factor in more than half of the country's homicides, suicides, and traffic accidents. Alcohol abuse also plays a role in many social and domestic problems, from job absenteeism and crimes against property to spousal and child abuse.

The immediate physical effects of drinking alcohol range from mild mood changes to complete loss of coordination, vision, balance, and speech—any of which can be signals of the temporary systemic poisoning known as **acute alcohol intoxication**, or drunkenness. These effects usually wear off in a matter of hours after a person stops drinking (see Hangover). Many law-enforcement agencies regard a .08 percentage of alcohol in the bloodstream as evidence of intoxication. Larger amounts of blood alcohol can impair brain function and eventually cause unconsciousness; an extreme overdose can be fatal.

Chronic alcoholism is a progressive, potentially fatal disease, characterized by an incessant craving for, increased tolerance of, physical dependence upon, and loss of control over drinking alcohol. The physical dependence on alcohol may or may not be obvious to other people. While some chronic alcoholics get very drunk, others exercise enough control to give the appearance of coping with everyday affairs in a near-normal way. However, alcoholism can lead to a number of physical ailments, including hypoglycemia, kidney disease, brain and heart damage, enlarged blood vessels in the skin, chronic gastritis, and pancreatitis (see Pancreatic Problems).

Alcoholism can also lead to impotence in men, damage to the fetus in pregnant women, and an elevated risk of cancer of the larynx, esophagus, stomach, pancreas, and upper gastrointestinal tract. Because alcoholics seldom have adequate diets, they are likely to have nutritional deficiencies. Heavy drinkers typically have impaired liver function, and at least 1 in 5 develops cirrhosis.

The alcoholic's continual craving for alcohol makes abstinence—an important goal of treatment—extremely difficult. The condition is also complicated by denial: Alcoholics employ a range of psychological maneuvers to blame their problems on something other than drink, creating significant barriers to recovery. Historically, alcoholic behavior was blamed on a character flaw or weakness of will; many authorities now consider chronic alcoholism a disease that can afflict anyone.

Virtually every culture has warned against overuse of alcohol, and some have prohibited it outright, rarely with lasting success. While laws and educational programs in the United States are designed to prevent alcohol abuse, commercial and social pressure continues to put people at risk. Alcoholism is particularly insidious among young people and the elderly, in part because the symptoms are not easily recognized until the affected person becomes truly alcohol dependent.

CAUSES

The cause of alcoholism seems to be a blend of genetic, physical, psychological, environmental, and social factors that vary among individuals. Genetic factors are considered crucial: A given person's risk of becoming an alcoholic is four to five times greater if a parent is alcoholic. Some children of alcohol abusers, however, overcome the hereditary pattern by becoming teetotalers.

TREATMENT

The goal of treatment is abstinence. Among alcoholics with otherwise good health, social support, and motivation, the likelihood of recovery is good: 50 to 60 percent remain abstinent at the end of a year's treatment, and a majority of those stay dry permanently. Those with poor social support, poor motivation, or psychiatric disorders tend to relapse within a few years of treatment. For these people, success is measured by longer

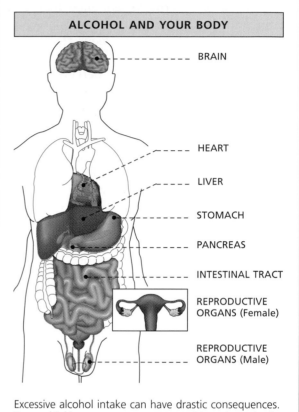

ALCOHOL AND YOUR BODY

BRAIN

HEART

LIVER

STOMACH

PANCREAS

INTESTINAL TRACT

REPRODUCTIVE ORGANS (Female)

REPRODUCTIVE ORGANS (Male)

Excessive alcohol intake can have drastic consequences. Heavy drinking can cause acute gastritis and can lead to pancreatitis. Long-term abuse can lead to cardiomyopathy (weakening of the heart), cirrhosis of the liver, and cancer of the upper intestinal tract. Chronic alcoholism is the second leading cause of brain damage and can also impair sexual function.

periods of abstinence, reduced use of alcohol, better health, and improved social functioning.

CONVENTIONAL MEDICINE

Treatment can begin only when the alcoholic accepts that the problem exists and agrees to stop drinking. He or she must understand that alcoholism is curable and must be motivated to change. Treatment has two stages: withdrawal—sometimes called detoxification—and recovery. Because withdrawal does not stop the craving for alcohol, recovery is often difficult to maintain. For a person in an early stage of alcoholism, withdrawal may bring anxiety and poor sleep. Withdrawal from long-term dependence may bring the uncontrollable shaking, spasms, panic, and hallucinations of delirium tremens (DT). If not treated professionally, people with DT have a mortality rate of more than 10 percent, so withdrawal from late-stage alcoholism should be attempted only at an inpatient center.

Treatment may involve one or more medications. Disulfiram interferes with alcohol metabolism so that drinking a small amount will cause nausea, vomiting, confusion, and breathing difficulty. Naltrexone reduces the craving for alcohol but is recommended only in comprehensive programs that teach patients new coping skills. Benzodiazepines are antianxiety drugs used to treat withdrawal symptoms such as anxiety and poor sleep, and to prevent seizures and delirium. They must be used with care, since they may be addictive. Tricyclic antidepressants may be used to control any resulting anxiety or depression, but because those symptoms may disappear with abstinence, the medications are usually not started until after detoxification.

Because an alcoholic remains susceptible to becoming dependent again, the key to recovery is total abstinence. Recovery typically takes a broad-based approach, which may include education programs, group therapy, family involvement, and participation in self-help groups.

ALTERNATIVE CHOICES

Once an alcoholic accepts his or her condition and stops using alcohol, a number of alternative therapies can help the recovery process.

ACUPUNCTURE

Treatment by a licensed acupuncturist is often found effective in relieving the symptoms of alcoholic withdrawal and is reported to prevent seizures, to help prevent relapse, and to increase the likelihood of a patient's completing a recovery program.

BODY WORK

Massage, as part of a physical therapy program, can ease recovery by relaxing the body and soothing the anxiety associated with withdrawal.

HERBAL THERAPIES

Ask an herbal therapist about taking milk thistle (*Silybum marianum*) to protect against, or even reverse, liver damage from alcohol abuse. The product is sold under the name silymarin in 70- to 210-mg capsules at health food stores.

For withdrawal symptoms, try infusing 2 tsp skullcap (*Scutellaria lateriflora*), lavender (*Lavandula officinalis*), or motherwort (*Leonurus cardiaca*) in water, and take three times a day. Some treatment centers use a sleep-mix tea made from equal parts chamomile (*Matricaria recutita*), hops (*Humulus lupulus*), skullcap, peppermint (*Mentha piperita*), yarrow (*Achillea millefolium*), and either catnip (*Nepeta cataria*) or valerian (*Valeriana officinalis*).

HYDROTHERAPY

Warm salted baths may be effective in drawing drugs and toxins from the body. Dissolve ½ cup sea salt or baking soda in a tub of warm water and soak in it 10 to 20 minutes every day.

MIND/BODY MEDICINE

Because alcoholics commonly use alcohol to deal with stress, various relaxation techniques, such as **massage** and **meditation,** may prove helpful. **Hypnotherapy** may help unlock psychological difficulties that underlie behavioral problems.

NUTRITION AND DIET

Poor nutrition goes with heavy drinking: Because an ounce of alcohol has more than 200 calories but no nutritional value, ingesting large amounts of alcohol tells the body that it doesn't need more food. Alcoholics are often deficient in vitamins A, B complex, and C; carnitine; magnesium, selenium, and zinc; as well as essential fatty acids and antioxidants. Restoring such nutrients—particularly thiamine (vitamin B$_1$)—can aid withdrawal and recovery. One study found that recovery programs were twice as effective when nutritional therapy was incorporated.

Some therapists think stabilizing blood sugar levels can help make treatment more successful. Recommendations include eliminating dietary sugar, even fruit juice, which has more sugar than whole fruit; reducing the amounts of simple carbohydrates in the diet, such as those found in white flour and instant potatoes; and increasing vegetable protein and the complex carbohydrates found in whole grains, beans, and vegetables.

AT-HOME REMEDIES

Abstinence is the most crucial—and probably the most difficult—step to recovery. To learn to live without alcohol, you must:

◆ Avoid people and places that make drinking the norm, and find new, nondrinking friends.
◆ Join a self-help group (see Support for Recovery, right).
◆ Enlist the help of family and friends.
◆ Replace your negative dependence on alcohol with positive dependencies such as a new hobby or volunteer work with church or civic groups.
◆ Start exercising. Exercise releases chemicals in the brain that provide a "natural high." Even a walk after dinner can be tranquilizing.

PREVENTION

Returning to drink is a major problem for recovering alcoholics; preventing this may be difficult, but it can be supported by continued therapy, positive motivation, and strong social support. Other ways to prevent relapse include changing routines, accepting a new sense of values, and avoiding activities or people associated with the drinking habit. For example, 90 percent of alcoholics smoke; alcoholics who stop smoking as well as drinking are more likely to achieve long-term abstinence—to say nothing of the other health benefits.

A SELF-SCREENING TEST

No single symptom defines alcoholism, but honest answers to the following questions will help you decide if you are at risk.

◆ Has a friend or relative ever suggested that you drink too much?
◆ Is it hard to stop drinking after you have had one or two drinks?

SUPPORT FOR RECOVERY

Despite the contention that alcoholism is a disease, not a weakness of will, the social stigma still lingers—especially for women. Many alcoholics deny that drinking is a problem, and family and friends who cover up an alcoholic's behavior only help stifle any incentive to reach out for help. It is vital for family and friends to learn about alcoholism and to motivate a loved one to seek help.

Group support helps many alcoholics lead normal, productive lives. About one million Americans are members of Alcoholics Anonymous (AA). For many, the positive peer pressure of AA is crucial to staying sober. Yet opinions differ about certain aspects of AA and similar groups. Some therapists are concerned because AA does not diagnose psychiatric disorders or provide medical evaluation. For those who object to the spiritual emphasis of AA's 12-step program, alternative groups such as Rational Recovery and Women for Sobriety are available.

◆ Have you ever been unable to remember what you did during a drinking episode?
◆ Do you ever feel bad about how much you drink?
◆ Do you get into arguments or physical fights when you've been drinking?
◆ Have you ever been arrested or hospitalized because of drinking?
◆ Have you ever thought about getting help to control or stop your drinking?

If you answered yes to one or more questions, you may have a serious alcohol problem. For your own good, it's time to discuss the situation openly with a physician or mental health professional. ■

ALLERGIES

SYMPTOMS

- Sneezing, wheezing, nasal congestion, and coughing indicate asthma, or drug or respiratory allergies.
- Itchy eyes, mouth, and throat are symptoms of respiratory allergies.
- Stomachache, frequent indigestion, and heartburn are signs of food sensitivities.
- Irritated, itchy, reddening, or swelling skin is associated with drug, food, and insect sting allergies.
- Stiffness, pain, and swelling of joints may indicate food or drug allergies.

CALL YOUR DOCTOR IF:

- you have violent stomach cramps, vomiting, bloating, or diarrhea; this could point to a serious food or other allergic reaction or food poisoning.
- breathing becomes extremely difficult or painful; you may be experiencing an asthma episode, another serious allergic reaction, or a heart attack. **Get emergency medical treatment.**
- you suddenly develop skin welts, accompanied by intense flushing and itching; your heart may also be beating rapidly. These symptoms may indicate the onset of anaphylactic shock, an extremely serious allergic reaction. **Get emergency medical treatment.** *(See also Shock in Emergencies/First Aid.)*

The term *allergy* applies to an abnormal reaction by your immune system to a substance that is usually not harmful. Allergies come in a variety of forms and vary in severity from mildly bothersome to life-threatening. An estimated one-fifth of the Western Hemisphere's population suffers from allergies. No one knows why some people develop them, but heredity seems to play a role in their development. Although allergies may flare up and subside throughout your life, people rarely acquire new ones past the age of 40.

The immune system protects the body from foreign substances—known as antigens—by producing antibodies and other chemicals to fight against them. Usually, the immune system ignores benign substances, such as food, and fights only dangerous ones, such as bacteria. A person develops an allergic reaction when the immune system cannot tell the good from the bad and releases a type of chemical called histamine to attack the harmless substance as if it were a threat. Histamine produces many of the symptoms associated with allergies. Substances that may trigger allergic reactions, known as allergens, range from pollen to pet dander to penicillin.

Most allergic reactions are not serious, but some, such as anaphylaxis, can be fatal *(box, page 108)*. Only a few allergies can be cured outright, but a variety of conventional and alternative treatments are available to relieve the symptoms. If your allergy is severe, it is vital that you visit a conventional medical doctor and get immediate treatment on an emergency basis.

CAUSES

Allergies come in many distinct forms and are typically grouped in general categories according to the types of substances that cause them or the parts of the body they affect.

Skin allergies: Contact dermatitis is caused by direct, topical exposure to a specific allergen; atopic dermatitis has no known cause, but it is usually hereditary. Hives, or urticaria, is an eruption of itchy, swollen, reddened welts that can last for minutes or days. Angioedema is characterized by a deeper swelling around the eyes and lips, and sometimes of the hands and feet as well. Both hives and angioedema stem from the body's adverse reaction to certain foods, pollen, animal dander, drugs, insect stings, cold, heat, light, or even emotional stress.

Respiratory allergies: Some 20 million Americans suffer from hay fever (allergic rhinitis). Typical symptoms include itchy eyes, nose, and roof of mouth or throat, along with nasal congestion, coughing, and sneezing. If you (or members of your family) have other allergies such as dermatitis or asthma, you are more likely to have hay fever. The terms *allergic rhinitis* and *hay fever* apply specifically to reactions caused by the pollens of ragweed, grasses, and other plants whose pollen is spread by the wind. But the same symptoms can be produced by other airborne substances that you inhale. These can include molds, dust, and animal dander. If, for example, you are allergic to pet dander (dead skin scales and saliva), being near a cat will make you sneeze, wheeze, and sniffle. Mold allergies are caused by airborne spores. Outdoor molds—alternaria and hormodendrum—thrive in warm seasons or climates, while indoor molds—penicillium, aspergillus, mucor, and rhizopus—grow year round in damp locations (basements and bathrooms, for example). Dust causes allergies because it harbors offenders such as pollen, mold spores, and microscopic dust mites; it may also contain irritating fibers from fabrics, upholstery, and carpets.

Asthma: Asthma has various causes, but the chief ones are allergies to pollen, mold spores, animal dander, and dust mites. *(See Asthma.)*

Food allergies: An estimated 70 percent of people with food allergies are under 30; most are children under the age of 6. It is sometimes difficult to pinpoint the specific allergens responsible for a food allergy, because reactions are often delayed or may be caused by food additives or even by eating habits. However, approximately 90 percent of food allergies are caused by proteins in cow's milk, egg whites, peanuts, wheat, or soybeans. Other common food allergens include berries, shellfish, corn, beans, yellow food dye No. 5, and gum arabic (an additive in processed foods). The classic symptoms of food allergies include stomach cramps, diarrhea, and nausea. In more severe cases, there may be vomiting, swelling of the face and tongue, and respiratory congestion, as well as dizziness, sweating, and faintness.

Drug allergies: The most common drug allergy is to drugs in the penicillin family. Other common drug allergens include sulfas, barbiturates, anticonvulsants, insulin, local anesthetics, and dyes injected into blood vessels for x-rays. Almost one million Americans have reactions to aspirin; these responses are not true allergies but rather "sensitivities."

Insect sting allergies: Some studies speculate that people who have other allergies (food, drug, or respiratory) may be more susceptible to insect sting allergies, which affect about 15 percent of the population. Venom in stings of bees, wasps, hornets, yellow jackets, and fire ants is a common allergen. *(See Insect and Spider Bites.)*

FOOD ALLERGY OR INTOLERANCE?

Two out of five Americans believe that they are allergic to certain foods, but fewer than 1 percent have genuine allergies; most are unable to tolerate certain foods, often because they lack an enzyme needed for proper digestion.

Some people are sensitive to lactose, a sugar found in milk; in general, however, they can tolerate dairy products such as yogurt, sour cream, and hard cheese. Some children cannot tolerate gluten, found in wheat products. Monosodium glutamate (MSG), a flavor enhancer, can cause flushing, headaches, and numbness. Sulfites, used as a preservative in many foods and wines, can cause sensitivity as well as trigger allergic reactions.

DIAGNOSTIC AND TEST PROCEDURES

After taking a full family and personal medical history, your physician will ask you a series of questions about your exposure and reactions to various allergens to eliminate and identify your allergies' causes. You may be asked to keep track of potential allergens and your allergic reactions for a week to aid in diagnosis. After this, your physician will choose a testing method.

The most common test for respiratory, penicillin, insect sting, skin, and food allergies is a skin test. A small amount of the allergen is placed on, or injected just underneath, the skin, and the physician watches for allergic symptoms. The symptoms—swelling, itchiness, and redness—generally appear within 20 minutes. Skin tests are not completely reliable, because if too much of the allergen is administered, even a nonallergic person may react. Also, extremely sensitive people may go into anaphylactic shock from skin tests. An alternative for respiratory allergies is RAST (for radioallergosorbent test), which measures the levels in the bloodstream of the antibodies associated with allergies.

TREATMENT

The best treatment for allergies is to avoid the substances that trigger them, but this can be difficult. The basic medications for allergies are antihistamines, which counteract the histamine chemicals that cause the allergic reactions. Prescription corticosteroid drugs may also be used for severe symptoms. In emergency situations—when anaphylactic shock occurs—injections of epinephrine are used to dilate bronchial passages. Immunotherapy, or allergy shots, may cure some allergies by introducing small amounts of the offending allergens in order to help the body learn to deal with them.

CONVENTIONAL MEDICINE

Skin allergies: Atopic and contact dermatitis can be treated with a variety of corticosteroids, usually hydrocortisone. Hives and angioedema often

W HAT TRIGGERS ANAPHYLACTIC SHOCK?

The most severe and dangerous of allergic reactions is anaphylaxis, or anaphylactic shock, which begins within minutes after exposure and advances quickly. Although any allergen can trigger anaphylactic shock, the most common are insect stings, certain foods (such as shellfish and nuts), and injections of certain drugs. Standard emergency treatment includes an injection of epinephrine to open up the airways and blood vessels; in severe cases, cardiopulmonary resuscitation (CPR) may be necessary. See Shock in Emergencies/First Aid.

need no medication, but severe cases may require prescription antihistamines, cimetidine, terbutaline, or oral corticosteroids.

Respiratory allergies: Hay fever is generally treated with over-the-counter antihistamines, but your doctor may prescribe other, more powerful drugs—such as cromolyn—if your symptoms are severe. The same treatments apply to other respiratory allergies, but if your symptoms are severe, your physician may prescribe corticosteroids, in nasal spray or oral form. Immunotherapy has a high success rate, curing 70 percent to 80 percent of people treated for respiratory allergies.

Food allergies: The best treatment for food allergies is avoidance. If your reactions to certain foods are irritating but not life-endangering, your doctor may prescribe antihistamines or topical creams to help relieve symptoms.

Drug allergies: The only effective treatment for drug allergies is avoidance. Skin rashes associated with drug allergies are generally treated with antihistamines; occasionally they are treated with corticosteroids.

Insect sting allergies: Avoidance is the best treatment, but immunotherapy may cure insect sting allergies. If you are extremely allergic and likely to go into anaphylactic shock, your doctor will prescribe an emergency kit, which you must carry with you at all times.

ALTERNATIVE CHOICES

Since allergies can be difficult to diagnose, and are in many cases incurable, alternative remedies for them have become quite popular. But if you have a severe allergy, or in case of an emergency, you must see a conventional physician.

ACUPRESSURE

To relieve symptoms associated with respiratory allergies, try Large Intestine 4, the highest spot of the area between the index finger and thumb; rub firmly for one minute, then repeat on the other hand. Do not use this point if you are pregnant. To fortify the immune system, firmly massage Triple Warmer 5, two finger widths from your wrist on the top of your forearm, specifically the area between the two arm bones.

AROMATHERAPY

To relieve nasal congestion, try mixing 1 drop of lavender (*Lavandula officinalis*) oil and 1 tsp of a carrier oil such as sweet almond or sunflower oil; massage into the skin around your sinuses once a day. Eucalyptus (*Eucalyptus globulus*), cedarwood, and peppermint (*Mentha piperita*) oils also act as decongestants; dab on a handkerchief and inhale.

CHINESE HERBS

Ephedra (*Ephedra sinica*) acts like the decongestant epinephrine, which opens up the lungs' airways when breathing is difficult. But be careful: Large quantities of this herb are equivalent to large quantities of the drug epinephrine and can have serious side effects. Do not use ephedra if you have high blood pressure or heart disease. Prepare an infusion by combining 5 grams ephedra, 4 grams cinnamon (*Cinnamomum cassia*) sticks, 1.5 grams licorice (*Glycyrrhiza uralensis*), and 5 grams apricot seed (*Prunus armeniaca*); let steep in cold water, then bring to a boil. Strain and drink hot.

HERBAL THERAPIES

Infusions of chamomile (*Matricaria recutita*), elder (*Sambucus nigra*) flower, eyebright (*Euphrasia officinalis*), garlic (*Allium sativum*), goldenrod (*Solidago virgaurea*), nettle (*Urtica dioica*), and yarrow (*Achillea millefolium*) have antimucus and anti-inflammatory effects.

HOMEOPATHY

For a runny nose, itchy throat, and sneezing, a homeopathic practitioner might suggest Arsenicum album (6c); for chronic thick mucus, Pulsatilla (6c); for a runny nose, sore upper lip, and itchy eyes, Allium cepa (6c).

NUTRITION AND DIET

Vitamin C and bioflavonoids (found in the white pith of citrus fruits) act as natural antihistamines, so you should increase your citrus intake or take 500 mg of vitamin C three times daily. Vitamins A and B complex are thought to be powerful stimulants to the immune system. Products made with bee pollen and royal jelly may alleviate or eliminate the symptoms of respiratory allergies but should not be taken if you are allergic to bee stings. For food allergies, read labels carefully and make sure you know what foods to avoid.

PREVENTION

Respiratory allergies: Install a high-efficiency air cleaner to help remove pollen and mold spores, and use an air conditioner in your home and car during warm seasons to keep pollen out; regularly clean damp areas with bleach to kill molds. Consider hiring a special cleaning service to rid furniture and upholstery of dust mites. Isolate (or, if you can stand it, get rid of) your pets and keep them outside as much as possible. Regular baths for your pet will help reduce dander.

Food allergies: Instead of dairy products, try tofu-based foods. Always check food labels for additives that are known allergens, such as yellow food dye No. 5 and gum arabic. ∎

ALZHEIMER'S DISEASE

SYMPTOMS

- mood changes: depression, paranoia, agitation, anxiety, selfishness, childish behavior.
- disorientation, confusion, inattention, loss of memory for recent events, inability to retain new information.
- increased tendency to misplace things.
- dizziness or impaired equilibrium.

CALL YOUR DOCTOR IF:

- a family member or friend exhibits signs of Alzheimer's disease over a period of time. Because the person may not be aware of having these problems, it is often up to others to help.

Alzheimer's disease, a progressive degeneration of brain tissue that primarily strikes people over age 65, is marked by a devastating mental decline. Intellectual functions such as memory, comprehension, and speech deteriorate. Attention tends to stray, simple calculations become impossible, and ordinary daily activities grow increasingly difficult, with bewilderment and frustration worsening at night. Dramatic mood swings occur—outbursts of anger, bouts of fearfulness, periods of deep apathy. The sufferer, increasingly disoriented, may wander off and become lost. Physical problems, such as an odd gait or a loss of coordination, gradually develop. Eventually, the patient may become totally noncommunicative, physically helpless, and incontinent. The disease is invariably fatal.

Alzheimer's can run its course from insidious onset to death in just a few years, or it may play out over a period of as long as 20 years; the average duration, however, is about 7 years. Among American adults, it is the fourth leading cause of death (after heart disease, cancer, and stroke). By the age of 80, about 1 person out of 3 has the disease. Women are twice as susceptible as men, and Caucasians are about four times as susceptible as African Americans.

CAUSES

Although many people develop Alzheimer's as they grow older, the disease is not a natural result of aging; it is an abnormal condition whose causes continue to be investigated.

The gradual loss of brain function that characterizes Alzheimer's disease seems to be due to two main forms of neural damage: Nerve fibers grow tangled, and protein deposits known as plaques build up in the affected tissue. Researchers are not yet sure why or how this tissue degeneration occurs, but some of the most promising recent research points to a normally occurring blood protein called ApoE (for apolipoprotein E), which is required for the transport of fatty substances in the body. As with all proteins, its form is genetically determined, and several different types have been identified—

some of them apparently associated with a higher risk of Alzheimer's. It may be that certain forms of ApoE lead to destruction of nerve cells in the brain. Another possibility is that the protein, perhaps working in combination with other substances, is involved in the formation of the plaques. Whether or not ApoE is part of the causative mechanism of Alzheimer's, genes almost certainly can play a role in the disease: A person with a parent who had Alzheimer's is known to be at higher risk.

Other causes have been proposed. One theory suggests that ingesting tiny particles of aluminum—from cookware, for example—may lead to Alzheimer's. Another proposes a link between plaque formation and free radicals—unstable, free-ranging molecules that can produce destructive chemical reactions. Both theories are controversial and unproved. Indeed, many researchers now consider the link between Alzheimer's and aluminum extremely questionable.

Another controversy centers on zinc. In a 1991 study, Alzheimer's patients were given zinc supplements because other studies suggested that zinc could help improve mental alertness in the elderly (zinc has also been shown to play a role in the functioning of memory). However, after only two days the patients' mental abilities deteriorated so rapidly that the study was considered too harmful for the subjects and was immediately abandoned. Three years later, laboratory tests showed that zinc could cause proteins to form clumps similar to the plaques found in the brains of Alzheimer's victims. But the connection between zinc and Alzheimer's remains unclear. For one thing, scientists remain unsure whether plaques cause Alzheimer's or are themselves a result of the disease; if the latter, zinc's ability to form plaques might be unrelated to what causes Alzheimer's in the first place.

In a minority of cases, trauma may be a contributing factor. About 15 percent of Alzheimer's sufferers have a history of head injury.

DIAGNOSTIC AND TEST PROCEDURES

Diagnosis by a professional is particularly important because a number of other ailments—many of which are treatable—share some symptoms associated with Alzheimer's disease. These include respiratory infections, inadequate nutrition, vitamin B_{12} deficiency, anemia, hypoglycemia, depression, and cerebral vascular insufficiency (decreased blood flow to the brain due to constricted arteries). An adverse reaction to prescribed medication, or a harmful combination of medicines, can sometimes cause Alzheimer's-like symptoms. Other diseases and conditions sometimes confused with Alzheimer's are Parkinson's disease, stroke, thyroid problems, brain tumors, advanced syphilis, and Huntington's chorea—an inherited degenerative nerve disease.

To check for Alzheimer's, the doctor will probably begin with physical and psychological tests designed to eliminate other possible causes of mental impairment. Verbal tests and interviews of the family are the usual next steps, but they will not produce a definitive diagnosis. Until recently, only a postmortem examination of brain tissue could yield absolute proof of Alzheimer's—the telltale evidence of nerve tangles, protein plaques, and general brain shrinkage from cell death.

Simple, accurate diagnosis has become possible with a newly developed procedure that involves no more than administering a certain type of eye drop. Apparently, Alzheimer's sufferers are extremely sensitive to the drug tropicamide, which is widely used by optometrists for the dilation of pupils. The dilation observed in individuals with the disease is three times as great as in healthy subjects. This seems to be true even before symptoms of the disease become apparent.

TREATMENT

Alzheimer's disease is incurable: Nothing can halt or reverse it. However, certain medications seem to slow its general progress to some degree in the early stages, and others can help with mood changes and other specific behavioral problems of the disease.

Caring for an Alzheimer's patient is often stressful for family members; support organizations can help caregivers cope with problems and feelings. Eventually, full-time nursing care will be necessary. Some families are able to provide this full-time care at home, while others turn to professional caregivers.

CONVENTIONAL MEDICINE

◆ In 1993 tacrine hydrochloride became the first drug approved by the FDA for treatment of Alzheimer's. In tests, it delayed progression of the disease by six months, and it improved mental functioning in cases that were not far advanced. The possible side effect of liver toxicity must be monitored weekly.

◆ Studies suggest that the experimental drug acetylcarnitine can bring temporary improvements in verbal ability, memory, attention span, and other mental functions among Alzheimer's patients.

◆ In one test, estrogen replacement therapy helped retard the onset of memory and reasoning deficiencies in 40 percent of female Alzheimer's patients.

◆ A number of drugs are prescribed for specific symptoms: haloperidol and thioridazine for aggressive behavior and agitation, sertraline for depression, and zolpidem and diphenhydramine for insomnia.

ALTERNATIVE CHOICES

As with conventional medicine, alternative therapies for the treatment of Alzheimer's cannot promise a cure, but in some cases they may help slow the progress of the disease or help address specific symptoms.

ACUPRESSURE

Not surprisingly, Alzheimer's patients easily become depressed and anxious. To help ease these burdens, practitioners suggest the acupressure techniques illustrated at right; they are specifically designed to promote relaxation and to serve as a general health tonic.

CHELATION THERAPY

Chelation therapy, which involves the nonsurgical removal of accumulated metals in the body,

ACUPRESSURE

1 Pressing Kidney 3, located on the inside of the ankle between the anklebone and the Achilles tendon, may help stimulate mental activity. Apply firm pressure and hold for one to two minutes, then repeat on the other foot.

2 Pressing Liver 2—on the top of the foot, in the web between the first and second toes—may help relieve irritability. Press steadily for one minute.

3 Pressing Spleen 3 may aid memory. The point is located on the inside of the foot, just behind the bulge made by the large joint of the big toe. Maintain a steady pressure for one minute, then repeat on the other foot.

4 Sleeping habits may be improved by pressing Heart 7, located along the crease on the inside of the wrist, directly in line with the little finger. Squeeze firmly between the thumb and index finger for one minute, then repeat on the other hand.

targets aluminum—believed by some researchers to have a causative role in Alzheimer's; it has been suggested that aluminum molecules link with calcium molecules to bind together the deposits called plaque. The chelation technique involves a series of intravenous injections of the amino acid ethylenediaminetetraacetic acid (EDTA), which is thought to loosen the hold of the calcium and capture the aluminum, later re-leasing it as waste. Studies have suggested that this therapy can slow the progress of the disease. It is controversial and may have potentially dangerous side effects, however. Consult your doctor before undertaking treatment.

HERBAL THERAPIES
Ginkgo biloba extract (GBE), from the ginkgo tree (*Ginkgo biloba*), is said to alleviate early symptoms of Alzheimer's—among them, deterioration of short-term memory, depression, absent-mindedness, anxiety, dizziness, inability to concentrate, confusion, and ringing in the ears. The recommended average dose is 40 mg, taken three times daily; look for capsules containing 24 percent ginkgo flavoglycosides. According to the proponents of this therapy, positive results are seen after four to six weeks.

HOMEOPATHY
To avoid overmedication with conventional drugs, consult a homeopath for remedies that may help in treating unusual or disruptive behavior; typically, you will see results within a week.

AT-HOME CARE
◆ To help an Alzheimer's patient cope with episodes of disorientation and mental lapses, promote a feeling of safety in every way possible: Maintain a stable, familiar living environment; stick to routine; when you must be absent, leave reminder notes and simple directions.
◆ Wandering and getting lost is a common problem with Alzheimer's patients; have the patient wear an ID bracelet with a phone number on it.
◆ To induce someone with Alzheimer's to talk more, go for a walk. Studies suggest that walking may stimulate areas of the brain linked to speech.
◆ To help an Alzheimer's patient develop a more positive outlook on the present, try eliciting reminiscences: Often, long-term memories are not initially impaired, and pleasant recollections can create feelings of happiness and

well-being. This can be effectively done in a group. Good nostalgia-promoting materials include old magazines, photo albums, and favorite family stories. Avoid pressuring the patient to remember. A subtle question or two may provide the key to a memory.
◆ See the Appendix for professional associations that may help you and the patient cope.

PREVENTION

No one knows for sure what causes Alzheimer's, so any preventive measures are highly speculative at best. But it's important to remember that even if Alzheimer's runs in your family, you will not necessarily develop it yourself. If you are concerned about the possibility that you might eventually develop Alzheimer's, your best strategy is to maintain a healthful lifestyle: Eat right and exercise regularly to keep your entire body—and especially the nerve cells in your brain—in good shape. In particular, avoid cigarette smoke and air pollution as best you can; this will help you minimize your exposure to free radicals, which some studies have implicated in the formation of nerve plaques.

Although some studies suggest a link between Alzheimer's and zinc, doctors do not recommend that you attempt to limit your daily intake; zinc is an essential mineral, and while you should avoid overdosing on zinc, you would do more harm than good by restricting your intake below the recommended daily allowance (15 mg for men, 12 mg for women). ∎

ANAL BLEEDING

Read down this column to find your symptoms. Then read across.

SYMPTOMS	AILMENT/PROBLEM
◆ bright red blood on stools or toilet paper; possibly, anal pain.	◆ Bleeding from the lower gastrointestinal tract, perhaps caused by hemorrhoids, anal fissure, diverticulosis, or vascular ectasia (blood vessels in the colon become distorted, then tangle and bleed)
◆ anal pain and itching; bright red bleeding from the anus; difficult, strained bowel movements but the bowels are never completely emptied.	◆ Anorectal stricture (a narrowing and tightening of the anal canal), caused by inflammation, scarring from a previous surgery, or laxative abuse
◆ recurrent watery or frequent stools that may contain blood (bleeding may be profuse); lower abdominal pain; weakness; nausea; vomiting; possibly, joint pain, skin sores in the anal region, and/or fever.	◆ Colitis, Crohn's disease, or gastroenteritis
◆ bright or dark red bleeding from the anus; pain around the navel.	◆ Meckel's diverticulum (a bulging pouch in the small-intestine wall); may lead to peritonitis or intussusception (in which the intestine folds into itself, causing blockage)
◆ frequent or watery stools; bright or dark red bleeding from the anus; rectal fullness; lower abdominal pain; possibly, vomiting.	◆ Rectal prolapse (part of the rectum falls through the anus)
◆ infrequent or hard stools; bright red blood and mucus in stools; rectal fullness; cramping in left abdomen.	◆ Proctitis (inflammation of the rectum), often due to infection
◆ vague abdominal and anal pain; anal itching or discharge; possibly, painless anal bleeding, or bright red stools, mucous anal discharge, and/or a lump near the anus.	◆ Polyps (tissue growths that protrude into the gastrointestinal tract), or colorectal cancer
◆ blood in stools; vomiting with blood; easy bruising; spiderlike blood vessels on the skin; fatigue; yellowish skin or eyes.	◆ Cirrhosis
◆ infant with dark red bloody stools that look like currant jelly; colic; shortness of breath; vomiting that may contain greenish yellow bile.	◆ Infant intussusception (see Meckel's diverticulum, above)

WHAT TO DO	OTHER INFO
◆ To help keep stools soft, which minimizes pain and bleeding, change to a high-fiber diet and drink at least eight glasses of water a day.	◆ Warm 15-minute sitz baths three times daily will relieve achiness.
◆ Take over-the-counter analgesics to alleviate pain; your doctor can dilate or surgically remove the scar tissue and/or the stricture area.	
◆ For gastroenteritis, fight dehydration (drink 8 to 10 glasses of water daily) and get plenty of rest. For colitis or Crohn's disease, avoid stressful situations and foods that disagree with you.	◆ For colitis, eating 1 clove of raw garlic (Allium sativum) daily may reduce cramping; drinking warm chamomile (Matricaria recutita) tea as often as desired can help the intestinal lining heal.
◆ Call your doctor without delay. You will probably need surgery to remove the diverticulum or any ulcerated area of the intestine.	◆ If your symptoms mimic appendicitis, you may have surgery to remove the appendix.
◆ Call your doctor without delay. Surgery is sometimes required for rectal prolapse.	
◆ See your doctor. Antibiotics can cure bacterial proctitis, and you can get symptom relief for the viral form.	◆ Potential causes include sexually transmitted diseases (especially the gonorrhea, chlamydia, and syphilis bacteria, and the herpes virus), laxative overuse, rectal injury, allergy.
◆ See your doctor without delay because of the possibility of cancer. Benign polyps may be surgically removed.	◆ Much serious anal bleeding is "occult," or hidden. If you are over 50, see your doctor for a test for occult bleeding every three years.
◆ **Get medical help immediately;** the bleeding can be life-threatening.	◆ Abstain from alcoholic beverages and any unnecessary medications. Sound nutrition is essential to stop the progression of cirrhosis.
◆ **Get medical help immediately** to prevent shock and/or death.	◆ Most cases occur in infants between 4 and 11 months old. Intussusception may recur and is second only to appendicitis in causing abdominal pain in children under age 13.

SYMPTOMS

- drops of bright red blood on bowel movement, toilet tissue, or clothing; occasionally the bleeding is more profuse.
- tearing or burning pain in the anal region during a bowel movement; dull ache may continue for several hours.
- a small piece of skin at the end of the fissure (called a "sentinel pile") that may show outside the anus.
- hard or infrequent stools, usually from deliberately retaining painful bowel movements.

CALL YOUR DOCTOR IF:

- you notice any anal bleeding. You may have a serious disorder, such as colorectal cancer, Meckel's diverticulum, or cirrhosis. Anal bleeding should never be ignored.
- he or she has confirmed you have an anal fissure, but after one month of treatment the fissure has not healed. There may be another reason for the fissure or for the poor healing, such as colorectal cancer.

An anal fissure, also called an anal ulcer, is a single shallow crack in the lining of the anus (the lowest region of your intestines, which also opens to the outside). A fissure begins just inside the anal opening and extends ¼ to ¾ inch along the anal wall.

An anal fissure can be excruciatingly painful. Passing stools irritates it, and the anal sphincter muscles, at the anal opening, may respond by going into spasm. These combined effects cause extreme pain that is made even worse if the stools are either hard or watery. Despite the pain, a fissure is not dangerous and will probably heal with simple treatment. Don't ignore it, however: If a fissure becomes chronic, scar tissue can form and impede bowel movements, and you may need surgery to correct the problem.

CAUSES

Often it isn't clear why an anal fissure has developed. Posterior fissures, along the back anal wall, are probably the result of straining with constipation; in passing large, hard stools, the anal lining stretches too much and breaks. Anterior fissures, along the front wall, are usually related to scar-tissue buildup from a previous surgery, or to the extreme pressure that the anal region endures during childbirth. Anal fissures can also be a side effect of another condition, such as proctitis (inflammation of the rectum), Crohn's disease, or colorectal cancer.

DIAGNOSTIC AND TEST PROCEDURES

Because any touch to this sensitive area can cause extreme pain, doctors try to do as little as possible to diagnose anal fissure and rule out serious disorders such as colorectal cancer, syphilis, tuberculosis, Crohn's disease, and AIDS. A visual examination—a close look at the anal region—is often all that is needed. Your doctor may insert a lubricated, gloved finger to manually examine the anus, or perhaps insert a small, thin instrument called an anoscope to get a clearer, closer view (using local anesthesia if necessary).

TREATMENT

Practicing good anal hygiene in order to avoid infection and keeping the stools soft to minimize pain and spasm will encourage a fissure to heal itself. Anal fissures, however, often reappear. Surgery is the only treatment known that can break this cycle, and thus it is the best choice of treatment for persistent fissures.

CONVENTIONAL MEDICINE

Anesthetic creams applied directly to the fissure are the first line of defense, along with warm sitz baths and dietary changes to avoid constipation. This combination is usually successful if the fissure is treated early. If a fissure doesn't respond to these therapies yet is not terribly severe, a physician may apply a local anesthetic and insert a gloved finger into the anus to dilate the anal sphincter. This decreases the pressure inside the anal canal, creating an environment more conducive to healing.

If the anal fissure is extraordinarily painful, resistant to other forms of treatment, or long-standing, surgery is the best option. This involves dividing the lower anal sphincter so it can't tighten and potentially cause fissures. The surgeon may also remove the fissure and the skin just around it, including the sentinel pile if one is present. This 20-minute outpatient procedure is performed under local or spinal anesthetic and is highly effective.

The fissure usually heals, and recurrence is unlikely. More than 90 percent of those who have surgery have no repeat fissure if they maintain a high-fiber diet afterward. It takes three or four days to recover, and you may have trouble controlling flatulence after surgery.

ALTERNATIVE CHOICES

You can often heal an anal fissure by regulating your bowel movements (see Constipation and Diarrhea) and keeping your stress and anxiety levels low. If you can maintain these lifestyle changes, it is unlikely the fissure will return.

HERBAL THERAPY

Dandelion (Taraxacum officinale) tea taken three times daily can help keep stools soft. Mix 2 or 3 tsp dandelion root with 1 cup water and simmer for 10 minutes.

HOMEOPATHY

For up to seven days, 12c of one of the following, taken four times daily, may help. If one remedy doesn't work, try another. Aesculus can help soothe burning anal pain accompanied by lower-back pain and large, dry, hard stools. Try Graphites for painful bowel movements with lumps and mucus. For sharp pains during and after constipated bowel movements that feel as if they tear the anus, use Nitric acid. When anal fissure pain is sharp and burning as though glass were in the anus, use Ratanhia.

AT-HOME REMEDIES

◆ Apply an over-the-counter cream containing 1 percent hydrocortisone or vitamins A and D just inside the anus. (Small rubber finger covers are available for this purpose.) The hydrocortisone can reduce swelling and pain, and the vitamin cream soothes pain and promotes healing. Suppositories move too far up into the rectum to help.

◆ Several times a day, sit in a warm sitz bath for 20 minutes. This relaxes the anal sphincter, reducing spasms and their associated pain.

◆ See Hemorrhoids for more suggestions.

PREVENTION

Prevention involves avoiding constipation and diarrhea through diet and exercise. Among other benefits, a healthy diet and regular exercise promote good bowel health and offer protection against anal fissures. ■

SYMPTOMS

- weakness, fatigue, and a general feeling of malaise; you may be mildly anemic.
- your lips look bluish, your skin is pasty or yellowish, and your gums, nail beds, eyelid linings, or palm creases are pale; you are almost certainly anemic.
- in addition to feeling weak and tired, you are frequently out of breath, faint, or dizzy; you may have severe anemia.
- your tongue burns; you may have **vitamin B$_{12}$ anemia.**
- your tongue feels unusually slick and you experience movement or balance problems, tingling in the extremities, confusion, depression, or memory loss; you may have **pernicious anemia.**
- other possible symptoms: headaches, insomnia, decreased appetite, poor concentration, and an irregular heartbeat.

CALL YOUR DOCTOR IF:

- you have the symptoms of **pernicious anemia;** this disorder can damage the spinal cord.
- you have been taking iron supplements and experience symptoms such as vomiting, bloody diarrhea, fever, jaundice, lethargy, or seizures; you may be suffering from **iron overload,** which can be life-threatening, especially in children.

To stay healthy, the organs and tissues of the human body need a steady supply of oxygen. Anemia, in which body tissues are deprived of oxygen, is caused by a reduction in the number of circulating red blood cells or by inadequate amounts of an essential protein called hemoglobin. The severity of anemia can range from mild to life-threatening.

Normally, the heart pumps oxygen-depleted blood to the lungs, where hemoglobin in the red blood cells binds to oxygen collected there; oxygen-rich blood then travels through the circulatory system to the rest of the body. Oxygen starvation occurs if the body lacks sufficient numbers of red blood cells, which survive for only about 120 days and must constantly be replaced. Anemia can occur if large amounts of blood are lost or if something interferes with the production of red blood cells or accelerates their destruction. Because hemoglobin is the main component of red blood cells and the carrier for oxygen molecules, anemia also occurs if the hemoglobin supply is insufficient or if the hemoglobin itself is dysfunctional.

In all, more than 400 different forms of anemia have been identified, many of them rare. An anemic person often appears pale and weak and may feel breathless, faint, or unusually aware of a pounding heart. The disorder may arise from a number of underlying conditions, some of which may be hereditary, but in many cases poor diet is to blame. Although some forms of anemia require supervised medical care, those stemming from improper nutrition can typically be treated at home once a physician has determined the cause.

CAUSES

Chronic blood loss, perhaps as a result of stomach ulcers, hemorrhoids, or gastrointestinal tumors, can bring on anemia, as can chronic alcohol abuse. More often, however, the problem can be traced to dietary deficiencies; indeed, anemia in alcoholics arises largely because they tend to prefer booze to food and often fail to eat properly. Anemia can also result when the digestive system loses its ability to absorb key vitamins and minerals.

Iron deficiency anemia, the leading form of anemia worldwide, occurs when the body does not store enough iron, the primary raw material of hemoglobin. Iron deficiency is usually a dietary problem, but in many cases other conditions complicate the picture. For example, women who lose excessive amounts of blood through heavy menstrual flows (see Menstrual Problems) may have a lower-than-average iron level. Women who are pregnant or nursing may also have low iron levels because of loss to the developing fetus or because of milk production. Iron deficiency anemia also afflicts patients who have had surgery to remove part of the stomach, thereby impairing the ability to absorb iron.

Megaloblastic anemias, in which red blood cells become unusually large, occur when the body lacks either folic acid or vitamin B_{12}, both critical to cell production.

Hemolytic anemias may arise when red blood cells have genetic defects that cause them to be destroyed prematurely, perhaps by infections. In some cases, the cells are destroyed by the body's own immune system. Some hemolytic anemias are inherited, while others are acquired. Thalassemia is an inherited type of hemolytic anemia that stems from the body's inability to produce sufficient amounts of hemoglobin. One kind of thalassemia, common to people of Mediterranean, African, or Middle Eastern origin, is marked by the production of red blood cells that are smaller and more fragile than normal. This type strikes only those people who inherit the responsible gene from both parents.

In sickle cell anemia, an inherited disease that disproportionately affects people of African and Mediterranean descent, the body produces red blood cells that have a crescent, or sickle, shape rather than the normal oval shape. The deformed cells cannot carry sufficient quantities of hemoglobin, nor can they squeeze easily through tiny blood vessels. Capillaries can become clogged by these abnormal red blood cells, sometimes leading to a life-threatening condition called a sickle cell crisis.

Of the megaloblastic anemias, the most common is the type caused by folic acid deficiency. People with this form of anemia usually aren't

THE IRON FACTS ABOUT SPINACH

Spinach, long heralded by mothers and Popeye the Sailor as a great source of iron, is in fact an iron-blocker. Technically speaking, the vegetable does contain a significant amount of iron. But, like butter beans, lentils, beet greens, and other leafy vegetables, spinach also contains phytate, a chemical that prevents iron from entering the bloodstream. So if your iron count needs a boost, try eating liver, which is high in available iron. Or garnish your spinach salad with slices of orange, as citrus fruits contain vitamins and acids that counteract the effects of phytate and promote iron absorption.

getting enough folic acid in their diet. While just one cup of spinach provides enough folic acid to meet the FDA's recommended daily allowance, this vitamin deficiency is still prevalent in the United States and throughout the world. For some people, the problem is caused not by dietary inadequacies but by an inability to absorb sufficient amounts of folic acid. Certain intestinal disorders, such as some inflammatory bowel diseases and Crohn's disease, as well as some drugs, including sulfasalazine (used to treat ulcerative colitis), can interfere with folic acid metabolism. Heavy consumption of alcohol can also lower blood levels of folic acid by interfering with proper nutrition and by hindering the digestive system's ability to absorb the vitamin.

Because most people, especially those who consume meat and eggs, get plenty of vitamin B_{12} from their diet, anemia linked to a vitamin B_{12} deficiency usually signals the body's inability to absorb the vitamin. This type of anemia can occur in people who have had surgery along the digestive tract. However, the most common form of

B$_{12}$ deficiency anemia, known as **pernicious anemia,** results when the stomach fails to produce a chemical that normally combines with vitamin B$_{12}$ to aid its absorption in the small intestine. Pernicious anemia is a rare condition that most commonly affects older people.

DIAGNOSTIC AND TEST PROCEDURES

Before beginning a treatment program, you need to find out what kind of anemia you have. The only way to know for sure is to have your doctor run tests on a sample of your blood. The results of these tests will quickly reveal whether your anemia is linked to a nutritional deficiency or to some other cause.

TREATMENT

Conventional remedies for anemia range from simple dietary changes and vitamin supplements to hormone treatments and, in severe cases, surgery. Some alternative practitioners approach the disorder through dietary modifications; others emphasize techniques to improve circulation and digestion.

CONVENTIONAL MEDICINE

Once blood tests reveal the underlying problem, treatment paths are well delineated. For anemia caused by a deficiency in iron or folic acid, your doctor will undoubtedly recommend dietary changes and possibly supplements. Because iron supplements can upset the stomach, you should get ones made from ferrous gluconate, which is easier on the digestive system than ferrous sulfate. In general, liquid solutions are less likely than tablets or pills to cause upset. Avoid enteric-coated supplements, since your body cannot absorb the iron as effectively. WARNING: Iron is extremely toxic in large quantities. Excessive use of supplements can lead to **iron overload**, possibly resulting in abdominal pain, nutritional imbalances, digestive problems, or even death, especially in children. Supplements pose a particular threat to people with the inherited disorder he-

mochromatosis, in which the digestive tract absorbs higher-than-normal amounts of iron. Be sure to consult your doctor or a professional nutritionist before taking iron supplements.

Since **vitamin B$_{12}$ anemia** is almost always linked to the body's inability to absorb the vitamin through the digestive tract, regular B$_{12}$ injections are the only recourse. Most people learn to self-administer B$_{12}$ injections at home.

In some cases of anemia caused by excessive blood loss, surgery is the only solution. To determine whether surgery is necessary, your doctor will run extensive tests to identify the cause of the bleeding. Some conditions—such as bleeding of the digestive tract, a frequent cause of iron deficiency anemia in men—can be corrected only through an operation. Doctors may also prescribe transfusions of red blood cells or injections of hormones to speed red blood cell production. (Supplements of hormones should be a last resort for women, as the drugs can produce unwanted side effects.) Severe cases of **thalassemia** may require lifetime blood transfusions, and treatment of other **hemolytic anemias** may involve surgery to remove the spleen.

ALTERNATIVE CHOICES

Some remedies treat anemia by promoting better circulation, others by increasing iron absorption, stimulating digestion, or adjusting the diet to include more iron- or vitamin-rich foods.

CHINESE MEDICINE

According to traditional Chinese medicine, anemia is a symptom of a weak spleen. A healthy spleen maintains the integrity of blood vessels and nourishes the blood itself, while a weak spleen produces deficient blood. Treatment would typically involve ways to stimulate the spleen, including **acupuncture** and **herbal therapies.** Research suggests that Asian ginseng *(Panax ginseng)* is useful as a general tonic to counteract anemia-induced fatigue. Dong quai *(Angelica sinensis),* another Asian herb used medicinally for thousands of years, might be prescribed for women with heavy menstrual flow. For anemic patients that have a sallow, yellowish complexion, a Chinese herbalist might recommend a combination of dong quai and Chinese foxglove root (*Rehmannia glutinosa*). For patients that have a stark white complexion, the remedy might be a mixture of ginseng and astragalus (*Astragalus membranaceus*).

HERBAL THERAPIES

In the history of folk medicine, bitter substances have always been thought to stimulate digestion and thereby promote the absorption of valuable nutrients. The bitter herb gentian (*Gentiana lutea*) is a popular remedy in Europe for a number of nutritionally based ailments, including anemia. Gentian can be brewed into a tea or ingested in the form of a commercially available alcoholic extract. Dandelion (*Taraxacum officinale*) is also thought to benefit people with anemia, simply because it is rich in vitamins and minerals. Other iron-rich herbs include parsley (*Petroselinum crispum*) and nettle (*Urtica dioica*). While many herbs used to treat anemia have anecdotal support, not all have been studied scientifically. Among those that have been shown to promote digestion are anise (*Pimpinella anisum*), caraway (*Carum carvi*), cumin (*Cuminum cyminum*), linden (*Tilia* spp.), and licorice (*Glycyrrhiza glabra*).

HOMEOPATHY

Homeopathy offers a number of remedies that may be helpful in treating anemia. Consult a professional homeopath for an evaluation that will determine which substances are most suitable for your condition.

NUTRITION AND DIET

Adjusting your diet is the easiest, most healthful, and longest-lasting way to combat any anemia linked to nutritional deficiency. A vast array of foods can boost your iron count, including enriched breads and cereals, rice, potatoes, carrots, broccoli, tomatoes, dried beans, blackstrap molasses, lean red meat, liver, poultry, dried fruits, almonds, and shellfish. Research indicates that iron from animal sources is absorbed more readily than plant iron. Evidence also suggests that vitamin C and copper help the body absorb iron, so drink citrus fruit juice with your meals and make sure that your daily multivitamin contains copper. Avoid caffeinated or carbonated beverages, antacids, calcium supplements, and black tea, all of which contain ingredients that interfere with iron absorption.

If you're low on folic acid, step up your consumption of citrus fruits, mushrooms, green vegetables, liver, eggs, milk, and bulking agents like wheat germ and brewer's yeast. Also, pumpkin is an excellent source of folate, which is the vitamin B complex component of folic acid. Keep in mind that folic acid is destroyed by heat and light, so fruits and vegetables should be eaten fresh and cooked as little as possible.

AT-HOME REMEDIES

◆ Your diet should include foods recommended on these pages. The specific choices should be dictated by the type of anemia you have.

◆ Keep track of the foods you eat and find out whether they are rich in iron, folic acid, or vitamin B_{12}. You might be surprised to learn that some of the foods you eat are preventing the absorption of needed nutrients. (*See "The Iron Facts about Spinach," page 119.*)

◆ Don't drink caffeinated tea, coffee, or cola with meals; caffeine inhibits iron absorption. The tannin in black tea has the same effect. However, you should drink citrus juices, because they are rich in vitamin C, which promotes iron absorption.

◆ Consider taking a daily multivitamin. However, be sure to consult a doctor before taking iron supplements; excess amounts of iron in your system can be harmful.

PREVENTION

◆ Avoid excessive consumption of alcohol. Chronic drinking can undermine proper nutrition and interfere with the digestive system's ability to absorb folic acid, necessary for the production of red blood cells.

◆ Take a daily multivitamin to maintain a healthful balance of vitamins and minerals. ■

SYMPTOMS

Although most aneurysms have no symptoms, in some cases the following symptoms may occur:

◆ Sudden and severe pain, often described as "ripping or tearing," or an unusual pulsing sensation, pain, or a lump anywhere in your body where blood vessels are located.

◆ Pain in the abdomen or lower back extending into the groin and legs may indicate an **abdominal aneurysm,** which can sometimes be seen or felt as a throbbing lump and may be accompanied by weight loss or loss of appetite.

◆ A pain in the chest, hoarseness, persistent coughing, and difficulty swallowing may indicate a **thoracic aneurysm.**

◆ A throbbing sensation or lump directly behind the knee may indicate a **peripheral aneurysm;** the knee is a common site for this type of aneurysm, especially in smokers.

◆ A severe headache, like none you've ever had before, accompanied by radiating neck pain, may indicate a **dissecting** or rupturing **berry aneurysm** in the head. Dissecting aneurysms, most commonly characterized by severe pain, can also occur elsewhere in the body and are always an emergency situation.

CALL YOUR DOCTOR IF:

◆ you suspect you have an aneurysm. Many aneurysms are serious and require a medical evaluation. An aneurysm that ruptures is potentially life-threatening.

An aneurysm is a permanent ballooning in the wall of an artery. The pressure of blood passing through can force part of a weakened artery to bulge outward, forming a thin-skinned blister.

Although any weak blood vessel can be affected, aneurysms usually form in the abdominal or thoracic portions of the aorta, the main blood vessel that carries blood from the heart, or in arteries nourishing the brain. Aneurysms in any of these places are serious, while those in peripheral arteries are often less hazardous.

The gravest threat an aneurysm poses is that it will burst and cause a stroke or life-threatening hemorrhage. But even if it doesn't rupture, a large aneurysm can impede circulation and promote unwanted blood-clot formation.

Detecting an aneurysm on your own is difficult since symptoms are rare. But certain people are at higher risk of developing aneurysms. Your best strategy is to know if you are at risk (see Causes, below), to be familiar with the symptoms of an aneurysm, and to take preventive steps.

CAUSES

Any condition that causes arterial walls to weaken or deteriorate can result in an aneurysm. The most common culprits are atherosclerosis and high blood pressure. Penetrating wounds and infections can also lead to an aneurysm. Some types, such as **berry aneurysms,** are the result of congenital, or inherited, weakness in artery walls.

TREATMENT

The only way to get rid of an aneurysm is to have it surgically removed—often a risky procedure, but highly effective when successful. Sometimes, however, surgery is impossible, or it may pose more danger than the aneurysm. Careful monitoring and drug therapy may then be the best course.

CONVENTIONAL MEDICINE

Your doctor will probably determine the size, type, and location of an aneurysm using any of various imaging techniques. This information will help determine the best course of treatment.

For inoperable aneurysms, you may be prescribed drugs that lower your blood pressure or reduce the force of your heart's contractions, thereby minimizing the risk of a rupture. But

even for an operable aneurysm, your doctor may first try drug therapy and advise a wait-and-see approach, with periodic testing to track the aneurysm's growth. You may need surgery if your doctor finds that the aneurysm has become dangerously swollen.

A surgeon can neutralize an aneurysm by inserting a clip that cuts off blood flow to the affected area. An aneurysm may also be removed and the section of artery replaced with a synthetic graft.

ALTERNATIVE CHOICES

The following treatments—all primarily intended to prevent aneurysms—should be pursued along with, not instead of, your doctor's orders.

HOMEOPATHY

For a small, relatively benign aneurysm or as a preventive remedy for someone at high risk of developing an aneurysm, a professional homeopath might recommend Baryta carbonica to tone and strengthen arterial walls.

MIND/BODY MEDICINE

Keeping your mind and body relaxed may prevent an aneurysm from worsening. Try exercises that you can do at home such as **yoga** or **meditation.**

NUTRITION AND DIET

Dietary changes that lower blood pressure and slow atherosclerosis may help prevent an aneurysm from developing. See entries on Atherosclerosis, Blood Clots, High Blood Pressure, and Cholesterol Problems.

PREVENTION

Know if you are at risk, and take appropriate steps to keep an aneurysm from forming. Especially if you have a family history of stroke or heart disease, make changes in your diet and lifestyle to improve your overall health. Exercise regularly, watch what you eat, and if you smoke, stop. ■

TYPES OF ANEURYSMS

SACCULAR
A saccular aneurysm is a balloonlike bulge in an artery wall. Usually caused by a congenital weakness in the wall's muscular middle layer, this type of aneurysm may contain a blood clot.

BERRY
Berry aneurysms, saccular types of aneurysms, are named for their small, round appearance. These bulges most often occur in branching arteries at the base of the brain.

FUSIFORM
Damage to the artery wall's inner and middle layers can cause a sausage-shaped swelling known as a fusiform aneurysm. High blood pressure and atherosclerosis are the primary causes of this type of aneurysm.

CYLINDROID
A cylindroid, or tubular, aneurysm is an elongated swelling that causes an abrupt change in an artery's normal diameter. Often the result of atherosclerosis or syphilis, a cylindroid aneurysm can develop along a length of artery.

A

SYMPTOMS

- pain that is crushing, constricting, strangling, suffocating, sharp, or burning; it is normally felt in the chest but may also occur in peripheral areas such as the jaw or abdomen. Location and specific sensations vary from person to person but are usually consistent from one attack to the next.
- pain that occurs with exertion and recedes with rest.
- weakness, sweating, shortness of breath, anxiety, palpitations, nausea, or lightheadedness—symptoms that may or may not be associated with an angina attack.

CALL YOUR DOCTOR IF:

- an attack lasts more than 15 minutes; this may be a heart attack. **Call 911 or your emergency number now.**
- you think this may be your first angina attack; you need to find out for sure.
- attacks have become more intense, frequent, prolonged, and unpredictable; these are signs of **unstable angina.**
- you are taking a beta blocker and experience distressing side effects.
- you are taking nitrate medication and become faint, dizzy, weak, pale, restless, or start vomiting or sweating excessively. These are signs of either oversensitivity or overdose.
- you are taking a calcium channel blocker and notice side effects such as stomach cramps, slow pulse, arrhythmia, headaches, constipation, swelling, faintness, or shortness of breath.

Angina is the heart's way of saying that it is not getting enough oxygen. This can be because coronary arteries—those that supply blood to the heart—are blocked or because the heart is being overworked and therefore needs more oxygen than usual.

The medical term angina pectoris literally means "a choking sensation of the chest." Usually, angina is a crushing or constricting pain that starts in the center of the chest, deep behind the breastbone, and may radiate to other parts of the body. Sufferers have said it feels like "an elephant sitting on my chest" or "a vise squeezing my chest."

Some people feel the pain of angina only in peripheral locations such as the jaw, abdomen, or arm. The pain can also be confused with indigestion because the tight, burning sensations are similar. Angina can also be misinterpreted as a heart attack; the pain is similar but does not last as long—usually no more than five minutes.

Of the many types of angina, **stable,** or **classical, angina**—triggered by exertion and receding with rest—is the most common. If you have stable angina, you should be able to predict what sort of activity will bring on an attack. Another type, **unstable angina,** is a more acute condition; it occurs unpredictably, even during rest, and should be interpreted as a warning sign of more serious heart trouble. A rare type called **variant angina,** which involves coronary artery spasms, is seen most often in women.

Angina affects some three million Americans. It is more prevalent in people over 30 and tends to strike men more than women; over age 65, however, more women are affected than men. Alone, angina causes no permanent damage because the heart is only temporarily deprived of oxygen. But if your angina worsens, you should know that you are at a greater risk of heart attack. Be especially concerned if you develop **unstable angina,** and consult a doctor.

CAUSES

The main underlying cause of angina is coronary artery disease, which stems from atherosclerosis

AREAS OF ANGINAL PAIN

Anginal pain can be distributed throughout the upper body in any of the following areas *(shown at left)* including the center and left part of the chest, the neck, and inside the left arm *(purple)*. Pain may also develop in the jaw *(green)*, right chest and arm *(pink)*, and between the navel and breastbone *(yellow)*; the shoulders may be affected as well. In some cases, pain occurs between the shoulder blades *(purple area in lower illustration)*.

of the coronary arteries—when the vessels become clogged or narrowed by fatty calcified deposits called plaques. Angina can also result from other diseases that tax the heart unduly, such as anemia, aortic valve disease *(see Heart Disease)*, heart arrhythmias, and hyperthyroidism *(see Thyroid Problems)*.

Stable angina is sometimes called "exertional" angina because it is triggered by activities that make the heart beat rapidly. Indeed, physical activity is the most frequent cause of attacks. Depending on the person, exertion that brings on an attack can mean anything from simple walking to heavy lifting or sexual activity. A large meal can also cause an attack, because digestion requires the heart to work. Other frequently cited triggers are emotional excitement and exposure to the cold, both of which stimulate the heart. In addition, more than 20 drugs have been known to spark angina, from over-the-counter decongestants and various prescription medications to illegal substances such as cocaine.

Certain risk factors for heart disease and coronary artery disease make the development of angina more likely. These include high blood pressure, stress, high cholesterol *(see Cholesterol Problems)*, smoking, obesity, diabetes, and a family history of heart disease. All of these risk factors are also linked to atherosclerosis.

DIAGNOSTIC AND TEST PROCEDURES

If you experience pain that might be angina, your doctor will give you a complete physical exam and various tests. A resting electrocardiogram (ECG) will usually be normal if you have angina, but the test may rule out other causes. You will likely undergo an exercise treadmill test, possibly combined with an imaging technique such as ultrasound or a radioisotope scan, which may reveal problems in the heart or arteries. If these tests indicate a possible problem, angiography will be performed to determine the location and extent of any blockages in coronary arteries.

TREATMENT

Drugs may alleviate angina symptoms, but fundamental changes in diet and lifestyle are an important part of any angina treatment program. Before taking any drug, review its properties and your medical history carefully with your doctor. Many drugs should not be mixed with other drugs or natural medicines, and you also need to be sure your doctor knows of any preexisting medical conditions you may have.

CONVENTIONAL MEDICINE

If you have angina, your doctor will undoubtedly mention the importance of an overall healthy lifestyle that includes proper diet, exercise, weight management, and no smoking.

Most angina patients also take prescribed medication. There are three main classes of angina drugs: nitrates, beta-adrenergic blockers, and calcium channel blockers. Physicians often use a combination of these to treat angina. Nitrates, which dilate coronary arteries and allow for greater blood flow, are a tried-and-true, inexpensive treatment. Nitroglycerin is by far the most widely used nitrate; it can be taken as often as needed and may provide relief within a few minutes. However, it also causes headaches in about half of all users. Beta-adrenergic blockers, which are used to reduce heart rate, lower blood pressure, and reduce cardiac oxygen consumption, are effective in combination with nitrates or alone. Calcium channel blockers quell coronary artery spasms, and some also slow heart rate. Patients with severe unstable angina are often treated initially with the anticoagulant heparin in conjunction with aspirin, nitrates, and beta blockers.

If drug therapy does not work or does not suffice, coronary artery angioplasty or bypass surgery may be considered. Angioplasty—a catheter technique that widens blocked arteries—has become a relatively routine procedure; bypass surgery, which diverts blood flow around clogged arteries, is reserved for very severe cases.

ALTERNATIVE CHOICES

Always consult a doctor if you think you have angina. The alternative therapies below may help relieve symptoms or prevent attacks, but they should be considered as complements to—rather than substitutes for—conventional medical care.

ACUPRESSURE

Applying pressure for at least one minute to points P 6 and Sp 6 may relieve angina symptoms. See pages 22–23 and page 127 for point locations.

AYURVEDIC MEDICINE

An Ayurvedic mixture of herbs and minerals known as Abana has been shown to significantly reduce the frequency and severity of angina attacks; consult a practitioner for the specific remedy.

CHELATION THERAPY

Although controversial, chelation therapy has been sought by thousands of angina sufferers. Its advocates claim that it is safer and cheaper than many conventional drug or surgical treatments—and just as effective. Critics insist that it undergo more rigorous scientific scrutiny before joining the ranks of standard treatment for angina and atherosclerosis. If you decide to try chelation therapy, be sure to seek out a practitioner certi-fied by one of the major American chelation societies. (See Atherosclerosis for a fuller explanation of chelation therapy.)

HERBAL THERAPIES

Hawthorn (Crataegus laevigata) is an excellent long-term tonic for angina because it simultaneously dilates coronary arteries and calms the heart. It is often an ingredient in herbal treatments for angina that a naturopath might prescribe.

HOMEOPATHY

For immediate relief during an acute attack, Cactus grandiflorus (30c) is recommended. Cactus may bring relief if, during an attack, your chest feels like it's bound with an iron band. Among the long-term remedies that might be prescribed by a homeopathic physician are Nux vomica and Arsenicum album.

LIFESTYLE

Certain air pollutants, particularly carbon monoxide, are known to aggravate and intensify angina. To avoid carbon monoxide, steer clear of tobacco smoke and stay inside on heavy smog days.

Avoid alcohol or drink only sparingly while on angina medication because of possible adverse reactions.

Gentle aerobic exercise is very beneficial for angina patients. Build stamina gradually, and exercise inside during cold weather. Be sure to consult your doctor before embarking on an exercise program.

MIND/BODY MEDICINE

If you find you have trouble controlling your emotions or stress levels, you must learn to relax. Many types of relaxation techniques—from **biofeedback** to **yoga**—could help tremendously. Choose a method you are comfortable with, and stick with it; the effectiveness of relaxation techniques varies from person to person and improves with time.

NUTRITION AND DIET

The principal goals of nutritional therapy for angina are to improve the blood flow to the heart and the energy metabolism of the heart so that it requires less oxygen. The main way to improve blood flow is to control atherosclerosis, and consuming less saturated fat and cholesterol is a critical first step. To improve energy metabolism, be sure to get enough magnesium in your diet or as part of a multivitamin supplement. You might also ask your doctor to recommend an appropriate supplement of L-carnitine and coenzyme Q10, nutrients found in the body that improve energy metabolism and are often depleted in heart disease patients. For more specific dietary tips, see Atherosclerosis, Blood Clots, Cholesterol Problems, and High Blood Pressure.

STRESS TEST

Exercising with angina is a tricky business. If done properly, it can help prevent angina from worsening; if done too ambitiously, it will aggravate the condition and could even be life-threatening. So how much is too much? If you want to start an exercise program, you should first undergo a stress test—also called an "exercise tolerance" or "treadmill" test. The test takes about half an hour. You will be fitted with electrodes on your chest and a blood-pressure cuff on your arm, and

will then start exercising on a treadmill or stationary bike; as time elapses, the workout becomes progressively more difficult. By monitoring your heart rate, blood pressure, and ECG tracings, your doctor will be able to determine your exertion limits. Armed with this knowledge, you can then plan a healthful exercise regimen.

AT-HOME REMEDIES

◆ If you have frequent angina attacks at night, try tilting the head of your bed up three or four inches. This lessens the work load on the heart from venous blood return.
◆ If you sense the onset of an attack while lying down, sit up and put your feet on the floor. If pain persists, take prescribed medication.
◆ An aspirin a day, with doctor's permission, can reduce the risk of heart attack and unstable angina.
◆ Spend at least an hour digesting heavy meals; exertion after eating is known to cause attacks.
◆ Stop smoking, as it greatly aggravates angina.
◆ Do not take birth-control pills if you have angina: Estrogens are associated with increased risk of blood clots.

PREVENTION

◆ Adopt a low-fat, low-cholesterol diet that will help keep arteries free of fatty deposits.
◆ Exercise! People who exercise are less likely to be overweight and less likely to develop atherosclerosis.
◆ Learn to control your emotions, rather than letting them control you. People who internalize stress are more likely to develop angina; many angina sufferers cite emotional outburst as a precipitator of attacks.
◆ If you smoke, quit. ■

ACUPRESSURE

1 To help calm nerves and reduce feelings of uneasiness, press Pericardium 6. Place thumb in center of inner wrist, two finger widths from the wrist crease and between the two bones of the forearm. Press firmly for one minute, three to five times; repeat on other arm.

2 Pressure on Spleen 6 may help regulate blood pressure. The point is four finger widths up from the inner anklebone, near the edge of your shinbone. Press gently with your thumb for one minute, then switch legs. Do not use this point if you are pregnant.

ANKLES, PAINFUL

Read down this column to find your symptoms. Then read across.

SYMPTOMS	AILMENT/PROBLEM
◆ pain following injury; ankle is not mis-shapen and can move and bear weight without severe pain.	◆ Soft-tissue injury, such as sprain, strain, or tear
◆ dull ache or pain, ranging from the heel through the back of the ankle and into the lower calf, especially when running or jumping; mild swelling or tenderness.	◆ Achilles tendonitis
◆ spontaneous onset of pain, redness, warmth, and swelling in ankle and/or other joints.	◆ Rheumatoid arthritis; bursitis
◆ spontaneous onset of pain, redness, warmth, and swelling in ankle and/or other joints; recent illness, such as sore throat, rash, or other infection; fever of 100°F or higher.	◆ Rheumatic fever; infectious arthritis
◆ gradual development of pain and stiffness in ankle, especially when the ankle is moved.	◆ Osteoarthritis
◆ sudden shooting pains in ankle; stiffness and tingling.	◆ Bone spur
◆ chronic pain in feet and legs, especially when walking; feet and legs feel cold.	◆ Poor circulation; peripheral vascular disease
◆ sudden onset of intense, throbbing pain in ankle; ankle swelling; feeling of heat in joint.	◆ Gout

WHAT TO DO	OTHER INFO
◆ See Sprains and Strains. If you are experiencing intense pain, you may have a severe sprain or a fracture that requires medical attention; call your doctor.	◆ Rest, ice, compression, and elevation—known collectively as RICE—are the initial treatment for most soft-tissue injuries. You may also need rehabilitation exercises.
◆ See Tendonitis. Rest the ankle, apply ice, and if needed, take pain-relieving medication. Wearing a half-inch lift or pad in the heel of your shoe may aid recovery.	◆ Osteopathy and chiropractic may be helpful. A doctor or physical therapist can prescribe stretching exercises. If the tendon is severed rather than inflamed, surgery is required.
◆ See Arthritis and Bursitis. Rest the ankle and apply ice for the first 24 hours, then heat. Take an anti-inflammatory drug for severe pain.	◆ Supplements of fish oil and vitamins C, B_6, and E may help relieve the pain of arthritis. Bursitis may respond to vitamin B_{12} injections.
◆ Call your doctor. You will need medical treatment, which is usually antibiotics and/or anti-inflammatory drugs. See Arthritis and Rheumatic Fever.	◆ Rheumatic fever is a serious complication of prior streptococcal infection. Infectious arthritis is usually a complication of another illness or injury.
◆ See Arthritis. Your doctor may prescribe an analgesic and exercises. Heat treatments, physical or occupational therapy, acupuncture, and yoga may be helpful.	◆ Osteoarthritis involves loss of bone tissue and wearing out of joints, which may be caused by either injury or aging.
◆ See Bone Spurs. Rest your ankle and take an anti-inflammatory drug. Try padding inside your shoe.	◆ These abnormal growths at the ends of bones are common in older people who have disk problems and in people who use their muscles extensively, such as athletes or dancers.
◆ Call your doctor to have the underlying cause (diabetes or vascular disease) diagnosed and treated. See Circulatory Problems.	◆ The risk factors associated with poor circulation include aging, obesity, lack of exercise, and smoking. Vitamin E and the herb ginkgo (Ginkgo biloba) may be helpful.
◆ See Gout. Seek medical care. Treatment usually consists of anti-inflammatory medication and the drugs colchicine, allopurinol, or probenecid. Gout attacks may be prevented with a low-purine diet.	◆ Gout is caused by excess uric acid in a joint. Vitamin C, cherries, and the herb devil's claw (Harpagophytum procumbens) may be helpful.

ANKLES, SWOLLEN

Read down this column to find your symptoms. Then read across.

SYMPTOMS	AILMENT/PROBLEM
◆ swelling occurring after injury; ankle is not misshapen and can move and bear weight without severe pain.	◆ Soft-tissue injury, such as sprain, strain, or tear
◆ spontaneous onset of swelling, pain, redness, warmth, and stiffness in ankle and/or other joints.	◆ Arthritis
◆ swelling after periods of standing; aching in lower leg, especially calf, that is worse at the end of the day; swelling and discoloration of veins in legs.	◆ Varicose veins
◆ swelling accompanied by weakness, fatigue, and/or dizziness; shortness of breath that worsens; cough.	◆ Congestive heart failure
◆ swelling in ankle accompanied by a hard, red, cordlike swelling of calf veins on the same leg; pain; redness; tenderness; itching.	◆ Phlebitis
◆ swelling while taking oral contraceptives or corticosteroid medications.	◆ Drug side effect
◆ swelling in a woman within a few days of her menstrual period; swelling not accompanied by pain.	◆ Premenstrual syndrome (PMS)
◆ painless swelling of ankles in a woman who is more than three months pregnant; swelling also occurs in face and fingers; weight gain of more than four pounds in the previous week.	◆ Pregnancy problem or preeclampsia

WHAT TO DO	OTHER INFO
◆ Apply cold compresses until the swelling goes down, then apply warmth. If you are experiencing intense pain, you may have a severe sprain or a fracture that requires medical attention. Call your doctor.	◆ Mild sprains are often compressed with an elastic bandage to reduce swelling. Severe sprains may require a cast or surgery.
◆ Rest the ankle, apply heat, and take an anti-inflammatory drug.	◆ Hydrotherapy, acupuncture, nutritional therapy, and homeopathy have been found to relieve symptoms in some people.
◆ Rest and elevate your feet. If the leg is significantly swollen or painful, or sores appear on the skin, call your doctor.	◆ Possible treatments include pain medications, elastic stockings, and injections of a drug that causes vein walls to cave in.
◆ **Call your doctor now.** If you are short of breath, **seek emergency medical care.** In addition to various heart medications, treatment usually involves resting with legs raised and wearing anti-embolism stockings. See Heart Disease.	◆ After conventional treatment has been established, nutritional and herbal therapy may be helpful in preventing the underlying heart disease from worsening.
◆ Call your doctor; a medical evaluation is necessary for diagnosis and treatment. Treatment usually involves rest, elevation of the leg, anti-inflammatory drugs, and possibly, antibiotics. If a blood clot has formed, you may be hospitalized and treated to ensure that the clot does not break off and travel to the lung.	◆ Warm compresses may ease inflammation for superficial phlebitis; elastic stockings or bandages may reduce swelling. Smokers should quit smoking.
◆ Call your doctor to discuss a possible change in medication.	
◆ Implement dietary changes and an exercise regimen.	◆ PMS is believed to be caused by a hormonal imbalance. Dietary changes, nutritional supplements, herbal therapy, and homeopathy may help reduce symptoms.
◆ **Call your doctor now.** You could have preeclampsia, a serious condition requiring immediate medical treatment. See Pregnancy Problems.	◆ Avoid standing for long periods, and rest with feet up. For preeclampsia, treatment includes rest, diuretics, and medication to lower blood pressure. In severe cases, hospitalization may be needed, with delivery of baby by induction or Cesarean section.

SYMPTOMS

- significant weight loss.
- fear of becoming fat, even when emaciated.
- excessive dieting and exercising.
- distorted body image.
- abnormal food preoccupations, such as counting all calories or obsessively studying cookbooks.
- constipation.
- dry, sallow skin.
- increase in facial and body hair; loss of some head hair.
- cessation of menstrual periods.
- suppression of sexual desire.
- hands and feet cold at normal room temperature.
- chronic insomnia; an unexplained increase or decrease in energy level.

CALL YOUR DOCTOR IF:

- your child or teenager is obsessed with dieting and continues to feel fat, usually after a major weight loss.
- your child chronically uses laxatives, diuretics, emetics, or diet pills.
- your child overexercises to lose weight.
- your child is preoccupied with food, calories, and food preparation.

Anorexia nervosa is an eating disorder centered on an overwhelming dread of becoming fat. The result of this unfounded fear is self-starvation and major weight loss; in addition to emaciation, the undernourishment may cause hormonal disturbances, anemia, irregular heartbeat, brittle bones, and many other problems.

Usually the condition occurs during early adolescence to young adulthood, although it may strike later. Some 90 percent of sufferers are female; about 1 percent of American women are afflicted. Anorexia is dangerous, and professional help should be sought early. Prompt treatment will usually keep the condition from progressing, but some cases are very resistant to treatment and may require hospitalization. As many as 15 percent of anorexics die from complications.

Although its focus is on food, anorexia is an illness of the mind. Often it begins with a relatively normal desire to lose a few pounds. But because dieting only temporarily relieves underlying psychological problems, it soon becomes compulsive; food intake is gradually minimized until eating is almost eliminated. The victim becomes obsessed with her body image and frequently sees herself as fat even though the opposite is true. Ironically, she ritualizes food preparation and consumption. She becomes fascinated with recipes and cooking yet will not eat the food herself, especially in the presence of others. She may intersperse fasting with periodic binging and purging *(see Bulimia)*, particularly when she is trying to regain normal eating habits. About half of all anorexics become bulimic at some point.

Anorexics tend to come from families that have high standards of achievement, and they are often perfectionists, compulsive in many aspects of their life, especially school. Denial often accompanies their intense focus on remaining thin: Anorexics will typically refuse to admit that anything is wrong, and they become angry or defensive at expressions of concern by others.

CAUSES

While some studies indicate that genes can play a predisposing role in anorexia, most researchers believe that psychological factors are key. Anorexics tend to have low self-esteem and feel undeserving of love. In adolescence, such feelings may be exacerbated by sexual changes, cultural messages that glorify thinness, and pressures or tensions within the family. Extreme fasting may be an anorexic's way of attempting to exert control over her life—not just shaping her appearance but also retarding maturation and sexual development.

DIAGNOSTIC AND TEST PROCEDURES

Although some screening measures—such as the Eating Attitude Test (EAT)—can help identify potential anorexics, the predominant indicator is emaciation for no evident physical reason other than fasting. Blood and urine should be thoroughly tested to rule out other possible causes of weight loss and, more important, to reveal hormonal imbalances and low levels of such important nutrients as potassium, zinc, and fatty acids. Zinc deficiency—common in anorexics, especially those who are vegetarians—may impair many of the body's biochemical actions, retarding growth and sexual development, and ultimately contributing to the anorexia itself. Because extreme hormonal and nutritional imbalances can lead to death, frequent monitoring is essential.

TREATMENT

Psychotherapy, regular medical monitoring, and nutritional guidance should be part of any treatment program for anorexia. Close cooperation

IMPORTANT!

As a parent or friend of someone coping with anorexia, avoid commenting about eating, weight, grooming, or school performance unless you are asked. Show her that you value her and others for their internal qualities, such as thoughtfulness and perceptiveness.

among all health professionals involved is important. All these professionals should be experienced specifically in treating eating disorders.

CONVENTIONAL MEDICINE

Treatment of anorexia will vary, depending on the stage at which it is recognized and the patient's willingness to cooperate. Hospitalization is usually necessary if the patient has lost more than 25 percent of normal body weight.

The primary focus of treatment is individual psychotherapy to uncover emotional problems and interpersonal difficulties that may underlie the disorder. Family therapy is also important if the patient is living at home, and behavior therapy can help change detrimental habits. In addition, a goal of a specific weight range should be set, and ongoing nutritional education and medical monitoring are important.

Supplements of zinc sulfate will redress any zinc deficiency. Other nutritional supplements, appetite enhancers, antidepressants, and anti-anxiety drugs are often prescribed as well.

ALTERNATIVE CHOICES

Alternative therapies may help with some of the symptoms of anorexia, and can serve as useful adjuncts to treatments that address nutrition and the emotional roots of the disorder.

HERBAL THERAPIES

See Anxiety for herbs that calm. To relax stomach muscles, try gentian (Gentiana lutea) or any other digestive bitter; make a tea by pouring boiling water over 1 to 3 tsp of dried herbs or a handful of fresh herbs. Steep for 10 to 15 minutes. Take a small cupful three or four times a day.

MIND/BODY MEDICINE

Yoga, t'ai chi, dance, and swimming are among the exercise or relaxation techniques that can reduce anxiety and increase body awareness.

EEG biofeedback can help bring anxiety and eating habits under control. Hypnotherapy may also be useful in exploring underlying emotional problems. ∎

A

- heart palpitations.
- sense of impending doom.
- inability to concentrate.
- muscle tension; muscle aches.
- diarrhea.
- chest pain.
- dry mouth.
- excessive sweating.
- undereating or overeating.
- insomnia.
- irritability.
- breathlessness; hyperventilation.
- loss of sex drive. *(See Impotence.)*

For school-age children:
- fear of being away from the family.
- refusal to go to school.
- fear of strangers.
- unnecessary worry.

CALL YOUR DOCTOR IF:

- your anxiety seems irrational or more extreme than the situation warrants.
- your anxiety inhibits normal activities.
- low-level anxiety persists for many weeks.
- your symptoms suddenly become severe or uncontrollable. You may be experiencing a panic attack.
- anxiety is accompanied by weight loss and bulging of the eyes; you may have thyroid problems.

Almost everyone feels anxious from time to time. When there is a threat of some kind, anxiety is normal—bound up with the way the body prepares to deal with danger: Adrenaline and cortisone are released in the bloodstream; heart rate quickens; breathing becomes shallow and rapid; muscles tense; sugar is released by the liver; and the mind goes on full alert. But when anxiety is not tied to an identifiable threat or is more severe and long-lasting than warranted, it is a clinical disorder, debilitating and disruptive.

Many different anxiety disorders are recognized. Among them are phobias (fear of certain situations, such as confining spaces, or of particular things, such as insects); panic attacks (a sudden onset of extreme fear or tension, for no evident reason); obsessive-compulsive disorder (persistent, irrational thoughts, such as a dread of infection, or repetitive behavior, such as checking that doors are locked); posttraumatic stress disorder (prolonged anxiety after a traumatic event); and generalized—or "free-floating"—anxiety (an inexplicable feeling of apprehension that may last for months).

Anxiety disorders can vary greatly in their severity; they may be mild or completely immobilizing. The incidence of the different disorders also varies: Phobias, panic attacks, and obsessive-compulsive disorder, for example, occur less frequently than generalized anxiety (which afflicts twice as many women as men). The disorders usually become noticeable during the teen years or early adulthood and are considerably more common among adults than children.

Some anxieties are very difficult to treat; others respond well to medications, psychotherapy, and alternative therapies. What does not work is self-treatment with alcohol or recreational drugs to alleviate the symptoms. Many sufferers choose this path, but ultimately it will only make the condition worse.

CAUSES

Anxiety can be caused by a recognizable stress—such as an accident, a death in the family, or the loss of a job; in such cases, adjustments to the situation, along with the passage of time, will have an ameliorating effect. In other cases, the stress is invisible—a buried memory of some unhappy or frightening facet of childhood, lurking below the surface of the conscious mind and revealing its presence in anxiety.

Genetic inheritance may predispose some individuals to anxiety: Studies of identical twins show that if one member of an identical pair suffers from anxiety, there is at least a 50 percent chance that the other will, as well. Food sensitivities may also contribute to anxiety, although more research must be done to certify this connection. In addition, anxiety frequently follows a sudden withdrawal from alcohol, tobacco, or other drugs.

DIAGNOSTIC AND TEST PROCEDURES

The first step is to rule out the possibility that the symptoms are being caused by an organic disease. Among the conditions that produce symptoms similar to those of anxiety are hyperthyroidism *(see Thyroid Problems);* hyper- or hypocalcemia (too much or too little calcium); coronary artery disease *(see Heart Disease);* tachycardia (rapid heart rate—*see Heart Arrhythmias);* and other heart problems. A thorough evaluation by your doctor will determine if any of these conditions are the cause.

If no organic culprit can be found and the symptoms seem out of proportion to any situation you are facing, the condition will be classified as an anxiety disorder.

TREATMENT

Anxiety can be treated with conventional medications, psychotherapy, and many alternative approaches. A combination of conventional and alternative methods is often effective.

CONVENTIONAL MEDICINE

Psychotherapy and psychoanalysis both aim at identifying conflicts and other stresses—perhaps long buried—that may lie at the roots of anxiety.

Behavior modification—a therapy that concentrates on changing patterns of behavior—can help the patient avert anxiety or better cope with it, as can cognitive therapy, which concentrates on changing ways of thinking.

Medication is useful for alleviating the symptoms of anxiety and is often prescribed in conjunction with other therapies. The most prominent of antianxiety drugs are those known as benzodiazepines; among them are lorazepam, diazepam, alprazolam, and clonazepam. They have drawbacks: Benzodiazepines sometimes cause drowsiness, irritability, dizziness, and dependency. Nonetheless, in recent decades they have largely replaced barbiturates, which not only pose a clear danger of addiction but also can be a threat with suicidal patients. Another antianxiety drug is buspirone. It has fewer side effects than the benzodiazepines but should not be taken if you have liver or kidney disease; also, check with your doctor before taking it during pregnancy or breast-feeding.

ALTERNATIVE CHOICES

Many alternative practices and treatments can relieve the symptoms of anxiety. **Meditation,** exercise (especially aerobic exercise), and **relaxation** techniques are among the most effective. Their usefulness varies from person to person, however. For example, people with physical symptoms—such as stomachache or sweating—do better with exercise, while those with mental symptoms benefit more from meditation or another form of mental relaxation.

Chinese and **Ayurvedic medicine** use various herbal preparations that can serve as a tonic for the whole system and diminish tension.

A gentle **massage** will help relax almost everyone.

ACUPRESSURE

A number of acupressure points are said to help calm the body and quiet the mind. Two are shown on page 137. For others, consult a practitioner. The effectiveness of particular pressure points is thought to depend on the underlying reasons for the anxiety.

ACUPUNCTURE

Weekly acupuncture treatments—also tailored to the cause of the anxiety—may be beneficial. Consult an acupuncturist experienced in treating mental states.

AROMATHERAPY

Aromatherapy is believed to be very effective with anxiety. Try essential oil of lavender, jasmine, or blue chamomile. Put a drop or two on a tissue and inhale it, or include the oils in a steam inhalation or a steamy bath. Or you can rub a drop into your temples.

BACH FLOWER REMEDIES

Developed at the turn of the 20th century by the British bacteriologist and homeopath Edward Bach, these remedies are used to treat a variety of psychological states. In all, there are 38 remedies, each specific to a particular emotional condition. Liquid in form, the remedies are made by soaking flowers on the top of a bowl of water in the sun for several hours; this procedure, according to practitioners, releases the flowers' energy into the water. Bach remedies can be bought at health food stores.

Agrimony and aspen are considered useful for mild to moderate cases of anxiety. Cherry plum used alone is said to be good for severe cases, or it can be used as part of the so-called rescue remedy—a combination of flowers recommended for all manner of anxiety-provoking situations, from a visit to the dentist to the shock felt after a car accident. Put 1 to 10 drops into a beverage or 1 drop directly on your tongue. Use as often as needed.

HERBAL THERAPIES

Chamomile *(Matricaria recutita)*, lemon balm *(Melissa officinalis)*, and linden *(Tilia* spp.) flowers are all considered mild relaxants and tranquilizers. Lemon balm is particularly good for digestive problems linked to anxiety. Skullcap *(Scutellaria lateriflora)* is somewhat stronger, while valerian *(Valeriana officinalis)*, hops *(Humulus lupulus)*, and passionflower *(Passiflora incarnata)* all have an even stronger effect on the central nervous system. These three help with insomnia and can be combined to advantage. However, hops should not be used with marked depression, and valerian—to be effective—must be used in fairly high dosage (½ to 1 tsp of the tincture). If the anxiety is associated with palpitations, use motherwort *(Leonurus cardiaca)*. If it is connected to high blood pressure, use cramp *(Viburnum opulus)* bark and linden blossoms. For all herbs, make an infusion by pouring boiling water over 1 to 3 tsp of the dried herbs or a handful of fresh herbs. Steep for 10 to 15 minutes. Take a small cupful three or four times a day.

You can buy the tincture of any of these herbs in a health food store; follow the directions on the bottle.

HOMEOPATHY

If the anxiety is the result of a sudden fright or shock, try Aconite. Ignatia is the "grief remedy," said to benefit someone who is upset by a sudden loss. Gelsemium is recommended for anticipatory and performance anxiety, such as stage fright or agoraphobia (a fear of public places). If none of these prove effective, seek out a homeopath. A skilled practitioner may be able to prescribe a mixture whose ingredients and strength are better suited to your anxiety.

MIND/BODY MEDICINE

A wide variety of mind/body treatments and practices can relieve anxiety. The key is to find the one or two that you prefer and to use them consistently. Among the useful meditation and relaxation techniques are progressive muscle relaxation, autogenic training, the **relaxation response,** transcendental **meditation** (TM), and Oriental exercise techniques such as **yoga, t'ai chi,** and **qigong.** For best results, meditation and relaxation practices should be undertaken daily or even twice a day.

Since anxiety is almost always accompanied by shallow breathing, deep breathing exercises are very helpful; it is impossible to be anxious when breathing deeply and slowly. Try the following form of **yoga** breathing: Lie on your back in a comfortable place. Breathe in slowly through your nose, using your diaphragm to suck air into your lungs while allowing your abdomen to ex-

ACUPRESSURE

1 Anxiety-induced sleeping problems may be improved by pressing Heart 7, located along the crease on the inside of the wrist, directly in line with the little finger. Squeeze firmly between the thumb and index finger for one minute, then repeat on the other hand.

2 To help calm nerves and reduce feelings of uneasiness, press Pericardium 6. Place your thumb in the center of your inner wrist, two finger widths from the wrist crease and between the two bones of the forearm. Press firmly for one minute, three to five times, then repeat on the other arm.

pand. (Put your hand on your abdomen just below the navel to make sure the abdomen is being pushed up and out by the diaphragm.) After the abdomen is expanded, continue to inhale as deeply as possible. When you breathe out, reverse the process: Contract the abdomen while exhaling slowly and completely. Repeat several times.

Therapeutic Touch (which does not involve direct touch) is particularly useful for bedridden patients and those with chronic diseases or injuries too sensitive for direct touch. In addition to relieving anxiety, Therapeutic Touch also diminishes pain. Call your hospital for the name of a nurse who practices it.

EEG **biofeedback**, used to retrain thought patterns, can be especially helpful with conditions that combine both physical and mental symptoms—as is the case with anxiety. In a series of sessions with a therapist, the patient watches his or her own brain-wave patterns on an electroencephalograph and gradually learns to control the waves. Practitioners estimate that after about a dozen sessions, the patient will be able to exert the control over mental activity without the help of the therapist or monitoring instrument.

Hypnotherapy is recommended for specific phobias such as fear of flying, stage fright, or fear of exams and sports contests. It also helps with general anxiety. Children and adolescents learn self-hypnosis far more quickly than adults, perhaps because they are so accustomed to using their imaginations. Hypnosis is not a magical or sinister process in which you are under the control of the hypnotist; instead, it is a form of concentration. All hypnosis is self-hypnosis; the hypnotist is there simply to teach you how to use the technique to best advantage. Hypnotherapy can frequently be enhanced if used in combination with biofeedback.

AT-HOME REMEDIES

◆ Daily exercise can be one of the most potent treatments for anxiety symptoms. If you find that exercise works for you, push yourself to go for brisk walks, or undertake an active sport that you enjoy.

◆ Magnesium supplements are helpful, especially if you suffer from muscle spasms. Take no more than 300 mg three times a day; too much magnesium can cause diarrhea.

◆ Avoid alcohol, and reduce or eliminate your consumption of sugar and caffeine.

◆ Trim a hectic schedule to its most essential items, and do your best to avoid activities you don't find relaxing.

◆ If you begin to hyperventilate, exhale into a paper bag and inhale the air within the bag. This increases the amount of carbon dioxide you are inhaling, which can reduce the urge to hyperventilate. Inhaling from a bag will help relieve any dizziness or tingling you might feel. ■

APPENDICITIS

SYMPTOMS

The classic symptoms of appendicitis include:

◆ dull pain near the navel or the upper abdomen that becomes sharp as it moves to the lower right abdomen. This is usually the first sign.
◆ loss of appetite.
◆ nausea and/or vomiting soon after abdominal pain begins.
◆ temperature of 99°F to 102°F.
◆ constipation or diarrhea with gas.

Almost half the time, other symptoms appear, including:

◆ dull or sharp pain anywhere in the upper or lower abdomen, back, or rectum.
◆ painful urination.
◆ vomiting that precedes the abdominal pain.

CALL YOUR DOCTOR IF:

◆ you have pain that matches the symptoms above. Acute appendicitis is a medical emergency that can be fatal. Prompt surgery is often essential. Do not eat, drink, or use any pain remedies, antacids, laxatives, or heating pads, which can cause an inflamed appendix to rupture.
◆ you have symptoms of appendicitis, but your appendix has already been removed. You may have pelvic inflammatory disease, colorectal cancer, diverticulitis, a tubal pregnancy, gastroenteritis, or problems with your colon. **Seek medical care immediately.**

Appendicitis is an inflammation of the appendix, a 3½-inch-long tube of tissue that extends from the large intestine. The appendix contains lymphoid tissue and may produce antibodies; however, no one is absolutely certain what its function is. One thing we do know: We can live without it, without apparent consequences.

Appendicitis is a medical emergency that requires prompt surgery to remove the appendix. Left untreated, an inflamed appendix will eventually burst, or perforate, spilling infection into the abdominal cavity. This can lead to peritonitis, a serious infection of the abdominal cavity's lining (the peritoneum) that can be fatal unless it is treated quickly with strong antibiotics.

Sometimes a pus-filled abscess forms outside the inflamed appendix. Fibrous scar tissue then "walls off" the appendix from the rest of the abdomen, preventing infection from spreading. An abscessed appendix is a less urgent situation, but unfortunately, it can't be identified without surgery. For this reason, all cases of appendicitis are treated as emergencies.

In the United States, 1 in 15 people gets appendicitis. Although it can strike at any age, appendicitis is rare under age 2 and most common between ages 10 and 30.

CAUSES

Appendicitis occurs when the tube-shaped appendix becomes blocked, often by fecal material, a foreign body, or cancer. Blockage may also be due to infection: Like other lymphoid tissue, the appendix swells in response to any infection in the body. As it expands, its opening gradually closes.

DIAGNOSTIC AND TEST PROCEDURES

Diagnosing appendicitis can be tricky. Time is critical, yet appendicitis symptoms are frequently vague, or extremely similar to other, less urgent ailments (including bladder infection, colitis, Crohn's disease, gastritis, gastroenteritis, and ovary problems). By gently pressing on your lower right abdomen, your doctor will feel for a hardened, inflamed appendix. Appendicitis can cause

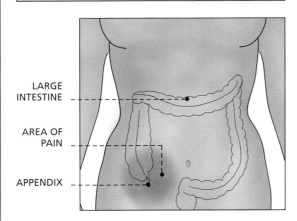

WARNING SIGNS

LARGE INTESTINE

AREA OF PAIN

APPENDIX

The appendix is a 3½-inch-long extension of the large intestine. If it becomes blocked or its opening to the intestine obstructed in some way, the appendix can become inflamed—the classic symptom of which is a persistent sharp pain in the lower right side of the abdomen (above).

rectal pain instead of abdominal pain, so your doctor will also examine your rectum by inserting a lubricated, gloved finger. A blood test will show if your white blood cell count is elevated, meaning your body is fighting infection. CT scans and ultrasound have proved fast and reliable—though not perfect—in revealing appendicitis.

TREATMENT

Surgery to remove the appendix, which is called an appendectomy, is the standard treatment for appendicitis.

CONVENTIONAL MEDICINE

If appendicitis is even suspected, physicians tend to err on the side of safety and quickly remove the appendix to avoid its rupture. If the appendix has formed an abscess, you may have two procedures: one to drain the abscess of pus and fluid, and a later one to remove the appendix.

Antibiotics are given before an appendectomy to fight possible peritonitis. General anesthesia is given, and the appendix is removed through a 4-inch incision. If you have peritonitis, the abdomen is also drained of pus. Within 12 hours of surgery you may get up and move around. You can usually return to normal activities in two or three weeks. If surgery is done with a laparoscope (a thin telescope-like instrument for viewing inside the abdomen), the incision is smaller and recovery is faster.

ALTERNATIVE CHOICES

If you have appendicitis you need a physician's care, but alternative therapies can be helpful in preparing for or recuperating from appendectomy.

ACUPRESSURE
Massaging the following points each day can help to speed your recovery from appendectomy. To improve appetite and intestinal function, massage Stomach 36 and Bladder 25; add Large Intestine 4 to calm pain; Liver 3 to reduce abdominal bloating; and Spleen 6 to promote overall healing. See pages 22–23 for information on point locations.

HOMEOPATHY
Taken before surgery, one dose of Phosphorus (30c) may help minimize nausea from the anesthesia; if needed, repeat every two hours after surgery until the nausea dissipates. After surgery, applying a solution of Hypericum and Calendula (4 drops of each, added to 1 cup water) three or four times daily can help your incision heal.

AT-HOME CARE
◆ Keep your incision clean to promote healing and avoid infection.
◆ Once your incision has closed, prick open a vitamin E capsule and apply the gel directly to your wound to minimize scarring. ■

ARM PAIN

Read down this column to find your symptoms. Then read across.

SYMPTOMS	AILMENT/PROBLEM
◆ moderate to severe pain following an injury; arm is not misshapen.	◆ Soft-tissue injury, such as a sprain or strain
◆ radiating pain in elbow or biceps when bending arm.	◆ Tendonitis
◆ gradually worsening pain in elbow, at bony protuberance, that may radiate down forearm into hand; pain follows chronic repetitive movement.	◆ Epicondylitis, commonly known as tennis elbow
◆ pain in arm or hand with weakness, numbness, or tingling; difficulty clenching the fist or grasping small objects.	◆ Carpal tunnel syndrome
◆ spontaneous onset of pain, redness, warmth, and swelling in elbow and/or other joints.	◆ Rheumatoid arthritis; gout; bursitis
◆ spontaneous onset of pain, redness, warmth, and swelling in elbow and/or other joints; fever and general malaise.	◆ Bone or joint infection, such as osteomyelitis or infectious arthritis
◆ arm pain with numbness or tingling; stiff neck; cracking sound when neck is moved.	◆ Cervical osteoarthritis (cervical spondylosis) or other problem involving neck bones
◆ pain accompanied by numbness or tingling that may radiate to the hand; reduced ability to pick up and hold objects with pinched fingers.	◆ Neuralgia
◆ pain that radiates from center of chest down left arm during exercise, then disappears after five minutes of rest.	◆ Angina
◆ persistent severe pain radiating from center of chest down left arm; nausea; shortness of breath.	◆ Heart attack

WHAT TO DO	OTHER INFO
◆ See Sprains and Strains.	◆ A homeopathic cream containing Arnica may be helpful.
◆ Apply ice and stretch the area.	◆ Osteopathy, chiropractic, or acupuncture may be helpful.
◆ Take a pain reliever if needed, rest the arm, and exercise it gently.	◆ Your doctor may advise use of a splint, heat therapy, or physical therapy. Acupuncture may help.
◆ Stop, limit, or modify the activity that brings on the discomfort. A wrist splint may be helpful.	◆ Pain may be temporarily relieved by shaking the hands vigorously or dangling the arms. Acupuncture, osteopathy, or chiropractic may be helpful.
◆ For pain relief, rest the arm; apply ice for the first 24 hours, then heat; and take an anti-inflammatory drug.	◆ Vitamins C, B$_6$, and E may help arthritis. Gout sometimes can be controlled by a low-purine diet but often requires medication to prevent recurrences.
◆ The usual treatment is joint aspiration— surgical cleansing—and antibiotics.	◆ If more than one joint is affected, you should be examined for rheumatic fever.
◆ See Arthritis.	◆ Spinal bones may be putting pressure on nerves in the neck.
◆ See Neuralgia.	◆ The cause may be cervical osteoarthritis. Acupuncture may help relieve pain.
◆ See Angina, Heart Attack, and Heart Disease. If you have angina, you will probably be treated with nitroglycerin. If this is the first time you have had this pain or if the pain does not abate when you stop exerting yourself, **call your doctor, 911, or your emergency number now.**	◆ Angina is a chronic condition. Alternative methods such as acupuncture, chelation therapy, or nutritional therapy may help.
◆ **Call your doctor, 911, or your emergency number now.** See Emergencies/ First Aid and Heart Attack.	◆ Medications, exercise, dietary changes, relaxation techniques, herbal therapies, and many other treatments may be used for preventive purposes or after conventional emergency treatment.

SYMPTOMS

- Pain and progressive stiffness without noticeable swelling, chills, or fever during normal activities probably indicate the gradual onset of **osteoarthritis.**
- Painful swelling, inflammation, and stiffness in the arms, legs, wrists, or fingers in the same joints on both sides of the body, especially on awakening, may be signs of **rheumatoid arthritis.**
- Fever, joint inflammation, tenderness, and sharp pain, sometimes accompanied by chills and associated with an injury or another illness, may indicate **infectious arthritis.**
- In children, intermittent fever, loss of appetite, weight loss, anemia, or blotchy rash on the arms and legs may signal **juvenile rheumatoid arthritis.**

CALL YOUR DOCTOR IF:

- the pain and stiffness come on quickly, whether from an injury or an unknown cause; you may be experiencing the onset of **rheumatoid arthritis.**
- the pain is accompanied by fever; you may have **infectious arthritis.**
- you notice pain and stiffness in your arms, legs, or back after sitting for short periods or after a night's sleep; you may be developing **osteoarthritis** or another arthritic condition.
- a child develops pain or a rash on armpits, knees, wrists, and ankles, or has fever swings, poor appetite, and weight loss; the child may have **juvenile rheumatoid arthritis.**

American workers lose more time to pain in the joints than to any other type of ailment. To the extent that our jobs and leisure activities become more sedentary, the likelihood of such ailments increases. Fortunately, many of the problems commonly labeled "arthritis" are easily healed or controlled, and the prospects of debilitating complications are far less than they were for our parents and grandparents.

Although the term is applied to a wide variety of disorders, arthritis means the inflammation of a joint, whether as the result of a disease, an infection, a genetic defect, or some other cause. Many people, however, perceive it as any kind of pain or discomfort associated with body movement, including such localized problems as low back pain, bursitis, tendonitis, and general stiffness or pain in the joints. *(See also Backache and Joint Pain.)*

For many—although by no means everyone—arthritis seems to be an inevitable part of the aging process, and there are no signs of real cures on the immediate horizon. On the positive side, advances in both conventional medical treatment and alternative therapies make living with arthritis more bearable.

MAJOR TYPES OF ARTHRITIS

Rheumatoid arthritis, sometimes called rheumatism or synovitis, tends to affect people over the age of 40, and women two to three times as frequently as men. It may occur in children, particularly girls from 2 to 5 years of age. It is characterized by inflammation and pain in the hands—especially the knuckles and second joints—as well as in the arms, legs, and feet, and by general fatigue and sleeplessness. It can also cause systemic damage to other parts of the body, including the heart, lungs, eyes, nerves, and muscles. The discomfort of rheumatoid arthritis can develop over weeks or months and tends to be most severe on awakening.

Rheumatoid arthritis in older people may eventually cause the hands and feet to become gnarled and misshapen as muscles weaken, tendons shrink, and the ends of bones become abnormally enlarged.

While there is no complete cure, treatment begun at the onset of the disorder relieves symptoms in most people. Symptoms may endure for five years or more, after which they tend to stabilize or decline. With early treatment, the likelihood of permanent disability is reduced in all but 5 to 10 percent of sufferers.

Juvenile rheumatoid arthritis, or Still's disease, is characterized by chronic fever and anemia. The disease can also have secondary effects on the heart, lungs, eyes, and nervous system. Arthritic episodes in children younger than the age of five can last for several weeks and may recur, although the symptoms tend to be less severe in recurrent attacks. Treatment is essentially the same as for adults, with heavy emphasis on physical therapy and exercise to keep growing bodies active. Permanent damage from juvenile rheumatoid arthritis is now rare, and most affected children recover from the disease fully without experiencing any lasting disabilities.

Infectious arthritis refers to various ailments that affect larger arm and leg joints as well as the fingers or toes. Arthritic infection is usually a complication of an injury or of another disease and is much less common than arthritic conditions that come on with age. Because the symptoms may be masked by the primary injury or illness, however, infectious arthritis may go unnoticed and, if left untreated, can result in permanent disability.

Osteoarthritis, or degenerative joint disease, refers to the pain and inflammation that can result from the systematic loss of bone tissue in the joints. It is the most common form of arthritis, particularly in the elderly. In osteoarthritis, the protective cartilage at the ends of bones in joints—especially in the spine and legs—gradually wears away. The inner bone surfaces become exposed and rub together. In some cases, bony spurs develop on the edges of joints, causing damage to muscles and nerves, pain, deformity, and difficulty in movement. *(See Bone Spurs.)*

Although the mechanism of osteoarthritis is unknown, some people appear to have a genetic predisposition to degenerative bone disorders. In rare cases, congenital bone deformation appears at an early age. Misuse of anabolic steroids, which are popular among some athletes, can

JOINT DEGENERATION

In a healthy joint, a tough, rubbery tissue called cartilage cushions the ends of the bones at contact points. A thin membrane called the synovium lines the entire joint cavity and secretes synovial fluid to lubricate the joint.

In rheumatoid arthritis, the synovial membrane becomes thickened and inflamed. The inflammation causes cartilage to break down at the pivot point of the joint, while excess synovial fluid causes the cavity to swell.

Osteoarthritis—also called wear-and-tear arthritis—results from gradual deterioration of cartilage in the joint after years of use. Without the protective cartilage, the bones begin to rub together, creating friction and pain.

BONE
CARTILAGE
SYNOVIAL FLUID
SYNOVIAL MEMBRANE
INFLAMED MEMBRANE
ERODED CARTILAGE

HEALTHY JOINT

RHEUMATOID ARTHRITIS

OSTEOARTHRITIS

A

also bring on early osteoarthritic degeneration.

In many people the onset of osteoarthritis is gradual and has no serious debilitating effect, although it can change the shape and size of bones. In other people, bony growths and gnarled joints may cause painful muscle inflammation or nerve damage, along with significant changes in posture and mobility.

Other arthritic conditions include ankylosing spondylitis (arthritis of the spine), bone spurs (bony growths on the vertebrae or other areas), gout (crystal arthritis), and systemic lupus (inflammatory connective-tissue disease). See also Back Problems, Bursitis, and Tendonitis, all of which can result from strain, injury, or other irritation.

CAUSES

Each of the three major types of arthritic condition has its own apparent causes:

Rheumatoid arthritis. The cause of rheumatoid arthritis is not fully understood. Some researchers think it may be some sort of autoimmune disorder *(see Immune Problems)*. Another theory suggests that it is an immune reaction to a viral infection somewhere in the body.

Infectious arthritis. This type of arthritis is caused by a bacterial or viral invasion of the joints and typically comes on the heels of another disease, such as staph infection, tuberculosis, gonorrhea, or Lyme disease.

Osteoarthritis. This common degenerative joint disease is part of the aging process. The condition may be associated with broken bones and can develop in young adults from wear and tear on the body's load-bearing joints, often as a result of intense athletic activity. In cases of osteoarthritis, the cartilage and bone cannot repair themselves sufficiently to keep up with the damage.

DIAGNOSTIC AND TEST PROCEDURES

In addition to symptom analysis, blood tests are commonly used to confirm **rheumatoid arthritis;** the majority of sufferers have antibodies called rheumatoid factors (RF) in their blood, although RF may also be present in other disorders.

X-rays are used to diagnose **osteoarthritis,** typically revealing shrunken joints or calcification at the ends of the bones. If your doctor suspects **infectious arthritis** as a complication of some other disease, testing a sample of fluid from the affected joint will usually confirm the diagnosis.

TREATMENT

Sometimes arthritic damage can be slowed or stopped, but in most cases the damage continues as the disease runs its course, regardless of whether drugs or other therapies are used to relieve the symptoms. Predictably, the duration and intensity of the actual pain and discomfort depend on the type of arthritis and the degree of severity. The process may take a few days in the case of minor joint problems in otherwise healthy adults, while in others it may last months or years. In older people with severe rheumatoid or degenerative conditions, for example, the effects may be lifelong.

CONVENTIONAL MEDICINE

In the case of localized pain, stiffness, and immobility, the typical three-stage therapy consists of medication to relieve pain and inflammation, rest to let injured tissues heal themselves, and exercise to rebuild mobility and strength.

To reduce pain and inflammation in mild cases of **rheumatoid arthritis** and **osteoarthritis,** your doctor will probably prescribe aspirin or another nonsteroidal anti-inflammatory drug (NSAID) such as ibuprofen. Physicians may combine these drugs with regimens of heat, rest and exercise, physical therapy, and physical aids such as canes or walkers. Controlled application of deep heat and ultrasound can also soothe affected joints.

In more advanced cases, your doctor may recommend corticosteroid injections to ease the pain and stiffness of affected joints. Depending on the individual, results range from temporary relief to long-lasting suppression of symptoms.

Early this century, researchers discovered that certain compounds containing gold, delivered orally or by injection, gave relief to some patients and total remission in others. Note, however, that because the side effects of gold therapy can range from minor skin rash to severe blood and kidney disorders, this therapy should be approached with caution.

In cases of arthritic complications from injury or infection, specific therapy will depend on the nature and seriousness of the underlying condition. The major concern is for healing the af-

WARNING!

BEWARE OF QUACK CURES

Because neither conventional nor alternative medicine can cure rheumatoid arthritis or osteoarthritis, unproven treatments abound. Over the years, arthritis sufferers have reported relief with remedies ranging from copper bracelets to laser treatments. While such therapies claim success in individual cases, you should exercise caution and a degree of skepticism when considering what's right for you.

In general, untested and unproven remedies that aren't injected or swallowed will probably do no harm. Invasive treatments may have dangerous side effects or cause other systemic problems, however. The results, if any, may not justify the money spent. The Arthritis Foundation estimates that people from every income bracket and education level spend more than a billion dollars every year on dubious arthritis treatments.

Your best defense against unscrupulous practices is to know as much as you can about your ailment and the risks and intended benefits of suggested treatments. Understanding the underlying causes of the disease and maintaining a healthy skepticism about claims for quick cures will help you avoid placing your health and your pocketbook at risk.

fected area before more serious complications occur. Treatment of **infectious arthritis** typically involves large intravenous doses of antibiotics as well as drainage of excess fluid from the joints.

Various forms of surgery may be needed to reduce the discomfort of arthritis or to restore mobility. Synovectomy is the removal of damaged connective tissue lining a joint cavity, and allows the body to regenerate new, healthy tissue in its place. This operation is most common in the knee. In cases of severe arthritic damage to the neck or foot, bones can be surgically removed or fused. Although movement is limited after such surgery, the operations relieve excruciating pain and help prevent further damage to nerves or blood vessels.

If arthritic pain and inflammation become truly unbearable, or arthritic joints simply refuse to function, the answer may lie in surgical replacement. Today, hip and shoulder joints—as well as smaller joints in elbows, knees, and fingers—can be replaced with reliable artificial joints made of stainless steel and plastic.

Because one of the most trying aspects of arthritis is learning to live with pain, many doctors recommend training in pain management, including cognitive therapy. Such programs focus on improving patients' emotional and psychological well-being by teaching them how to relax and conduct their daily activities at a realistic pace. Learning to overcome mental stress and anxiety can be the key to coping with the physical limitations that may accompany chronic rheumatoid arthritis and osteoarthritis. Cognitive therapy may include various techniques for activity scheduling, imaging, relaxation, distraction, and creative problem solving.

ALTERNATIVE CHOICES

Because medical science has not found any full cures for the various kinds of arthritis, many people turn to alternative treatments to ease their pain and disability. While few alternative approaches can definitively be substantiated in controlled studies of their effectiveness, research indicates that some of these methods can play a significant role in treating arthritic ailments. **Meditation,** self-hypnosis, **guided imagery,** and

A

relaxation techniques, for example, can have positive effects in controlling chronic arthritis pain. Arthritis sufferers should be extremely cautious, however, about practices that claim to "cure" the disease. Furthermore, what appears to work for one person under a given set of circumstances may not work at all for someone else.

ACUPRESSURE AND ACUPUNCTURE
Some arthritis patients find that these therapies, administered by a trained practitioner, offer effective relief from the pain of **rheumatoid arthritis** or **osteoarthritis** for several weeks or months.

BODY WORK
In combination with other treatments, soft-tissue massage around affected joints or compassionate touching by a physician or other practitioner can have a comforting, reassuring effect on those who suffer from arthritis. Manipulation by a trained therapist constitutes passive exercise for people unable to perform vigorous exercise. In addition to making a patient feel better physically, sympathetically administered touch therapy can help soothe the emotional effects of chronic illness. Studies suggest that relieving stress and tension has a positive influence on the body's hormonal balance.

CHIROPRACTIC
After diagnostic examination, testing, and appropriate conventional therapy, a chiropractor may manipulate the spine and other arthritic joints to relieve pain and help reestablish normal use.

HERBAL THERAPIES
Among the various remedies herbalists recommend to relieve pain is a 5-ml tincture made from 2 parts willow (*Salix* spp.) bark and 1 part each of black cohosh (*Cimicifuga racemosa*) and nettle (*Urtica dioica*), taken three times a day. To relieve muscle tension, rub a tincture of lobelia (*Lobelia inflata*) and cramp (*Viburnum opulus*) bark on the affected area.

HOMEOPATHY
For chronic **osteoarthritis** and **rheumatoid arthritis,** constitutional remedies will be prescribed af-

YOGA TECHNIQUES

1 To loosen the joints of the hand, use the **Spider Push-Up.** Press your fingertips together firmly, palms two to three inches apart. Push your palms toward each other while keeping your fingertips touching. Do this 20 times.

2 To ease stiff finger joints, do the **Thumb Squeezer.** Curl your fingers into a fist around your thumb, gently squeeze, then slowly release. Do this 10 times with each hand.

3 The Dog and **Cat** help stretch your hips and back. On your hands and knees in the table position, inhale as you lower your back and lift your head and buttocks (Dog). Then exhale as you arch your back and drop your head and buttocks (Cat). Repeat 9 times.

4 Do the **C** exercise on your hands and knees. Exhale and swing your head and buttocks as far to the left as you can. Breathe deeply as you hold this position for 10 seconds; exhale as you slowly straighten your back. Repeat to the right. Do this 10 times.

ter consultation with a trained homeopathic practitioner. Homeopathic remedies to relieve immediate pain and joint stiffness may include Rhus toxicodendron or Bryonia.

HYDROTHERAPY

Swimming or other water exercise, preferably in a heated pool, allows arthritis patients to work on movement of affected joints and improve muscle strength; the water helps support the body and reduce the stress of gravity.

NUTRITION AND DIET

Avoiding specific foods can stop arthritic symptoms tied to allergies, especially to grains, nuts, meats, eggs, and dairy products. Use trial and error, preferably under the supervision of an allergist.

Some practitioners recommend cutting out plants in the nightshade family: tomato, potato, eggplant, and pepper. They believe the alkaloids in these foods inhibit formation of the collagen that makes up cartilage.

Low-fat, low-protein vegetarian diets may ease the pain and inflammation of **rheumatoid arthritis.** Positive results are reported from elim-

inating partially hydrogenated fats and polyunsaturated vegetable oils, and supplementing the diet with flax oil, sardines, and other oily fish as a source of omega-3 fatty acids.

Vitamin therapy may relieve certain arthritic symptoms. Beta carotene (vitamin A) has an antioxidant effect on cells, neutralizing destructive molecules called free radicals. Vitamins C, B$_6$, and E, as well as zinc, are thought to enhance collagen production and the repair of connective tissue. Vitamin C may also be advised for people taking aspirin, which depletes the body's vitamin C balance. Niacin (vitamin B$_3$) may also be helpful, although excessive use may aggravate liver problems. Always take vitamin supplements under professional guidance, since overdoses of some vitamin compounds can have side effects or undesirable interactions with drugs.

Some therapists recommend cherries or dark red berries to stimulate the production of collagen, essential to cartilage repair.

YOGA

A number of yoga positions *(opposite)* may have beneficial effects on arthritis.

AT-HOME REMEDIES

Heat and rest—traditional remedies for arthritic pain—are very effective in the short term for most people with the disease. Overweight sufferers should begin weight reduction, especially when arthritis strikes the lower back and legs.

If arthritic pain comes on unexpectedly, supplement an over-the-counter painkiller with dry heat from a heating pad or moist heat in the form of a hot bath or a hot-water bottle wrapped in a towel. Regular exercise is important to keep the joints mobile. People with weakened, badly deformed fingers from **rheumatoid arthritis** benefit from specially designed utensils and door and drawer handles; people suffering weakness in the legs and arms from **osteoarthritis** can use special bathroom fixtures, especially tub rails and elevated toilet seats. ∎

SYMPTOMS

- restlessness or insomnia.
- increasing, but relatively painless, tightness in chest.
- mild to moderate shortness of breath.
- when breathing, a wheezing or whistling sound that can range from faint to clearly audible.
- coughing, sometimes accompanied by phlegm.

CALL YOUR DOCTOR IF:

- you or another person is experiencing an episode of asthma for the first time; asthma is a chronic condition and can be quite serious if not treated properly.
- the prescribed asthma medicine does not work in the time it is supposed to; you need a new prescription, or you may be suffering from a severe episode.
- you or the person with asthma has a suffocating feeling, making it difficult to talk; nostrils flare, the skin between the ribs appears sucked in, and the lips or the skin under the nails looks grayish or bluish. These are all signs of extreme oxygen deprivation. **Get immediate emergency treatment.**

Asthma is a chronic respiratory disease that, like bronchitis and emphysema, causes a tightening of the chest and difficulty in breathing. In the case of asthma, however, these symptoms are not always present. They come in episodes set off by various environmental or emotional "triggers," such as pollen, animal dander, tobacco smoke, and stress. Some people with asthma experience only mild and infrequent episodes; for them the condition is an occasional inconvenience. For others, episodes can be frequent and serious, requiring emergency medical treatment. If you have asthma, you should be monitored by a physician regularly, and you must seek immediate medical intervention for a serious episode. By identifying your triggers, you can learn to lessen the intensity and frequency of asthma attacks and perhaps even avoid them completely.

Asthma is not a problem with breathing in, but with breathing out. During an asthma episode, muscle spasms and swelling bronchial tissues narrow the lungs' tiny airways, which then become clogged with excess mucus. Stale air gets trapped in the bottom of the lungs, forcing you to use the top part to gasp for air. Mild and moderate episodes consist of short incidents of breathlessness and wheezing. In severe cases, the lungs' airways become so narrow and clogged that breathing is impossible.

An episode may pass quickly or last more than a day. Sometimes symptoms recur suddenly and with surprising intensity. This "second wave" attack can be more severe and dangerous than the initial episode and may last days or even weeks.

A fairly common disease, asthma affects somewhere between 15 million and 16 million Americans. More prevalent in children than in adults, asthma is the leading cause of school absenteeism and pediatric hospital admission. Although asthma is seldom fatal, it is quite serious. If you have asthma, you should seek the help of a doctor before trying alternative therapies.

CAUSES

Asthma has no single cause; rather, episodes can be brought on by a variety of factors working alone or in combination. Allergies are the primary offenders. Between 50 percent and 90 percent of people with asthma have allergies. The most common allergens, or allergy-causing substances, are pollen, grass, dust, mold, tobacco smoke, and animal dander. When inhaled, these substances can trigger the release of histamine and other body chemicals, causing an allergic reaction and asthma episodes. Other allergens include chemical fumes; aspirin or aspirin-like compounds, such as phenylbutazone, indomethacin, ibuprofen, and other nonsteroidal anti-inflammatory drugs (NSAIDs); and sulfites, high concentrations of which are found in some foods and liquids *(see Prevention, page 151)*. Another factor in allergy-related asthma is heredity: Scientists have discovered a gene that appears to make people susceptible to the disease.

Lung infections can also induce asthma. Bronchiolitis, a viral respiratory infection that usually affects children aged two and younger, is a common cause of childhood asthma. Adults may develop asthma as a result of an upper respiratory infection, such as bronchitis. Other asthma triggers include exercise, emotional stress, and environmental stresses such as air pollution.

DIAGNOSTIC AND TEST PROCEDURES

To determine if you have asthma, your doctor will probably administer a pulmonary function test, which measures the strength of your exhalation. Normally, a person without asthma can exhale about 75 to 85 percent of the air in the lungs within a second, emptying them within three seconds. However, it takes a person with asthma six or seven seconds to expel all the air from the lungs. The pulmonary function test used most often is called a peak flow test, which takes readings as you exhale into a device called a peak flow meter. Your doctor can prescribe a peak flow meter for you, so that you can monitor your condition at home.

TREATMENT

If you have asthma, you should see a doctor regularly; for severe episodes, conventional medical treatment is always necessary. However, a number of alternative treatments can be helpful when used in conjunction with conventional therapy.

CONVENTIONAL MEDICINE

Following a diagnosis of asthma, your first step should be to work with your doctor to develop a treatment plan. As part of this plan, the physician might ask you to keep a daily diary, noting environmental and emotional factors that bring on asthma episodes. This not only will help the doctor monitor the disease but will help you recognize and avoid your asthma triggers.

To treat asthma medicinally, doctors generally prescribe bronchodilators, drugs that help dilate the lungs' constricted airways. These medications are available in two forms: inhaled and oral. Inhaled bronchodilators, which come in aerosol or metered-dose inhaler form, resemble epinephrine (the synthetic version of the hormone adrenaline produced by the body). Doctors usually prefer inhaled bronchodilators, such as

ASTHMATIC AIRWAYS

TRACHEA

HEALTHY BRONCHIOLE

OBSTRUCTED BRONCHIOLE

Air travels down the trachea and into the lungs through branching tubes called bronchioles, which normally are lined with a thin mucous membrane. For people with asthma, certain conditions or inhaled substances can act as "triggers," prompting the release of chemicals that cause the bronchioles to constrict and produce too much mucus. The clogged airways trap air and make breathing difficult.

A

isoproterenol, metaproterenol, isoetharine, and albuterol, because they are delivered directly to the lungs, and because they use 1,000 times less medicine than oral forms. Generally, one or two "puffs" relieve the wheezing and chest tightness associated with mild to moderate episodes. WARNING: Bronchodilators are potent drugs. If overused, they can cause dangerous side effects, such as high blood pressure.

Oral bronchodilators, which include theophylline, metaproterenol, albuterol, and terbutaline, are available in liquid, tablet, or capsule form. They are frequently prescribed for people who cannot tolerate inhaled medication or who suffer from chronic asthma. In severe cases, corticosteroids may be prescribed, but a doctor needs to monitor this treatment carefully because of serious side effects. Emergency situations may require an injection or inhaled dose of epinephrine to help open the lungs' airways.

If your asthma has been caused by allergies (especially to pollen or stinging insects), your doctor might suggest immunotherapy. By gradually exposing your body to a certain allergen through a series of injections, immunotherapy can help your immune system build up defenses; over time, your allergic reactions may lessen or disappear entirely.

ALTERNATIVE CHOICES

Many people have reported success with alternative asthma treatments, but even advocates recommend these methods only as complements to conventional therapies. Remember: Once diagnosed, asthma should be monitored by a physician, and serious episodes always require conventional medical attention.

ACUPRESSURE

Applying gentle pressure to certain body points may help relieve some of the discomfort of asthma. Reaching over your left shoulder with your right hand, press firmly on the part of your back in between the left shoulder blade and spine (point BL 13); take five deep breaths, then repeat on the other side. Or put your fists on your chest, thumbs pointing upward, and feel for the sensitive spot next to the breastbone, just underneath the collarbone (point KI 27). Press firmly for two minutes. *(See pages 22–23 for more information about point locations.)*

ACUPUNCTURE

Several medical studies suggest that acupuncture may help alleviate the symptoms of asthma. The procedure should be carried out only by a licensed acupuncturist.

AROMATHERAPY

Essential oils such as eucalyptus *(Eucalyptus globulus)*, hyssop *(Hyssopus officinalis)*, aniseed *(Pimpinella anisum)*, lavender *(Lavandula officinalis)*, pine *(Pinus sylvestris)*, and rosemary *(Rosmarinus officinalis)* may help ease breathing and relieve nasal congestion. Inhaled through the nose, a few drops of one of the oils or a mixture of several dabbed on a handkerchief or tissue can help ease breathing during a mild episode of asthma. If you feel congested at other times (not during an episode), mix a few drops of essential oil in a sink full of hot water, cover your head with a towel, and inhale the fragrant steam through your nose.

CHINESE HERBS

The Chinese herb ephedra *(Ephedra sinica)* is a potent bronchodilator. CAUTION: Large quantities of this herb can have the same effect as large quantities of epinephrine; do not use it if you have high blood pressure or heart disease. Prepare an infusion by combining 5 grams ephedra, 4 grams cinnamon sticks *(Cinnamomum cassia)*, 1.5 grams licorice *(Glycyrrhiza uralensis)*, and 5 grams apricot seed *(Prunus armeniaca)*. Steep the mixture in cold water, then bring to a boil. Drink it hot.

HERBAL THERAPIES

Elecampane *(Inula helenium)*, a root that acts as a soothing expectorant, may help clear the body of excess mucus. To prepare an infusion, shred the root to yield 1 tsp and add a full cup of cold water; let the infusion stand for 10 hours, then strain and drink it hot three times daily. An infusion made from mullein *(Verbascum thapsus)* is recommended for soothing the mucous membranes, especially during nighttime episodes.

HOMEOPATHY

Homeopaths offer a variety of treatments for asthma symptoms. Following are just a few: To help calm restlessness and anxiety, take Arsenicum album (30c) as required. For symptoms that worsen at night or during cold weather, or that come on very suddenly, take Aconite (6c) as required. For symptoms exacerbated by dampness, take Natrum sulphuricum (6c) as required. For more remedies, consult a licensed homeopath.

REFLEXOLOGY

Massage the skin between the big toe and second toe on both feet; this area is said to correspond to your throat and lungs. Then, flexing so the toes are spread apart, massage the ball of the foot, the area said to correspond to the lungs and chest.

YOGA

Yoga can help you learn to breathe deeply and to relax, thereby helping you deal more effectively with stress, a common trigger for asthma. *(See Wheezing for exercises.)*

PREVENTION

◆ Learn to identify your triggers: Keep a diary detailing all the environmental and emotional factors that affect you every day over the course of several months. When you have an asthma attack, go back to your diary to see which factor, or combination of factors, might have contributed to it.

◆ Monitor the shifts in your lung capacity at home using a peak flow meter, a device that your doctor can prescribe for you. Alerted to reductions in your ability to exhale, you can take precautions and lessen the severity of an asthma episode.

◆ Avoid foods and drinks that have high concentrations of sulfites, such as beer, wine, wine vinegar, instant tea, grape juice, lemon juice, grapes, fresh shrimp, pizza dough, dried fruits (such as apricots and apples),

canned vegetables, instant potatoes, corn syrup, fruit topping, and molasses. Some nutritionists recommend that you also steer clear of foods that cause excess mucus production, such as milk.

◆ A daily dose of B-complex vitamins (50 to 100 mg) and magnesium (400 to 600 mg) may help reduce the frequency and severity of asthma episodes.

Asthma MYTHS AND FACTS

MYTH: *Asthmatics shouldn't exercise.*
FACT: *Exercise is as important for people with asthma as it is for anyone else. Equipped with the proper medication, people with asthma can exercise normally. Note: Many doctors recommend swimming for people with asthma, as humidity helps ease breathing. But the chlorine in swimming pools may cause an allergic reaction, triggering an asthma episode.*

MYTH: *You'll grow out of it.*
FACT: *This is both true and false. Although about half of the people who had asthma when they were between the ages of 2 and 10 seem to "outgrow" the disease, in many cases it recurs when they hit their thirties. It's also possible to develop asthma as an adult even if you did not have it as a child.*

MYTH: *Allergic mothers shouldn't breast-feed.*
FACT: *Infants who are breast-fed are less likely to become allergic than those who are not.* ■

SYMPTOMS

In its early stages, atherosclerosis has no obvious symptoms. Damaged or partially blocked blood vessels may cause one or more of the following:

- dull, crampy pain in your buttock, thigh, and calf muscles during exertion. This may be a sign of atherosclerosis in the pelvic region or leg.
- sudden onset of localized paralysis, tingling, or numbness in a limb; partial vision or speech loss. These symptoms may indicate **cerebral atherosclerosis,** which can lead to stroke.
- angina, a feeling of tightness or heavy pressure in the chest. This may signal atherosclerosis in the coronary arteries.

CALL YOUR DOCTOR IF:

- you experience angina pain for the first time, or angina attacks progress from predictable to unstable. Either event is a serious condition that needs immediate medical attention.
- you have discolored, ulcerous skin and sudden sharp pains in the legs or feet when you are at rest. This may indicate severe atherosclerosis and possibly a circulatory blockage that needs treatment to prevent gangrene.
- you notice unexplained loss of balance, coordination, speech, or vision. Any such loss indicates a temporary halt in the flow of blood to the brain, a situation that can result in stroke if left unattended.

Atherosclerosis—also known as arteriosclerosis or hardening of the arteries—is an inflammatory disease that results in scarring of the artery walls, primarily from long-term buildup of fatty deposits and calcifications. Atherosclerosis is one of the most common cardiovascular diseases and is so prevalent in developed countries that many Americans assume it is a natural consequence of aging. Overwhelming evidence links atherosclerosis closely to diet and lifestyle, suggesting that it can be prevented or slowed, and in some cases, even reversed.

Depending on the location and degree of arterial damage, atherosclerosis can lead to kidney problems, high blood pressure, stroke, and other life-threatening conditions. Atherosclerosis tends to target the aorta—the body's largest artery, which leads from the heart—and arteries leading to the brain, the lower limbs, and the kidneys. Damage to arteries carrying blood to the legs and feet makes walking painful; severely restricted circulation to the limbs can cause skin ulcers and even gangrene (tissue death). Blockage in the coronary arteries, which feed oxygen-rich blood directly to the heart muscles, is known as **coronary artery disease** or **coronary heart disease.** This disorder and its complications—angina, heart arrhythmia, and heart attack—are the leading causes of death in the U.S. and most of Europe.

CAUSES

Arterial deposits begin as thin, fatty streaks on an arterial wall. In a person with a healthy lifestyle, the streaks may come and go. But if a person's arteries are damaged—typically from high blood pressure, stress, or smoking—the inner surface of the walls can start to deteriorate. To compensate, the artery grows new tissue that may create tiny bumps or scars. Cholesterol, white blood cells, and other deposits can start to accumulate within these bumps, forming plaque that clogs the arteries. Eventually, calcium deposits and scar tissue surround the soft plaque, making the arteries hard and inelastic. Because atherosclerosis progresses slowly—usually over many years—it is commonly thought of as an affliction of the el-

HARDENING OF THE ARTERIES

NORMAL ARTERY — CLOGGED ARTERY

ENDOTHELIUM

MUSCLE

INFLAMED WALL

PLAQUE

Inside a normal artery, a layer of muscle surrounds the endothelium, the smooth inner lining through which blood flows *(above, left)*. In some people the endothelium can develop streaks or bumps of fat deposits. Over time, continued accumulation of fatty deposits results in inflammation of the artery wall. Eventually, a hard, calcified plaque can develop that may obstruct blood flow *(above, right)*.

derly. However, studies show that arterial deposits can begin in childhood, with significant plaque formation by the time a person is 30.

While the stages of atherosclerosis are well established, the reasons for its development are less clear. People with a high level of blood cholesterol—especially low-density lipoprotein (LDL) cholesterol—are at risk for developing atherosclerosis. LDL cholesterol—the kind that forms arterial plaque—can react with unstable chemical compounds called free radicals in a complicated process that degrades both the transport mechanism for moving cholesterol through the bloodstream and the tissue lining of arterial walls. Nonetheless, most people with high cholesterol do not develop atherosclerosis, and many people with atherosclerosis have normal cholesterol levels. *(See Cholesterol Problems.)*

Artery walls can become damaged by high blood pressure, by the carbon monoxide in tobacco smoke, and by stress. For example, one study in a war-torn country found that citizens exposed to ongoing battle had greater plaque buildup than those out of harm's way.

While virtually everyone can expect to de-

velop arterial deposits to some degree over time, other factors influence susceptibility to actual atherosclerosis:

◆ **Age.** Atherosclerosis tends to affect people over 35, although it can begin much earlier.
◆ **Gender.** Premenopausal women are less likely than men of the same age to have atherosclerosis, but after menopause the risk is about equal.
◆ **Heredity.** A family history of atherosclerosis increases the risk of developing the disease.
◆ **Obesity.** Obese people are more likely to have atherosclerosis, probably because as a group they tend to have high cholesterol and high blood pressure. *(See Obesity.)*
◆ **Lifestyle.** Lack of exercise is associated with atherosclerosis and the eventual onset of coronary heart disease.

DIAGNOSTIC AND TEST PROCEDURES

Doctors usually look for characteristic symptoms of arterial blockage in various parts of the body as indications of atherosclerosis. To determine the precise location and extent of blockage, your doctor may order an angiogram, which highlights arterial plaque on an x-ray.

TREATMENT

After addressing any obvious symptoms, the first step in treating atherosclerosis is to eliminate or reduce risk factors for the disease, for example by lowering the amount of saturated fat in the diet to prevent further plaque buildup. If you have high blood pressure you should take steps to regulate it, such as losing weight, exercising regularly, and reducing stress. People with diabetes must control their blood sugar levels. Smokers should quit.

CONVENTIONAL MEDICINE

No drug treats atherosclerosis directly, although various medications may be prescribed to treat contributing conditions such as high blood pressure, blood clots, or cholesterol problems. Sever-

A

al surgical procedures have been developed to restore damaged arteries: Portions of a diseased artery can be opened and obstructing plaque deposits removed, or a damaged section of artery can be replaced.

One of the more common procedures is bypass surgery, in which blood is rerouted around a blockage using either grafted or synthetic blood vessels. Balloon angioplasty is a nonsurgical technique that opens arteries by splitting and flattening plaques against vessel walls *(right)*. Various other techniques use catheterization, lasers, and stents—tiny pieces of woven wire mesh—to restore blocked blood vessels to an acceptably functioning state.

ALTERNATIVE CHOICES

Since diet and lifestyle are significant factors in both the development and the prevention of atherosclerosis, alternative therapies offer a range of choices to keep the ailment at bay.

AYURVEDIC MEDICINE

Ayurvedic therapy combines diet, herbal remedies, relaxation, and exercise. Consult a specialist for a comprehensive program of treatment.

CHINESE HERBS

Numerous Chinese herbal combinations are recommended for atherosclerosis, including siler *(Ledebouriella divaricata)*, platycodon *(Platycodon grandiflorum)*, and bupleurum *(Bupleurum chinense)* in an appropriate combination. Consult a practitioner of Chinese medicine.

HERBAL THERAPIES

Herbal remedies to combat atherosclerosis are typically intended to reduce existing plaques or to improve blood-vessel integrity so plaques are less likely to form. Hawthorn *(Crataegus laevigata)* is considered one of the best plaque fighters, because of its reputation for strengthening arteries. Its flowers, leaves, and berries can be brewed as tea, and it is also available in extract and tincture form. For herbs that may provide relief from discomfort associated with atherosclerosis of the lower limbs, see Circulatory Problems.

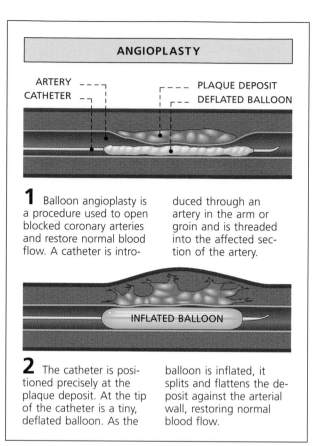

ANGIOPLASTY

ARTERY ---- CATHETER

PLAQUE DEPOSIT ---- DEFLATED BALLOON

1 Balloon angioplasty is a procedure used to open blocked coronary arteries and restore normal blood flow. A catheter is introduced through an artery in the arm or groin and is threaded into the affected section of the artery.

INFLATED BALLOON

2 The catheter is positioned precisely at the plaque deposit. At the tip of the catheter is a tiny, deflated balloon. As the balloon is inflated, it splits and flattens the deposit against the arterial wall, restoring normal blood flow.

HOMEOPATHY

Various long-term remedies may be prescribed by a licensed homeopath for treating atherosclerosis. Diagnosis and prescriptions will vary according to the homeopath's evaluation of the patient.

LIFESTYLE

The benefits of lifestyle improvement have been demonstrated in a yearlong program designed for heart disease patients, conducted by Dr. Dean Ornish, that involved strict vegetarianism, exercise, and stress reduction. At the end of the trial, a measurable reversal of plaque buildup in the coronary arteries was reported in 82 percent of participants.

MIND/BODY MEDICINE

Since stress is believed to accelerate the rate at which atherosclerosis develops, therapeutic relaxation techniques may help prevent or retard its progress. A number of approaches can help you relax, including **yoga, meditation, guided imagery,** and **biofeedback.**

NUTRITION AND DIET

Diet and lifestyle changes, if started early and maintained aggressively, may be enough to prevent or even reverse atherosclerosis. First, your diet should be not only low in cholesterol and saturated fat, but high in antioxidants, which neutralize free radicals believed to aggravate tissue damage. The key antioxidants are vitamins E and C, beta carotene (vitamin A), and selenium, which can be toxic in high dosages. Be careful about taking any vitamin indiscriminately, however: Too much vitamin D, for example, may actually accelerate calcification of arterial plaques. To be safe, seek advice from a doctor or nutritionist.

Some evidence suggests that garlic (*Allium sativum*), eaten in large quantities, deters oxidation of cholesterol. Grape-skin extracts and gugulipid (*Commiphora mukul*), an herb from southern India, are reputed to reduce plaque deposits. Alfalfa (*Medicago sativa*) and bromelain, a pineapple enzyme, are reported to have done the same in animals and may work on humans.

Numerous studies over the past 30 years have indicated moderate alcohol consumption—a glass or two of wine a day—may protect against atherosclerosis and coronary artery disease. One study suggests that flavonoids in grape skins, which give red wine its color and flavor, inhibit buildup of fatty deposits.

For more nutritional information, see Cholesterol Problems and Blood Clots.

PREVENTION

Atherosclerosis develops when genetic predispositions meet known risk factors head-on. If you have a family history of atherosclerosis, the prudent course of action is to accept what you cannot change and change what you can.

◆ Adopt a low-fat, low-salt, high-fiber diet. Take extra pains to avoid foods high in saturated fat and cholesterol.

◆ If you smoke, quit.

◆ Know your blood pressure. If it's high, get it down. (*See High Blood Pressure.*)

◆ Get moderate exercise—a 30-minute walk, swim, or bicycle ride—several times a week, and daily if possible.

◆ Find a relaxation program that you enjoy, and incorporate it into your daily routine.

◆ If you have a high-risk family history, be sure to get checked regularly by a cardiologist.

CHELATION THERAPY: THE JURY IS STILL OUT

Every year thousands of people in the U.S. look to chelation therapy for treatment of atherosclerosis—more people than have bypass surgery. Chelation involves injecting a chemical called EDTA into the bloodstream. One theory holds that chelation removes the calcium in arterial plaque; another suggests that EDTA works as an antioxidant.

While chelation therapy has proved beneficial for ailments like lead poisoning, its use as a cardiovascular treatment remains controversial. Advocates tout chelation as a safe, relatively inexpensive, and effective alternative to other treatments. Critics cite the lack of reliable scientific testing and claim that chelation is ineffective or potentially dangerous (early trials sometimes caused kidney damage).

Treatment typically requires from 10 to 40 sessions and may cost thousands of dollars. Until chelation therapy survives at least one rigorous scientific study, physicians will undoubtedly remain divided over its merits. Once science provides answers, chelation therapy will become either a standard recommendation of every cardiologist or a therapeutic relic. ■

SYMPTOMS

- itchy, scaly, red rash that usually starts between the toes; if untreated, develops into cracked, blistered skin that may become infected.
- dry, flaking skin on the soles of the feet.
- unpleasant foot odor.
- whitish, brittle, flaky toenails.

CALL YOUR DOCTOR IF:

- the rash does not respond to treatment with over-the-counter antifungal medication or other at-home measures in four to six weeks; or if the condition becomes incapacitating. You need a medical diagnosis and prescription medication.
- the rash develops blisters, intense redness, painful swelling, or pus; or if you develop a fever. These are signs of a secondary bacterial infection, which requires treatment with oral antibiotics.
- your toenails become brittle or discolored, usually whitish. This form of athlete's foot is difficult to eradicate and usually requires long-term medical treatment to prevent recurrence.

Athlete's foot is a common fungal infection, and you don't have to be an athlete to get it. This annoying ailment occurs most often in men and boys, but it is common enough in women and girls, too. Virtually unheard of in ancient Greece and Rome, when people went barefoot or wore sandals, athlete's foot is a by-product of a society that keeps its feet enclosed in shoes most of the time.

CAUSES

The various kinds of fungi that cause athlete's foot belong to a group called dermatophytes, which also cause jock itch. The fungi thrive in closed, warm, moist environments and feed on keratin, a protein found in hair, nails, and skin. Athlete's foot is mildly contagious; it can be spread through direct contact with the infection and by skin particles left on towels, shoes, and floors of shower stalls and around swimming pools. Although walking barefoot in the shower at the gym or around the pool may increase your chance of contracting athlete's foot, you are more likely to develop the infection from not changing sweaty socks and shoes. The risk of developing athlete's foot can also depend on your susceptibility. For example, people who have taken an antibiotic for two weeks or longer are at greater risk because the drug not only fights infection but can kill beneficial bacteria that help keep the athlete's foot fungus from spreading. *(See Yeast Infections.)*

TREATMENT

You should treat athlete's foot at the first sign of itchy feet or redness between your toes. Most cases of athlete's foot can be cured with over-the-counter antifungal powder and basic good hygiene. Wash and dry your feet thoroughly morning and evening, change your socks or stockings daily, and don't wear the same shoes day after day. Sprinkle antifungal powder on your feet and in your shoes daily.

Make sure your feet get plenty of air. If you can't go barefoot or wear sandals, wear cotton socks and shoes made of a natural, porous material such as leather or fabric, not water-resistant synthetics. If not treated properly and promptly, the infection can be very persistent. Even when treated with antifungal drugs, the infection may take several weeks to disappear.

CONVENTIONAL MEDICINE

For cases that resist at-home treatment, your doctor may prescribe 1 percent terbinafine ointment. The medication is expensive, but terbinafine treatment can lead to complete cure in a week. Doctors prescribe oral antifungal drugs for athlete's foot only when topical remedies fail, since the treatment may have serious side effects, such as liver toxicity. Typical oral medications are ketoconazole and griseofulvin. The same treatment options apply to athlete's foot affecting the toenails.

ALTERNATIVE CHOICES

AROMATHERAPY

To combat infection, put 5 drops of tea tree oil (*Melaleuca* spp.) in your bathwater. To relieve itching, try 2 drops of peppermint (*Mentha piperita*) oil and 4 drops of chamomile (*Matricaria recutita*) oil in the bathwater.

HERBAL THERAPIES

Soak your feet for half an hour in a solution of 6 tsp goldenseal (*Hydrastis canadensis*) to a pint of water; you can also powder your feet with goldenseal. Or rub tea tree oil (*Melaleuca* spp.) on the affected area daily. Try other herbal baths and ointments, following label directions: Myrrh (*Commiphora molmol*) is said to fight fungus; lavender (*Lavandula officinalis*) may reduce inflammation; calendula (*Calendula officinalis*) cream is recommended to heal cracked skin.

HOMEOPATHY

To soothe inflammation, try an over-the-counter preparation containing Calendula. A professional homeopath may recommend Graphites for a condition with weeping skin.

AT-HOME REMEDIES

Soak your infected feet in warm, salted water (1 tsp salt per cup) for 5 to 10 minutes every day. Dry your feet thoroughly, then apply a baking soda paste between your toes, or dab on an aluminum chloride solution, available from your local pharmacy. You may prefer using an over-the-counter antifungal powder, cream, or spray. The most effective products contain undecylenic acid or the antifungal drugs clotrimazole or miconazole. As long as the area is not blistered or cracked, remove flakes of dead skin with a soft brush before using a topical powder or ointment. Do not tear off flaking skin; you may break nearby healthy skin and spread the infection.

Use the same topical treatment for athlete's foot of the toenails, but don't expect fast action. Keep your nails short, and clean out debris under and around infected nails using a smooth wooden toothpick or matchstick rather than a nail file that might scratch or break the skin.

PREVENTION

Your coach and the school nurse were on the right track when they made you wear shower shoes in the locker room and around the pool. But we now know that susceptibility is as big a factor as actual contact with the fungus. Cut your risk by keeping your feet clean, dry, and powdered with an over-the-counter fungicide. Other sensible steps:

◆ Wear cotton socks, and shoes that breathe; shoes that keep water out also keep sweat in.

◆ Never share shoes, socks, or towels.

◆ If you get athlete's foot, wash your socks and towels in the hottest water possible—or boil them.

◆ Be doubly cautious of your feet if you take an antibiotic for two weeks or more. The medication can kill beneficial bacteria that normally control the fungus that causes athlete's foot. ■

A

SYMPTOMS

- Pain, discomfort, restricted movement, tenderness, and possible swelling may be indicative of some form of muscle or ligament injury, such as a sprain or strain.
- Pain, swelling, tenderness, and deformity may indicate a **fracture.**
- Pain, restricted movement, misshapen appearance, and swelling in a joint are symptoms of a **dislocation.**
- Localized pain just below the kneecap may be a sign of patellar tendonitis. In adolescents, the condition may indicate Osgood-Schlatter disease if accompanied by swelling.
- Pain in the elbow, often accompanied by tenderness in the inner or outer portion of the elbow and forearm, and possibly a weak and painful grasp, may indicate **epicondylitis.**

CALL YOUR DOCTOR IF:

- your muscles gradually become weak for no apparent reason; you may have a neurological problem or another disorder of immediate concern.
- you experience chronic muscle cramps. Although most often benign, this may be a sign of serious problems such as blood clotting, restricted blood flow, or nerve damage.
- you think your swelling or puffiness is caused by a fracture, dislocation, ligament or muscle tear, or cartilage damage. If not treated by a physician in a timely manner, the affected area could suffer permanent damage.

Every family has seen its share of injuries tracing to athletic endeavors or, ironically, the pursuit of physical fitness. For the most part, athletic injuries are a result of stress put on bones or muscles. Most common are injuries to soft tissue—muscles, tendons, and ligaments.

A **dislocation** occurs when two bones are jolted apart at a joint and is often accompanied by a ligament tear in the joint. The pain is caused by the severe stretching of soft tissues.

A **fracture** is either simple (closed)—in which the broken bone remains beneath the skin surface and does minimal damage to surrounding tissues—or compound (open)—in which the bone protrudes through the skin. The ankle, hand, wrist, and collarbone are common sites of fracture.

Shoulder injuries are common in sports that require throwing motions or intense contact. Dislocations are most common in the shoulder joint. **Acromioclavicular joint (AC) separation** occurs when the ligaments that support the collarbone are torn. The rotator cuff is where four muscles meet and attach to the humerus; overuse of the shoulder may inflame or tear tendons in the area, causing **rotator cuff tendonitis.**

CHILD SPORTS INJURIES: WHAT PARENTS SHOULD KNOW

- *Each year during the high-school football season there are an estimated one million injuries; wrestling, soccer, and basketball also carry a high risk of injury.*
- *Children are at a higher risk of injury than adult athletes because those playing together may be at vastly different weights, stages of development, and strengths. Try to ensure that participants in a group are at a similar level of physical development.*

Epicondylitis affects the elbow and typically occurs in sports requiring frequent wrist manipulation and forearm rotation. The lateral (affecting the outer elbow) form is tennis elbow. Medial epicondylitis involves the inner elbow.

Lower-back injuries, such as muscle tears, are common in sports that involve a lot of bend-ing. The high velocity and full contact nature of hockey and football frequently cause neck and spine injuries, such as a **herniated disk,** in which an intervertebral disk protrudes from the spinal column *(see Disk Problems).*

Intense leg movement, including twisting and spreading, may tear the adductor muscle **(groin strain),** which connects the leg with the pubic bone.

The knees are involved in some of the most common lower-body injuries. Continual jumping may result in tearing of the tendon just below the kneecap, or patella, causing **patellar tendonitis,** or jumper's knee. The knees may also suffer from other injuries, such as tears of the meniscus, a piece of cartilage in the knee joint between the femur and tibia.

The sudden tearing of muscle fibers that may occur after excessive athletic activity and the consequent accumulation of fluid in the muscle that causes pain, tenderness, and local swelling characterize a **charley horse.**

Increased interest in jogging and cross train-ing has resulted in a parallel rise in leg injuries, including shin splints, tendonitis, and **stress fractures,** especially in the tibia or fibula bones. If continually exposed to stress from prolonged standing, running, or walking, a stress fracture may result in a larger fracture.

The foot often falls victim to injury because it must support the weight of the entire body. **Plantar fasciitis** often affects inexperienced runners, causing pain along the inner heel and along the arch of the foot, sometimes accompanied by stiffness and numbness in the heel. A similar problem, **march fracture,** develops in the bones of the foot when extreme stress (running, walking) is continually placed on the ball of the foot.

CAUSES

An **AC separation** results from sudden impact on the side of the shoulder or on an outstretched arm. Wear on the rotator cuff, causing **rotator cuff tendonitis,** may occur if you continually engage in sports that require overhead motion like that in a tennis serve. Medial **epicondylitis** is caused by traumatic, repetitive arm motion, as

---

COMMON SPORTS INJURIES

The highlighted areas below show some of the sites of common injuries sustained from sports or other physical activity. The best way to prevent an athletic injury is to be in good physical condition and to stretch for several minutes before and after exercising. Never attempt to "play through" pain—doing so may cause more extensive injury and lengthen the time needed for complete healing.

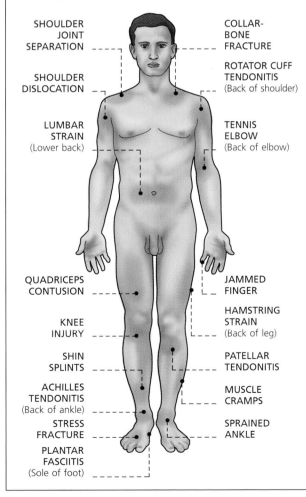

SHOULDER JOINT SEPARATION

SHOULDER DISLOCATION

LUMBAR STRAIN (Lower back)

QUADRICEPS CONTUSION

KNEE INJURY

SHIN SPLINTS

ACHILLES TENDONITIS (Back of ankle)

STRESS FRACTURE

PLANTAR FASCIITIS (Sole of foot)

COLLAR-BONE FRACTURE

ROTATOR CUFF TENDONITIS (Back of shoulder)

TENNIS ELBOW (Back of elbow)

JAMMED FINGER

HAMSTRING STRAIN (Back of leg)

PATELLAR TENDONITIS

MUSCLE CRAMPS

SPRAINED ANKLE

A

when pitching in baseball. Sudden, violent twisting of the elbow or continual pulling and strain on the forearm muscles can cause the condition.

A **charley horse** is usually caused by a sudden, acute strain in the leg, but mineral deficiency, hormone imbalance, calcium deposits in the muscles, or dehydration can also be causes. Muscle imbalance, a poorly aligned leg, or running on a hard road with improper footwear may cause a **stress fracture.** Tight hamstrings may contribute to lower-back problems, and tight Achilles tendons may precede cases of tendonitis of the foot and ankle.

DIAGNOSTIC AND TEST PROCEDURES

Basic assessment of an injury begins with your medical history and a physical exam. X-rays may be ordered to examine your bones for possible **fractures, dislocations,** and other injuries. A bone scan is a highly sensitive test that may detect **stress fractures** that might not show up in x-rays.

Arthroscopy, ultrasound, and magnetic resonance imaging (MRI) are generally used on joints. Arthroscopy employs a tiny camera inside a very small tube, called an arthroscope, to examine the interior of your joints; it is useful in both diagnosing and repairing some joint injuries (for example, cartilage fragments can be removed through the tube). Ultrasound scanning uses sound waves to generate an image that your doctor can view on a screen. An MRI produces excellent images of soft tissue, enabling diagnosis of damage to muscles, ligaments, and tendons.

TREATMENT

Treatment for sports injuries aims to relieve pain, repair or realign bones, and restore your body to its full athletic ability.

CONVENTIONAL MEDICINE

Most minor soft-tissue injuries are best treated with RICE: rest, ice, compression, and elevation. (See Sprains and Strains.)

Injuries such as tendonitis and **plantar fasci-**

GROWING PAINS

Osgood-Schlatter disease is a condition associated with sudden growth spurts in adolescence (usually in boys ages 10 to 14). It is characterized by pain and swelling below the kneecap, where the patellar tendon attaches to the shinbone. The quadriceps muscle, located at the front of the thigh, continually pulls on the affected tendon, causing the disorder. The condition persists for six months to a year and usually clears up completely without treatment, but as long as your child suffers from symptoms, running, jumping, and squatting should be kept to a minimum, if not eliminated.

itis usually require rest and a rehabilitation program to maintain flexibility and strength. Aspirin or ibuprofen may help reduce the pain and inflammation that accompany these conditions.

Depending on the severity of the pain, your physician may treat your **epicondylitis** with an injection of a corticosteroid, with nonsteroidal anti-inflammatory drugs (NSAIDs) such as ibuprofen, or with aspirin. An elbow cuff and physical therapy may also be indicated (see Tennis Elbow).

For acute pain as a result of an **AC separation,** codeine may be prescribed for the first couple of days. Thereafter, aspirin and a nonsteroidal anti-inflammatory drug may be taken for chronic pain. Your physician may immobilize the injured area with a sling.

If possible, the displaced bones of a dislocation are manipulated back into place. If this is not feasible, you may need surgery, after which the joint is immobilized until it is stable.

If necessary, a fracture is treated by reduction, a procedure in which the broken bone ends are manipulated so that they abut each other in their original position. The procedure may be done surgically or without cutting the skin. More serious fractures are repositioned and held in place with metal pins or by screws, plates, and rods placed permanently in or on the bone.

A **march fracture** is customarily treated by placing the foot in a plaster cast or a rigid boot; you must rest it for three to six weeks.

ALTERNATIVE CHOICES

ACUPUNCTURE
Administered by a professional, acupuncture may be helpful in treating athletic injuries and soothing the body after strenuous training. It has been shown to reduce pain and swelling and should be applied as soon as possible after injury occurs.

BODY WORK
Massage relieves aches and pains, is especially helpful for tendonitis and **epicondylitis,** and can lessen the onset of muscle soreness. Administered by a professional, the **Alexander technique, Rolfing,** and the **Feldenkrais method** may be useful.

Knead the area of a **charley horse,** rubbing in the direction of the muscle fibers.

HOMEOPATHY
Arnica (12c) may be taken every 10 minutes for 1 to 2 hours, until the shock of fracture passes, and then every 8 hours for the next two to three days. Taken every 8 to 12 hours for up to three days, Ruta (12c) may aid healing after a dislocation. The symptoms of a sprained ankle may be eased with Rhus toxicodendron (12c), taken four times a day for as long as a week.

HYDROTHERAPY
Water is the perfect place for athletes recovering from injuries to work out. Aquatic movement provides muscle resistance without straining joints.

LIFESTYLE
Heat before exercise can loosen joints and soft tissue. Various types of braces and supports worn during exercise can protect joints and soft tissue and stabilize an uncomfortable joint or tendon. Consult your doctor or a physical therapist. To avoid ankle injuries, always wear appropriate shoes with ample protection and support.

NUTRITION AND DIET
Many experts advise athletes to maintain a high-carbohydrate, low-fat diet to increase energy levels and promote muscle strength.

Taken orally or topically, vitamin E may guard against muscle damage during exercise. Magnesium helps maintain muscle flexibility, which lessens susceptibility to injury.

For bone fractures, vitamin B complex and zinc may help.

AT-HOME REMEDIES
◆ Replacing fluids lost through perspiration with a carbohydrate-electrolyte sports drink helps prevent cramping.
◆ Ice packs reduce swelling; a bag of frozen vegetables can be a makeshift ice pack. Do not use chemical cold packs; they are much colder than water packs. Place a damp towel around your pack so that it is not directly on your skin.
◆ A warm compress may relieve muscle pain, especially before massage and stretching.
◆ To relieve cramping, elevate the affected area to direct blood flow toward the heart.
◆ If muscles are sore the day after a tough workout, soak in a hot tub and rest the affected area.

PREVENTION

Before you begin a sport or exercise routine, have a physical exam, especially if you are over 40.

Sports injuries usually result when the muscles are poorly conditioned. You should have a 10-minute warmup session—running in place or doing jumping jacks—before an athletic activity to increase your body temperature and diminish chances of muscle injury. Stretching after your workout will prevent soreness the next day.

Engage in your sport or exercise at least three times a week to maintain proper conditioning. ■

SYMPTOMS

Keep in mind that attention deficit disorder (ADD) is often misdiagnosed. Because so many of the symptoms are related to child development, they can be normal at one age and not at another; moreover, they may be appropriate to one child and not to another of the same age. However, ADD does exist, and it can be treated. In many cases, a child will show signs of the disorder in early childhood—even in infancy—but go undiagnosed until first or second grade, when the demands of schoolwork make them more apparent.

Symptoms include:
- habitual failure to pay attention.
- difficulties with schoolwork.
- excessive distractibility.
- an inability to organize, even with activities that are enjoyed.
- impulsiveness.
- hyperactivity—fidgeting and running about.
- excessive talking and frequent interrupting.

CALL YOUR DOCTOR IF:

- your child shows symptoms of ADD. Because the disorder is difficult to assess, you may want to consult more than one professional; a second opinion is particularly important because of evidence that ADD is sometimes diagnosed in children who do not have the genuine disorder. It is essential that those consulted have experience with ADD.

Difficulty in paying attention—the defining sign of attention deficit disorder (ADD)—is among the most common developmental problems of childhood, affecting about 20 percent of all schoolchildren, according to some estimates. (Other estimates, however, suggest a lower figure of 5 to 7 percent.) Five times as many boys suffer from ADD as girls, and the disorder can persist through adolescence, with some symptoms continuing into adulthood. Great progress has been made in treatment in recent decades. At the same time, though, much about this condition remains uncertain or ill-defined, leading to popular overuse of the term: Professionals report that it has become fashionable, especially among teenagers or their parents, to blame ADD for what may simply be negligent performance.

Most ADD children are of normal or high intelligence. Their activity levels may be normal, lower than normal (hypoactivity), or higher than normal (a version that has its own diagnostic label: attention deficit hyperactivity disorder, or ADHD). An ADD child may also have a specific learning disability that prevents him from taking in and sorting out information in the same way other children do. His brain is unable to process the messages his ears, eyes, or muscles give him.

CAUSES

Although the causes of ADD are poorly understood, biological inheritance appears to be important in many cases: The disorder seems to run in families. A number of nongenetic factors can also play a causative role. Among them: drug or alcohol abuse or other problems in a mother's pregnancy, birth trauma, early child abuse, brain injuries from accidents, meningitis, encephalitis, low-level lead poisoning (see Environmental Poisoning), and psychological disorders.

In the late 1970s and early 1980s, some researchers thought ADD was caused—or intensified—by sugar and artificial food additives. This theory is now controversial, but some studies still show that specific foods such as chocolate, wheat, cow's milk, and oranges may exacerbate the condition in some hyperactive children.

DIAGNOSTIC AND TEST PROCEDURES

A battery of tests—sometimes including positron emission tomography (PET) scans—are given to assess a child's neurological and psychological status. They should be administered by a pediatrician with a special interest in school problems. Tests include:

◆ a medical and social history of both the child and his family.
◆ a physical exam and neurological assessment including screenings of vision, hearing, and verbal and motor skills, as well as tests for blood levels of lead, a mineral that has been implicated in hyperactivity.
◆ a quantitative evaluation of intelligence, aptitude, personality traits, and processing skills.

You may also be advised to check with an allergist if any sensitivities are suspected.

TREATMENT

The best treatment is thought to be a combination of medication and psychological therapies. Close cooperation among therapists, physicians, teachers, and parents is very important, and team meetings are useful.

CONVENTIONAL MEDICINE

Although there is considerable controversy about their possible overuse, stimulants such as amphetamines or, more usually, methylphenidate (better known by the brand name Ritalin) are the medications often prescribed for ADD. (Strange as it seems, stimulants often calm hyperactivity.) A physician needs to monitor the dosage closely (about twice a month), both to check for the right level and to watch for side effects. Since the benefits of a Ritalin dose last only about four hours, two or three tablets may be needed each day.

Of the psychological therapies, behavior modification may be best, particularly if the therapist helps parents learn some of the techniques for behavior control. It is often given in conjunction with specific educational interventions, such as help with learning skills. Psychotherapy is a valuable option, particularly if the child suffers from low self-esteem.

ALTERNATIVE CHOICES

Several different alternative therapies may prove helpful, among them **homeopathy;** consult a homeopath for guidance. EEG **biofeedback** also shows promise as a means of behavior modification.

NUTRITION AND DIET

Although the effectiveness of dietary restrictions is controversial, some doctors recommend a high-protein, low-carbohydrate, sugar-free diet. Some children may also benefit from the B-vitamin supplements niacin (B_3), pyridoxine (B_6), and possibly thiamine (B_1). The stimulant caffeine—ingested at the rate of 150 to 300 mg per day—can be helpful. Depending on the results of your child's tests for mineral blood levels, he may need supplements.

AT-HOME MANAGEMENT

◆ Join a support group. Connect with the national organization Children and Adults with Hyperactivity and Attention Disorders (see Appendix).
◆ Because an ADD child may process directions and other information in faulty ways, he is apt to be bombarded with corrections, leaving him with a low opinion of himself. Do whatever you can to promote your child's self-esteem.
◆ Praise and reward good behavior promptly.
◆ Be consistent with discipline, and make sure baby-sitters follow your methods.
◆ Make instructions simple and specific ("Brush your teeth; now, get dressed"), instead of general ("Get ready for school").
◆ Encourage your child's special strengths, particularly in sports and out-of-school activities.
◆ Have set routines for meals, sleep, play, and TV.
◆ Don't let homework monopolize all of his time after school; play and exercise are important.
◆ Simplify your child's room. Store toys out of sight. ■

BACKACHE

Read down this column to find your symptoms. Then read across.

SYMPTOMS	AILMENT/PROBLEM
◆ soreness after overexertion or injury; soreness that develops during the night; soreness that radiates to buttocks or thighs.	◆ Back muscle strain
◆ pain, stiffness, and tenderness in the back, buttocks, or thighs; difficulty moving or bending the back.	◆ Osteoarthritis of the spine, also called spondylosis
◆ sudden onset of pain; pain may shoot down one leg after lifting heavy objects, strenuous exercise, twisting, sneezing, or coughing; bending forward at the waist increases pain; lying down eases pain.	◆ Herniated disk (also called prolapsed disk); ruptured disk; or slipped disk
◆ chronic low-back pain that comes and goes for months or years.	◆ Misalignment of the spine
◆ sharp pain in a specific place along the spine.	◆ Osteoporosis
◆ pain in the lower back in a woman who is more than four months pregnant.	◆ Pregnancy problem
◆ pain in the lower back; fever of 100°F or above; painful urination; nausea or vomiting.	◆ Kidney infection
◆ chronic pain and stiffness that seem worse in the morning; person with the pain is between the ages of 20 and 40.	◆ Ankylosing spondylitis
◆ pain in back, buttocks, thighs, and/or calves when walking or climbing stairs; pain is relieved by standing still or sitting.	◆ Spinal stenosis
◆ back pain, especially at night, that is unrelieved by lying down.	◆ Possibly, a tumor

- See Back Problems and Sprains and Strains. Rest for a few days; use pain relievers if necessary.

- Physical therapy may include the application of heat and cold, gentle massage, and exercises to prevent future problems.

- See Arthritis. Take an anti-inflammatory drug for pain relief. Rest, heat, exercise, and physical therapy may be helpful.

- This condition may be caused by strain, injury, or aging.

- See Back Problems and Disk Problems. Treatment may include pain relievers, bed rest, physical therapy, and wearing a supportive collar.

- Disk problems may lead to other problems, such as sciatica or bowel or bladder incontinence. Chiropractic and acupuncture may help. If part of the disk is pressing on a nerve, surgery may be needed.

- See Back Problems.

- The underlying cause may be poor muscle tone in the abdomen or back, obesity, or osteoarthritis.

- Hormone replacement therapy may be recommended for postmenopausal women, to prevent further bone loss.

- This condition is most common in women over 60 and people confined to bed or a wheelchair. Patients are encouraged not to smoke or drink alcohol, to eat less animal protein and fat, to obtain sufficient calcium, and to do weight-bearing exercise.

- Learning how to lift properly, wearing supportive shoes, improving posture, and sleeping on a firm mattress may help.

- Acupressure, massage, or chiropractic may be helpful.

- **Call your doctor now.** A kidney infection requires immediate treatment with antibiotics.

- Be sure to take the antibiotics for the full length of the prescription.

- Usual treatment is anti-inflammatory drugs, physical therapy, massage, and prescribed exercises.

- Treatment is essential to prevent progression to fusion of the joints and a rigid spine.

- Call your doctor. Losing weight and doing abdominal exercises may help. Surgery is required in some cases.

- The pain is caused by a narrowing of the spinal canal at a point where a nerve passes. Modifying the posture may help.

- **Call your doctor without delay.** A medical evaluation is necessary for diagnosis and treatment.

- A tumor may be benign or malignant. By the time it causes pain, it is probably sizable. Cancer of the back is more likely in someone who already has cancer elsewhere.

B

SYMPTOMS

- persistent aching or stiffness anywhere along your spine, from the base of the neck to the hips.
- sharp, localized pain in the neck, upper back, or lower back, especially after lifting heavy objects or engaging in other strenuous activity.
- chronic ache in the middle or lower back, especially after sitting or standing for extended periods.

CALL YOUR DOCTOR IF:

- you feel numbness, tingling, or loss of control in your arms or legs; you may have damaged your spinal cord.
- the pain in your back extends downward along the back of the leg; you may be suffering from sciatica.
- the pain increases when you cough or bend forward at the waist; this may be the sign of a herniated disk (see Disk Problems).
- the pain is accompanied by fever; you may have a bacterial infection.
- you have dull pain in one area of your spine when lying in or getting out of bed, especially if you are over 50; you may be suffering from osteoarthritis (see Arthritis).

Back problems are the most common physical complaints among American adults. Nonspecific back pain is a leading cause of lost job time, to say nothing of the time and money spent in search of relief. And it's all because of one characteristic that makes us different from other animals—our upright posture.

The spinal column is an extraordinary mechanism, providing the stability we use to stand upright and the flexibility we need for active movement. The spine, or backbone, is actually a stack of 24 individual bones called vertebrae. A healthy spine is S-shaped when viewed from the side, curving back at the shoulders and inward at the neck and small of the back. As well as being the body's main structural member, it houses the spinal cord—the intricate sensory network that runs through the vertebrae to transmit feeling and control movement throughout the entire body.

The main reason late-20th-century Americans suffer from back problems is that we are increasingly defying our evolutionary heritage and becoming sedentary creatures. The upright posture is designed for walking, and for most of human history that's what people did. Only in this century, with the advent of motor vehicles, have most people gone from place to place while sitting down. In much the same way, our work habits are changing. Most of our ancestors worked standing up—hunting, gathering, working on farms or at workbenches. Today, a high proportion of people spend the better part of their working day sitting at desks, at work stations, or in cars and trucks. These recent but momentous changes in human behavior have had a profound—and largely negative—impact on human physiology.

People who walk a lot or do physical labor develop good muscle tone in their backs and legs. People who sit most of the day lose that muscle tone, and their backs are the first place to show it. To compensate, many of us turn to exercise programs: In some instinctual way, we are hearing our bodies cry out for the old ways that demanded more activity. If you are a healthy, active adult and your normal activities keep you on the go, you may not need a special exercise routine; if you work in a sedentary job or if you aren't building several hours of walking or other physi-

WHERE IT HURTS

Back pain can have many causes. Pain caused by **osteoarthritis (1)** can occur anywhere along the spine. The larger back muscles can be affected by **fibrositis (2)**. Pain in the loin area on either side of the spine may indicate a **kidney infection (3)**. Damage to spinal disks, joints, ligaments, or muscles can be responsible for **lower back pain (4)**. A fall or other injury can cause pain in the **coccyx (5)**. Pain radiating from the buttock down the back or outside of the leg may be **sciatica (6)**.

cal activity into your weekly routine, you should exercise regularly, with emphasis on toning up those muscles that keep your back strong.

CAUSES

Back problems rank high on the list of ailments that are self-inflicted. Most of our back troubles happen because of bad habits, generally developed over a long period of time: poor posture; overexertion in work and play; sitting incorrectly at the desk or the steering wheel; pushing, pulling, and lifting things carelessly. Sometimes the effects are immediate, but in many cases back problems develop over time. The most common type of back pain comes from straining the bands of muscles surrounding the spine. Although such strains can occur anywhere along the spine, they happen most often in the curve of the lower back; the next most common place is at the base of the neck.

Sometimes, however, backache occurs for no apparent reason. Nonspecific backache may develop from weakened muscles that cannot handle everyday walking, bending, and stretching. In oth-

er cases, the discomfort seems to come from—or is aggravated by—general tension, lack of sleep, or stress, much like a tension headache. A condition called fibrositis causes chronic backache from localized muscle tension, which may in turn be psychosomatic in origin. Whether the muscle strain is from lifting heavy objects or something as innocuous as a sneeze makes little difference to the sufferer—the pain can be agonizing.

Pregnancy commonly brings on back pain, as the developing fetus, hormonal changes, and attendant weight gain put new kinds of stresses on a pregnant woman's spine and legs. Injuries from contact sports, accidents, and falls can cause all manner of problems, from minor muscle strains to severe damage to the spinal column or to the spinal cord itself.

DIAGNOSTIC AND TEST PROCEDURES

Unless you are totally immobilized from a back injury, your doctor will probably test your range of motion and nerve function, and may use palpation to locate the area of discomfort. Blood and urine tests will make sure the pain is not due to an infection or other systemic problem. X-rays are useful in pinpointing broken bones or other skeletal defects, and can sometimes help locate problems in connective tissue. To analyze soft-tissue damage, computed tomography (CT) or magnetic resonance imaging (MRI) scans may be necessary. To determine potential abnormalities affecting nerve and muscle stimuli, an electromyogram (EMG) can be useful.

TREATMENT

Because back problems stem from a variety of causes, some of which may not be readily apparent, conventional medical treatment and alternative therapies share a common pattern of pain relief, rest, and suitable restoration of movement.

CONVENTIONAL MEDICINE

The basic treatment for relieving back pain from strain or minor injury is immediate bed rest with an ice pack and aspirin or another nonsteroidal anti-inflammatory drug (NSAID) to reduce pain and inflammation. After the inflammation subsides, applying heat can soothe and restore muscles and connective tissue.

When back pain becomes truly immobilizing, the doctor will probably prescribe an appropriate over-the-counter or prescription painkiller and possibly a muscle relaxant. Some muscle relaxants such as methocarbamol or cyclobenzaprine may cause nausea, disorientation, and drowsiness as side effects, but such medications are usually recommended only for a few days. To relieve inflammation and inhibit the patient's pain perception in severe cases, therapy may include an injection of a local anesthetic such as lidocaine in combination with a corticosteroid into the tissue around the affected area or into trigger points elsewhere in the body. For relief of chronic back pain, low doses of antidepressant medications are sometimes prescribed.

Long-term bed rest is no longer considered necessary for most cases of back pain. Indeed, the lack of activity may actually contribute to recurring back problems. In most cases, you will be expected to start normal, nonstrenuous activity within 24 to 72 hours, after which controlled exercise or physical therapy should begin. Physical therapy treatments may employ massage, ultrasound, whirlpool baths, controlled application of heat, and specifically tailored exercise programs to help patients regain full use of the back.

In addition, some physicians—especially those in sports medicine—advocate using a transcutaneous electrical nerve stimulator (TENS). Electrodes taped to the body carry a mild electric current that helps relieve pain. After appropriate training, patients can use a TENS on their own to help speed recovery of strained or moderately injured backs.

Surgery for nonspecific back pain is a last resort. In cases of persistent pain from extreme nerve damage, rhizotomy—surgically severing a nerve—may be necessary to stop transmission of pain to the brain. Rhizotomy can correct the symptoms caused by friction between the surfaces in a spinal joint, but it doesn't address other problems such as herniated disks.

ALTERNATIVE CHOICES

Alternative therapies can be directed toward relieving the immediate discomfort of a back problem as well as conditioning and strengthening the body to prevent recurrence.

ACUPRESSURE

To relieve lower-back pain, apply 60 seconds of thumb pressure on either side of the spine just above the top of the pelvic bone, then massage at this point, as well as at the hip and knee joints.

ACUPUNCTURE

Some people troubled by back problems praise acupuncture for pain relief. In the hands of a trained acupuncturist, needle therapy is believed to redirect energy flow and balance throughout the body, not simply to relieve immediate or chronic back pain. Therapy involves inserting needles into points in specific muscles and on the ear to relieve blockages in the energy channels associated with back pain. Acute problems can be relieved in 1 to 4 sessions, while chronic pain problems typically require 12 or more treatments.

BODY WORK

Massage of the muscles along both sides of the spine helps relieve tension and restore mobility, especially in areas that feel tight or hard. To avoid potential damage to the spinal cord, a trained physical therapist or massage therapist is careful not to exert direct pressure on the vertebrae themselves.

The **Alexander technique** and the **Feldenkrais method** are useful for corrective whole-body positioning, not simply to correct posture but to relieve chronic tension and stress.

CHIROPRACTIC

Relief of back problems is the chiropractor's stock in trade: It is estimated that more people see chiropractors for back problems than for all other ailments combined. Chiropractic spinal manipulation has been recognized by the U.S. Agency for Health Care Policy and Research as an effective therapy for acute low-back pain.

Traditional chiropractic therapy relies on spinal manipulation to correct subluxations, or misaligned vertebrae, which may be responsible for problems anywhere along the spine. By helping restore motion to poorly functioning vertebrae, chiropractic therapy diminishes the accompanying pain and muscle spasm.

Chiropractors who use mixed therapies may rely on x-rays and other conventional diagnostic methods to treat back pain, combining spinal manipulation with muscle massage, ultrasound stimulation of deep tissue, nutritional recommendations, and exercise. For people wary of becoming dependent on painkillers and muscle relaxants for chronic back problems, modern chiropractic treatment offers a drug-free option to pain relief.

HERBAL THERAPIES

For general pain relief, drink infusions of white willow *(Salix alba)* or vervain *(Verbena officinalis)*. For inflammation, try teas brewed from lobelia *(Lobelia inflata),* yarrow *(Achillea millefolium),* cramp *(Viburnum opulus),* or white willow. Valerian *(Valeriana officinalis),* available as a tincture and in capsules, is particularly recommended as a muscle relaxant and sedative.

HOMEOPATHY

Over-the-counter remedies reported to help nonspecific back problems include Arnica for bruised or sore muscles, Bryonia and Rhus toxicodendron for sharp pain that gets worse when you move, and Nux vomica for persistent backache.

MIND/BODY MEDICINE

Biofeedback therapy, using carefully monitored low-level electrical impulses, is reported to help back-pain sufferers. The special equipment translates muscle tension into audible signals. Patients learn to slow the signals and relax the muscle. **Guided imagery** treatments may have similar results without the use of electronic equipment.

OSTEOPATHY

Osteopathic treatment is likely to combine drug therapy with spinal manipulation or traction, followed by physical therapy and exercise. More and more doctors and physical therapists are using spinal manipulation techniques as part of back-pain therapy. The U.S. government has recognized spinal manipulation by osteopaths and chiropractors as being highly effective in treating many back problems.

PREVENTION

The most important preventive measure for lower-back pain is practicing good posture when standing and sitting.

First, analyze your posture by standing with your heels against a wall. Your calves, buttocks, shoulders, and the back of your head should touch the wall, and you should be able to slip your hand behind the small of your back. Then step forward and stand normally: If your posture changes, correct it right away. If you stand for long periods at work, wear flat shoes with good arch support and get a box or step about six inches high to rest one foot on from time to time.

Your sitting posture may be even more important. A good chair bottom supports your hips comfortably but doesn't touch the backs of your knees. Your chair back should be set at an angle of about 10 degrees and should cradle the small of your back comfortably; if necessary, use a wedge-shaped cushion or lumbar pad. Your feet should rest flat on the floor. Your forearms should rest on your desk or work surface with your elbows almost at a right angle.

When you have to lift heavy objects, don't bend at the waist. Squat with your legs, keep your back upright as you grasp the object, and stand upright again. Let your legs do the lifting, not your back. A nonprescription back brace may also give support and prevent back strain; its main benefit is that it won't let you bend over at the waist. Use a back brace sparingly: Long-term use can make you dependent on it and may eventually lead to weaker—not stronger—back muscles. ■

Most adults and many children have occasional bad breath, and some people are convinced they have it when they don't. Fear of bad breath has spawned a vast industry that promotes toothpastes, mouthwashes, and other products that promise to vanquish odors. For most of us, good oral hygiene and a balanced diet are all that's necessary for fresh-smelling breath, although in some cases bad breath—or halitosis—can signal serious health problems.

CAUSES

Plaque—a sticky coating of food particles, saliva, and bacteria on the teeth—is a major cause of bad breath. Residual traces of coffee, alcoholic drinks, tobacco smoke, and highly spiced or strong-smelling foods can also contribute to mouth odor. A regular flow of saliva helps clean the mouth, so a dry mouth after a night's sleep may smell stale. Not eating at all can cause stale breath because eating stimulates saliva flow. But when saliva collects in the mouth—particularly in depressions at the back of the tongue—and is digested by oral bacteria, powerful odors can result.

Bad breath can be caused by indigestion and such disorders as tooth decay, gum problems, and postnasal drip. Some diseases cause foul breath, including lung and gastrointestinal ailments, cancer, diabetes, kidney disease, tuberculosis, sinusitis, and strep throat. Taking certain drugs, especially some antidepressants, may cause dry mouth and bad breath. In rare cases, particularly in toddlers, prolonged bad breath may indicate a foreign body lodged in the nose. Anyone who has persistent bad breath that doesn't seem related to oral hygiene or temporary indigestion should ask a doctor about the potential cause.

TREATMENT

Good oral hygiene will take care of most bad breath. Brush and floss your teeth at least twice a day, especially after meals when food particles may be trapped in your mouth. Baking soda can substitute for toothpaste; it's a good cleanser and also deodorizes the breath. Eliminating strong-smelling food can help reduce the problem, as can stimulating the flow of saliva *(see Nutrition and Diet, right)* and drinking plenty of water. Mouthwashes, mints, and chewing gum are only temporary cover-ups for bad breath.

CONVENTIONAL MEDICINE

Plaque buildup is a major cause of bad breath, so have your teeth cleaned by a dental professional regularly. Chronic bad breath should be diagnosed and treated by a doctor or dentist.

ALTERNATIVE CHOICES

HOMEOPATHY

If your breath is particularly bad on awakening, after meals, or after drinking alcohol, try Nux vomica or Kali phosphoricum. Both are available over the counter; follow dosages on the labels.

HERBAL THERAPIES

An infusion of echinacea *(Echinacea* spp.), myrrh *(Commiphora molmol),* bloodroot *(Sanguinaria canadensis),* and peppermint *(Mentha piperita)* can be used as everyday mouthwash. To help sweeten the breath, try tea brewed from fenugreek *(Trigonella foenum-graecum)* or peppermint *(Mentha piperita).* Preparations containing

▎S IT REALLY THAT BAD?

Unfortunately, the person with bad breath is often the last to know. If you aren't sure whether or not you have bad breath, ask your best friend—or your dentist. Or try this self-test: Cup your hands over your mouth, exhale deeply, then inhale through your nose to smell your breath.

cloves, aniseed, and fennel *(Foeniculum vulgare)* also are popular.

NUTRITION AND DIET

A high-fiber diet with plenty of whole grains, fresh fruit, and raw, leafy vegetables helps good digestion and reduces the chance of bad breath. Eating apples, oranges, and celery can help by cleaning the teeth, dispersing bacteria in the mouth, and stimulating saliva flow. Try chewing fresh parsley or peppermint leaves, a method used by ancient Romans to sweeten their breath.

AT-HOME REMEDIES

There's no substitute for good oral hygiene. Brush your teeth with circular—not back-and-forth—movements, then floss thoroughly between your teeth all the way around your mouth.

Cleaning the tongue, which many people neglect, is very important: Use your toothbrush to brush the top of the tongue as far back as possible. A tongue blade, a device used in the Middle East and India to scrape the tongue, may be helpful. Several American companies make them, or you can try a store that sells Asian or Middle Eastern products. A soupspoon will work just as well; gently draw the inverted bowl of the spoon over your tongue to scrape off any residue. But be careful: Don't push the brush, spoon, or scraper so far back that you start to gag.

After cleaning, rinse your mouth with water. In fact, taking a few sips of water, swishing it around your mouth, and spitting it out is a good idea when brushing isn't possible. As on-the-spot breath fresheners, try mints, mouthwash, or chewing gum that contains chlorophyll, but don't rely on them to replace good oral hygiene.

PREVENTION

If you're worried about bad breath, avoid highly spiced or strong-smelling foods such as onions, hot peppers, garlic, pastrami, salami, pepperoni, and anchovies. They not only smell strong themselves but may be hard to digest, bringing on stomach gas, which can contribute to bad breath. ■

- an inflamed, sometimes painful, reddish patch of skin, especially on the shoulder blades, spine, lower back, hip joints, knees, ankles, or heels of a bedridden or wheelchair-bound person.
- a raw, open sore in any of the areas noted above, caused by the top layer of skin having cracked and peeled away; open bedsores can quickly become ulcerated.

CALL YOUR DOCTOR IF:

- a person is going to remain bedridden or immobile for an extended period, cannot move or is very weak, and is beginning to develop bedsores. The person may need regular attendance by a nurse or other trained healthcare provider.
- the sore produces a discharge, which may contain pus or become foul smelling; or if the sore turns black. This indicates an infection or tissue death; **get immediate medical attention.**

Anyone who cares for an immobile person at home understands the curse of bedsores. Even hospital and nursing home staffers may not be able to keep their patients from developing these irritating and sometimes debilitating skin injuries. More than a million Americans get bedsores each year, two-thirds of them being bedridden people over the age of 70.

CAUSES

A bedsore begins as a tender, inflamed area caused by unrelieved pressure on a bony, weight-bearing area of the body; it can quickly turn into a painful skin ulcer that usually heals slowly. The likely pressure points are the ankles, knees, heels, shoulder blades, and—particularly in wheelchair patients—the spine, hips, and lower back. The pressure need not be present for extended periods to cause inflammation; in some cases, bedsores form in a matter of hours. Patients with diabetes or other conditions that promote skin breakdown and infection are at risk, as are those who are underweight, paralyzed, or suffering from poor circulation, heart problems, spinal cord injury, or atherosclerosis.

TREATMENT

CONVENTIONAL MEDICINE

At most hospitals and nursing homes, the standard treatment for bedsores is to clean the wound with a saline solution or hydrogen peroxide, remove any dead skin, and cover the area with a dressing that does not stick to the damaged skin. Dead tissue may need to be removed with a fine scalpel. In severe cases, when an ulcerated bedsore is deep and difficult to stabilize, plastic surgery or skin grafts may be required to restore damaged areas.

Unfortunately, some injuries and conditions prevent bedridden patients from being moved at all. Even those who can be shifted regularly risk tearing delicate skin if they are pulled over the sheets. One option for such patients is to improve

MOVING A BEDRIDDEN PERSON

To prevent bedsores from becoming ulcerated, two people should move a bedridden patient every two waking hours. First, sit the patient up with legs bent. The movers face the head of the bed and sit on either side of the patient with one leg on the bed. Each reaches under the patient's legs and grasps the other's forearm *(top)*.

With their inside shoulders under the patient's armpits, the movers put their free hands on the bed for support *(bottom)*. Together they lift the patient and gently move him to a new position, adjusting the bedding as necessary.

their circulation, either by massage or by controlled, low-level electrical stimulation.

ALTERNATIVE CHOICES

Various alternative treatments can soothe inflammation and relieve pain, but they cannot replace the essential steps of moving a bedridden person often and improving the individual's diet.

HERBAL THERAPIES

Herbal treatments may relieve the discomfort of bedsores and may help fight infection. To ease minor inflammation, apply a marsh mallow *(Althaea officinalis)* root ointment; or try a poultice made from equal parts of powdered slippery elm *(Ulmus fulva)* bark, marsh mallow root, and echinacea *(Echinacea* spp.) blended with a small amount of hot water. Two drops of essential tea tree oil *(Melaleuca* spp.) in a cup of water makes an infection-fighting rinse.

NUTRITION AND DIET

Patients with bedsores need to drink plenty of water to prevent their skin from becoming dry and

vulnerable to pressure. Certain vitamins and minerals, especially vitamins A, C, E, and B complex, and zinc, promote skin growth and repair. Vitamin C in particular has been shown to be effective in healing bedsores. But because some vitamins can be toxic in large doses—especially to people whose bodies are weakened by disease or injury—taking any vitamin or mineral supplements must be supervised by the attending physician.

AT-HOME CARE

Caring for invalids at home—especially aging loved ones—can be a daunting task. Some helpful tips for making each day tolerable:
◆ Make sure the person confined to bed or a wheelchair moves his body as often as possible when awake, but at least every two hours. If he can't move around on his own, others should move his body for him.
◆ Cushion the person's feet, knees, spine, and shoulders with soft pillows or cloth-covered foam pads, and adjust them frequently for comfort.
◆ Never pull or slide the person over bedclothes, because the friction may cause further skin damage. Always use the two-person lifting technique *(above, left)*.

PREVENTION

When it comes to bedsores, prevention is clearly worth more than any cure. Wheelchair-bound or bedridden people should shift their positions regularly. They should be bathed frequently and dried thoroughly, and their skin should be lubricated with a mild, nonirritating lotion. They should have clean, dry, tight-fitting, unstarched cotton sheets; loose-fitting clothes; plenty of air circulation; a healthy diet; and some sort of regular exercise—even if a caregiver has to move their limbs.

To cushion sensitive areas, try an "eggcrate" foam mattress overlay, a water-filled mattress, or a sheepskin pad over the bedsheets. Consider a variable-pressure mattress with separate sections that can be inflated and deflated independently to adjust pressure on the patient's body. ■

173

SYMPTOMS

It is not unusual for children under the age of six to have trouble controlling their bladders at night. You should be concerned about bedwetting only if:

◆ your child is older than six and has never been dry at night or continues to wet the bed twice a month or more.

◆ your child suddenly starts wetting at night after a period of having been dry through the night.

CALL YOUR DOCTOR IF:

◆ your efforts to help your child learn to stay dry through the night are not working, or your child wants additional help in managing the situation.

◆ your child is wetting the bed and has frequent or painful urination, dark brown urine (a sign of bleeding), abdominal pain, or fever; these symptoms may indicate a urinary tract or bladder infection.

◆ your child experiences side effects that affect his behavior or interfere with his sleep after starting a course of prescribed medication to treat bedwetting. Many drugs used in treatment cause these types of side effects.

The most important thing to remember about bedwetting is that it is a benign disorder and not a willful act. Punishment is never an answer. Between five million and seven million children suffer from bedwetting; the majority are boys.

Don't be unduly concerned about bedwetting unless your child is older than six. Before then, your child's body may not have developed enough to control bladder actions at night. Time usually cures the problem: Most children resolve any difficulties on their own by the age of seven.

CAUSES

Why bedwetting occurs is not fully understood, although most cases seem to result from some kind of developmental delay. Some experts think bedwetting is purely a behavioral issue, others believe its origins are physiological, and still others think both physiological and behavioral factors play a role. Only 2 percent of cases can be traced to neurological problems (often caused by structural spinal abnormalities) or specific diseases such as diabetes or bladder infections.

Alternative therapists believe that a misalignment of muscles and joints around the pelvis can affect the activity of the sphincter muscle that controls urine release.

Any new, stressful situation may cause a child to revert to bedwetting. Once your child adjusts to the situation, the problem should resolve itself. If your child does not improve, the treatments listed here should help. In addition, you will want your child to talk through his fears.

TREATMENT

CONVENTIONAL MEDICINE

To rule out a disease-related problem, your pediatrician will perform a blood or urine test. If the test reveals diabetes or an infection, your pediatrician will treat that condition first. The doctor will also test your child to rule out nervous system problems.

There are three primary ways to treat bedwetting in an otherwise healthy child: waiting for spontaneous resolution, employing behavioral conditioning, and undertaking drug therapy.

Waiting, though often the preferred course, may make your child anxious. However, if he is old enough to benefit from motivational counseling—to learn about the condition and participate in its management—he and the rest of your family will be better able to cope. One form of motivation is to have your child place a star on a chart or calendar to mark dry nights.

Behavioral conditioning—utilizing a device with a sensor that detects wetness and sets off an alarm—has proved very effective. The child begins associating bladder distention with being awakened and in time "learns" to awaken before losing control.

Drug therapy is considered less effective because most children relapse after stopping medication. It has its place, however. For short-term help—when your child sleeps at a friend's, for example—desmopressin, an antidiuretic, works well. Doctors are moving away from the antidepressant imipramine because of side effects.

ALTERNATIVE CHOICES

ACUPRESSURE
According to proponents of acupressure, daily application of deep thumb pressure in an upward motion to the following points may help: Conception Vessel 4, Kidney 3, Spleen 6. See pages 22–23 for point locations. Also, try holding Heart 7, the point in the hollow of your child's wrist just below the little finger, for up to one minute and then switch sides.

BODY WORK
Shiatsu and **reflexology** may be helpful in bedwetting caused by a neurological problem. Consult a trained therapist for help.

EXERCISE
Bladder-stretching exercises may help your child increase bladder capacity. Once a day your child should hold his urine as long as possible past the first indication that his bladder is full. You and your child should measure the voided urine daily to see if capacity is increasing. Have your child practice this for up to three months to give this technique an opportunity to work.

HOMEOPATHY
Because bedwetting is a chronic problem, you need to seek help from an experienced homeopath. Common remedies include Equisetum, Causticum, Lycopodium, and Pulsatilla.

MIND/BODY MEDICINE
Hypnotherapy can be effective with children who are highly motivated. With the help of a trained professional, your child will master a series of action statements that he will say before going to bed, such as: "When I need to urinate, I will wake up all by myself and go to the bathroom."

NUTRITION AND DIET
Sometimes bedwetting is associated with food allergies. Try eliminating milk products, citrus fruits, and chocolate—foods most frequently linked to allergies—from your child's diet.

OSTEOPATHY
If exercises or behavior-based treatments don't work, consult an osteopath for manipulation of your child's lower back and pelvic area to modify possible structural problems.

WAYS TO COPE
◆ Teach an older child how to change his own bed. Set out clean pajamas and sheets in his room each night. You will help him avoid embarrassment and give him a sense of being in control if he no longer has to rely on you.

◆ If you are using an alarm device for behavioral conditioning, avoid nylon sheets and pajamas; nylon induces sweat, which can set off the alarm.

◆ Prevent the mattress from getting wet by using a plastic-lined mattress cover (which may cause the child to sweat) or, better yet, provide him with a smaller, rubberized, felt-covered pad that he can place over the wet area on the bed after an accident. ■

In most cases, a bee or wasp sting causes only minor symptoms at the site of the sting, including:

- pain.
- swelling.
- redness.
- itching or burning.

Allergic reactions may produce extensive swelling. Allergies are also responsible for an even more serious, and potentially fatal, condition called **anaphylactic shock.** *(See Emergencies/First Aid: Shock.)* Multiple stings can produce a toxic reaction, with the same symptoms:

- rapid swelling around the eyes, lips, tongue, or throat.
- difficulty breathing.
- wheezing or hoarseness.
- itching, cramping, or numbness that is severe.
- dizziness.
- a reddish rash, or hives.
- stomach cramps.
- loss of consciousness.

CALL YOUR DOCTOR IF:

- ◆ you are stung and develop any of the symptoms of anaphylactic shock listed above. **Get medical help now.**
- ◆ you are allergic to bee or wasp stings and you are stung. You are at risk of anaphylactic shock, even if your reaction to previous stings was mild; you may need emergency treatment. (See your doctor to determine if you are allergic.)

The venom from a bee or wasp sting causes local swelling, pain, and redness, which usually go away within several hours. Some people who are allergic to the venom experience larger local reactions, with more extensive swelling.

For about 3 percent of people, however, a sting can trigger a life-threatening allergic reaction called anaphylaxis (from the Greek for "nonhealing"). Painful hives and swelling may progress rapidly to block off airways, causing circulatory collapse and, sometimes, death. In the United States, about 50 people die each year from sting-induced **anaphylactic shock,** primarily people over 40 with preexisting heart disease. If you are stung by a swarm of 50 to 100 bees, the effect can be similar to that of anaphylactic shock.

The only insects with true stingers belong to the order Hymenoptera, including the Apidae (honeybees and bumblebees) and Vespidae (wasps, yellow jackets, white-faced hornets, and yellow hornets). The stinging mechanism, located in the female's abdomen, consists of a stinger attached to a venom-filled sac. The honeybee's stinger has multiple barbs so that it usually remains in the wound, causing the bee's death. Wasps, whose stingers do not have barbs, can sting more than once.

CAUSES

The venom of Hymenoptera contains toxins and inflammatory agents that cause the local pain and swelling that go away after a few hours. Some people, however, are allergic to elements in the venom and have more severe reactions, which can range from extended swelling to potentially fatal anaphylactic shock. The process of sting-induced allergies is poorly understood. Like other allergies, sting allergy appears to run in families. But scientists still don't understand why only 60 percent of allergic adults and only 8 percent of allergic children suffer shock when stung.

A person may be stung many times and have only normal reactions, then suddenly one sting will produce a strong allergic reaction. Doctors are not sure why a person suddenly develops such sensitivity or why the sensitivity may last fewer than 3 months or more than 25 years.

DIAGNOSTIC AND TEST PROCEDURES

Your doctor can determine if you are allergic to bee and wasp stings with a simple skin test, using purified, freeze-dried venom. However, only about 20 percent of people with a positive skin test suffer severe reactions to a real sting.

TREATMENT

For most stings, minimal treatment, such as a cold compress or ice pack, is sufficient. If you have multiple stings or a severe allergic reaction, you need medical help at once.

CONVENTIONAL MEDICINE

For pain, take aspirin or acetaminophen. For strong reactions, try diphenhydramine or another nonprescription antihistamine. For children, use cough medicine containing antihistamine (avoid aspirin because of the risk of Reye's syndrome).

For **anaphylactic shock,** the usual treatment is the bronchodilator epinephrine. You may give yourself an injection from a bee-sting kit; but after the injection, see a doctor promptly for further treatment. (Note: Bee-sting kits are designed for adults; for children, read the directions.)

ALTERNATIVE CHOICES

HERBAL THERAPIES

Apply aloe *(Aloe barbadensis)* or the fresh bruised leaf or juice of plantain. Or apply calendula *(Calendula officinalis)* ointment four times a day.

HOMEOPATHY

A homeopath may recommend applying a few drops of Pyrethrum tincture, available over the counter, to a sting. For swelling, take Apis (30c) every 30 minutes to 2 hours.

AT-HOME REMEDIES

If the stinging apparatus remains in the skin, scrape it away with a knife or fingernail; if you

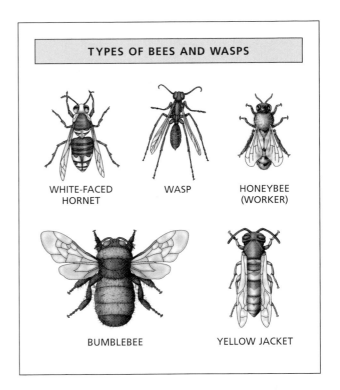

TYPES OF BEES AND WASPS

WHITE-FACED HORNET   WASP   HONEYBEE (WORKER)

BUMBLEBEE   YELLOW JACKET

use tweezers, you may squeeze more venom into the skin. For bee stings, a paste of baking soda will ease the itching. Wasp stings are alkaline and can be neutralized by vinegar or lemon juice. If you're far from home, apply mud; as it dries, it will draw out some of the toxin.

PREVENTION

To avoid sting-induced shock if you are allergic, carry a bee-sting kit (be sure you know how to administer a self-injection). You should also wear a Medic Alert bracelet or necklace describing your allergy.

If you have had a severe reaction to a sting and a positive venom skin test, venom immunotherapy—a series of weekly injections of venom—is highly effective at preventing anaphylaxis.

Reduce your chances of being stung by avoiding brightly colored, white, or pastel clothing. Don't use cosmetics or perfume with floral scents. Food odors attract insects, especially yellow jackets, so be alert when you are cooking or eating outdoors. ∎

- bruising and swelling of the eyelid and soft tissue around the eye, sometimes accompanied by broken blood vessels in the white of the eye. The discoloration starts out purple or blue; as the bruise heals, it may turn green or yellow before disappearing, usually in about a week.

- a pair of black eyes occurs simultaneously; you should be examined by a doctor for possible skull fracture.

Any of the symptoms below may indicate damage to the eyeball, which should be evaluated and treated by a doctor or an ophthalmologist:
- your eyeball hurts.
- you have an open cut around the eye.
- you have blurred vision, multiple images, or floating spots.
- you see blood or other fluid in front of the iris of the eye.
- you experience unusual sensitivity to light or other vision changes.

Like many bruises, a "shiner" may be nothing to worry about and will heal of its own accord in a few days. In some cases, however, a black eye is a sign of more serious injury to the eye or the skull. Any damage to the eyeball that causes it to become red and swollen must be evaluated by an ophthalmologist or other physician; an eye injury could involve a detached retina or lead to glaucoma. A fracture in the ring of bones around the eye may trap muscle or soft tissue and can impair vision; surgery may be required to correct the condition. (See also Eye Problems, Vision Problems.)

CAUSES

Most black eyes are the result of a blow that causes bleeding beneath the skin, producing the characteristic blue-black discoloration. A skull fracture can cause black eyes, in which case both eyes are usually affected. People with sinusitis from allergies sometimes get "allergic shiners"—darkening under the eyes caused by inflamed and engorged blood vessels.

TREATMENT

Applying something cold to a black eye works in two ways: It helps to reduce swelling and to constrict blood vessels, which in turn stops the internal bleeding. Putting a cold steak on a black eye is a needlessly expensive variation; you can save money by using an ice pack or a package of frozen vegetables, which works just as well.

Besides cold treatment, there's not much that can be done for a black eye except to avoid doing anything that could cause further injury, such as putting pressure on the swollen eye or trying to force it open. If you need a pain reliever, take an analgesic such as aspirin or ibuprofen, either of which will also help reduce inflammation.

CONVENTIONAL MEDICINE
A doctor will recommend applying an ice pack or a cloth soaked in ice-cold water and wrung out.

Hold the ice pack or cold compress to the eye for up to 10 minutes, being careful not to apply pressure. You might try putting crushed ice in a plastic bag and taping it to the forehead. Repeat the cold treatment for 5 to 10 minutes every hour for 24 hours or as long as swelling is present.

If the eyeball itself is damaged or if vision is affected, your doctor or ophthalmologist will determine the nature and extent of the injury and give appropriate treatment. If the eye is protruding from the eye socket, surgery may be necessary.

ALTERNATIVE CHOICES

Until the beginning of this century, leeches were used to suck blood from around a black eye. That treatment actually did relieve the pressure, but it's thankfully a thing of the past. Today other nonmedical remedies may be helpful.

HERBAL THERAPY

You may want to gently apply a compress made with chamomile (Matricaria recutita). Chamomile is said to reduce the fragility of tiny capillaries and to serve as an anti-inflammatory agent.

HOMEOPATHY

A homeopath may recommend various over-the-counter remedies for black eye; be sure to follow label instructions carefully. Arnica (12x) may

C A U T I O N !

DON'T BLOW YOUR NOSE

If you have a black eye, blowing your nose may rupture more blood vessels around the damaged facial tissue. If the injury that caused your black eye also fractured the bone of the eye socket, the pressure of blowing your nose could cause additional damage to an already unstable eyeball. Also, never try to force open an eyelid that is swollen shut; doing so could further injure the skin or the eye.

help speed the reabsorption of escaped blood. If skin is unbroken, Arnica cream around the eye may help reduce bruising. If bruising is slow to clear and pain is relieved only by cold, try Ledum (12x), three doses a day for four days. If bones around the eye are very sore or the eyeball itself is injured, Symphytum (12x), three doses a day, up to four days, may help relieve the pain. For severe shooting or radiating pains around the eye, Hypericum (12x) once an hour for up to four hours may help relieve pain and speed healing.

NUTRITION AND DIET

A good balanced diet with plenty of protein, vitamins, and minerals is important in the healing of any injury. In particular, bromelain, the enzyme in raw pineapple, may help reduce bruising. Eat fresh pineapple or take bromelain capsules, available in health food stores.

AT-HOME REMEDIES

For a black eye that is not severely damaged, applying ice and taking a painkiller are probably all that's necessary. Boxing trainers minimize facial swelling by using a gadget that looks like a small metal iron but is cold. You can get the same effect with a cold can of soda or a bag of frozen vegetables. Be sure the can or the bag is clean, and hold it lightly against the cheek or forehead, not the eye itself.

Be careful not to go overboard with cold treatment. Even though the swelling may be painful, it is one of the body's healing responses. You want to control excessive swelling without inhibiting the repair process. Your own good sense will tell you how much cold is too much. Most swelling reactions to mild injuries last only a few hours, so you shouldn't need an ice pack after the first day. If the pain and swelling persist after an hour or two of intermittent cold application, the injury is significant and should be seen by a doctor. ∎

SYMPTOMS

In its early stages, bladder cancer may not have obvious symptoms; in later stages symptoms may include:

◆ bloody urine, ranging in color from faintly rusty to deep red, sometimes containing blood clots. Blood traces, invisible to the naked eye, may show up in tests of urine samples.

◆ frequent urinary tract infections, painful urination, and a need to urinate often.

◆ weight or appetite loss.

◆ abdominal or back pain, persistent low-grade fever, anemia.

CALL YOUR DOCTOR IF:

◆ you have any of the symptoms listed above; although they may not be cancer related, you should be screened for bladder cancer.

The bladder is a pouch in the urinary tract that stores urine after it is produced by the kidneys. The bladder is lined with specialized transitional cells, and when it is irritated, extra layers of transitional cells develop. This process increases the likelihood of a transitional cell turning cancerous, then multiplying to create a malignant tumor. Malignant tumors begin as small, superficial lumps on the inner wall of the bladder. The cancer spreads by penetrating bladder muscle, infiltrating surrounding fat and tissue, and—if untreated—eventually invading the bloodstream and lymphatic system.

The earlier the cancer is detected, the more localized it will be and the more effective the treatment. Thanks to improved procedures for early detection, five-year survival rates for this disease improved from 50 percent in the 1960s to over 70 percent in the 1990s. While bladder tumors often recur, prompt detection means they can be stopped while they are still superficial. The average age for getting bladder cancer is 68. Men are more susceptible to the disease than women, and Caucasians more susceptible than African Americans. Bladder cancer accounts for about 5 percent of cancers in the United States, or about 50,000 cases a year.

CAUSES

Chronic irritation of the bladder increases the risk of cancer. People with congenital disorders of the bladder, chronic bladder infections, or persistent cystitis—inflammation of the bladder—are more susceptible, as are people with histories of benign bladder tumors.

More than most cancers, bladder cancer is associated with exposure to cancer-promoting chemicals, or carcinogens. For example, cigarette smokers have three times more risk than nonsmokers of developing bladder cancer because of specific carcinogens in tobacco smoke. Painters, truckers, leatherworkers, machinists and metalworkers, rubber and textile workers, and people exposed to industrial dyes are at increased risk. People who have been treated with radiation or alkylating chemotherapy agents are also at higher risk. Consumption of nitrates in smoked and cured meats may also be associated with bladder cancer, as may consumption of caffeine and saccharin, but the connection is so weak that some researchers question the risk at all.

DIAGNOSTIC AND TEST PROCEDURES

The bladder can be viewed through a fiberoptic tube known as a cystoscope. If the doctor detects a tumor, a tiny tissue sample is taken through the tube and examined in the laboratory. Should the tumor be malignant, the treatment will depend on how far, if at all, the cancer has spread. Blood and urine studies and x-rays of the bladder, ureters, kidneys, and other organs provide information about tumor size, location, and the degree or amount of spread.

TREATMENT

There is no acceptable primary treatment for cancer other than medical care by a certified oncologist. Alternative therapies outside mainstream medicine may help ease the pain of the disease and the side effects of conventional treatment, but none is a proven cure for cancer. See Cancer for more information about treatment.

CONVENTIONAL MEDICINE

If detected early, superficial malignancies can usually be treated successfully by transurethral resection (TUR). In this procedure the surgeon inserts a small tube into the bladder and removes the tumor surgically or burns it out with heat or a laser beam. Combined with chemotherapy or radiation therapy, TUR may also be successful against more invasive bladder cancer. Immunotherapy with the bacillus Calmette-Guérin (BCG) vaccine is beneficial in 60 percent of cases. Injecting BCG into the bladder after the tumor has been removed significantly reduces the chance of the cancer's recurring.

Invasive cancers may require radical cystectomy, or bladder removal. The surgeon then diverts the urinary tract and creates an opening, or stoma, through which urine is passed. Patients once had to wear external urine pouches, but new techniques synthesize internal pouches from intestinal tissue. Bladder removal may also mean removing the reproductive organs in women and the prostate and seminal vesicles in men. Although this procedure renders men impotent and women infertile, men can have penile implants to overcome impotence, and women can remain sexually active.

After surgery, a combination of radiation and chemotherapy may be necessary to deter recurrence. Anyone who has had bladder cancer should have regular follow-up tests, since tumors often recur. If the cancer has metastasized, or spread beyond the urinary tract, surgery is not usually considered. Chemotherapy is the primary treatment for recurrent and metastatic cancer.

COMPLEMENTARY THERAPIES

Several scientific studies suggest that certain vitamins and minerals are beneficial in both treatment and prevention of bladder cancer. Patients receiving BCG immunotherapy may have better results with megadoses of vitamins A, B_6, C, and E, as well as zinc. Research also suggests reduced incidence of bladder cancer among people with adequate vitamin B_6, beta carotene, and selenium in their diets.

PREVENTION

To prevent bladder cancer, your best bet is to steer clear of possible carcinogens. For starters, don't smoke. Eat smoked or cured meats only occasionally and prepare fresh rather than processed foods. If you work around carcinogenic chemicals, follow safety guidelines to avoid undue exposure. And if you feel you may be at risk for bladder cancer, arrange regular screenings with your doctor to ensure early detection. ■

BLADDER INFECTIONS

SYMPTOMS

- a burning sensation when urinating; this is the most common sign of a bladder infection, but any pain or difficulty in urination may also indicate the condition.
- frequent urge to urinate.
- urine with a strong, foul odor.
- in the elderly: lethargy, incontinence, mental confusion.

In severe cases, these symptoms may be accompanied by fever and chills, abdominal pain, or blood in the urine.

CALL YOUR DOCTOR IF:

- the burning sensation persists for more than 24 hours after you begin trying self-help treatments. Untreated, bladder infections can lead to more serious conditions.
- painful urination is accompanied by vomiting, fever, chills, bloody urine, or abdominal or back pain; it may indicate potentially life-threatening kidney disease, a bladder or kidney tumor, or prostate infection. **Seek medical help immediately.**
- the burning is accompanied by a discharge from the vagina or penis, a sign of sexually transmitted disease, pelvic inflammatory disease (PID), or other serious infection. See your doctor without delay.
- you experience any persistent pain or difficulty with urination; this may also be a sign of sexually transmitted disease, a vaginal infection, a kidney stone, enlargement of the prostate *(see Prostate Problems),* or a bladder or prostate tumor. See your doctor without delay.

Bladder infections—generally termed cystitis, which means inflammation of the bladder—are common in women and very rare in men. In fact, about half of all women get at least one bladder infection at some time in their lives. Although doctors are not sure exactly why women have many more bladder infections than men, they suspect it may be because women have a shorter urethra, the tube that carries urine out of the bladder. This relatively short passageway—only about an inch and a half long—makes it easier for bacteria to migrate into the bladder. Also, the opening to a woman's urethra lies close to both the vagina and the anus, giving bacteria from those areas access to the urinary tract.

Bladder infections are not serious if treated promptly. But recurrences are common in susceptible people and can lead to kidney infections, which are more serious and may result in permanent kidney damage. So it's very important to treat the underlying causes of a bladder infection and to take preventive steps to avoid recurrences.

In elderly people, bladder infections are often difficult to diagnose because the symptoms are less specific and are frequently blamed on aging. Older people who suddenly become incontinent or who begin acting lethargic or confused should be checked by a doctor for a bladder infection.

CAUSES

Most bladder infections are caused by various strains of *Escherichia coli (E. coli)*, the bacteria commonly found in the intestines. Women sometimes get bladder infections as a direct result of intercourse, which can push bacteria up into the bladder through the urethra. Some women contract the infection—dubbed "honeymoon cystitis"—almost every time they have sex. Women who use a diaphragm as their primary method of birth control are also particularly susceptible to bladder infections, perhaps because the device presses on the bladder and keeps it from emptying completely. Bacteria then rapidly reproduce in the stagnant urine left in the bladder. Pregnant women, whose bladders become compressed as the fetus grows, are prone to infections for the same reason. Some people develop symptoms of a bladder infection when no infection actually exists. These disorders are usually benign but are difficult to treat.

While they can be quite uncomfortable and potentially serious if complications set in, the bladder infections that most women get clear up quickly and are relatively harmless. In men, however, a bladder infection is almost always a symptom of an underlying disorder and is generally regarded as cause for more concern. Often the infection has migrated from the prostate or some other part of the body, signaling problems in those locations. Or it may indicate the presence of a tumor or other obstruction that is interfering with the urinary tract. Some studies have shown that uncircumcised boys are at somewhat greater risk of contracting a bladder infection during their first year of life because bacteria may collect under the foreskin.

In recent years, an increasing number of bladder infections in both men and women have been linked to two sexually transmitted bacteria, chlamydia and mycoplasma. And both home and hospital use of catheters—tubes inserted into the bladder to empty it—can also lead to infection.

DIAGNOSTIC AND TEST PROCEDURES

Bladder infections usually can be diagnosed readily with a urine test. If you are experiencing persistent or frequent infections, or if an anatomical defect is suspected as the cause of the problem, your physician may also want you to undergo cystoscopy, a diagnostic procedure in which a lighted tube inserted through the urethra is used to examine the inside of the bladder. And to make sure your kidneys have not been affected, your physician may order an intravenous pyelogram (IVP), a special x-ray technique for viewing kidneys, or an ultrasound scan to produce an image of the entire urinary tract system.

TREATMENT

Mild bladder infections often clear up quickly in response to simple home remedies. But if you ex-

perience no relief within 24 hours, you should consult a physician for more aggressive treatment. Delay in clearing your body of the infection can lead to more serious problems.

CONVENTIONAL MEDICINE

Bladder infections are treated with a wide variety of antibiotics to clear up the infection; with phenazopyridine, which is often given to relieve the pain and burning; and by increased intake of fluids to flush out the urinary tract. The antibiotic your physician prescribes and the number of days you will need to take it will depend on the type of bacteria that are causing the infection. Although some studies indicate that uncomplicated infections require only one to three days of treatment, your physician may prefer to treat you for a longer period of time in order to ensure that all of the bacteria are eradicated. Elderly people and those with a chronic underlying health condition, such as diabetes or HIV infection, are often prescribed a longer course of antibiotics—sometimes up to 14 days.

After the treatment has run its course, you may be asked to come in for a follow-up urine test to make sure your bladder is free of all signs of infection. People with frequently recurring bladder infections are often prescribed low daily doses of antibiotics for an additional six months or longer. Patients whose infections are related to sexual activity may be given a small dose of antibiotics to take each time they have intercourse. Some doctors prescribe the hormone estrogen, either as a topical cream or in pill form, to prevent recurrences in postmenopausal women. For cases where the infection is the result of a blockage or obstruction, such as a kidney stone or an enlarged prostate, surgery may be required.

ALTERNATIVE CHOICES

If begun promptly at the first hint of burning during urination, alternative means of treatment can be successful in getting rid of a bladder infection. But if these methods do not bring relief within 24 hours, you should call your doctor for antibiotic treatment. Consult with your doctor if you wish

B

to continue with alternative methods while on the antibiotics to speed up the recovery process.

ACUPUNCTURE

Acupuncture treatment may help prevent recurrences of bladder infections. Consult a professional acupuncturist.

CHIROPRACTIC

Adjusting the bones and joints around the pelvis can act to strengthen the bladder muscles, helping to ward off recurrences of the infection. An **osteopath** can also provide this treatment.

HERBAL THERAPIES

Some herbs have been found useful in both clearing up bladder infections and easing the burning that accompanies them. Perhaps the best known is cranberry, which, recent scientific studies show, has a remarkable ability to combat bladder and other urinary tract infections *(box, opposite)*.

Another herb useful in treating bladder infections is nettle *(Urtica dioica)*, which has been shown to have anti-inflammatory properties. Mix 1 tsp dried, crushed nettle leaves or root in 1 cup boiling water. Allow the infusion to cool, then drink 1 tbsp every hour or two—up to 1 cup a day.

The evergreen shrub uva ursi *(Arctostaphylos uva-ursi)*, or bearberry, which acts as a diuretic and an anti-inflammatory medication, has a long history as a folk remedy for bladder infections. Soak fresh leaves in brandy or other liquor for a few hours, then add to boiling water—about 1 tsp leaves per cup of water. If you have dried leaves, you can boil them directly in the water without a preliminary alcohol soak.

Women who are prone to bladder infections after sexual activity can help prevent recurrences by washing their perineal area with a medicinal solution of the herb goldenseal *(Hydrastis canadensis)* before and after intercourse. Mix 2 tsp of the herb per cup of water, bring to a boil, and simmer for 15 minutes. Cool to room temperature before using.

HOMEOPATHY

Depending on the symptoms, homeopaths recommend a number of different remedies to help relieve the pain of a bladder infection. Here are three of the most commonly prescribed:

◆ If the urge to urinate is very strong and the burning is intense, Cantharis.
◆ If you experience painful cramping with urination or your urine is very dark or bloody, Mercurius corrosivus.
◆ For women whose infections are brought on by sexual contact, Staphysagria.

Take these remedies hourly until symptoms disappear. If you experience no relief after 24 hours, seek professional help.

HYDROTHERAPY AND AROMATHERAPY

Hot sitz baths can help relieve the symptoms of a bladder infection. Adding certain pungent herbal oils to the bathwater creates a soothing, fragrant steam that aromatherapists believe makes the treatment particularly effective. Try putting in a few drops of the essential oils of juniper berry, eucalyptus, sandalwood, pine, parsley, cedarwood, chamomile, or cajuput.

You can also try a massage oil made with 1 oz vegetable oil and 5 drops each of any com-

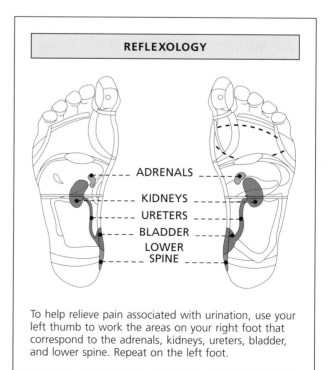

REFLEXOLOGY

ADRENALS
KIDNEYS
URETERS
BLADDER
LOWER
SPINE

To help relieve pain associated with urination, use your left thumb to work the areas on your right foot that correspond to the adrenals, kidneys, ureters, bladder, and lower spine. Repeat on the left foot.

CRANBERRY JUICE: A PROVEN FOLK REMEDY

For centuries, Native Americans used crushed cranberries as a treatment for bladder and other urinary tract infections. Controlled studies now give scientific support to that ancient remedy. The research suggests that the berries' proficiency in fighting off infection is due to their high level of hippuric acid, a substance that inhibits the growth of E. coli bacteria and keeps them from adhering to the lining of the bladder.

To treat an existing bladder infection and to help prevent future ones, drink 12 to 16 oz of cranberry juice each day. Or, if you prefer, take cranberry capsules; follow the directions on the package. You can also try alternating cranberry juice with blueberry juice, which appears to have similar infection-fighting properties.

bination of the herbs mentioned. Massage daily, rubbing the oil over your lower back, abdomen, stomach, and hips.

NUTRITION AND DIET

Both conventional and alternative practitioners agree that drinking plenty of fluids to keep you urinating frequently and to flush out your urinary tract thoroughly is one of the most effective means of combating a bladder infection—whatever its cause. However, you should avoid beverages that might irritate the urinary tract and aggravate the burning. Culprits include alcohol, coffee, black tea, chocolate milk, carbonated beverages, and citrus juices. Until clear of the infection, you should also avoid potentially irritating foods such as citrus fruits, tomatoes, vinegar, sugar, chocolate, artificial sweeteners, and heav-

ily spiced dishes. Wait 10 days after the burning is gone before reintroducing these foods and drinks—one at a time—into your diet.

Supplements of vitamin C (500 mg every two hours) and vitamin A (25,000 IU each day) may also aid recovery. But check with your doctor before taking the supplements. Vitamin C increases the acidity of urine, which hampers the growth of bacteria but can also interfere with the action of some antibiotics, making them less effective.

AT-HOME REMEDIES

◆ Take aspirin or ibuprofen to reduce inflammation and burning.
◆ Drink cranberry juice daily.

PREVENTION

◆ Practice good bathroom hygiene. Clean the anal area thoroughly after a bowel movement. Women should wipe from front to back to avoid spreading fecal bacteria to the urethra.
◆ Urinate as soon as possible when you feel the urge, and make sure you empty your bladder completely each time.
◆ Wear cotton underwear and loose, nonbinding clothing that does not trap heat and moisture in the crotch.
◆ Drink plenty of liquids.

Women:
◆ Empty your bladder as soon as possible after intercourse to wash out any bacteria that may have been pushed into the urethra.
◆ Avoid using perfumed soaps, bubble baths, scented douches, and vaginal deodorants. These contain substances that can irritate the urethra and make it more vulnerable to infection.
◆ If you use a diaphragm for birth control, make sure it fits properly, and don't leave it in too long. ■

SYMPTOMS

◆ one or more bubbles of skin filled with clear fluid, ranging from pinpoint size to more than one-half inch in diameter. Depending on the cause, blistering may be accompanied by pain, inflammation, and itching.

CALL YOUR DOCTOR IF:

◆ the blistering is the result of contact with chemicals, and your skin continues to burn after flushing the area with water or saline solution. You need medical attention to counteract the irritating agent. *(See Emergencies/First Aid: Burns.)*

◆ the blistering results from a burn that has penetrated beyond the surface layer of skin. Some second-degree burns and all third- and fourth-degree burns are medical emergencies. *(See Emergencies/First Aid: Burns, and the Burns entry.)*

◆ your blister discharges white, yellow, or green pus, rather than clear fluid. The discharge is almost surely the result of an infection.

Most blisters form as a reaction to irritation or other damage to the skin from an external source, although some can result from a disease or other ailment. A single blister is usually the result of friction or a minor burn, typically on the hands, feet, or other exposed areas. Clusters of blisters may result from extensive burns, contact dermatitis, insect bites, viral infections, drug or chemical reactions, or autoimmune disorders.

CAUSES

Friction: Blisters can be caused by excessive rubbing of exposed skin, such as a tool handle against the hand or a new pair of shoes against the ankle. Unlike corns and calluses, which develop from prolonged rubbing, friction blisters come from brief, intense contact.

Burns: Flames, steam, or contact with a hot surface can raise blisters, as can excessive sunburn or exposure to other types of radiation.

Contact dermatitis: Skin may blister when it comes in contact with chemical irritants, cosmetics, and many plant and animal toxins. *(See Dermatitis, Poison Ivy, Insect and Spider Bites, Bee and Wasp Stings.)*

Drug reactions: Many people develop blisters as a reaction to taking certain oral and topical drugs. The most common agents are penicillins and the ACE inhibitor captopril. Before prescribing any new drugs, a doctor should ask you about any drug reactions you may have had in the past.

Autoimmune disorders: Of the various autoimmune disorders known to cause blistering, three are most prevalent. **Pemphigus vulgaris,** a potentially fatal skin disorder, causes blisters in the mouth that sometimes spread to the head and other parts of the body; the painful blisters become raw and crusted before bursting. **Bullous pemphigoid** causes less severe eruptions that heal faster and are not life-threatening; this condition is seen chiefly in the elderly. **Dermatitis herpetiformis** causes small, itchy blisters; it is a chronic condition that usually starts in early adulthood.

Infection: Blisters are a common symptom of many infectious illnesses, including chickenpox, cold sores, herpes simplex, shingles, and impetigo.

TREATMENT

Most blisters caused by friction or minor burns do not require a doctor's care. New skin forms underneath the affected area and the fluid is simply absorbed. Soothe ordinary friction blisters with vitamin E ointment or an aloe-based cream. Do not puncture a blister unless it is large, painful, or likely to be further irritated. If you have to pop it, use a sterilized needle or razor blade; put the point or edge in a flame until it is red hot, or rinse it in alcohol. Wash the area thoroughly, then make a small hole and gently squeeze out the clear fluid. A dab of hydrogen peroxide can help protect against infection. If the fluid is white or yellow, the blister is infected and needs medical attention. Do not remove the skin over a broken blister; the new skin underneath needs this protective cover. For blisters caused by chemical contact, disease, or an autoimmune disorder, see a doctor.

CONVENTIONAL MEDICINE

While many blisters heal on their own, a few types require special care. Blistering caused by toxic agents or disease must be treated not only to relieve immediate discomfort but also to address the underlying cause. Some cases of **pemphigus,** for example, can be treated with oral corticosteroids on an outpatient basis; others require both corticosteroids and antibiotics under hospital supervision.

ALTERNATIVE CHOICES

If your blister is purely pressure- or burn-related, various ointments and rinses can be effective in relieving minor discomfort. To make good use of other therapies, you must first determine the underlying cause of the blistering.

HERBAL THERAPIES

Two drops of chamomile *(Matricaria recutita)* oil in half a cup of water makes an excellent antiseptic to be used under a protective dressing. Blisters caused by herpes simplex respond to licorice *(Glycyrrhiza uralensis)* ointment.

HOMEOPATHY

Calendula ointment is a soothing, antiseptic dressing for all types of blisters. Cantharis (12x) taken three or four times a day may help relieve the pain of a burn. Rhus toxicodendron (12x) taken three or four times a day may relieve blistering from contact dermatitis and cold sores.

AT-HOME REMEDIES

◆ If you have a blister from friction or a minor burn, apply petroleum jelly to keep the skin soft. An ordinary adhesive bandage will keep a small blister protected; cover a large blister with a gauze pad and adhesive tape.

◆ When a blister breaks, wash the area with soap and water, then apply a mild antiseptic such as hydrogen peroxide. Cover with a bandage during the day to protect the new skin from friction and dirt. You can remove the bandage at night and expose the new skin to air so it hardens faster.

◆ If your skin is blistered by chemical contact, flush it immediately with plenty of water or a saline solution. If pain or itching persists, or if large blisters develop, call a doctor.

◆ Forget the old folk remedy about putting butter on burns and vinegar on blisters; both can aggravate the skin and may actually cause infection.

PREVENTION

◆ Jobs you do only occasionally, such as shoveling snow or raking leaves, are great for raising a blister or two; be sure to wear work gloves.

◆ Break in new shoes gradually, and put petroleum jelly or an adhesive bandage on areas that take the rub—before the blister happens.

◆ Wear socks with heels, not tube socks, which bunch up and cause blisters. Acrylic and other synthetic-fiber socks are good low-friction choices, but because they don't breathe as well as natural fibers, you should wash and dry your feet after wearing them to prevent athlete's foot. ■

SYMPTOMS

Blood clots normally produce no obvious symptoms. Complications from abnormal clots may cause various conditions and disorders.

- Sudden and isolated pain in an arm or leg—sometimes followed by skin discoloration, tingling, numbness, or a cold feeling just below the site of pain—suggests a large clot blocking blood circulation. If left untreated, gangrene (tissue death) could result.
- A hard, bluish lump in a vein may be caused by a large blood clot.
- Sudden partial or complete blindness in one eye may be due to a blood clot blocking a retinal artery.
- Violent dizziness, or vertigo, that impairs your ability to stand or walk may be caused by a small blood clot blocking a cerebral artery.

CALL YOUR DOCTOR IF:

- you suffer from angina or have any symptoms associated with stroke. The cause may be abnormal blood clotting.
- you experience sudden or persistent sensory impairment. Among the potential causes that should be investigated is blockage of a blood vessel.

Your blood flows freely through arteries as thick as your thumb and capillaries thinner than a hair. At the first sign of injury or trauma, blood thickens, or clots, and stanches its own flow at the site of the wound. Clotting is desirable, even vital, when a blood vessel is injured, but clot formation inside healthy blood vessels is abnormal and potentially life-threatening. Such clots are frequent complications of heart disease or venous diseases such as phlebitis.

A clot that forms in the heart or a blood vessel and stays there is called a **thrombus.** Tiny thrombi develop on blood vessel walls to heal minute injuries, then normally dissolve. If they don't dissolve, they not only can slow circulation but also can break loose or break apart and flow with the blood. A clot that travels and then becomes lodged at some point in a blood vessel is called an **embolus.** Emboli are less common than thrombi but potentially more dangerous.

The threat posed by an abnormal blood clot depends on both its size and its location. An obstructive clot in a cerebral artery, for example, can cause stroke. Blood clots in the arteries supplying the heart—the coronary arteries—are the major cause of heart attack. Tiny blood clots in arteries of the eye can lead to loss of vision. An embolus in the lungs that blocks a pulmonary artery can cause severe shortness of breath and even death.

CAUSES

Blood will coagulate inside blood vessels if vessel walls are damaged or if circulation becomes unusually sluggish, as in atherosclerosis. *(See also Circulatory Problems.)* Diseases such as phlebitis inflame the walls of blood vessels and promote abnormal clots. Clotting from sluggish blood flow is a common complication of bed rest and may even be brought on by lots of long-distance flying or driving. Pelvic vein thrombosis is an occasional complication of childbirth and is usually associated with uterine or pelvic infections.

Abnormal clotting is sometimes linked to a congestive heart muscle disease that prevents the heart from pumping blood effectively. In addition, blood may clot if it is diseased or altered by certain conditions. A blood disorder called thrombo-cythemia, for example, causes increased production of platelets, the tiny blood cells that help clotting, resulting in overclotting. Factors that may contribute to clot formation include smoking, use of oral contraceptives, poor nutrition, obesity, varicose veins, and many other diseases.

TREATMENT

CONVENTIONAL MEDICINE

In some circumstances, drug therapy is prescribed to reduce the risk of abnormal clotting. A doctor may prescribe aspirin for patients at risk for embolisms or thrombosis. During critical care, streptokinase may be used to dissolve existing clots in areas such as the heart or lungs. After surgery, intravenous heparin may be used to prevent clotting or inhibit deep vein thrombosis. Blood clots may be removed during cardiovascular surgery, but surgery merely to remove clots is justified only in acute cases, such as impending tissue death.

ALTERNATIVE CHOICES

If you take anticoagulant drugs, ask your doctor about potential contraindications before starting any herbal or vitamin therapies.

BODY WORK

If the source of clotting is in your legs and is caused by poor circulation, **massage** therapy can be beneficial. If you have phlebitis, massage should always be done by a trained therapist to avoid dislodging a clot in a blood vessel.

HERBAL THERAPIES

Cayenne (*Capsicum frutescens*) and ginkgo (*Ginkgo biloba*) are thought to dissolve fibrin, a protein active in clot formation. Turmeric (*Curcuma longa*), bilberry (*Vaccinium myrtillus*), ginger (*Zingiber officinale*), grape-skin extract, and gugulipid, an extract of myrrh (*Commiphora molmol*), are believed to reduce platelet stickiness. Garlic (*Allium sativum*) and onion (*Allium cepa*) are said to do both, as is bromelain, a pineapple enzyme.

BITES THAT CURE

Vampire bat saliva, leech saliva, and copperhead venom sound like ingredients in a witch's brew, but they may wind up saving human lives. Scientists have found enzymes in all three fluids that keep blood from clotting. The enzymes give the leech and vampire bat ample time to feed on their victims' blood; for the snake, they help venom spread quickly through the victim's bloodstream. For the rest of us, synthesized versions of the same enzymes could mean new antidotes for potentially harmful blood clots.

NUTRITION AND DIET

If you want to condition your blood naturally, some authorities recommend eating more fish, believing that some fish oils make blood platelets less sticky. Certain vitamins and minerals may also act as natural anticoagulants. Ask your doctor or licensed nutrition therapist about supplemental vitamin E and magnesium to prevent abnormal clots from forming.

PREVENTION

◆ Eat a balanced diet low in saturated fats and high in fruits, vegetables, and natural fiber.
◆ Exercise regularly to stimulate circulation and keep extra pounds at bay.
◆ Some doctors recommend daily doses of aspirin for patients at risk of abnormal clotting. But because aspirin is a powerful drug, never take it on a regular basis without a doctor's prescription.
◆ If scheduled for surgery, ask your doctor about administering heparin during and after the operation. If possible, gentle exercise during recuperation will promote good circulation. ∎

SYMPTOMS

While recovering from surgery, an infection, or a wound, a person may suffer blood poisoning or septic shock. Symptoms are described below.

◆ High fever and chills, rapid breathing, headache, and nausea may indicate an attack of blood poisoning, or **septicemia.**

◆ Severe chills, low blood pressure, loss of appetite, and possibly loss of consciousness are potential signs of **septic shock**.

◆ Red lines extending from a boil can be a sign of blood poisoning.

CALL YOUR DOCTOR IF:

◆ your symptoms suggest blood poisoning; you should have immediate medical attention to stop the spread of infection and to prevent **septic shock.**

◆ you experience severe chills, have a noticeable drop in blood pressure, and your skin becomes pale, cold, and clammy. You may be going into **septic shock** and need emergency medical attention.

Blood poisoning, or **septicemia,** is a serious secondary infection that occurs when bacteria from an infected site somewhere on your body invade your bloodstream. *(See Infections.)* If bacteria continue to multiply without being stopped by your immune system, you run the risk of **septic shock,** a potentially life-threatening condition.

Blood poisoning occurs most frequently in people who have just had surgery or other invasive treatment and in people whose immune systems are weakened by an acute or chronic ailment. Both blood poisoning and septic shock require immediate treatment to stop the spread of infection and to ensure full recovery.

CAUSES

Blood poisoning is almost always a complication of an infection and occurs when bacteria escape from the primary site and enter the bloodstream. Both the bacteria that cause the infection and endotoxins released by your body's immune system to battle those bacteria impede the blood flow to your body tissues. This triggers fever and chills—the characteristic symptoms of acute **septicemia.** If the poisoning is not brought under control by the body's immune system or by medical intervention, **septic shock** begins.

Although blood poisoning can result from infected surgical incisions, wounds, or burns, other types of infection can release enough bacteria into your blood to create septicemia. Such conditions may range from urinary tract infections or pneumonia to boils and abscessed teeth or gum problems. Unfortunately septicemia is on the rise in hospitals: As the number of patients undergoing invasive procedures for testing and surgery increases, the bacteria responsible for septicemia are continually evolving new strains that are immune to conventional antibiotics.

In rare cases, blood poisoning develops from eating unpasteurized dairy foods, including certain soft cheeses, that contain the bacterium *Listeria monocytogenes.* Eating raw oysters or other seafood that is infected with the bacterium *Vibrio vulnificus* can result in lethal septicemia for members of certain high-risk groups, such as people with liver disease, iron imbalances, and weakened immune systems.

DIAGNOSTIC AND TEST PROCEDURES

If your doctor thinks you have blood poisoning, your symptoms will be evaluated and your blood tested to identify the bacteria responsible. If symptoms indicate septic shock, you will be hospitalized; your blood will be tested for bacteria, blood gas levels, and other indicators; and you may need an electrocardiogram (ECG) to check for irregular heartbeat patterns.

TREATMENT

If you have blood poisoning or septic shock, full recovery demands professional medical treatment. Alternative treatments may help to speed your recovery and increase your resistance to bacterial infection in the future.

CONVENTIONAL MEDICINE

Once the bacteria that have caused the blood poisoning are identified, your physician will give you oral or intravenous antibiotics to fight the infection and may choose to drain and disinfect the infected area. If you develop septic shock, you will need emergency treatment and intravenous antibiotics, which may include penicillins, cephalosporins, or aminoglycosides. Until you recover completely, you will probably need to stay in a hospital so that you can be monitored for potential complications.

ALTERNATIVE CHOICES

Although you must have immediate medical treatment for blood poisoning and septic shock, alternative therapies may assist recovery and strengthen the immune system to help prevent recurrence.

HERBAL THERAPIES

To stimulate the bacteria-destroying function of your white blood cells, simmer 2 tsp echinacea (*Echinacea* spp.) in a cup of water for 15 minutes; drink a cupful three times a day. Eat garlic (*Allium sativum)* for its antibacterial and antiviral action, or take three garlic capsules three times daily.

PREVENTION

◆ If you develop a mouth infection, see your dentist for treatment or referral to a specialist. To speed recovery from an abscessed tooth, apply a warm-water compress, eat soft foods, floss, and rinse regularly with warm salt water.

◆ If you develop a boil, place a warm-water compress on it for 20 to 30 minutes three or four times daily until it bursts; this may take up to a week. Apply compresses for three days or until the boil is completely drained of pus.

◆ If the boil becomes infected or if red lines extend from it, see your doctor. An infected boil can cause septicemia, and squeezing an infected boil can spread the infection. ■

ACUPRESSURE

Pressure on Spleen 10 may stimulate your immune system. Bend your knee and locate the point two thumb widths from the top and in line with the inner edge of the kneecap, on the bulge of the muscle. Press with your thumb one minute. Repeat on the other leg.

To help fight blood infection, put your thumb on Spleen 6, four finger widths above your right inner anklebone, near the edge of your shinbone. Press gently with your thumb for one minute, then switch legs. Do not use this point if you are pregnant.

SYMPTOMS

- a distinctive, sweaty odor, especially from the armpits, groin, and feet; usually considered unpleasant.
- any unusual odor emitted from body tissues, different from a sweaty smell, but not necessarily unpleasant.

CALL YOUR DOCTOR IF:

- the odor persists after washing, using deodorants, or trying other treatments. Body odors that are unlike the easily recognizable odor of perspiration can be signs of systemic disorders. For example, a smell like nail polish remover may indicate diabetes; an ammonia-like smell may be a sign of liver disease.

Americans have an aversion to body odor. It is the source of much self-consciousness and locker-room humor. It also supports a huge industry selling soaps, fragrances, deodorants, and antiperspirants to a willing public. Many cultures, however, don't understand the problem. They consider body odors normal, acceptable, even erotic.

Body odor is a general term for what happens to sweat and other skin secretions when they are acted upon by naturally occurring bacteria. Two types of glands produce sweat, the eccrine glands and the apocrine glands. The eccrine glands are dispersed throughout the body but are concentrated in the armpits, palms of the hands, soles of the feet, and the forehead. When the body is overheated—from hot weather, physical exertion, or fever—the eccrine glands help regulate body temperature by expelling a solution of water and salts that evaporates and cools the skin.

The apocrine glands are concentrated in the armpits and around the groin. These glands develop during puberty and have nothing to do with temperature regulation; instead, they respond to such conditions as sexual arousal, nervousness, and anger, as well as to heat and exertion. The sweat they produce is rich in organic substances that attract bacteria and produce a strong odor. Scientists believe that such odors may have been recognized as sexual signals by our ancient ancestors, just as they are in most animals.

CAUSES

By itself, sweat doesn't have an odor. Only after sweat is acted upon by naturally occurring bacteria on the skin does a person develop what we all recognize as a sweaty smell. The smell is especially noticeable in the feet, armpits, and groin, because those areas have a high concentration of sweat glands. Also, shoes and clothing trap perspiration, encouraging bacterial activity.

Eating certain foods and taking certain drugs can also cause distinctive smells; the cancer-fighting medication tamoxifen, for instance, may induce a distinctive odor. Proteins and oils from foods such as onions and certain spices may cause you to give off their characteristic smells. Deficiencies in certain nutrients, such as zinc, may also contribute to body odor. Women are sometimes troubled by odors associated with menstruation, but most of these can be prevented with good hygiene.

Body odor that smells fruity—or like nail polish remover, ammonia, or maple syrup—may indicate the presence of a disease or metabolic problem. Disorders that may produce unusual body odor include fungal infections, liver disease, kidney disease, diabetes, and various gastrointestinal problems. A person who has a persistent, nonsweaty smell should be checked by a doctor to diagnose and treat the underlying cause. *(See Sweating, Excessive.)*

TREATMENT

The most effective way to rid your body of odors is to wash with soap and water, sometimes more than once a day. To help control the bacterial activity responsible for a sweaty smell, wash with an antibacterial soap. Deodorants containing mild antibacterial agents and scents help to slow bacterial action and cover up underarm odor, but they don't stop perspiration. To do that, you have to use an antiperspirant that blocks eccrine glands and suppresses their function. If you choose an antiperspirant, be patient; it must be used daily for about a week to provide maximum effectiveness.

You should be aware that antiperspirants contain metallic salts that can be absorbed by the skin and may cause irritation. If that happens, discontinue use and try another product, preferably one with different active ingredients. Many authorities discourage the use of antiperspirants altogether. They contend that people should not try to prevent or reduce sweating at all, since it is one of the body's natural processes.

CONVENTIONAL MEDICINE

To control unusually persistent, profuse sweating, a condition called **hyperhidrosis,** a doctor may recommend a prescription antiperspirant contain-ing a high concentration of an ingredient such as aluminum chloride. These products must be used with care because they can cause skin irritation.

ALTERNATIVE CHOICES

Tablets containing chlorophyll, a natural plant product, are sold as a deodorant that can be taken orally. Dusting the underarms and toes with baking soda, a good natural deodorant, also helps absorb odor. Crystallized mineral salts to control body odor are sold in health and cosmetic stores.

HERBAL THERAPIES

Preparations containing essential oils of rosemary (*Rosmarinus officinalis*) and thyme (*Thymus vulgaris*) are recommended as herbal deodorants and can be used as antibacterial washes.

NUTRITION AND DIET

Excessive sweating may be linked to a zinc deficiency. Taking a 30- to 60-mg zinc supplement daily may help resolve the problem.

AT-HOME REMEDIES

◆ Bathe, shower, or wash yourself thoroughly every day. Use a mild underarm deodorant or antiperspirant if you wish, or sprinkle baking soda under your arms and between your toes after drying off.

◆ Change, wash, and dry-clean your clothes often, especially underwear, socks or stockings, and anything worn next to the skin. In hot weather, avoid tight clothing and wear sandals, with or without socks.

◆ Cotton clothes and leather shoes let perspiration evaporate faster than synthetic materials.

◆ Excessive body hair helps to retain sweat and bacteria, so one way to minimize body odor is to shave under the arms. ■

BOILS

SYMPTOMS

- The first stage of a boil is an inflamed, painful, sometimes throbbing nodule under the skin, most often appearing on the face, neck, buttocks, armpits, or—rarely—a woman's nipple.
- After several days, the boil develops into a raised, reddish sore with a white or yellow center; it may be extremely painful because of pus buildup under the skin.
- A clump of boils is called a **carbuncle;** a boil on the eyelid is a sty.

CALL YOUR DOCTOR IF:

- the boil causes excessive pain; you may want a doctor to lance and drain it.
- the inflammation is accompanied by a fever, or the boil appears on your lip, nose, cheeks, forehead, or spine; any infection in those locations places you at risk of a secondary infection, by spreading bacteria internally through the bloodstream to the spine or the brain.
- you think you have a **carbuncle.** This is a serious condition that should be treated with antibiotics.
- You have a boil that is very tender, particularly if it has red lines radiating from it, or if you have fever and chills; the infection may have spread.

A boil, or **furuncle,** may look like a nasty pimple but in fact is the result of a staph infection that has invaded a blocked hair follicle or, occasionally, an oil gland. *(See Acne.)* In the beginning a boil is red and tender; after a week to 10 days pus collects under the skin, causing the center of the boil to take on a whitish color. Pus is actually a mass of white blood corpuscles—which the body's immune system has sent to fight the infection—mixed with bacteria and dead skin cells. The boil can become quite swollen and painful before the skin breaks, the pus drains, and the sore clears. A **carbuncle** is a collection of boils. Before the advent of antibiotics earlier in this century, a carbuncle was considered a potentially life-threatening condition.

CAUSES

The staph bacteria that cause boils typically enter the body through cuts, scratches, and other breaks in the skin. Various factors can cause people to be predisposed to boils, including immune problems; diabetes; exposure to certain industrial chemicals; overuse of corticosteroids; treatment of skin lesions with petroleum-based products; and general poor health, hygiene, or nutrition.

TREATMENT

Most boils can be treated at home simply by washing the infected area with antibacterial soap and applying hot compresses, which help bring the boil to a head. Over-the-counter topical antibiotics are also effective in limiting the spread of bacterial infection. Do not squeeze or lance the boil yourself; most boils burst of their own accord after about two weeks. When they do, wash the area gently until no more pus appears, then cover with an adhesive bandage to avoid reinfection and to prevent drained pus from reaching other skin areas and spreading the infection. Be sure to wash your hands thoroughly, and disinfect towels.

CONVENTIONAL MEDICINE

If the pain is severe, or if a boil refuses to break, a doctor can lance and drain it under sterile conditions. To treat a severe outbreak, a doctor may prescribe an oral antibiotic such as erythromycin or dicloxacillin.

ALTERNATIVE CHOICES

Boils have plagued humans for centuries, and humans have countered with all sorts of remedies. Use caution when trying alternative remedies on your skin, because the wrong treatment may actually aggravate an infection.

AYURVEDIC MEDICINE

Boiled onions—wrapped in a cloth to protect your skin—are said to help bring a boil to a head.

CHINESE HERBS

Chinese herbal medicine focuses on reducing heat in the body, which is thought to cause boils. Try drinking tea made from dandelion *(Taraxacum mongolicum),* chrysanthemum flower *(Chrysanthemum indicum),* or violet *(Viola yedoensis).*

HERBAL THERAPIES

Herbal remedies for boils abound. To fight inflammation, you can choose among an over-the-counter ointment made with marsh mallow *(Althaea officinalis),* a poultice of slippery elm *(Ulmus fulva),* and a tincture of blue flag *(Iris versicolor)* or myrrh *(Commiphora molmol).*

To fight infection, apply tea tree oil *(Melaleuca spp.)* to the boil four to six times a day. Essential oils of bergamot *(Citrus bergamia),* lavender *(Lavandula officinalis),* chamomile *(Matricaria recutita),* and sage *(Salvia officinalis)* are also recommended for their antibacterial properties. Goldenseal *(Hydrastis canadensis)* contains an alkaloid known as berberine, for which bacteria-fighting properties are claimed; mix with distilled witch hazel *(Hamamelis virginiana)* to use as a wash.

HOMEOPATHY

If a boil comes up suddenly and is very red and hot, Belladonna (12x) three to four times daily may slow or halt the infection. For very painful boils try Hepar sulphuris, and for those that heal slowly use Silica, in the same potency and frequency.

NUTRITION AND DIET

Poor diet and certain nutritional deficiencies can suppress the body's immune system. Besides recommending a diet high in fresh fruits and vegetables, a nutritionist may suggest eating more garlic *(Allium sativum)* for its antiseptic properties, and foods high in zinc to enhance the immune system. You can accomplish this through your diet, or you can take up to three garlic capsules and a 45-mg zinc supplement daily.

AT-HOME REMEDIES

◆ Warm compresses or a warm Epsom salt bath will help draw the pus out of a boil.
◆ Men who get boils on the face should wash with antibacterial soap before shaving, and apply antibacterial cream when they finish.
◆ Resist the urge to lance or break a boil yourself; the result could be a severe secondary infection. Most boils break of their own accord; in some cases the boil heals without breaking and disperses under the skin.

PREVENTION

Breaks in the skin make a person susceptible to the infections that cause boils. Shaving nicks can cause them; so can contact sports, manual labor, insect bites, and a host of other everyday activities. Some tips:
◆ Wash regularly and take care of minor skin injuries promptly.
◆ Never share towels, bed linens, clothes, or athletic equipment with someone who has a boil or other infection. That person's clothes, bed linens, and towels should be washed daily in very hot water with detergent or bleach.
◆ Never squeeze a boil. The pus can spread the infection and cause complications, such as secondary infection or a **carbuncle**. ∎

SYMPTOMS

- a hard lump felt on the surface of a bone that may or may not be painful.
- pain or swelling in bones and joints, often more intense at night, and not necessarily associated with movement; the pain may be dull and constant, or may be felt only when pressure is applied.
- spontaneous bone fractures.
- fever, weight loss, fatigue, and impaired mobility, which sometimes occur in late stages of bone cancer.

Benign bone tumors are usually painless.

CALL YOUR DOCTOR IF:

- you have any of the symptoms described above, particularly an unexplained lump on a bone or chronic pain in bones or joints. You should be tested for bone cancer.
- you have persistent, unexplained back pain. You may simply have a back problem or backache; but if the symptoms do not respond to treatment, you may want to ask your doctor about being examined for a tumor in the spine.
- you suffer one or more bone fractures for no apparent reason. After treatment for the fracture, you may want to ask your doctor about being tested for **osteosarcoma** or osteoporosis.

Most primary bone tumors—those that originate in bone, cartilage, or other bone tissue—are benign, not cancerous. Primary bone cancer is rare, accounting for less than 1 percent of all cancers diagnosed in the U.S. each year. Far more common are secondary cancers that spread to bones from cancers in other parts of the body.

Primary bone cancer generally attacks young people, especially those who are unusually tall for their age. Of the main types, **osteosarcoma** accounts for nearly 60 percent of all primary bone cancers; it tends to affect teenagers, whose bones are in a stage of rapid growth. **Ewing's sarcoma** originates in bone marrow and occurs most often in children between the ages of 5 and 9 and in young adults between the ages of 20 and 30. **Chondrosarcoma** originates in cartilage and tends to attack middle-aged adults; other, less common types of bone cancer that occur in adults include fibrosarcoma, malignant giant cell tumor, and chordoma.

Primary bone cancer can be a lethal disease, but improved methods of detection and treatment have raised the five-year survival rate to more than 70 percent. The likelihood of cure depends largely on how early a tumor is detected and how rapidly the particular cancer tends to spread. The survival rate for secondary bone cancer varies. Benign tumors normally pose no long-term health risk.

CAUSES

In most cases of primary bone cancer, specific causes cannot be identified, but some cases may have genetic links. Certain chromosome abnormalities and a handful of rare, genetically linked diseases have been associated with bone cancer. Cancer is more likely to occur in bones that have been fractured or infected in the past. Exposure to specific carcinogens, such as chemicals in some kinds of dyes and paints, may increase the risk of bone cancer slightly. High-dose radiation and certain chemotherapeutic agents—particularly the so-called alkylating agents—may also be associated with some types of bone cancer.

DIAGNOSTIC AND TEST PROCEDURES

When symptoms suggest bone cancer, a doctor will run blood tests to eliminate other possible causes. X-rays and other imaging tests are used to identify bone tumors, and a biopsy is taken for a positive diagnosis. If a tumor is cancerous, tests are run to check for metastasis—the spread of cancer cells from one part of the body to another.

TREATMENT

When cancer is diagnosed, there is no acceptable substitute for conventional medical treatment. Alternative therapies may complement, but cannot replace, conventional care.

CONVENTIONAL MEDICINE

When possible, bone tumors are removed surgically. If the cancer is in an arm or a leg, the tumor can be removed without amputation in about 90 percent of cases; the surgeon then reconstructs the bone using a metal prosthesis. If amputation is unavoidable, the patient is usually fitted with an artificial limb.

Patients who have had bone cancer surgery are encouraged to begin physical therapy as soon as possible in order to overcome stiffness, improve mobility, and—if necessary—learn how to use their new artificial limb.

Radiation therapy and chemotherapy may be given before surgery to reduce the size of the tumor, and radiation may be used after surgery to kill stray cancer cells. Both radiation and chemotherapy are also used to treat inoperable bone cancers. Together they may keep the cancer from spreading but rarely bring about a full cure. Some doctors are experimenting with supplemental immunotherapy so that lower doses of radiation and chemotherapy can be given without compromising the overall effectiveness of treatment. For further information on these experimental treatments, see Cancer.

COMPLEMENTARY THERAPIES

Many alternative therapies have been shown to alleviate stresses associated with cancer and its treatment. Some body-work therapies, such as the **Feldenkrais** and **Aston-Patterning** methods, may be particularly beneficial to people adjusting mentally and physically to using an artificial limb. For further information on all complementary cancer therapies, see Cancer.

PREVENTION

Always heed safety warnings when using paint, solvents, pesticides, household cleaners, and other products that may contain carcinogenic chemicals. If you have ever been treated with radiation in the past, be alert for bone cancer symptoms and see a doctor at once if they occur. ∎

BONE SPURS

- stiffness or pain in the neck or back.
- "pins-and-needles" tingling in the neck, arms, or hands.
- dizziness, headache, difficulty in maintaining balance.
- sharp pain when putting weight on one or both feet.

CALL YOUR DOCTOR IF:

- back pain persists more than two or three days after taking an over-the-counter pain reliever and resting your back; you may have a degenerated disk.
- you experience intense shooting pain in the neck or back with even slight movement; you may have a bone spur pinching a nerve.

Almost everyone has waked up with a stiff neck or a backache at one time or another, especially after an injury or strenuous physical activity. Occasionally, however, you may experience sudden shooting pains that are not linked to a particular event. Problems like these often go away on their own, but sometimes they are signs of a more serious condition, such as arthritis.

A potential cause of such pains can be spurs, arising from abnormal growth in the ends of bones, especially in the spine or extremities. Bone spurs may cause excruciating pain when they interfere with nerves or muscles during normal activity.

CAUSES

Bone spurs are the result of changes over time to the ends of the bones that meet in joints, particularly the vertebrae that make up the spinal column. The fibrous cushions, or disks, between vertebrae tend to toughen and shrink with age *(see Disk Problems)*. Meanwhile, the tough, elastic cartilage at the ends of the bones progressively hardens.

As the space between the vertebrae becomes narrower, the bone tends to compensate for the loss by growing knobby enlargements, commonly called bone spurs. These growths are often seen in older people who have disk problems, but they also can occur in young adults—especially athletes, dancers, or laborers—who put unusual stress on muscles, ligaments, and tendons.

Unlike the rounded ends of bones in normal joints, spurs do not develop a layer of protective cartilage. In some cases, the new bony surfaces eventually smooth themselves through normal movement. But when they don't, bone spurs can rub against other bony surfaces, nerves, or blood vessels, causing pain and inflammation. When such bony growths appear in the upper vertebrae of the neck, the condition is called cervical osteoarthritis. Bony spurs can also be a cause of sciatica. A particularly bothersome condition occurs when a spur develops in the foot *(right)*, causing pain when standing or walking.

DIAGNOSTIC AND TEST PROCEDURES

Since back pain can have various causes, the usual test for complications due to spinal bone spurs is an x-ray or a CT scan of the affected area of the spine. Magnetic resonance imaging (MRI) or electromyography (EMG) is often used to check for impairment of nerves or muscles.

TREATMENT

The discomfort caused by bone spurs can be alleviated through rest, good back support, and drug therapy.

CONVENTIONAL MEDICINE

Your doctor will probably prescribe aspirin, ibuprofen, or another anti-inflammatory painkiller. To restrict movement and take pressure off a pinched nerve, you may have to wear an orthopedic collar or back brace. Only in severe cases is surgical removal of bone spurs necessary, but even relief through surgery may be temporary, since spurs can grow back.

HEEL PAIN

HEEL BONE

BONE SPUR

Bone spurs frequently develop at the base of the heel, where they can irritate nerves or tissue and cause pain with every step. Spurs in the foot are usually the result of unusual stress that prompts the normally smooth heel bone to sprout a knobby protrusion.

If a spur develops on a weight-bearing bone in the foot, the doctor may recommend a foam rubber pad for your shoe, with a hole cut directly under the spur to relieve pressure.

ALTERNATIVE CHOICES

Alternative therapies focus on pain relief and body work to improve range of movement.

CHIROPRACTIC

Chiropractic manipulation may help relieve the pain caused by a degenerative problem in the vertebrae. A chiropractor may also use physical therapy to relieve the discomfort of a heel spur.

HOMEOPATHY

For localized neck and back discomfort, a homeopath will typically prescribe a remedy based on whether the pain results from weather conditions, emotional stress, or mechanical strain. Before treating long-term conditions, the practitioner may conduct an analysis of the patient's genetic and psychological makeup.

YOGA

A trained instructor can prescribe effective **yoga** positions to relieve stress on affected areas and promote general relaxation and strengthening.

AT-HOME REMEDIES

When minor back pain strikes, take an over-the-counter painkiller. After inflammation has subsided, apply a heating pad or a hot-water bottle wrapped in a towel. Sleep on a firm mattress with a board under it, or on the floor with pillows beneath your head and calves.

PREVENTION

◆ Use your joints properly.
◆ Engage in moderate total-body exercises such as walking, bicycling, swimming, and tennis.
◆ Lose excess weight. ∎

BOWEL MOVEMENT ABNORMALITIES

Read down this column to find your symptoms. Then read across.

SYMPTOMS	AILMENT/PROBLEM
◆ passing hard and/or infrequent stools or straining to have a bowel movement.	◆ Constipation
◆ watery and/or frequent bowel movements.	◆ Diarrhea
◆ worms in the stool, perhaps appearing as light-colored threads; possible itching in the anal area.	◆ Pinworm, roundworm, or tapeworm infection
◆ alternating hard/infrequent and watery/frequent stools.	◆ Irritable bowel syndrome; colon tumor; diabetes; alternating use of laxatives and antidiarrheal drugs
◆ extremely foul-smelling, large stools; weight loss despite good appetite; abdominal pain.	◆ Pancreatic problems, possibly associated with celiac disease
◆ any visible blood in the stools.	◆ Many possibilities, including hemorrhoids, anal fissure, and colorectal cancer
◆ persistent thin, ribbonlike stools; possible anal bleeding.	◆ Possibly, colorectal cancer
◆ maroon-colored or black, tarry, metallic-smelling stools; possible abdominal pain.	◆ Bleeding from the upper or middle gastro-intestinal tract, caused by any of a number of ailments or use of certain medications
◆ stools that are either too hard or too watery; abdominal pain; flatulence; nausea; vomiting; fever.	◆ Appendicitis
◆ black or dark-red stools; vomiting with blood; easy bruising; spiderlike blood vessels on the skin; fatigue; yellowish skin and eyes; weight loss or gain; distended abdomen.	◆ Cirrhosis
◆ pale or chalky stools; dark-orange to tea-colored urine; yellowish skin and eyes; dull abdominal pain, fever, shaking, chills.	◆ Bile duct blocked by a gallstone; gallbladder disorder; liver disorder

WHAT TO DO	OTHER INFO
◆ Change to a high-fiber diet and drink at least eight glasses of water each day.	◆ Over 30 possible causes: irritable bowel, anal fissure, depression, and inactivity.
◆ Drink fluids copiously to replace those being lost. If diarrhea persists beyond 48 hours, call your doctor.	◆ More than a dozen causes, including flu and food poisoning.
◆ See your doctor; prescription medication can cure the infection.	◆ Wormwood (Artemisia absinthium) taken three times daily in a pill or a tea (pour 1 cup boiling water over $\frac{1}{2}$ tsp wormwood; steep for 10 minutes) is reported to cure many worm infestations.
◆ If you frequently use laxatives and anti-diarrheal drugs, gradually reduce your use until you can stop; otherwise, call your doctor without delay for proper diagnosis.	◆ Laxatives can mimic the abdominal pain of irritable bowel syndrome or a colon tumor. See Colorectal Cancer.
◆ See your doctor soon. You may need to eliminate all gluten-containing foods from your diet.	◆ If celiac disease prevents absorption of iron, vitamin B_{12}, or folic acid, take supplements.
◆ Call your doctor today—immediately if patient is a child or if bleeding is profuse.	◆ Never ignore anal bleeding; it can indicate colorectal cancer.
◆ Call your doctor today; an early and accurate diagnosis is essential.	◆ Treated early, colorectal cancer is curable; untreated, it can be fatal.
◆ Call your doctor today for a proper diagnosis; report any prescription or over-the-counter medications you are taking.	◆ A home test kit can determine if blood is in stools; maroon color may be from eating red foods such as beets.
◆ **Call your doctor or seek emergency care now.**	
◆ **Call your doctor or seek emergency medical help now;** cirrhosis may be life-threatening.	◆ Avoid alcohol, high-fat foods, and all drugs (except those your doctor prescribes) to enhance liver function.
◆ Adopt a low-fat diet. If abdominal pain is severe or any fever is present, see your doctor immediately. See Gallstones, Hepatitis.	◆ Vitamin K supplements may help alleviate symptoms.

Most brain tumors do not show symptoms until they attain a certain size.

Symptoms associated with increased pressure on the brain from a tumor include:
- persistent headaches that get worse over a period of weeks and are often more intense when lying down.
- vomiting, sometimes but not always accompanied by nausea.
- sudden onset of seizures.
- inexplicable changes in personality or mental ability.

Symptoms that vary according to the type and location of the tumor include:
- sudden vision loss, speech problems, or other changes in the senses.
- localized weakness or paralysis, especially in the limbs.
- impaired memory.
- loss of coordination or balance.

CALL YOUR DOCTOR IF:

- you experience any of the symptoms described above. Although other ailments can cause similar symptoms, persistent headaches that occur with vomiting, convulsions, or progressive loss of speech, sight, hearing, feeling, or limb function may indicate a brain tumor.

Primary brain cancer—cancer that originates in the brain itself—is rare, accounting for only 1 percent of all cancers and about 2.5 percent of all cancer deaths. However, one in four patients with cancer elsewhere in the body eventually develops metastatic, or secondary, brain cancer. Brain cancer can occur at any age, but most often it strikes young children and middle-aged adults.

Brain tumors whose cells do not spread are considered benign, in contrast to malignant tumors, or cancers, whose cells multiply uncontrollably and can spread throughout the body. But no brain tumor is harmless: Anything that takes up space in the skull, even a noncancerous growth, can exert pressure on delicate brain tissue, produce severe pain, cause irreversible neurological damage, and threaten life. The symptoms and prognosis for recovery vary according to the location of the tumor and the type of brain cells involved.

CAUSES

The causes of primary brain cancer are unknown. Sometimes it runs in families, implying a genetic link. Other research suggests ties to chemicals such as vinyl chloride, certain herbicides and pesticides, or overexposure to electromagnetic fields. A few rare diseases, such as tuberous sclerosis and multiple intestinal polyposis, are also associated with brain cancer (see Colorectal Cancer).

DIAGNOSTIC AND TEST PROCEDURES
Diagnosis of a brain tumor begins with a complete physical examination and neurological testing. Computed tomography (CT) and magnetic resonance imaging (MRI) scans will locate and identify a tumor. If taking a tissue biopsy is feasible, it can confirm or rule out the presence of cancer cells. X-rays and other tests determine whether cancer exists elsewhere in the body.

TREATMENT

While research for a cure continues, there is no acceptable substitute for conventional medical

TUMORS IN THE BRAIN

MENINGIOMA

GLIOBLASTOMA
MULTIFORME

Several kinds of tumors can develop in the brain. Meningiomas occur in the protective membrane covering the brain, not in brain tissue itself. They are usually benign and can often be removed surgically. Glioblastoma multiformes are malignant tumors that form directly in cerebral tissue. They are usually inoperable.

treatment for cancer. Although many alternative therapies—those outside mainstream medicine—can enhance the benefits of standard care, none is a proven cancer cure. Alternative cancer therapies should be considered potential complements to, but not replacements for, conventional care.

CONVENTIONAL MEDICINE

Curing brain cancer depends on where the tumor is located and how far the malignancy has spread. Advances in computer-assisted surgery now let surgeons treat cancers that were once considered inoperable. Whenever possible, a brain tumor is treated surgically. If it can be removed, the patient may recover fully. After surgery, radiation therapy and sometimes chemotherapy are prescribed to make sure stray cancer cells are killed. But some brain tumors are located too deep in the brain to be removed even partially without causing severe brain damage. In such cases, treatment is limited to chemotherapy and a refined radiation therapy that trains laser beams on the tu-

mor. Neither is likely to provide a cure, but they may slow the growth of cancer cells, control symptoms, and prolong the patient's life.

When cure is impossible, the main goals of treatment are to provide comfort and preserve neurological function. Various drugs, including analgesics, anticonvulsants, and corticosteroids, may be given to relieve pain, control seizures, and reduce brain swelling. Because tumors often cause residual brain damage, a patient may require physical or mental rehabilitative therapy.

For further information on radiation, chemotherapy, and other treatments, see Cancer.

COMPLEMENTARY THERAPIES

While many brain cancer sufferers can handle everyday activities, the strain of the disease and the side effects of radiation and chemotherapy may eventually be debilitating. A number of alternative therapies can provide relief from such stresses, among them **hydrotherapy, Therapeutic Touch, yoga, guided imagery, meditation,** and **biofeedback.** Various forms of body work, including **massage** and **reflexology,** may also help.

GENE THERAPY

Foreign genes—not scalpels or laser beams—may prove to be the ultimate weapon against brain cancer, if promising test results are confirmed. Scientists at the National Institutes of Health have been refining a type of gene therapy that kills brain cancer cells by altering them genetically. This ingenious therapy is designed to make cancer cells vulnerable to a cell-destroying drug, while leaving healthy brain cells alone and intact. When the therapy was tested on rats, tumors virtually disappeared in 11 of 14 animals. In the first human trial, tumors shrank significantly in 5 of 8 patients, all of whom had previously failed to respond to conventional treatment. While further testing and refinement are needed, this new gene therapy may hold great promise for the future. ∎

SYMPTOMS

In early stages, breast cancer usually has no symptoms. As a tumor progresses, you may note the following signs:

◆ swelling in the armpit.

◆ pain or tenderness in the breast.

◆ a lump in the breast; often the first apparent symptom of breast cancer, breast lumps are usually painless, although some may cause a prickly sensation. Lumps are usually visible on a mammogram long before they can be seen or felt.

◆ a noticeable flattening or indentation on the breast, which may indicate a tumor that cannot be seen or felt.

◆ any change in the contour, texture, or temperature of the breast; a reddish, pitted surface like the skin of an orange is symptomatic of advanced breast cancer.

◆ a change in the nipple, such as an indrawn or dimpled look, itching or burning sensation, or ulceration; scaling of the nipple is symptomatic of **Paget's disease,** a localized cancer.

◆ unusual discharge from the nipple that may be clear, bloody, or another color—usually caused by benign conditions but possibly due to cancer.

CALL YOUR DOCTOR IF:

◆ one or both breasts develop an abnormal lump or persistent pain, or look or feel abnormal. The cause could be something other than cancer but should be identified.

◆ you have swollen lymph glands in your armpits. Any such swelling could be associated with cancer.

Each month, a woman's breasts go through temporary changes associated with menstruation, and a lump may form. While 90 percent of these are not cancerous, any lump should be examined immediately. Lumps are most common in the lobules—small sacs that produce milk—or the ducts that carry milk to the nipple, but they occasionally start in nonglandular tissue. The two main categories of breast cancer are **lobular** and **ductal carcinomas.** Each has many subtypes.

Breast cancer usually begins with formation of a small, localized tumor. Some tumors are benign, meaning they do not invade other tissue; others are malignant, or cancerous. The potential for a malignant tumor to metastasize, or spread, is common to all cancer. Once such a tumor grows to a certain size, it is more likely to shed cells that spread to other parts of the body through the bloodstream and lymphatic system. Different types of breast cancer grow and spread at different rates; some take years to spread beyond the breast, while others move quickly.

Men can get breast cancer, but they account for less than half a percent of all cases. It is the most common cancer among women, who share a lifetime risk of one in nine. It constitutes one-sixth of all U.S. cancer cases and one-third of all cancers in women. It trails only colorectal and lung cancers as a cause of cancer death. Two of every three female breast cancer patients are over 50, and most of the rest are between 39 and 49.

Fortunately, breast cancer is very treatable if detected early. Localized tumors can usually be treated successfully before the cancer spreads; 9 cases out of 10 have a 5-year survival rate. Once the cancer begins to spread, getting rid of it completely is more difficult, although treatment can often control the disease for years. Improved screening procedures and treatment options mean that at least 7 out of 10 women with breast cancer will survive more than 5 years after initial diagnosis, and fully half will survive more than 10 years.

CAUSES

Although the precise causes of breast cancer are unclear, we know what the main risk factors are.

Still, most women considered at high risk for breast cancer do not get it, while many who do have no known risk factors. Among the most significant factors are advancing age and a family history of breast cancer. Risk increases slightly for a woman who has had a benign breast lump and increases significantly for a woman who has previously had cancer of the breast or the ovaries.

A woman whose mother, sister, or daughter has had breast cancer is more likely to develop the disease, particularly if more than one so-called first-order relative has been affected. Researchers have now identified a gene that they think is responsible for familial breast cancer: About 1 woman in 200 carries it. Having the gene predisposes a woman to breast cancer, but does not ensure that she will get it.

Generally, postmenopausal women—which usually means those past age 50—are more likely to get breast cancer than premenopausal women, and statistics suggest that African American women are more likely than Caucasians to get breast cancer before menopause.

A link between breast cancer and hormones is gradually becoming clearer. Researchers think that the greater a woman's exposure to the female hormone estrogen, the more susceptible she is to breast cancer. Basically, estrogen tells cells to divide; the more the cells divide, the more likely they are to be abnormal in some way—possibly becoming cancerous. A woman's exposure to estrogen and progesterone rises and falls during her lifetime, influenced by the age she starts and stops menstruating, the average length of her menstrual cycle, and her age at first childbirth. A woman's risk for breast cancer is increased if she starts menstruating before age 12, has her first child after 30, stops menstruating after 55, or has a menstrual cycle shorter or longer than the average 26 to 29 days. Taking hormones in the form of birth-control pills or hormone replacement therapy may also increase risk, although the evidence is inconclusive. Heavy doses of radiation therapy may also be a factor, but low-dose mammograms pose almost no risk.

The diet–breast cancer link is still debated. Obesity is a noteworthy risk factor, and drinking alcohol regularly may promote the disease. Many

YOGA EXERCISE AFTER BREAST SURGERY

1 Scar tissue resulting from breast cancer surgery may limit your range of arm motion. To keep the scar tissue and muscles stretched and strong, try **Climbing the Wall.** Begin by standing about a foot from a wall with your feet slightly apart and placing both hands on the wall.

2 Slowly slide both hands up the wall as far as you can, but stop immediately if you feel any pain. Repeat five times a day, with the goal of raising both arms above your head. As with any post-surgical exercise, always have your physician's approval and guidance.

studies have shown that women whose diets are high in fat are more likely to get the disease. Researchers suspect that if less than 20 percent of a woman's daily calories come from fat, her diet may protect her from developing breast cancer.

DIAGNOSTIC AND TEST PROCEDURES

Breast cancer responds to treatment best when it is detected early. In addition to having an annual medical checkup, all women should conduct monthly breast self-examinations (see Breast Problems). A baseline mammogram—a low-dose x-ray of the breast—is recommended for women between the ages of 35 and 40. Most women should also get a mammogram every other year beginning around age 40 and every year beginning at age 50. Women at risk for breast cancer should consult their doctor for the best schedule. Any risk of developing cancer from mammography is clearly offset by the benefits: Breast lumps can be identified on a mammogram up to two years before they can be felt.

Several tests can help distinguish a benign lump from a malignant tumor. Feeling the lump may provide clues: A benign cyst may feel like a round, slippery bean, whereas a tumor may feel

B

thicker and may cause dimpling of the skin above it. Because malignant and benign lumps tend to have different physical features, imaging tests such as mammography and ultrasonography can often rule out cancer. The only way to confirm cancer is to perform needle aspiration or a biopsy and to test the tissue sample for cancer cells.

In the event of malignancy, you and your doctor need to know how far along the cancer is. Various tests are used to check for the presence and likely sites of metastasis. Cancer cells can be analyzed for the presence or absence of hormone receptors, to find out if the cancer is likely to respond well to hormone therapy. Other tests can help predict the likelihood of metastasis and the potential for recurrence after treatment.

TREATMENT

If you have breast cancer, do what you can as soon as you can to get rid of it. But before making treatment decisions, research your options. Ask questions of your doctor, other specialists, and people who have had the disease, and seek a second opinion at a major cancer treatment center. Find a doctor you trust, and don't rush your decision. A brief delay between diagnosis and treatment will not compromise the effectiveness of treatment.

CONVENTIONAL MEDICINE

The options for treating breast cancer depend on how advanced the cancer is, how old the patient is, and how healthy she is otherwise. If possible, breast cancer is treated surgically, followed usually by some combination of radiation therapy, chemotherapy, or hormone therapy.

The standard surgical procedure for breast cancer was once **radical mastectomy**—total removal of the breast and the surrounding fat, muscle, and lymph nodes. For many women whose breast cancer is detected early and is still localized, **lumpectomy**—removal of the cancerous lump and the lymph nodes under the arm—is now the preferred treatment. Followed by appropriate radiation therapy, chemotherapy, and hormone therapy, lumpectomy has proved as effec-

RECONSTRUCTIVE BREAST SURGERY

Lumpectomy is not disfiguring the way breast surgery once was, but even mastectomy need not be permanently disfiguring. While some women choose to wear a prosthesis after a mastectomy, others opt for reconstructive surgery. For three decades, the most common reconstructive surgery involved implanting a silicone-filled prosthesis behind skin or muscles in the chest wall. Some women claim to have developed debilitating immune disorders from leaking silicone implants, and in 1992 such implants were removed from the market. Since then, several scientific studies have found no link between immune disorders and silicone breast implants, although they have confirmed lesser, yet undesirable, side effects. Saline-filled implants are now widely used. Surgeons can also transfer tissue from the abdomen, back, or elsewhere to construct artificial breast replacements. The cosmetic results are impressive, but the surgery is costly and complex, produces additional scarring, and may cause weakness in the area from which tissue is removed.

tive as radical mastectomy for early breast cancer and is much less disfiguring.

Faced with surgery, some women choose **modified radical mastectomy** over lumpectomy and radiation therapy. In this procedure the tumor and surrounding breast tissue are removed, but most of the muscle on the chest wall is left intact—which is less disfiguring than radical mastectomy.

For breast cancer that has metastasized and for recurrent breast cancer, radiation therapy and chemotherapy are the primary modes of treatment. Hormone therapy may also be beneficial for cancers that are hormone responsive; of the estrogen-suppressing drugs in use, tamoxifen is most widely used. Meanwhile, researchers are exploring treatment of breast cancer with various forms of immunotherapy; by manipulating the body's immune system, they hope to improve its natural resistance to cancer.

For further information on radiation, chemotherapy, and other treatments, see Cancer.

COMPLEMENTARY THERAPIES

As with any cancer, there is no acceptable alternative to conventional medical treatment. The therapies listed should be considered preventive measures or complementary options to be pursued in conjunction with standard medical care.

LIFESTYLE

Regular aerobic exercise may offer some protection against a woman's developing breast cancer. Studies have found that women who exercised vigorously and often were at least half as likely as nonexercisers to get breast cancer. Exercise can also help breast cancer patients better tolerate the side effects of radiation or chemotherapy.

MIND/BODY MEDICINE

Relaxing the mind can certainly help alleviate the mental and physical stresses of cancer. Besides pursuing such individual mind/body approaches as **meditation** or **yoga,** many people benefit from structured support-group therapy. One retrospective study over 10 years of 86 women with metastatic breast cancer showed that those who participated in support-group therapy and self-hypnosis while receiving conventional treatment felt better and lived 18 months longer on average than those who got conventional care alone.

NUTRITION AND DIET

Your diet can play an important role in breast cancer prevention. In principle, dietary fats may increase your risk of developing breast cancer, and fruits, vegetables, and grains may help to reduce the risk. It's a good idea to make whole-milk dairy products, meat, and foods fried at high tempera-

tures occasional treats rather than staples. You can enliven your menus by sampling different kinds of fresh fruits and vegetables and basing new dishes on whole grains and legumes. This way, you're bound to get plenty of body-cleansing fiber, along with vitamins and minerals thought to protect against breast cancer, specifically vitamins A, C, D, and E, and calcium, selenium, and iodine. Some doctors recommend that breast cancer patients and survivors take antioxidant supplements.

Certain plant foods contain phytoestrogens, weak plant estrogens that may be particularly useful against hormone-sensitive breast cancers. In theory, phytoestrogens block the uptake of normal estrogen in breast tissue. Withholding estrogen may reduce the likelihood of cancer and, if malignancy exists, may reduce the rate at which cancer cells multiply. Wheat, soybeans, olives, plums, carrots, apples, yams, and coconuts are among the foods that contain phytoestrogens.

AT-HOME CARE

After breast surgery, a regular routine of simple exercises *(page 205)* will help to restore your mobility and reduce muscle stiffness. To minimize potential discomfort from radiation therapy, avoid wearing a bra or clothes that may irritate the area, keep your skin clean and well aired, and use only those skin lotions, creams, and deodorants recommended by your doctor.

PREVENTION

◆ Check your breasts once a month, have a thorough medical checkup once a year, and have mammograms annually if you are age 50 or older. Start mammograms earlier if you have a family history of breast cancer.
◆ Make fruits, vegetables, grains, and fish the mainstays of your diet.
◆ If you practice contraception, ask your doctor about the pros and cons of estrogen-based birth-control pills.
◆ If you are at high risk for breast cancer, talk to your doctor or gynecologist about managing menopause symptoms without estrogen pills. ■

(see below and page 210).

SYMPTOMS

- pain or a feeling of fullness in one or both breasts, most likely caused by premenstrual swelling.
- pain accompanied by redness and warmth or a discharge from the nipple; this may indicate an infection. Discharge can also signal a benign growth or breast cancer.
- a lump that is movable and feels unattached to the chest wall; you may have a **cyst** or a **fibroadenoma.**
- a lump that is hard, is not movable, or feels attached to the chest wall, with or without pain, perhaps with dimpling or puckering of the breast; this may be a sign of breast cancer.

CALL YOUR DOCTOR IF:

- you notice any kind of new or unusual lump in your breasts, especially one that remains throughout your menstrual cycle. Although most lumps are harmless, in rare instances they may signal infection or cancer. Have your doctor check any lump.

The female breast is an organ that changes with puberty, with the monthly menstrual cycle, and with pregnancy; it also continues to change with age. Most changes in your breast are perfectly normal and no cause for concern. However, you may experience any of several conditions that require medical attention. Chief among these are **breast pain** and masses or **lumps** *(see below and page 210).*

Starting at puberty, you should examine your breasts every month, so that you are familiar with their structure and can detect any new masses or lumps. Premenstrual changes can cause temporary thickening that disappears after the period, so it is best to check your breasts about a week after your period. If you are no longer menstruating, examine your breasts monthly on a day you will remember, such as the day corresponding to your birthday.

Mammograms—detailed x-ray pictures of the breasts—can reveal tumors too tiny to be felt by hand. There is disagreement and no small controversy as to when a woman should begin getting routine mammograms: Some doctors say between ages 35 and 40; others say not until age 50. A typical pattern is every other year beginning around age 40, then increasing the frequency to once a year at age 50. If you have a family history of breast cancer, especially in your mother or sister, your physician may advise a different schedule.

BREAST PAIN

Breast pain can have many causes, including the normal swelling of breast tissue during the menstrual cycle. Other causes include infection or injury; growths, including cancer; and perhaps diet.

The general swelling of breast tissue with the menstrual period can be painful, but it is not dangerous, and no treatment is necessary if you can tolerate the discomfort. Each monthly cycle brings about hormonal changes, including increases in estrogen and progesterone, that bring more fluid into the breasts, expanding tissue, stretching nerve fibers, and producing pain. Some women experience this painful swelling just before their periods, with symptoms subsiding near the end of the menstrual flow. Others experience it as a side effect of birth-control pills.

Another possible reason for breast pain is decreased progesterone levels during the menstrual cycle. Several studies have shown a correlation between cyclic breast pain and low progesterone levels.

Trauma and infection in the breast produce the same symptoms you would see elsewhere in your body, except that in your breast, infections tend to become walled off from surrounding tissue, producing small abscesses. This may give them the appearance of cysts. Infections occur almost exclusively in breast-feeding mothers. If you suspect you have an infection, see your doctor.

Cysts may produce pain *(see Lumps, page 210)*, but breast cancer rarely does—although pain does not rule out the possibility of cancer.

TREATMENT

Practitioners of both conventional and alternative medicine use diet and nutrition to prevent and treat monthly swelling of the breasts. Both would encourage you to maintain a healthy weight and eat a balanced diet as good preventive medicine. Because salt can contribute to fluid retention and thus worsen symptoms, you should restrict your salt intake near your period. For some women, eliminating caffeine and related substances, such as methylxanthines (found in chocolate and tea), can alleviate breast pain. Both conventional and alternative practitioners may suggest wearing a bra, even 24 hours a day, to reduce breast movement and lessen the discomfort until the tenderness passes.

CONVENTIONAL MEDICINE

In recent years, some conventional doctors have suggested vitamin E supplements, in daily doses of up to 800 IU, to treat breast pain not caused by cancer. In addition, a conventional physician may suggest relieving pain with an analgesic such as aspirin or ibuprofen.

If these treatments don't help, your doctor may prescribe treatment with a hormone such as danazol, which has been shown to help relieve breast pain. You might also be given progesterone, since some studies suggest a lack of progesterone may contribute to breast pain. The anticancer drug tamoxifen is also prescribed. If one of these drugs doesn't work or gives you troublesome side effects, your doctor may switch you to another. However, do not use these drugs if you are trying to become pregnant.

All of the hormone treatments above have side effects; those of danazol, a male hormone, include headache, nausea, menstrual irregularity, and weight gain, as well as masculinization (increased hair growth and, rarely, deepening of the voice) that may not be reversible. Your doctor may be reluctant to use tamoxifen because of uncertainty about its long-term effects on cancer risk, bone density, gynecological growths, and blood clots. In fact, most patients can get relief without strong drugs; the greatest benefit comes from eliminating caffeine.

Breast infections are treated with antibiotics. If an abscess exists, your doctor may also make a small incision to drain it. If this doesn't work, minor surgery is the next step.

ALTERNATIVE CHOICES

In addition to the dietary changes and supplements cited above, alternative-medicine practitioners frequently treat breast pain with higher doses of nutritional supplements and with herbs.

HERBAL THERAPIES

Evening primrose oil *(Oenothera biennis)*, although not approved in the United States for treating breast pain, is used in Europe and has proved effective. You can take a 500 mg capsule three times a day, every day if necessary. This treatment has fewer side effects than the hormone therapies often prescribed in conventional medicine.

NUTRITION AND DIET

Vitamin E effectively relieves breast pain. How it does this is unclear, but researchers do know that this vitamin affects blood clotting; if you are

Check your breasts monthly, 7 to 10 days after your menstrual period ends. (It's easiest in the shower, using soap to smooth your skin.) Look for dimpling, then try either the spiral or grid method below, using light pressure to check for lumps near the surface and firm pressure to explore deeper tissues. Squeeze each nipple gently; if there is any discharge—especially if it is bloody—consult your doctor.

1 With either the spiral or the grid method, begin by raising your arm, and always use the flat surface of your fingers. Apply light pressure by barely depressing the surface of your skin *(left);* this will enable you to feel for any tiny lumps near the surface.

2 To apply firm pressure, press deeply into the tissue, again using the flat surface of your fingers. Be aware of any sensitive areas, unusual lumps, or thickened tissue.

3 To use the spiral method, begin at the top of your breast near your armpit and follow the pattern illustrated at left. Apply light pressure first as you work in toward the nipple. Repeat the same pattern using firm pressure.

4 To use the grid method, imagine the pattern of squares illustrated at left, and follow the direction indicated by the arrows. Make a tiny spiral in each square, using first light pressure, then firm pressure.

taking a blood thinner, consult your doctor before taking any vitamin E. Alternative practitioners sometimes recommend dosages up to 1,200 IU, but many women find relief with only 400 IU a day.

Because fat in the diet is associated with estrogen production, you can reduce estrogen levels in your body by eating a low-fat diet.

AT-HOME REMEDIES

For pain relief, try applying a warm castor-oil pack to your breast. Saturate a flannel cloth with high-grade castor oil, put it on the breast, and cover it with plastic wrap and a towel; apply heat to the pack with a heating pad or hot-water bottle for 20 to 30 minutes.

LUMPS

Breast lumps come in many forms, including **cysts, adenomas,** and **papillomas.** They differ in size, shape, and location, as well as in causes and treatment. About half of all women have lumpy breasts, or fibroadenosis, which is sometimes associated with hormonal changes related to the menstrual cycle. Most lumps are benign and do not signal cancer; however, any time you find a new or unusual lump, have your doctor check it to make sure it is not cancerous or precancerous. For more information, see Breast Cancer.

Researchers are studying the incidence of breast lumps in women taking birth-control pills or using hormone replacement therapy (HRT). In HRT, women take varying amounts of the hormones estrogen and progestin to alleviate the symptoms of menopause and to reduce the risk of cardiovascular disease. While the evidence is inconclusive, your doctor may have concerns about HRT and breast lumps. An additional concern is that using HRT changes breast structure, increasing the breast density and making mammograms harder to read and evaluate. This could make detecting cancer more difficult.

Cysts, which can be large or small, are benign fluid-filled sacs. They sometimes occur cyclically, and they may be painful. The best tool for distinguishing a cyst from a solid tumor is ultrasound; a needle biopsy may also be done.

With the cessation of menstruation at menopause, many cystic lumps diminish or disappear; therefore, you should immediately have your doctor check any lumps that form after menopause.

Fibroadenomas are the most common benign breast tumors seen in women under age 40 and are occasionally seen in adolescents. Fibroadenomas are usually round, several centimeters across, and mobile. They can be positively identified only by biopsy, which is recommended for anyone over age 20.

Nipple adenomas are tumors of the nipple area. They vary in appearance, sometimes recur after surgical removal, and are sometimes but not usually associated with cancer.

An intraductal **papilloma** is a relatively uncommon small growth in the lining of the milk ducts near the nipple. Usually seen in women over 40, papillomas produce a discharge, which may be bloody.

TREATMENT

CONVENTIONAL MEDICINE

For breast lumps, treatment and diagnosis are frequently related. For example, your doctor may insert a needle into a **cyst** and draw out fluid, both to examine the fluid and to eliminate the cyst. If the fluid is clear and the cyst disappears, your doctor will probably diagnose it as a benign cyst and undertake no further treatment. Many physicians take the added precaution of having the fluid checked by cytology—a pathologist's examination of the cells. If a lump does not disappear and is still present after your next menstrual period, your doctor will want to re-examine you.

If the fluid extracted from a suspected cyst is bloody or if little or no fluid can be extracted, this is a cause for concern, and a biopsy may be indicated to check for cancer.

Fibroadenomas can be diagnosed only by biopsy. Surgical removal, usually in a same-day surgical procedure, is considered the only treatment.

Nipple adenomas are surgically removed because they are sometimes associated with breast cancer. Intraductal **papillomas** are surgically removed before they grow enough to block the milk ducts.

Some conventional doctors recommend eliminating caffeine to shrink breast cysts, but the only study completed on caffeine's effect showed no connection. Some studies have suggested (although none has proved) a link between dietary fat—especially saturated fat—and benign lumps, as well as breast cancer. Limiting fat may help shrink or eliminate lumps.

ALTERNATIVE CHOICES

Alternative medicine emphasizes prevention as an effective way to manage breast problems. Diet and nutritional supplements are the first line of defense.

HERBAL THERAPIES

Evening primrose oil *(Oenothera biennis)*—500 mg two or three times a day—may be helpful in reducing breast lumps.

NUTRITION AND DIET

Although no studies have proved that diet causes breast tumors, some do suggest a relationship. Many practitioners of alternative medicine urge eliminating caffeine and recommend taking 400 to 1,200 IU of vitamin E, plus no more than 150 mcg (micrograms) a day of selenium. Caution: Selenium can be toxic in higher doses; you should use it only under the supervision of your healthcare practitioner. ■

BREATHING PROBLEMS

Read down this column to find your symptoms. Then read across.

SYMPTOMS	AILMENT/PROBLEM
Breathing problems can be indicative of a wide variety of ailments. The symptoms listed below are intended as a general guide to several broad categories. For more information on specific sets of symptoms, see the entries listed in the next column.	
◆ shortness of breath, hyperventilation, or wheezing after mild or no exercise.	◆ Stress; allergies; asthma; emphysema; pneumonia; heart attack; lung cancer
◆ coughing accompanied by yellowish or greenish phlegm.	◆ Acute or chronic bronchitis
◆ coughing accompanied by frothy white, pink, rust-colored, or bloody phlegm.	◆ Heart disease; pneumonia; tuberculosis; lung cancer; lung abscess; pulmonary edema
◆ dry cough with pain in chest.	◆ Heart disease; lung cancer; pleurisy; pneumonia; reaction to heart medication

WHAT TO DO	OTHER INFO
◆ **Call 911 or your emergency number now** if you suspect a heart attack. See also Emergencies/First Aid: Heart Attack.	◆ If you suspect that your shortness of breath is caused by stress due to poor physical shape or to anxiety, you can remedy the problem by exercising regularly and practicing mind/body techniques such as yoga or meditation.
◆ See Bronchitis. Your doctor will prescribe antibiotics if the cause is a bacterial infection.	◆ If the cough is accompanied by a fever and has lasted only a few days, you probably have acute bronchitis. If the cough has persisted for several weeks, and you smoke, you may have chronic bronchitis.
◆ **Call your doctor now.** Treat coughs accompanied by this type of sputum as medical emergencies.	◆ Frothy white or pinkish sputum is nearly always a sign of heart disease, while rust-colored phlegm points to pneumonia. Strenuous coughing can rupture small blood vessels in the back of your throat and cause bleeding, but you should still see a doctor immediately if you are coughing up bloody sputum.
◆ Call your doctor for a proper diagnosis.	◆ If a dry cough comes on very suddenly in a child, it may mean that a small object is lodged in the throat. See Emergencies/First Aid: Choking. Also, the class of heart medications known as angiotensin-converting enzyme (ACE) inhibitors can produce the side effect of a dry cough in some people.

BRONCHITIS

SYMPTOMS

Acute Bronchitis:
- hacking cough.
- yellow, white, or green phlegm, usually appearing 24 to 48 hours after a cough.
- fever, chills.
- soreness and tightness in chest.
- some pain below breastbone during deep breathing.

Chronic Bronchitis:
- persistent cough producing yellow, white, or green phlegm (for at least three months of the year, and for more than two consecutive years).
- wheezing, some breathlessness.

CALL YOUR DOCTOR IF:

- your cough is so persistent or severe that it interferes with sleep or daily activities; you could be damaging sensitive air sacs in your lungs.
- your symptoms last more than a week, and your mucus becomes darker, thicker, or increases in volume; most likely, you have an infection requiring antibiotics.
- you display symptoms of acute bronchitis and have chronic lung or heart problems or are infected with the virus that causes AIDS; respiratory infections can leave you vulnerable to more serious lung diseases, such as pneumonia.
- you have great difficulty breathing. This symptom, sometimes mistakenly associated with bronchitis, could signal asthma, emphysema, tuberculosis, heart disease, a serious allergic reaction, or cancer.

Bronchitis is an upper respiratory disease in which the mucous membrane in the lungs' upper bronchial passages becomes inflamed. As the irritated membrane swells and grows thicker, it narrows or shuts off the tiny airways in the lungs, resulting in coughing spells accompanied by thick phlegm and breathlessness. The disease comes in two forms: acute and chronic.

Acute bronchitis is responsible for the hacking cough and phlegm production that sometimes accompany an upper respiratory infection; in most cases the infection is viral in origin, but sometimes it is caused by bacteria. If you are otherwise in good health, the mucous membrane will return to normal after you've recovered from the initial lung infection, which usually lasts for several days.

Chronic bronchitis, like the lung disease emphysema, is a serious long-term disorder that requires regular medical treatment. People who have chronic bronchitis tend to be obese and lead sedentary lives, and most are heavy smokers; they typically have emphysema as well, which accounts for some of the overlapping symptoms.

If you are a smoker and come down with acute bronchitis, it will be much harder for you to recover. Even one puff on a cigarette is enough to cause temporary paralysis of the tiny hairlike cells in your lungs that are responsible for brushing out debris, irritants, and excess mucus. If you continue smoking, you may do sufficient damage to these cells, known as cilia, to prevent them from functioning properly, thus increasing your chances of developing chronic bronchitis. In some heavy smokers, the membrane stays inflamed and the cilia eventually stop functioning altogether. Clogged with mucus, the lungs are then vulnerable to viral and bacterial infections, which over time distort and permanently damage the lungs' airways.

Acute bronchitis is very common among both children and adults. Although the disorder often can be treated effectively without professional medical assistance, you will need to see a doctor for a prescription of antibiotics if the underlying lung infection is bacterial. If you suffer from **chronic bronchitis,** you are at risk for developing cardiovascular problems as well as more serious lung diseases and infections, so you should be monitored by a doctor.

CAUSES

Acute bronchitis is generally caused by lung infections; approximately 90 percent of these infections are viral in origin, 10 percent bacterial. **Chronic bronchitis** may be caused by one or several factors. Repeated attacks of acute bronchitis, which weaken and irritate bronchial airways over time, can result in chronic bronchitis. Industrial pollution is another culprit. Chronic bronchitis is found in higher-than-normal rates among coal miners, grain handlers, metal molders, and other people who are continually exposed to dust. But the chief cause is heavy, long-term cigarette smoking, which irritates the bronchial tubes and causes them to produce excess mucus. The symptoms of chronic bronchitis are also worsened by high concentrations of sulfur dioxide and other pollutants in the atmosphere.

DIAGNOSTIC AND TEST PROCEDURES

Tests are usually unnecessary in the case of **acute bronchitis,** as the disease is easy to detect on examination. Your doctor will simply use a stethoscope to listen for the rattling sound in your lungs' upper airways that typically accompanies the problem. If your symptoms persist for a week or more, your doctor may also take a culture of the phlegm you produce when you cough, to determine if you have a bacterial or viral infection. In cases of **chronic bronchitis,** the doctor will almost certainly augment these procedures with an x-ray of your chest to check the extent of the lung damage, as well as with pulmonary function tests to measure your lung capacity.

TREATMENT

Conventional treatment for both acute and chronic bronchitis may consist of antibiotics and a prescription cough syrup. In severe cases of chronic bronchitis, supplemental oxygen may be

THE BRONCHIAL TUBES

NORMAL BRONCHIAL TUBE

MUCOUS MEMBRANE

CLOGGED BRONCHIAL TUBE

EXCESS MUCUS

Air flows down the windpipe and into the lungs through branching conduits called the bronchial tubes, or bronchioles, which normally are lined with only a thin mucous membrane. In bronchitis, however, this membrane becomes inflamed, resulting in stepped-up mucus production. Over time, excess mucus can clog the bronchioles, cutting off air flow to the lungs. Coughing is the body's way of ridding the lungs of this mucus buildup.

necessary. Alternative choices, by and large, help relieve the accompanying discomfort but do not treat infections.

CONVENTIONAL MEDICINE

If your **acute bronchitis** is caused by a bacterial infection, your doctor probably will prescribe antibiotics, which should help clear up the symptoms in several days. Even if the cause is viral, your doctor may prescribe antibiotics as a preventive measure, because your lungs are susceptible to bacterial infections in their weakened state. The productive (phlegm-producing) coughing that comes with acute bronchitis is to be expected and, in most cases, encouraged; coughing is your body's way of getting rid of excess mucus. However, if your cough is truly disruptive—that is, it keeps you from sleeping or is so violent it becomes painful—or nonproductive (dry and raspy sounding), your doctor may prescribe a cough suppressant. In most cases, you should simply do all the things you normally would do for a cold: Take aspirin for fever and drink lots of liquids.

If you have **chronic bronchitis,** your lungs are

vulnerable to infections. Unless your doctor counsels against it, get a yearly flu shot as well as a vaccination against pneumonia. The pneumonia vaccine is typically a one-shot procedure: One vaccination should protect you for life against all the common strains of the disease. Only in very rare cases is a second shot required.

Do not take an over-the-counter cough suppressant to treat chronic bronchitis unless your doctor directs you to do so. As with acute bronchitis, the productive coughing associated with chronic bronchitis is helpful in ridding the lungs of excess mucus. In fact, your doctor may even prescribe an expectorant if your cough is relatively dry. However, if you notice any changes in the color, volume, or thickness of the phlegm, you may be coming down with an infection. In that case, your physician may prescribe a week-long or 10-day course of broad-spectrum antibiotics, which fight a range of bacteria.

If you are overweight, your doctor may insist that you diet to avoid putting excessive strain on your heart. Many doctors also prescribe bronchodilators, drugs that help dilate the lungs' constricted airways. For people with chronic bronchitis, inhaled bronchodilators, available in aerosol or metered-dose inhalers, are generally preferred over oral medications. In most cases, one or two puffs will relieve the breathlessness that accompanies chronic bronchitis. Special circumstances may require a greater dosage, but you should never increase your intake unless instructed to do so by your doctor. Bronchodilators are potent drugs; overuse can cause dangerous side effects, such as high blood pressure.

If your body's ability to transfer oxygen from your lungs into the bloodstream is significantly handicapped, your doctor may prescribe **oxygen therapy,** either on a continuous or on an as-needed basis. Oxygen-delivering devices are widely available. If you use an oxygen tank at home, be sure to take special care not to expose the apparatus to flammable materials (alcohol and aerosol sprays, for example) or to sources of direct heat, such as hair dryers or radiators.

If you smoke, your doctor will urge you to quit. Studies show that people who kick the habit even in the advanced stages of chronic bronchitis not only can reduce the severity of their symptoms but also can increase their life expectancy.

ALTERNATIVE CHOICES

A number of alternative therapies can be used to complement—but never to replace—a conventional doctor's care. These remedies may help ease some of the symptoms of acute and chronic bronchitis, but they do not treat infections.

ACUPUNCTURE

Studies suggest that acupuncture may relieve the symptoms associated with bronchitis. The technique should be performed only by a licensed acupuncturist.

AROMATHERAPY

Essential oils such as eucalyptus (*Eucalyptus globulus*), hyssop (*Hyssopus officinalis*), aniseed (*Pimpinella anisum*), lavender (*Lavandula officinalis*), pine (*Pinus sylvestris*), and rosemary (*Rosmarinus officinalis*) may help ease breathing and relieve nasal congestion. Inhaling deeply through your nose, breathe the aroma from a few drops of one or more of these oils dabbed on a handkerchief, or sniff directly from the bottle. Try mixing a few drops of essential oil in a sink full of hot water; cover your head with a towel and breathe in the fragrant steam.

CHINESE HERBS

The Chinese herb ephedra (*Ephedra sinica*) is a potent bronchodilator. CAUTION: Large quantities of this herb have the same effect as large quantities of the hormone epinephrine; do not use ephedra if you have high blood pressure or heart disease. Prepare an infusion by combining 5 grams ephedra, 4 grams cinnamon sticks (*Cinnamomum cassia*), 1.5 grams licorice (*Glycyrrhiza uralensis*), and 5 grams apricot seed (*Prunus armeniaca*). Steep the mixture in cold water, then bring it to a boil. Drink it hot.

HERBAL THERAPIES

A wide variety of herbs act as soothing expectorants, making them appropriate in the treatment of bronchitis. A sampling of therapies follows; for more, seek the advice of a professional herbalist or homeopath.

In the case of **acute** or **chronic bronchitis,** the herb coltsfoot *(Tussilago farfara)* may relax constricted or spasming bronchial tubes and gently help to loosen phlegm. To prepare an infusion, add a cup of boiling water to 1 or 2 tsp of coltsfoot; let the infusion steep for 10 minutes. Drink it as hot as possible, three times daily. Mullein *(Verbascum thapsus),* believed to have an anti-inflammatory effect on mucous membranes, can also be prepared as an infusion by following the directions above.

To treat **acute bronchitis,** use the same directions to prepare an infusion from the herb hyssop *(Hyssopus officinalis),* which may encourage sweating (thus lowering fever) and lessen inflammation. Herbal expectorants appropriate for **chronic bronchitis** include aniseed *(Pimpinella anisum),* elecampane *(Inula helenium),* and garlic *(Allium sativum).*

HOMEOPATHY

For **acute** and **chronic bronchitis,** take the following three times a day, for up to four days: To treat fever, cough, and tightness in the chest, use Aconite (6c). For loose white phlegm, cough, and irritability, use Kali bichromicum (6c). For loss of voice, cough, thirst, and sore throat, use Phosphorus (6c).

NUTRITION AND DIET

To strengthen the immune system and protect against infection, nutritionists often recommend vitamins A, B complex, C, and E, along with the minerals selenium and zinc. Some experts suggest that you also avoid mucus-producing foods, found mainly in the dairy group (although goat's milk generally causes less mucus production than cow's milk), as well as in refined starches (white-flour–based products) and processed foods.

AT-HOME REMEDIES

For acute bronchitis:
Throughout the duration of your infection, stay at home and keep warm. You don't necessarily need to stay in bed, but don't overextend yourself. Consider using a vaporizer, or try inhaling steam over a sink full of hot water.

For chronic bronchitis:
Avoid exposure to paint or exhaust fumes, dust, and people with colds. Consider using a vaporizer or inhaling steam over a sink full of hot water. Dress warmly in cold, dry weather. ■

STEAMING TOWARD RECOVERY

Humidity is helpful in treating both acute and chronic bronchitis, as moisture in the air can loosen phlegm inside the lungs and make it easier for you to expectorate. To be effective, however, humidifying devices must be used properly.

The warm steam distributed by vaporizers works well when used in a relatively small space, such as a bathroom; in an average-size room, most vaporizers aren't powerful enough to generate the density of steam necessary to be truly helpful. Be sure to clean the vaporizer regularly for the duration of your infection, to prevent the distribution of germs.

Some devices can actually be hazardous to your health. Cold humidifiers, used frequently in homes with dry air, must be cleaned daily with bleach; otherwise, they can spread germs and encourage mold or mildew growth, increasing your chances of developing lung infections.

- recurrent episodes of binge eating and purging.
- unrealistic fear of becoming fat.
- weight fluctuation (although relatively normal weight may be maintained).
- food cravings.
- overuse of laxatives.
- depression.
- tooth enamel erosion, gum infections, cavities, and tooth discoloration (caused by stomach acids from frequent vomiting).
- gastrointestinal upset.

CALL YOUR DOCTOR IF:

- you find yourself secretly binging, then vomiting or using laxatives.
- you avoid eating in front of other people.
- your child has an unreasonable fear of being fat and thinks she's fat when she's not.
- your child avoids eating with others or frequents the bathroom immediately after meals.

Bulimia is an eating disorder that, like anorexia nervosa, is psychological in origin and can have dire physical consequences. While anorexics simply starve themselves, bulimics binge on food and then purge by self-induced vomiting. Bulimics also frequently use diet pills, laxatives, and diuretics to reduce their weight. The purging may serve two purposes: preventing weight gain and also temporarily relieving depression and other negative feelings.

Like anorexia, bulimia mostly afflicts young women. Because binging and purging are practiced in secret, the incidence of the disorder is uncertain, but researchers estimate that as many as one-fifth of all U.S. women in high school and college display at least temporary bulimic symptoms. The average age of onset is 18.

Bulimia can occur on its own or intermittently with anorexia. In the intermittent pattern—which occurs in about 1 case out of 5—a young woman will not eat for some time, setting herself up for a binge; she may use appetite suppressants in the noneating phase. Despite their overlap, the two disorders are associated with some different personality traits: Anorexics are apt to suppress all urges, including sexual ones; bulimics, on the other hand, tend to indulge their cravings, impulsively getting into trouble with drugs, sexual promiscuity, shoplifting, or binge buying.

A bulimic's overall health depends on how often she binges and purges. She may vomit occasionally (once a month) or very frequently (many times a day). Physical repercussions include swelling of the stomach or pancreas, inflammation of the esophagus, enlarged salivary glands, and tooth decay and gum disease from vomiting stomach acids. Frequent vomiting also depletes the water and potassium in bodily tissues, causing abnormal heart rhythms, muscle spasms, and even paralysis. In severe cases, some of these physical problems can lead to death. Another danger is suicidal depression.

Bulimia is a real illness and usually cannot be controlled voluntarily by its sufferers without professional help. Admonitions from family and friends to stop are at best useless, at worst counterproductive.

CAUSES

Pressures and conflicts within the family are thought to be the primary cause of bulimia. A bulimic is apt to be an overachiever and perfectionist who feels she can't live up to her parents' expectations. She has low self-esteem and often suffers from depression. She may have been physically or sexually abused as a child: About half of all bulimics report a history of abuse.

TREATMENT

Psychotherapy—often combined with antidepressants—is the primary treatment, together with nutritional counseling. Be sure to find a psychologist or psychiatrist experienced in dealing with eating disorders. The same is true for nutritional counseling, whether the patient sees the family doctor or another health professional. Clinics that specialize in eating disorders can often provide psychiatrists, psychotherapists, and nutritionists. All therapists involved should work in close cooperation with one another.

CONVENTIONAL MEDICINE

Psychological treatments for bulimia may involve individual, family, or group psychotherapy. Behavior or cognitive therapies are also often prescribed. Behavior therapy focuses on altering habits (binging and purging, in this case); sessions are usually devoted to analyzing the behavior and devising ways to change it, and the patient follows specific instructions between sessions. Cognitive therapy also concentrates on habitual behavior; it aims at exploring and countering the negative thoughts that underlie destructive habits. Individual or group psychotherapy focuses on the underlying emotional experiences and relationships that have caused the bulimia.

Antidepressants, used in conjunction with psychological therapies, are now a mainstay in bulimia therapy. Selective serotonin reuptake inhibitors, such as sertraline and fluoxetine, appear to be more helpful than tricyclic antidepressants, such as amitriptyline and imipramine.

ALTERNATIVE CHOICES

Most alternative therapies for bulimia do not address the root causes of the disorder, but they can be helpful in relieving some of the physical distress resulting from it. It is important to consult practitioners who are experienced in dealing with eating disorders.

HERBAL THERAPIES

Use any herbal therapies that reduce anxiety or depression. To soothe stomach pains or mouth inflammation, try marsh mallow (*Althaea officinalis*) root or slippery elm (*Ulmus fulva*) powder. (*See also Canker Sores and Gastritis.*)

HOMEOPATHY

Homeopathic medicine offers potentially beneficial prescriptions for eating disorders. In difficult cases, where conventional medicine has not been successful, consider seeking out a homeopath who has experience in treating bulimia.

MIND/BODY MEDICINE

Body exercises such as **yoga, t'ai chi, qigong,** and dance can help bulimics with their problems of body image. Reprogramming mental processes to gain control over the binge-and-purge cycles is another approach. Either **hypnotherapy** or EEG **biofeedback** may help. Be sure to interview hypnotherapists or biofeedback practitioners about their experience in treating eating disorders.

NUTRITION AND DIET

A nutrient-dense, sugar-free diet may help reduce binge eating. Also eliminate alcohol, caffeine, flavor enhancers, most salt, and cigarettes. Eat a balanced diet, supplemented daily with vitamin C (1,000 mg), vitamin B complex (50 mg), and a multivitamin/multimineral supplement. ■

◆ an angular protrusion at the side of the foot behind the big toe, sometimes accompanied by hardened skin or a callus.
◆ swelling, redness, unusual tenderness, or pain at the base of the big toe and in the ball of the foot, especially if the area becomes shiny and cool to the touch.

◆ you have persistent pain when walking normally in otherwise comfortable, flat-soled shoes; you may be developing bursitis or a bone spur in your foot.

A bunion is an unnatural bump or bend in the bone that forms the ball of the foot at the base of the big toe. The result is an unsightly swelling at the inside of the foot, sometimes pushing the big toe inward so it overlaps one or more other toes. A similar condition on the little toe is called a bunionette.

Because a bunion occurs at the joint where the toe bends in normal walking, your entire body weight rests on it at each step. While most bunions don't affect normal walking, they can be extremely painful.

CAUSES

Foot problems typically develop in early adulthood, becoming more pronounced as the foot spreads with aging. In many people, bunions are hereditary and occur along with other problems associated with weak or poor foot structure, as well as with corns and calluses, bone spurs, and bursitis. Bunions sometimes develop with arthritis and can be associated with other progressive deformation of bones in the foot.

Bunions can also be brought on by years of wearing tight, poorly fitting shoes—especially high-heeled, pointed shoes styled more for fashion than for comfort and good support. As the bones gradually assume an unnatural shape, pressure on the other bones of the foot can lead to bursitis.

DIAGNOSTIC AND TEST PROCEDURES

Most of the time, bunions are so obvious from the pain and the unusual shape of the toe that further diagnosis is unnecessary. Even so, a doctor will usually take x-rays to determine the extent of the deformity and to see if orthopedic shoes or surgery is needed.

TREATMENT

Relieving a bunion's discomfort generally consists of steps to reduce pain and inflammation, followed by measures to prevent recurrence.

BUNION

JOINT	
BUNION	
BURSA	

Weakness in the structure of the foot, exacerbated by poorly fitting shoes or some sports, can force the large joint of the big toe outward, resulting in a knobby protrusion called a bunion. Pain occurs when the bursa, a fluid-filled sac overlying the joint, becomes inflamed and swollen.

CONVENTIONAL MEDICINE

Your doctor may recommend aspirin or another over-the-counter pain remedy, or may prescribe a specific medication to relieve the swelling and inflammation. A heating pad or warm footbath may also help relieve the immediate pain and discomfort, as may an analgesic cream containing capsaicin, a chili-pepper extract.

If your bunion isn't persistently painful and you catch it early, wearing well-made, well-fitting shoes may be all the therapy you need. Most doctors don't advise bunion pads, splints, or other shoe inserts, which can exert pressure elsewhere on the foot and aggravate foot problems.

In some cases, an orthotic specialist can prescribe shoes with specially designed insoles and uppers that take the pressure off affected joints and help the foot regain its proper shape.

Most physicians are reluctant to recommend surgery for bunions, since many patients remain dissatisfied with the results. Done in a hospital under local anesthesia, a bunionectomy realigns the metatarsal bone behind the big toe by cutting the ligament at the joint. Wires may be tem-

porarily inserted to keep the bones in line, and excess bone may be removed.

ALTERNATIVE CHOICES

Various therapies for reducing pain and inflammation can be used effectively on bunions.

BODY WORK

In certain cases, especially if bone degeneration is not advanced, **Rolfing** and Reiki techniques have been reported to alleviate the discomfort.

CHIROPRACTIC

Professional manipulation can help change the positioning of deformed bones. Practitioners can also help lessen the pain of bunions by having patients alter the way they walk.

HOMEOPATHY

Following an analysis of your overall situation, a homeopath can prescribe remedies that may relieve the pain of a bunion and may stabilize bone degeneration.

AT-HOME REMEDIES

◆ When a bunion causes sore feet, a hot compress or a good soak in warm water will ease the pain.
◆ Sacrifice a pair of old but comfortable shoes: Cut away the leather or fabric upper—not the sole—to take pressure off a bunion.

PREVENTION

Because bunions develop slowly, taking precautions as your feet grow in childhood and early adulthood can pay off later in life. Closely monitor the shape of your feet as they develop, especially if foot problems run in your family. Exercising your feet can strengthen them, particularly if you learn to pick up small objects with your toes. Wear shoes that fit properly and that do not cramp or pinch your toes. Women should avoid shoes with high heels or pointed toes. ■

B

SYMPTOMS

If the burn is:

- red, tender, and possibly swollen and blistering, it is probably a **first-degree burn** (which can include sunburn).
- red, painful, and blistering, it is probably a **second-degree burn** (which can include severe sunburn).
- severely painful, the burned skin looks white or charred and blood vessels are exposed, or nerve damage is so substantial that there is no pain, it is probably a **third-degree burn.**
- characteristic of a third-degree burn, and muscle or bone is exposed, it is a **fourth-degree burn.**

CALL YOUR DOCTOR IF:

- you have a large first-degree burn.
- you have a second-degree burn on your hands, face, feet, groin, buttocks, or a major joint, or the burn is larger than three inches in diameter; or you have a third- or fourth-degree burn. You may suffer from shock, low blood pressure, and rapid pulse, and the area could become infected. **Get medical help immediately.**
- you have a chemical burn. This type of burn can cause serious secondary symptoms such as seizures and loss of consciousness. **Get medical help immediately.**
- you have an electrical burn. This type of burn can also cause injuries that might not be apparent. All electrical burns should be checked by a doctor.

See also Emergencies/First Aid: Burns.

The skin is sensitive, living tissue composed of three primary layers: the epidermis, the dermis, and subcutaneous tissue. Any exposure to heat above 120°F will damage its cells and cause some degree of burning. Every year in the United States two million people are burned: 300,000 seriously, 70,000 requiring admission to a hospital, and 6,000 fatally. Children and the elderly are more susceptible to more serious forms of burning because their skin is thinner.

Minor burns include **first-degree burns,** limited **second-degree burns,** and sunburns (which may be classified as first- or second-degree burns depending on severity). **First-degree burns** affect the top layer of skin, the epidermis. Such burns are generally not serious and heal quickly. Within two days the damaged skin from a first-degree burn will peel away. **Second-degree burns** affect the epidermis and some of the underlying dermis layer of skin. Unless a second-degree burn covers a large area or has developed a secondary infection (which may be avoided with proper treatment), it is not serious and will heal in a short time.

Major burns include widespread **second-degree** and all **third-** and **fourth-degree burns.** Third- and fourth-degree burns are always serious and involve all three layers of skin. The area may appear white, or blackened and charred. Such severe burns affect fat tissue and nerves. **Fourth-degree burns** penetrate to muscle and bone.

Electrical burns can be deceiving. Although burning of the skin may be minimal, interior damage can be extensive and may include damage to

Dᴏɴ'ᴛ ʙᴜᴛᴛᴇʀ ᴛʜᴀᴛ ʙᴜʀɴ

Don't try to soothe any kind of burn by putting butter or margarine on it. Such greasy substances can actually hold heat in the wound and slow down healing; they can also lead to infection.

LEVELS OF SKIN DAMAGE

HAIR

EPIDERMIS

DERMIS

SUBCUTANEOUS LAYER

MUSCLE

BONE

HAIR FOLLICLE

1ST-DEGREE

2ND-DEGREE

3RD-DEGREE

4TH-DEGREE

First-degree burns damage the thin epidermal layer and usually heal quickly. Second-degree burns damage some of the dermis, but not enough to destroy hair follicles and cells that generate new skin. Third-degree burns penetrate the subcutaneous layer, usually requiring skin grafts for new growth. Fourth-degree burns, by far the most severe, destroy the skin and damage muscle and bone.

the heart. High-voltage electric shock can cause cardiac arrest. *(See Emergencies/First Aid: Cardiac and Respiratory Arrest and Electric Shock.)*

TREATMENT

For any type of burn, immediate, aggressive treatment, whether conventional or alternative, is essential to speed healing and recovery.

CONVENTIONAL MEDICINE

After at-home first-aid treatment has been applied to minor burns, any persisting pain may be alleviated with aspirin or acetaminophen. If your burn requires medical treatment, your doctor will cover the area with an antibacterial dressing or leave it exposed to promote healing (in which case the burn must diligently be kept clean). Avoid breaking blisters; exposure of the tissue underneath increases your likelihood of infection. Analgesics may be prescribed, or antibiotics if there are signs of infection. Any shock resulting from major burns will be treated with the administration of intravenous fluids. Severe major burns may require skin grafting or plastic surgery for repair and to avoid extensive scarring.

ALTERNATIVE CHOICES

All major burns should be treated by a medical professional. In addition to the therapies mentioned below, Chinese herbs, homeopathy, aromatherapy, and Ayurvedic medicine may also be helpful in treating minor burns.

HERBAL THERAPIES

The juice from an aloe *(Aloe barbadensis)* plant may reduce pain, promote healing, and prevent infection in minor burns. Herbalists believe that honey is an effective healing agent. Spread a thin layer on your minor burn, cover with a loose dressing, and repeat daily until healed.

MIND/BODY MEDICINE

In some cases of major burns, concentrated healing thoughts and a positive attitude toward recovery have minimized symptoms such as pain, inflammation, and scarring. The most dramatic results have occurred when this technique has been applied within a few hours of injury.

AT-HOME REMEDIES

Flush minor burns with running water, then apply a cool compress. When your burn begins to heal, pierce a vitamin E capsule and rub the liquid onto the affected area to help prevent scarring. If your burn is major, drink lots of fluids during recovery; such burns cause loss of body fluids.

PREVENTION

Burns are frequently caused by preventable accidents in the home. Each floor should have a working smoke detector, and a fire extinguisher should be kept in the kitchen. All detectors and extinguishers should be tested at least annually. When cooking, turn pot handles to the inside of the stove, and if you have small children in the home, place covers over all unused electrical outlets. ■

BURSITIS

SYMPTOMS

- pain, inflammation, and swelling in the shoulders, elbows, hips, knees, or joints of the hands or feet, particularly during stretching or extension when exercising, lifting, or otherwise pushing the joint beyond its normal limits.
- restricted range of motion in a joint, with or without immediate pain.

CALL YOUR DOCTOR IF:

- pain in a joint persists more than a few days; you may be experiencing tendonitis, a strained ligament or tendon, or the onset of arthritis.
- swelling persists after taking a painkiller or anti-inflammatory agent as prescribed; you may need to have a physician drain fluid from the affected joint or to undergo corticosteroid treatment.

Wherever your bones, tendons, and ligaments move against each other, particularly near joints, the points of contact are cushioned by small fluid-filled sacs called bursae. By reducing friction, each of the more than 150 bursae in your body helps joints operate smoothly through the full range of natural movement.

When a joint is overused, or when it stays under pressure or tension for extended periods of time, a nearby bursa can become inflamed. The sac fills with excess fluid, causing pressure on surrounding tissue. The immediate signal is pain, often accompanied by inflammation, swelling, and tenderness in the area.

One of the most common sites for bursitis to strike is the shoulder, which has the greatest range of motion of all the body's major joints. The pain is generally felt along the outside top of the shoulder. The discomfort of bursitis tends to be most severe after a night's sleep and will typically subside somewhat with normal activity. Other places that are prone to bursitis are the elbows, hips, and knees.

Bursitis is associated with strenuous activity, particularly among manual workers and athletes, as well as in otherwise sedentary people who push their bodies past reasonable limits. While you may be tempted to "tough out" the pain, it's not a good idea. Chronic bursitis left untreated can lead to the formation of calcium deposits in normally soft tissues, sometimes causing permanent reduction of motion in the affected joint.

CAUSES

The immediate cause of bursitis is typically an injury to or sustained pressure on a joint, resulting in inflammation of the bursal sac. Professional and amateur athletes alike recognize bursitis in the form of the sore shoulder that comes from running, throwing, and jumping, or the exaggerated arm swings used in tennis, baseball, and bowling. Heavy lifting, repetitive motion, or working for extended periods in unusual positions can also bring on a bursitis attack.

B

TREATMENT

Although bursitis generally disappears in a few days or weeks, you must take measures to avoid further strain or injury.

CONVENTIONAL MEDICINE

Initial treatment typically consists of aspirin or over-the-counter nonsteroidal anti-inflammatory drugs (NSAIDs). These pain relievers also tend to reduce inflammation. Heat and ultrasound can help relax the joint and promote tissue repair.

Diathermy (deep-heat therapy), under the direction of a sports physician, licensed physical therapist, or trainer, not only can relieve the discomfort and inflammation of bursitis but also can soothe tense muscles, nerves, and tendons.

Bursitis may recur, particularly if you engage regularly in strenuous exercise or physical labor. In such cases your doctor may prescribe corticosteroid treatment, in the form of either oral medication, topical creams, or injections to the affected joints. In severe cases, it may be necessary to draw fluid from inflamed and swollen bursae with a hypodermic syringe to relieve the pressure. In persistent conditions, bursae can be surgically removed.

ALTERNATIVE CHOICES

Bursitis tends to heal itself with rest, but in the meantime the pain and inflammation can be relieved through a variety of remedies.

ACUPUNCTURE

Treatment by a trained acupuncturist can bring quick relief of bursitis pain.

BODY WORK

An injured or strained joint needs rest and immobilization for natural healing to occur. In the short term, **massage** of the affected area stimulates circulation and relaxes surrounding muscles. After the initial therapy, exercise—such as **yoga**—is a practical long-term method of loosening and strengthening affected joints.

CHIROPRACTIC

Following conventional methods of pain relief, a chiropractor can use mobilization techniques to restore a joint's active range of motion.

HERBAL THERAPIES

To increase blood circulation, reduce inflammation, and alleviate muscle tension, an herbalist might recommend a 5 ml tincture of the following herbs, taken orally three times a day: 2 parts each of willow (*Salix* spp.) bark, cramp bark (*Viburnum opulus),* and celery (*Apium graveolens)* seed, along with 1 part prickly ash (*Zanthoxylum americanum).*

Mix equal parts lobelia (*Lobelia inflata)* and cramp bark to make a tincture that you can rub into your muscles as needed to ease the tension associated with bursitis pain.

HOMEOPATHY

After evaluating the nature of the bursitis pain, a homeopath may prescribe regimens of Belladonna, Bryonia, or Rhus toxicodendron.

NUTRITION AND DIET

Vitamin C (ascorbic acid), vitamin A, and zinc are recommended for making tissue-building collagen and for repairing injured tendons and bursa tissue. Good dietary sources of vitamin C are citrus fruits and potatoes; cod-liver oil is a good source of vitamin A. In addition, vitamin E is considered effective in promoting the healing of damaged tissue. Follow the recommendations of a trained dietitian for amounts and duration when taking vitamin supplements. Another approach reported to be helpful in recurring cases of bursitis involves vitamin B_{12} injections, administered by a licensed healthcare practitioner.

PREVENTION

Warming up before strenuous exercise and cooling down afterward is the most effective way to avoid bursitis and other strains affecting the bones, muscles, and ligaments. ∎

SYMPTOMS

In its early stages cancer usually has no symptoms, but eventually a malignant tumor will grow large enough to be detected. As it continues to grow, it may press on nerves and produce pain, penetrate blood vessels and cause bleeding, or interfere with the function of a body organ or system. The following symptoms may signal the presence of some form of cancer:

- change in the size, color, shape, or thickness of a wart, mole, or mouth sore.
- a sore that resists healing.
- persistent cough, hoarseness, or sore throat.
- thickening or lumps in the breasts, testicles, or elsewhere.
- a change in bowel or bladder habits.
- any unusual bleeding or discharge.
- chronic indigestion or difficulty swallowing.
- persistent headaches.
- unexplained loss of weight or appetite.
- chronic pain in bones.
- persistent fatigue, nausea, or vomiting.
- persistent low-grade fever, either constant or intermittent.
- repeated instances of infection.

CALL YOUR DOCTOR IF:

- you develop symptoms that may signal cancer, are not clearly linked to another cause, and persist for more than two weeks. You should schedule a medical examination. If the cause of your symptoms is cancer, early diagnosis and treatment will offer a better chance of cure.

Throughout our lives, healthy cells in our bodies divide and replace themselves in a controlled fashion. Cancer starts when a cell is somehow altered so that it multiplies out of control. A tumor is a cluster of abnormal cells: Most cancers form tumors, but not all tumors are cancerous. Benign, or noncancerous, tumors—such as freckles and moles—stop growing, do not spread to other parts of the body, and do not create new tumors. Malignant, or cancerous, tumors crowd out healthy cells, interfere with body functions, and draw nutrients from body tissues. Cancers continue to grow and spread in a process called metastasis—eventually forming new tumors in other parts of the body.

The term "cancer" encompasses more than 100 diseases affecting nearly every part of the body, and all are potentially life-threatening. The four major types are **carcinoma, sarcoma,** lymphoma, and leukemia. **Carcinomas**—the most commonly diagnosed cancers—originate in the skin, lungs, breasts, pancreas, and other organs and glands. **Lymphomas** are cancers of the lymphatic system. **Leukemias** are cancers of the blood and do not form solid tumors. **Sarcomas** arise in bone, muscle, or cartilage, and are relatively rare. (*See entries for specific types of cancers.*)

Cancer has been recognized for thousands of years as a human ailment, yet only in the past century has medical science understood what cancer really is and how it progresses. Cancer specialists, called oncologists, have made remarkable advances in cancer diagnosis, prevention, and treatment. Today, more than half of all people diagnosed with cancer are cured. However, some forms of the disease remain frustratingly difficult to treat. For those people who cannot be cured, modern treatment can significantly improve quality of life and may extend survival.

CAUSES

The fundamental cause of all cancer is a change, or mutation, in the nucleus of a cell. For a healthy cell to turn malignant, its genetic code must be reprogrammed for constant, uncontrolled cell division. Substances that either start or promote

THE SEVEN WARNING SIGNS

To remember the seven early warning signs of cancer (as designated by the American Cancer Society), think of the word CAUTION:

C *hange in bowel or bladder habits*

A *sore that does not heal*

U *nusual bleeding or discharge*

T *hickening or lump in the breast or elsewhere*

I *ndigestion or difficulty swallowing*

O *bvious change in a wart or mole*

N *agging cough or hoarseness*

the process are called carcinogens, and there are many types. Scientists theorize that about 10 million of the 300 trillion cells in a human body die and are replaced every second. With such a high rate of cell activity, the potential for occasional malignant cell mutation is high. In a healthy person, special cells from the body's immune system can somehow recognize mutant cells and destroy them before they multiply. Nevertheless, some mutant cells may occasionally evade such detection and survive, causing cancer.

Because the causes of cancer are complicated, experts speak in terms of "risk factors." Any habit, trait, or use of a substance that increases the odds of getting cancer is a risk factor, and the risk for nearly all cancers increases with age. Inherited, or familial, predisposition is a risk factor, although its influence varies from case to case. Researchers continue to identify genes that, when flawed, strongly predispose a person to getting a particular type of cancer. Such genetic predisposition is considered an influential risk factor but by no means guarantees that the person will develop the cancer.

Environmental risk factors relate to where and how we live. Most common cancers are linked to one of three environmental risk factors:

smoking, sunlight, and diet. Smoking is linked to cancer of the lung, head-and-neck area, bladder, kidney, stomach, cervix, and pancreas, as well as to some leukemias. Excessive exposure to sunlight is linked to skin cancer. Dietary factors are associated with some cancers of the gastrointestinal tract, and may be linked to others, such as cancer of the breast, prostate, and uterus. Eating habits suspected of promoting cancer include overconsumption of alcohol, fat, and foods that have been smoked, cured, pickled, or charred. Lack of dietary fiber or antioxidant vitamins and minerals is also believed to be a risk factor.

Many substances in the environment have been identified as carcinogens, but in most cases a very high level of exposure is needed to cause cancer. Environmental carcinogens include various chemicals, gases, and other substances found in air, water, foods, pesticides, tobacco smoke, cleaning products, paints, and many industrial settings; excessive ionizing radiation—the type in x-rays, nuclear radiation, and radioactive waste; and certain viruses, such as the HIV, hepatitis B, papilloma, and Epstein-Barr viruses. Although stress and certain personality types have been suggested as cancer risk factors, there is no hard scientific evidence to confirm such ideas.

All these factors may contribute to cancer causation, yet cancer is not caused by any single factor. Cancer results from a "multifactor hit" of age, inherited predisposition, general health, and carcinogenic exposure. For example, some people exposed to particular carcinogens will develop cancer, while others, exposed just as intensely to the same carcinogens, will not. And as far as we know, most people who get a particular form of cancer are not strongly predisposed genetically to the specific disease. Thus, everyone's cancer risk profile is complex and unique.

DIAGNOSTIC AND TEST PROCEDURES

The earlier cancer is diagnosed and treated, the better the chance of its being cured. Some types of cancer—such as those of the skin, breast, mouth, testicles, prostate, and rectum—may be detected by routine self-examination or other screening measures before the symptoms become serious. Most cases of cancer are detected and diagnosed after a tumor can be felt or when other symptoms develop. In a few cases cancer is diagnosed incidentally as a result of diagnosis or treatment for other medical conditions.

Diagnosis begins with a thorough physical examination and a complete medical history. Lab studies of blood, urine, and stool can detect abnormalities that may indicate cancer. When a tumor is suspected, imaging tests such as x-rays, computed tomography (CT), magnetic resonance imaging (MRI), ultrasound, and fiberoptic scope examinations help doctors determine its location and size. To confirm the cancer diagnosis, a biopsy is performed: A tissue sample is surgically removed from the suspected malignancy and studied under a microscope to check for cancer cells.

If the diagnosis is positive (meaning cancer is present), other tests are performed to provide specific information about the cancer; this essential follow-up phase of diagnosis is called staging. The most important thing doctors need to know is whether cancer has spread from one area of the body to another. If your initial diagnosis is made by a primary care physician, or if symptoms persist even though you are told that you do not have cancer, seek a second opinion. In any event, before the actual treatment begins, it is extremely important that you get a confirming opinion by a doctor who specializes in cancer treatment.

TREATMENT

A comprehensive cancer program combines both curative and supportive treatment. Curative treatment attempts to terminate or slow the disease with some combination of surgery, radiation therapy, chemotherapy, and possibly hormone therapy or immunotherapy. When cancer is no longer detected, a patient is said to be in remission. Generally, patients who remain cancer free for five or more years are considered cured. Some cancers cannot be cured, but all can be treated, and in most cases the patient will improve.

Supportive treatment by nurses and other professionals accompanies cancer treatment. The goal is to relieve pain and other symptoms; maintain general health; and provide emotional, psychological, and logistical support to patients and their families. Similar supportive treatment is available to rehabilitate patients after curative treatment. Supportive therapy such as hospice care for cancer patients nearing the end of their lives provides relief from pain and other irreversible symptoms. Most mainstream care is geared toward providing supportive treatment through the broad resources of a cancer treatment center. The best complementary cancer therapies, which are generally provided outside a hospital, also provide excellent supportive care.

CONVENTIONAL MEDICINE

Goals of treatment vary according to how advanced a cancer is at diagnosis and whether it is considered curable. If cure seems likely, the patient is treated aggressively in the hope of long-term remission and cure. Cancer not considered curable can still be treated in an effort to prolong life and help make the patient comfortable.

The three standard cancer treatments are **surgery, radiation,** and **chemotherapy.** Each is designed to remove or kill the malignant cells and can be used either to effect a cure or to relieve severe symptoms. Surgery and radiation destroy cancer cells locally, while chemotherapy uses drugs to kill cancer cells that spread through the body. Surgery can treat localized tumors successfully but only rarely cures metastatic cancer. Radiation and chemotherapy are used mainly to reduce tumor size before surgery, as well as to minimize the chance of recurrence after surgery and to treat metastatic cancer.

Because chemotherapy and radiation can affect healthy as well as diseased cells, they typically cause side effects. With chemotherapy, side effects may include nausea, vomiting, fatigue, temporary hair loss, mouth sores or dryness, difficulty swallowing, diarrhea, and increased vulnerability to infection. Radiation may have some of the same effects, depending on the area of the body that is irradiated. Medication and other complementary therapy can help curb side effects during treatment, and most side effects disappear when the treatment is concluded.

BEWARE OF CANCER QUACKERY

Sadly, the sale of bogus cancer treatments to vulnerable people is a multi-billion-dollar-a-year business. To protect yourself from cancer quackery, be an educated consumer. Research unproven therapies critically, skeptically, and thoroughly. Do not accept anecdotes and testimonials in place of scientific proof. Interview critics as well as supporters. Ask the following questions when assessing a treatment—and get satisfactory answers:

◆ Has it been objectively shown in peer-reviewed scientific literature to be safe and effective?

◆ Does its potential for benefit outweigh its potential for harm?

◆ Is it logical and understandable? If it relies on a secret formula or technique, avoid it.

◆ Does the practitioner claim that the treatment is experimental, yet still ask you to pay for it? If so, it's probably a scam.

◆ Does the practitioner have legitimate degrees and licenses from accredited institutions?

◆ Does the practitioner claim to be a victim of a conspiracy by the mainstream medical community? If so, look into such charges further rather than accept them as adequate explanations for lack of proof or endorsement.

◆ Do you have any doubts? If so, resolve them before you spend any money or begin treatment.

Hormone therapy is standard treatment for some types of cancer that grow faster in the presence of particular hormones—for example, cancer of the breast, prostate, or uterus. By blocking either the production or the action of the hormones, this therapy slows tumor growth and may extend survival for several months or even years.

Although still largely experimental, **immunotherapy** is emerging as another mode of cancer treatment, with the goal of destroying cancer cells without affecting healthy cells. It does not attack cancer cells directly but employs various techniques to manipulate the body's immune system into fighting cancer more aggressively. **Gene therapy**—a promising subcategory of immunotherapy—manipulates genetic material inside either cancerous cells or the immune cells intended to attack them, in order to make the cancer cells easier targets. Immunotherapy and other experimental treatments generally are reserved for patients with metastatic or recurrent disease who do not respond well to standard treatment.

Patients who have practiced good nutrition tend to respond better to treatment, with fewer side effects. Because weight loss and malnutrition may become problems for cancer patients, clinical nutrition programs are fundamental parts of mainstream care. Most hospitals also offer support groups or individual counseling to help patients deal with mental and emotional difficulties.

As cancer advances, pain may become a significant problem. Fortunately, moderate to severe cancer pain can be managed effectively with prescription medication, such as codeine and morphine. Addiction does not occur with drugs given for advanced care, and research shows that people with reduced pain respond better to treatment and enjoy better quality of life.

COMPLEMENTARY THERAPIES

Alternative and unconventional treatments for cancer are numerous and varied. While some legitimate therapies offer real support, many questionable therapies have no benefits, may be dangerous, and may harm patients by delaying appropriate care. Even the most promising unconventional therapies do not cure cancer and should never replace standard treatment. Instead, supportive therapies should complement conventional care.

Appropriate complementary therapies improve quality of life and may relieve physical and emotional stress. The act of seeking complementary therapy is beneficial in its own right: It gives patients a sense of control over their illness and the opportunity to play a role in their own care. Before trying any complementary cancer therapy, research it thoroughly to make sure it is potentially beneficial and absolutely safe. Then check with your doctor to be sure it will not compromise standard treatment.

ACUPUNCTURE
Acupuncture has proved to relieve pain associated with many major illnesses. Although scientific study has not fully documented its effectiveness in treating cancer pain and side effects such as nausea and vomiting, it is a safe therapy that many cancer patients find beneficial.

BODY WORK
By promoting relaxation, body-work therapies such as **massage, qigong,** and **reflexology** ease muscle tension and may alleviate other symptoms such as nausea and chronic pain. Because many body-work therapies provide comforting physical contact, they can lessen the anxiety, depression, and isolation that cancer patients often feel.

CHINESE HERBS
Some cancer sufferers report relief from pain, nausea, and vomiting using traditional Chinese medicine. Most practitioners recommend herbal remedies not to cure cancer but to relieve side effects of conventional treatment. Researchers are studying plants used in traditional Chinese medicine to identify constituents that may combat cancer cells directly or stimulate the immune system to do so, among them astragalus *(Astragalus membranaceus),* dong quai *(Angelica sinensis),* and Asian ginseng *(Panax ginseng).*

EXERCISE
Exercise can help control fatigue, muscle tension, and anxiety. Patients tend to feel better if they do exercises such as walking or swimming, which calm the mind as well as strengthen the body.

HERBAL THERAPIES
Thousands of herbs are used by folk healers worldwide to treat cancer, but no herbal remedy cures cancer, despite claims to the contrary. Some nontoxic herbs can be used to relieve symptoms and support general health, but because some herbs contain toxic ingredients, check with your doctor before taking any herb to relieve cancer symptoms.

HOMEOPATHY
Homeopathic remedies do not treat cancer directly, but some can alleviate side effects of radiation and chemotherapy. Consult a professional homeopath for safe and appropriate remedies.

MIND/BODY MEDICINE
Some mind/body therapies work to improve quality of life through behavior modification; others encourage expression of emotions. Behavior therapies such as **guided imagery,** progressive muscle **relaxation, hypnotherapy,** and **biofeedback** are used to alleviate pain, nausea, vomiting, and the anxiety that may occur in anticipation of or after cancer treatment. Individual or group counseling and art or music therapy let patients confront problems and emotions caused by cancer and receive support from fellow patients. Patients who pursue these types of therapies tend to feel less lonely, less anxious about death, and more optimistic about recovery.

NUTRITION AND DIET
Scientific evidence suggests that nutrition can play a role in cancer prevention. But no diet has been shown to slow or reverse cancer—and no diet cures cancer. Vitamins, minerals, and other nutrients may inhibit cancer by neutralizing carcinogens, ensuring proper immune function, or preventing tissue and cell damage. Researchers are particularly interested in antioxidants—vitamins A (particularly beta carotene), C, and E, and selenium—but are also studying folic acid, vitamin B_6, magnesium, zinc, and coenzyme Q10, among others.

Because too much of some vitamins can be harmful, many experts are cautious about dietary supplements. Instead, they advise a varied diet that includes lots of fresh fruits, vegetables, and whole grains; avoids processed, smoked, cured, fried, or barbecued foods; emphasizes lean cuts of meat and low-fat seafood; and minimizes sugar, fats, and alcohol.

Many customized diets for cancer emphasize vegetarianism, and patients who follow a nutritionally sound vegetarian diet tend to feel better. Unfortunately, many anticancer diets also promote fasting, purging, and taking supplemental "immune-boosting" vitamins, minerals, and other concoctions that do not treat cancer and may be both harmful and expensive. As a rule, patients should avoid any diet that claims to cure cancer, advocates abandoning standard treatment, causes severe weight loss or weakness, requires severe food restriction, or costs a lot of money.

CONTROVERSIAL CANCER TREATMENTS

The search for new cancer treatments is a vigorous and highly controversial branch of medical research. All treatments must be thoroughly tested and proved effective before they are authorized for general use. Supporters of some experimental treatments claim remarkable recoveries; critics insist that objective trials, not anecdotal claims, are the only true measure of their worth.

The following treatments have their share of advocates but have thus far been deemed ineffective or unproven in independent tests and clinical trials: hydrazine sulfate, studied by Dr. Joseph Gold as a cancer therapy since the 1970s; Dr. Stanislaw Burzynski's treatment with antineoplastons, originally synthesized from human urine; the "immuno-augmentative therapy" of the late Dr. Lawrence Burton; Dr. Emanuel Revici's "biologically guided chemotherapy"; Dr. Gaston Naessens's "714X" therapy; and shark cartilage supplements.

AT-HOME CARE

Relieving side effects of treatment:

◆ After radiation therapy, be gentle to your skin. Do not scrub it, expose it to sunlight, or wear tight clothing. Aloe vera ointment is gentle and soothing, and you can ask your radiation oncologist about other nonirritating lotions.
◆ Eat light snacks throughout the day rather than three heavy meals. Also try eating food cold or at room temperature to avoid nausea.
◆ If your treatment involves lowering your white blood cell count, steer clear of sick people; tell your doctor about any fever or unusual symptoms.

Relieving pain:

◆ In addition to taking prescribed medication, try relaxation techniques such as **yoga, meditation,** or **massage** given by a friend or spouse.

Other tips:

◆ Join a cancer support group.
◆ Get plenty of rest.
◆ Rather than feeling compelled to maintain a "positive attitude," express your emotions honestly. Don't worry if you sometimes feel depressed or afraid: These are normal and legitimate reactions that will not make your cancer worse.
◆ Fill your days with activities you enjoy. Reading a good book, listening to music, and talking with friends are simple pleasures, but surprisingly therapeutic.
◆ Contact the American Cancer Society and the National Cancer Institute for free information about cancer prevention, diagnosis, treatment, and tips for managing cancer symptoms. *(See the Appendix.)*

PREVENTION

◆ Do not smoke or use chewing tobacco.
◆ Stay out of the sun. Use sunscreen outdoors to protect your skin from ultraviolet rays.
◆ Follow the diet tips under **Nutrition and Diet.**
◆ Drink alcohol only in moderation.
◆ Exercise regularly to keep your body active.
◆ Get regular screening for cancer as part of your annual physical checkup.
◆ If your work exposes you to known carcinogens, be sure to follow all safety guidelines.
◆ To limit exposure to carcinogenic chemicals at home, avoid aerosol cleaning products; clean up spills and wash hands after using cleaning products; wear gloves when using pesticides; and open doors and windows to allow fumes to escape when using chemicals, stains, or paints indoors.

SYMPTOMS

- small, painful, craterlike ulcers that appear singly or in clusters on the inside of the mouth, usually lasting 5 to 10 days. The sores are grayish white or pale yellow with red borders; they may occur on the inside of the cheeks and lips, on the tongue, at the base of the gums, or on the soft palate.
- tingling or burning in the mouth; this sensation often occurs 6 to 24 hours before sores appear.

CALL YOUR DOCTOR IF:

- your canker sores are extremely painful; your doctor can give you medication to alleviate pain.
- the sores last more than 14 days; this may indicate a more serious condition that needs treatment.
- you have persistent multiple mouth sores, which may indicate an underlying problem, such as a drug reaction or, in rare cases, oral cancer or leukemia.

Canker sores, also known as aphthous ulcers, are annoying infections of the mouth that afflict up to 50 percent of Americans each year. They appear most commonly in adolescents, whose immune systems are not fully developed, and in women just before the onset of menstrual periods. In fact, women are twice as likely as men to get them. If your parents suffered from canker sores, you have a 90 percent chance of developing them. Often canker sores occur when you are under stress or run down.

Traumatic ulcers, which are caused by injuries, result in similar sores. These injuries are often caused by rough dentures, a slip of the toothbrush, or hot food.

CAUSES

No one knows what causes most canker sores, or why women are more likely to get them. Their appearance, however, often seems related to stress. Some doctors think that canker sores may result from deficiencies in iron, folic acid, vitamin B_{12}, or a combination. Canker sores may also be caused by an immune system defect, such as a food allergy. Canker sores are not thought to be contagious.

TREATMENT

Canker sores generally go away by themselves, and in most cases, you can safely ignore them. Over-the-counter remedies may help the healing process. Some alternative therapies reduce stress and soothe the inflamed area. If a sore is extremely painful or doesn't clear up, see your doctor.

CONVENTIONAL MEDICINE

Many physicians suggest the use of over-the-counter ointments to relieve the discomfort of a canker sore. Look for a medicine that contains glycerin, which protects the sore, and peroxide, which fights bacteria. If your sore does not respond to over-the-counter or at-home treatments, your doctor may prescribe a medication containing diphenhydramine to dry up the sore and lidocaine to relieve pain. If you have an infection, your doctor may treat it with an antibiotic such as tetracycline. If the sore is the result of another medical condition, such as a food sensitivity, the underlying condition should be diagnosed and treated.

ALTERNATIVE CHOICES

Alternative therapies are aimed both at healing sores and at preventing them from recurring.

ACUPRESSURE

To relieve stress, press Gall Bladder 21, the highest point of the shoulder muscle, midway between the outer tip of the shoulder and the spine. If you do this as soon as you notice a tingling in the mouth, before a sore develops, it may help reduce its severity. See pages 22–23 for more information on point location.

AROMATHERAPY

Aromatherapists recommend applying antiseptic oils of myrrh *(Commiphora molmol),* tea tree *(Melaleuca* spp.), and geranium *(Pelargonium odoratissimum).* You may also rinse your mouth four times a day with ½ cup water mixed with 1 drop each of the oils of geranium and lavender *(Lavandula officinalis).*

CHINESE HERBS

A practitioner of Chinese medicine may create an herbal formula to strengthen your entire system, heal sores, and prevent them from recurring.

HERBAL THERAPIES

To heal sores and prevent them from recurring, drink dandelion *(Taraxacum officinale)* tea or take capsules of 500 to 1,000 mg of the powdered root three times a day for six weeks. You may also apply compresses made from teas of calendula *(Calendula officinalis),* goldenseal *(Hydrastis canadensis),* or myrrh *(Commiphora molmol).*

MIND/BODY MEDICINE

Canker sores are often brought about by stress. Learn to **meditate,** listen to **guided-imagery** cas-settes, and visualize yourself as a healthy, relaxed person. The most important thing is to find a relaxation technique you enjoy and will keep doing.

NUTRITION AND DIET

If you're prone to develop canker sores, avoid coffee, spices, citrus fruits, and other foods that may irritate your mouth.

If your sores are caused by a vitamin or mineral deficiency, supplements of vitamins C and B complex, as well as folic acid, iron, and zinc, may help. If you suffer from recurrent mouth ulcers caused by a food sensitivity, avoid the foods that set off the allergic reactions.

AT-HOME REMEDIES

◆ Rinse your mouth four times a day with a combination of 2 oz hydrogen peroxide, 2 oz water, and 1 tsp each of salt and baking soda. Do not swallow.

◆ Rinse your mouth with milk of magnesia to coat sores.

◆ Try mouthwashes that contain the pain-relieving medication chlorhexidine.

◆ Cover the ulcer with a wet tea bag; the tannin will help dry up the sore.

◆ Use over-the-counter salves containing glycerin and peroxide.

◆ Try stress-relieving acupressure exercises.

PREVENTION

◆ Brush your teeth with disinfecting baking soda.

◆ Eat 4 tbsp live-culture yogurt a day; it contains bacteria that can keep your system healthy.

◆ Avoid foods that are spicy, salty, or acidic.

◆ Take vitamin and mineral supplements C, B complex, folic acid, iron, and zinc.

■

SYMPTOMS

- a tingling or numb feeling in the hand, usually just in the thumb and first three fingers.
- shooting pains in the wrist, forearm, and sometimes extending to the shoulder, neck, and chest, or foot.
- difficulty clenching the fist or grasping small objects.
- sometimes, dry skin and fingernail deterioration.

CALL YOUR DOCTOR IF:

- you feel pain in your wrist, hand, or fingers after a fall or other accident; you may have a broken bone.
- your hands or fingers feel painful and stiff, especially if the joints become swollen; you may be suffering from a form of arthritis.
- the skin on your hands and fingers becomes white and then bright red, especially in cold weather; you may be in the early stages of Raynaud's syndrome.
- pain in the hands and fingers is more intense at night; this may signal late-onset diabetes.

Carpal tunnel syndrome (CTS) is one of several names for painful and disabling injuries to the thumb and fingers, and sometimes to the wrists, elbows, and other joints. Your doctor may call it **cumulative trauma disorder, occupational neuritis, repetitive stress injury (RSI),** or **overuse injury.** The warning signs are tingling and numbness in the affected joints—typically the fingers—especially after the regular workday, or when you're ready to go to sleep, or on wakening.

Left untreated, the symptoms progress to persistent pain and aching in other areas such as the hands and arms. CTS can eventually lead to the inability to grip things firmly and to use your hands in a normal way. If you experience similar tingling and numbness in your feet, ankles, and lower legs, the condition is called **tarsal tunnel syndrome.**

Many people think CTS came in with the computer keyboard. In fact, injuries to the carpal tunnel and other major nerve passages have been around a long time; but with so many fingers tapping away at computer keyboards, the problem is more widespread than ever. The same symptoms can develop from any repetitive manual activity.

CTS and other forms of RSI are most common in middle age and tend to affect women more than men, especially if the women are overweight, pregnant, or menopausal. Whether the causes are systemic or the result of repetitive stress, most injuries to the carpal and tarsal tunnels are easily prevented and entirely correctable if recognized early. The critical factor in injuries involving repetitive stress is for the patient to stop or change the activity that brings on the discomfort. Failure to do so can result in permanent, irreversible damage to the nerves and muscles in the hand, wrist, or other parts of the body.

CAUSES

Repetitive stress injuries can happen to anyone whose work calls for long periods of steady hand movement, from musicians to meat cutters. They tend to come with work that demands repeated grasping, turning, and twisting; they are especially likely if the work requires repeated twisting or involves repetitive vibration, as in hammering nails or operating a power tool. Stressful hand, arm, and neck positions—whether from working at a desk, long-distance driving, or waiting on tables—only aggravate the potential for damage.

A number of sports can bring on repetitive stress injuries: Rowing, golf, tennis, downhill skiing, archery, competitive shooting, and rock climbing are just a sampling of activities that stress the hand and wrist joints. Injuries and ailments that cause swelling or compression of soft tissue on nerves, such as sprains, leukemia, and rheumatoid arthritis, can lead to stress injuries. Diabetes, thyroid problems, and other systemic disorders are also associated with discomfort from stressed nerves, as is the fluid accumulation that sometimes accompanies pregnancy. Some authorities believe that a pyridoxine (vitamin B_6) deficiency can also induce the symptoms.

DIAGNOSTIC AND TEST PROCEDURES

Your doctor will first check for swelling, inflammation, weakness, poor reflexes, and limited range of movement in the hand and arm. Numbness will affect the thumb, first two fingers, and inside of the ring finger; the little finger usually is not affected. The Tinel's sign test, which involves tapping the front of the wrist, will cause numbness in the forearm of an RSI sufferer.

The classic procedure for identifying RSI is the Phalen wrist flexion test—sometimes called the reverse prayer test: Holding the hands together back to back, with fingernails touching, induces tingling in a patient suffering from RSI. The doctor may want to confirm the condition by inducing pain or numbness with compression, using a blood-pressure cuff inflated above systolic pressure on the forearm. To check for potential abnormalities in the joint itself, a physician may call for an x-ray, magnetic resonance imaging (MRI), nerve-conducting velocity (NCV) studies, or an electromyograph (EMG).

TREATMENT

An instinctive reaction to numbness or tingling in the fingers is to drop the hands to the sides and shake the wrists and fingers. This natural response often provides immediate relief and—if the symptoms occur only occasionally—may be all that's needed. But if you continue doing the activity that brings on tingling and numbness, the symptoms will continue, and you can suffer permanent damage to the affected nerves. The following treatments, ranging from conservative to radical, can help prevent, counteract, or cure that damage.

CONVENTIONAL MEDICINE

You can expect your doctor to recommend rest, cool baths, or cold compresses, and to show you how to use a splint to keep your wrist from bending, especially while sleeping. You may need to wear the wrist splint for a week or two, but normally it does not keep you from using the hand. In some cases, however, the doctor may recommend that you stop typing or doing hand/finger work until the symptoms subside. You can also change your hand position on the job, use a wrist support in front of your computer keyboard, take frequent breaks to relieve stress, and do regular

THE WRIST

MEDIAN NERVE

CARPAL BONES

The wrist is a complicated, vulnerable joint. The median nerve—which runs from the forearm to the fingertips and controls movement of the fingers and thumb—passes through a tunnel formed by carpal bones and a tough layer of ligaments. If the median nerve is stressed or pinched, your fingers feel numb or tingly and you may lose feeling in your hand.

hand and arm exercises. The doctor may also recommend treatment for arthritis, obesity, or other associated disorders.

To relieve long-term pain, the doctor may prescribe aspirin or another nonsteroidal anti-inflammatory drug (NSAID) such as ibuprofen. Cortisone cream, or other externally applied analgesic preparations, can be helpful in relieving pain and counteracting the dry skin and cracked nails that sometimes accompany RSI. Corticosteroid injections can help reduce inflammation in severe cases. If the symptoms occur during pregnancy or are associated with obesity, you may be given a diuretic to get rid of excess fluid in the soft tissues.

To rebuild strength and normal movement, you may need physical therapy involving deep soft-tissue massage, stretching, and gentle range-of-motion exercises. To activate the body's own painkilling mechanisms, your doctor may recommend that you use a self-administered transcutaneous electric nerve stimulation (TENS) device, which sends low-intensity electrical pulses to the affected area.

If you have had persistent or intermittent symptoms of carpal tunnel syndrome for a year or more—or if you have a pinched or entrapped nerve—more aggressive medical intervention may be necessary. In some cases, your forearm and hand may have to be immobilized in a cast for several weeks. As a last resort, you may need surgery to relieve pressure on the nerve and remove any scar tissue. While the surgery is generally an outpatient procedure, recovery may take from several weeks to a month or more.

ALTERNATIVE CHOICES

Nonconventional treatments for carpal tunnel syndrome complement the need to reduce inflammation, rest the damaged wrist, and take the necessary steps to correct the habits or activities that caused the problem in the first place.

ACUPUNCTURE

Acupuncture may provide symptomatic pain relief by stimulating healthy circulation, calming nerves, and releasing the body's own painkilling

agents. In addition to inserting needles around the sore wrist, an experienced acupuncturist may treat the back, shoulders, and neck. Chinese herb therapy is often recommended as a complement to acupuncture.

BODY WORK

A physical therapist may offer a combination of **massage, hydrotherapy,** low-level electrical stimulation, and ultrasound to help reduce inflammation and swelling. Massage combined with ultrasound stimulates blood circulation while relaxing muscles and reducing tension, not only in the affected area but in the entire body.

Exercises that strengthen the hand and wrist can be useful in preventing further stress injuries. If the injury was caused by repetitive stress, a few minutes of warmup exercises before beginning work and regular tension-relieving exercises throughout the workday can have a positive, preventive effect.

CHIROPRACTIC

Conventional chiropractic therapy will look beyond the wrist itself to spinal adjustment of the neck and upper back to restore normal nerve activity. Some chiropractors will also adjust the wrist and elbow and may advise ultrasound, massage, and nutritional therapy.

HERBAL THERAPY

Make a soothing compress by grating 1 to 2 oz of fresh ginger (Zingiber officinale) and making an infusion with half a cup of hot, but not boiling, water. Dip a soft, folded cloth into the infusion and apply the compress to the affected area, covering it with a dry cloth to retain the heat.

HOMEOPATHY

Over-the-counter homeopathic remedies may provide relief of carpal tunnel symptoms: Arnica (6x to 30c) for swelling and bruising caused by overuse or misuse of the joints; Ruta (6x to 12x) for tendon inflammation; and Rhus toxicodendron (6x) for pain. If these remedies do not relieve symptoms within a week, see a licensed homeopath for a more specific analysis and remedies appropriate to your condition.

NUTRITION AND DIET

Supplemental vitamin E in amounts up to 800 IU daily is reported to help reduce tissue inflammation. Vitamin C supplements up to 1,000 mg may be beneficial in tissue restoration. Vitamin B$_6$, or pyridoxine, is reported to help nerve inflammation and enhance blood circulation, and serves as a mild diuretic. Because high-protein diets inhibit the absorption of B$_6$, reduce your protein intake. Start with 50 mg a day, or try a vitamin B complex supplement; symptoms should ease within the month.

Cutting down on sugar and sweets in general may be helpful, since a diet high in refined sugar is thought to weaken the body's ability to combat inflammation.

OSTEOPATHY

Osteopathic physicians may recommend manipulation of the joint and surrounding soft tissue to improve circulation and nerve function, as well as appropriate drugs.

YOGA

If you are suffering from carpal tunnel syndrome or other stress-related problems, yoga positions that relax the neck and back may be advisable. Avoid hand and neck stands, as well as positions that include arm twists, any of which could harm already sensitive nerves.

AT-HOME REMEDIES

A few simple exercises and a cold pack may be the most effective on-the-spot treatment for reducing the discomfort and numbness of a repetitive stress injury. For most of us, the quickest source of cold is a few ice cubes or a pack of frozen vegetables wrapped in a towel. Use the cold pack for about an hour at a time, 10 minutes on the affected area and 10 minutes off.

An effective exercise you can do anytime and anywhere is opening and closing your fist a dozen or more times. Other quick hand routines:
◆ With palms facing each other, press your fingertips together 20 times, rest, then repeat.
◆ Holding your hands over your head, rotate them at the wrists clockwise for 20 seconds, then do the same exercise counterclockwise.
◆ Strengthen hand and forearm muscles with a spring-style or foam-rubber grip exerciser.

For **tarsal tunnel syndrome,** some people find that walking barefoot whenever possible alleviates the discomfort and helps prevent recurrence.

PREVENTION

The natural position of the hand in most normal activities is straight or slightly bent at the wrist, with the thumb more or less in line with the forearm. Bending the hand forward or backward at the wrist for extended periods stresses the carpal nerves, so learn to keep your wrist and hand as straight as possible as you work.

If your job calls for repetitive hand or finger work, take breaks and exercise your hands and wrists every hour. If you work at an office keyboard, use a wrist support to help prevent unnatural bending and make sure your desk and chair height are correct for your stature.

Interior architects and designers now realize that the science of ergonomics—human engineering—is essential not just to make the home and workplace efficient, but to maintain the well-being of the inhabitants. Fortunately, ergonomically designed offices and factories are fast becoming the norm.

Finally, if carpal tunnel symptoms begin, don't work through the pain. Get a professional diagnosis and follow the recommendations. ■

C

SYMPTOMS

Because everyone's eyesight changes later in life, and because cataract development is usually a gradual process, your first symptom may be having trouble passing the vision test when renewing your driver's license or having a regular eye exam. Physical symptoms include:

- hazy vision that might be worse in bright light.
- impaired vision at night; difficulty in discerning movements, details, or objects.
- blinding or uncomfortable glare from automobile headlights or bright sunlight.
- seeing halos around lights.
- unexpected improvement in near vision.
- double or triple vision in one eye only.
- a milky white or opaque appearance to the normally transparent lens of the eye (advanced case).
- painful inflammation and pressure within the eye (very advanced case).

CALL YOUR DOCTOR IF:

- you have any of the above symptoms or if your vision deteriorates or becomes distorted in any way. Cataracts are not visible to a casual observer until they are quite advanced, so it is essential that you see an ophthalmologist for evaluation.

The lens of the human eye focuses light so that you can see objects clearly at various distances. It must remain transparent for clear vision. The clouding of this lens is called a cataract. As the developing cataract blocks or distorts the light entering the eye, you will experience a gradual, persistent, painless blurring of vision, as though you were looking through a haze.

Cataracts are the leading cause of blindness, accounting for almost 20 million cases worldwide and at least 40,000 cases in the United States. Despite these numbers, the disease is actually one of the less serious eye disorders, because surgery can restore the lost sight in most cases. Yet in the U.S. alone, some 5,000 people go blind each year because of ignorance, fear, or refusal to undergo a relatively painless operation.

CAUSES

Cataracts are the result of changes in the chemical structure of proteins in the cells of the lens. The usually clear protein becomes cloudy, primarily as a result of the protein's aging over the course of a lifetime; about 75 percent of all cataracts arise from this natural aging. Called **senile cataracts,** they are most prevalent in people over the age of 70.

A variety of ordinary stresses can contribute to senile cataracts. One major factor is exposure to sunlight, particularly ultraviolet B (UVB) radiation, which reacts with the lens protein. Other risk factors, according to some specialists, are cigarette smoke, air pollution, vitamin deficiencies, and heavy alcohol consumption.

The most common type of senile cataract, and one with a surprising side effect, is known as **nuclear sclerosis,** in which the cataract develops in the nucleus (center) of the lens. During the early stages of cataract formation, the lens swells slightly, which increases its focusing power and improves near vision to such an extent that some people find they can suddenly read without eyeglasses. But the improvement doesn't last long; as clouding increases, vision deteriorates again.

Cataracts may also develop as a secondary effect of other eye ailments such as glaucoma or

THROUGH A LENS DARKLY

NORMAL EYE

IRIS
PUPIL
CATARACT

EYE WITH CATARACT

In a normal eye, the lens is clear and appears black in the center of the pupil *(top)*. As a person ages, natural changes in the lens fibers cause a clouding of the lens known as a cataract, which in severe cases appears opaque in the pupil *(bottom)*. Progressive clouding leads to blurred, dim, hazy vision. Fortunately, surgery can correct most cataracts and restore near-normal vision.

of systemic diseases such as diabetes mellitus. Other causes include physical injury to the lens, large amounts of radiation, chemical and drug toxicity, and hereditary disorders.

DIAGNOSTIC AND TEST PROCEDURES

By shining a penlight on your pupil, your doctor may detect the cataract. Using special instruments and techniques, your ophthalmologist will identify its precise character, location, and extent.

TREATMENT

At present the only corrective treatment for a developed cataract is surgery. However, both conventional and alternative therapies are seeking ways to prevent cataract formation.

CONVENTIONAL MEDICINE

Cataract surgery is one of the most successful of all operations. More than 500,000 cataract operations are performed each year in the United States, and approximately 95 percent of the patients report improved vision.

The operation, usually performed under local anesthesia on an outpatient basis, is safe, fast, and nearly painless. The clouded lens may be removed through a small incision made at the outer edge of the cornea or with an ultrasonic needle called a phacoemulsifier using a technique that reduces the size of the incision, making sutures unnecessary. The next step often is the implantation of a clear plastic replacement lens. In cases where lens removal is not followed by an artificial lens implant, strong or thick corrective eyeglasses or contact lenses are necessary.

Following surgery, you will usually wear a protective eye shield or glasses during the day and an eye shield at night. To prevent infection and reduce inflammation, your physician may recommend that you apply antibiotic and steroid ointments or drops to your eye.

Over time, 20 to 50 percent of patients experience a recurrence of visual clouding caused by a cellophane-thin membrane that sometimes develops behind the artificial lens implant. The membrane can be easily removed by laser.

PREVENTION

The single most important thing you can do to prevent cataract development is to avoid bright sunlight outdoors by wearing sunglasses that filter out UVB. Dark glasses that do not filter out UVB can actually increase your risk, because your pupils widen to adjust to the decreased light, thus exposing your eyes to more of the dangerous UVB radiation.

Some ophthalmologists think that antioxidants, which reduce free radicals (unstable chemical compounds) that can damage lens protein, offer protection against cataract development by lessening or retarding protein deterioration in the lens brought on by environmental factors. Naturopaths recommend a diet high in fruits and vegetables containing antioxidants such as beta carotene (vitamin A), selenium, and vitamins C and E, including citrus fruits, spinach, sweet potatoes, carrots, and broccoli. ∎

SYMPTOMS

- abdominal pain and swelling.
- flatulence and a bloated feeling.
- diarrhea.
- pale, foul-smelling stools that may float in water, sometimes with yellow fat globules floating on the surface of water in the toilet.
- fatigue, loss of appetite, and eventual loss of weight.
- itchy, blistering skin on elbows and knees in people with dermatitis herpetiformis.
- in children, delayed growth and muscle weakness.
- in infants, signs of extreme gastrointestinal distress within a few weeks after starting to eat cereal.

CALL YOUR DOCTOR IF:

- you have celiac disease and you begin to have new abdominal pain, diarrhea, or weight loss; these could be early signs of intestinal cancer.
- your infant does not appear to improve within a few days after cereal is eliminated from the diet.

Celiac disease—sometimes called celiac-sprue—is a sensitivity of the small intestine to gluten, a protein found in most cereal grains but not in corn and rice. The intolerance to gluten irritates the small intestine and leads to deterioration of the tiny fingerlike villi (essential for the absorption of food) on the mucous lining.

The term *celiac* simply refers to the abdominal cavity, but the disease can have complications beyond the stomach and intestines. Women with untreated celiac disease often fail to conceive and, if they do, tend to miscarry more frequently than the normal population. Even after treatment, conception may not occur for 18 months or more. The disease can cause impotence in men, who may take up to two years to regain full sexual potency after starting treatment.

Celiac disease often appears in infancy or early childhood but may occur at any age. It seems to have a strong genetic component and affects twice as many women as it does men, especially women of northern European ancestry. In Iceland, for example, where virtually the entire population is Scandinavian, 1 out of 300 infants has the disease, but it is relatively rare in the more varied population of the United States.

Most people with celiac disease accept a life-long ban on baked goods, pasta, and other foods made from whole-grain or processed wheat flour. Celiac patients who fail to eliminate gluten from their diets are 10 to 15 percent more likely than the norm to develop cancer of the small intestine.

CAUSES

Sensitivity to gluten seems to be hereditary and frequently affects siblings, but its exact cause is unknown. Some research suggests it stems from a deficiency of an enzyme that digests gluten. Other research points to a defect in the immune system that causes certain cells to attack the intestinal mucous membrane when gluten is in the diet.

DIAGNOSTIC AND TEST PROCEDURES

To diagnose celiac disease, your doctor may first test your blood for antibodies that will be present if you are sensitive to gluten. The doctor may order a barium x-ray to detect abnormalities on the intestinal lining. A final diagnosis requires a biopsy so that a tiny sample of the intestinal lining can be examined under a microscope.

TREATMENT

Corrective treatment for celiac disease is almost entirely dietary, and in most cases the patient responds without the need for additional measures.

CONVENTIONAL MEDICINE

Primary treatment consists in changing your diet. Your doctor will direct you to eliminate foods that contain wheat, rye, barley, and oats. You can probably eat foods made with corn, rice, and millet, and with gluten-free wheat, which some patients tolerate well. A dietitian can identify products that contain gluten in unlikely forms such as soy sauce and modified food starch, which is added to a number of packaged foods. In families known to carry celiac disease, breast-feeding babies for at least four months and not giving them wheat products until they are a year old lower their chances of developing the disease.

Until the intestine is well on its way back to health, doctors frequently advise celiac patients to avoid fatty foods and dairy products, which are relatively difficult to digest. If you are constipated because you're not getting enough fiber on the gluten-free diet, your doctor may suggest you try a spoonful of rice bran mixed with juice or fruit. If you have lost weight and appear very ill, your doctor may prescribe steroids, such as prednisone, to help the intestine heal.

ALTERNATIVE CHOICES

The information that follows includes suggestions for relieving uncomfortable symptoms and complementing the gluten-free diet.

NUTRITION AND DIET

You may need supplemental folic acid, vitamin A, and zinc to speed healing and maintain a healthy gastrointestinal tract. Papain, a protein-digesting enzyme, may help you digest any gluten that sneaks into your diet; take 500 to 1,000 mg daily with meals.

REFLEXOLOGY

For celiac-associated diarrhea, a reflexologist will massage areas on the bottoms of the feet associated with the ascending colon, transverse colon, diaphragm, liver, and adrenal glands. *(See page 25 for area locations.)*

YOGA

To tone the intestinal tract, practitioners recommend the following exercise: Sit on the floor with legs outstretched. Place the sole of your right foot on your inner left thigh, with your right knee on the floor. Place your left foot on top of your right thigh. Straighten your spine, neck, and head. Hold the pose for 60 seconds, then switch sides. Do as often as possible, up to 15 times a day.

HERBAL THERAPIES

Slippery elm *(Ulmus fulva)* bark has long been used to soothe the bowels. Mix ¼ tsp of the powder in a cup of warm water and drink promptly, four times a day. A teaspoon of meadowsweet *(Filipendula ulmaria)* infused in a cup of warm water may soothe the bowels and reduce the likelihood of diarrhea.

AT-HOME REMEDIES

People rarely "grow out of" celiac disease. The key to controlling the illness is to stop eating foods made from or containing gluten, which means cutting out all wheat, rye, and barley, and usually oats. Some patients need dietary supplements to offset deficiencies in iron and folic acid caused by the disease. If the gluten-free regimen is strictly followed, people usually begin feeling better within days. Complete recovery may take several months, as the intestines regain their normal lining. Thereafter, most people can digest any food permitted in the gluten-free diet. ■

SYMPTOMS

In its early stages, cervical cancer causes no pain or other symptoms. The first identifiable symptoms of the disease are likely to include:

- watery or bloody vaginal discharge, sometimes heavy and foul smelling.
- vaginal bleeding after intercourse, between menstrual periods, or after menopause; menstrual periods may be heavier and last longer than normal.

If the cancer has spread to nearby tissues, symptoms may include:

- difficult urination and possible kidney failure.
- painful urination, sometimes with blood in urine.
- dull backache or swelling in the legs.
- diarrhea, or pain or bleeding from the rectum upon defecation.
- fatigue, loss of weight and appetite, and general feeling of illness.

CALL YOUR DOCTOR IF:

- abnormal bleeding, vaginal discharge, or any other symptoms last more than two weeks without explanation. You should have a complete gynecological examination that includes a Pap smear.
- NOTE: Any vaginal bleeding after menopause should be brought to your doctor's attention right away. The cause may simply be vaginal dryness or a benign uterine polyp, but vaginal bleeding is the most common symptom of cervical and uterine cancer. (See also Cervical Problems.)

The cervix is the narrow neck of a woman's uterus, just above the vagina. More than 9 out of 10 cervical cancers originate in surface cells lining the cervix. In some women, healthy cells enter an abnormal phase called **dysplasia;** although these cells are not cancerous, they can become so. When dysplastic cells turn malignant, the first detectable stage is **carcinoma in situ.** As cancer cells multiply, some may invade the lining of the cervix itself, spread to nearby tissue, and enter the bloodstream or lymphatic system.

Just as it usually takes many years for **dysplasia** to become **carcinoma in situ,** it often takes months or even years for cervical cancer to become invasive. For this reason, and because of the Pap smear—a highly effective, widely available screening test—cervical cancer is one of the least threatening kinds. When caught early, it is curable; even in advanced cases, the chance of surviving at least five years, with likelihood of full cure, is still better than 60 percent. Only when the cancer spreads to distant organs does prognosis for five-year survival dip below 20 percent.

Dysplasia is most likely to occur in women between the ages of 25 and 35, **carcinoma in situ** between ages 30 and 40, and invasive cancer between ages 40 and 60. Cervical cancer constitutes about 2.5 percent of all cancers afflicting American women; each year some 55,000 cases of **carcinoma in situ** and about 15,000 cases of invasive cancer are diagnosed.

CAUSES

Four out of five cervical cancer cases are linked to sexually transmitted viral infections, such as genital herpes and a few of the 60 or so human papilloma viruses (HPV) that often cause genital warts. But many women who have a sexually transmitted viral infection do not develop cervical cancer, while others who get cancer have never had such infections. Women who began having sexual intercourse before age 18, have had multiple sex partners, have had several full-term pregnancies, or have a history of sexually transmitted disease are most likely to develop **dysplasia** or cervical cancer. Apparently genetic makeup and other factors are also part of the complex interactions that cause cervical cancer.

Cervical cancer is also more common among women who smoke. Many researchers doubt that smoking causes cervical cancer on its own but feel that it may heighten one's vulnerability to other illnesses, such as viral infections. Women whose immune system is severely suppressed by other diseases, by treatments, or by organ transplants are more vulnerable to cervical cancer, as are women whose mother took diethylstilbestrol (DES) while pregnant; DES is a drug once prescribed to prevent miscarriage but no longer marketed. Women who are obese or who use birth-control pills may be at slightly increased risk.

DIAGNOSTIC AND TEST PROCEDURES

Every woman should have an annual pelvic exam and Pap smear, which tests a cervical cell sample for abnormalities. Together these procedures detect cervical cancer 95 percent of the time, often long before the disease produces symptoms. If your Pap smear is abnormal, your doctor may prescribe antibiotics and test you again, since a minor infection can affect the results. If the second test is abnormal, your doctor will visually examine your cervix and take a tissue sample of any apparent abnormality for biopsy. If the biopsy confirms cancer, further tests will determine whether the disease has spread. These tests might include x-rays of the bladder, rectum, bowels, and abdominal cavity; blood and urine tests; and liver and kidney function studies. If you have ever had a sexually transmitted viral infection, your doctor will need to know what strain you were infected with to determine the most appropriate treatment for the cervical cancer.

TREATMENT

Most cases of cervical cancer are cured or controlled by a combination of surgery, chemotherapy, and radiation therapy. A variety of alternative therapies might prove useful in easing side effects and improving overall health. See Cancer for more information on therapies.

CONVENTIONAL MEDICINE

Women with genital warts and mild **dysplasia** should be carefully monitored for signs of cancer but usually require no immediate treatment. **Carcinoma in situ,** severe **dysplasia,** and mildly invasive cancers are normally treated surgically. Superficial tumors can be treated with radiation but are more often removed with a scalpel, a laser beam, controlled freezing, or cauterization.

If cancer has advanced deep into the cervix or spread to neighboring organs, hysterectomy—removal of the cervix, uterus, and possibly other organs—is imperative. If cancer spreads beyond the pelvic area, radiation therapy and perhaps chemotherapy may relieve symptoms and suppress the spread but rarely result in cure. Any woman who has had **dysplasia** or cervical cancer should see her doctor regularly for at least five years after treatment to check for recurrence.

COMPLEMENTARY THERAPIES

One promising field of cancer prevention research is **nutrition and diet.** Some evidence suggests that folic acid and beta carotene help ward off precancerous and cancerous conditions of the cervix. Patients undergoing radiation therapy may benefit from supplements of vitamin B_6. Ask your doctor about other dietary recommendations or nutritional supplements.

PREVENTION

◆ If you are a woman over age 18, or are under 18 and sexually active, have a pelvic exam and Pap smear yearly. If your Pap smear is normal several years in a row, your doctor may recommend the test less often.

◆ If you practice contraception, consider barrier or spermicidal contraceptives, which—according to one study—may lower the risk of cervical cancer compared with hormone-based contraceptives.

◆ If you have more than one sexual partner, be sure to use condoms to protect yourself from sexually transmitted diseases. ■

SYMPTOMS

- vaginal discharge that is green, gray, white, or yellow.
- pain during intercourse.
- vaginal bleeding, sometimes during or after intercourse.
- unusually heavy menstrual periods.
- crampy pelvic pain or a feeling of heaviness.

Many cervical problems have no symptoms.

CALL YOUR DOCTOR IF:

- you have a smelly or colored discharge; you may have an infection.
- you have bleeding between your periods or after menopause; you may have an infection, hormone problem, **cervical polyps, cervical erosion, uterine fibroids,** or uterine cancer *(see Uterine Problems).* You should seek a medical diagnosis as soon as possible.

The cervix is the knoblike lower portion of the uterus that connects the uterus to the vagina. At its center is a small opening, known as the cervical os, that provides an exit for uterine tissue and blood during menstruation and allows sperm to enter. On the uterine side of the os is the cervical canal, a narrow, inch-long passageway leading into the uterus. During childbirth the cervix thins and gradually opens, or dilates, to allow for the delivery of the child.

The part of the cervix that protrudes into the vagina is covered with pink tissue called squamous cell epithelium. The part that extends into the cervical canal is covered with red, mucus-producing tissue called columnar epithelium. The place where these two parts meet is known as the squamocolumnar junction.

Inflammations of the cervix, both acute and chronic, are known by the general term **cervicitis.** The main symptom of cervicitis is abundant vaginal discharge that is grayish, green, white, or yellow, depending on the type of infection. Other symptoms may include pain during intercourse. Some women with cervicitis experience backache or a feeling of pelvic heaviness caused by the drainage of the infection-fighting lymph nodes along the ligaments in the back that support the uterus.

Two other common conditions of the cervix are **cervical eversion** and **cervical erosion.** Cervical eversion occurs when the red columnar cells lining the inner cervical canal begin to form on the outer vaginal part of the cervix. This condition is common among teenagers and women who are pregnant or on birth-control pills. Cervical erosion occurs when the pink squamous cell tissue of the cervix has been worn away, leaving red exposed sores on its surface. Many women with cervical eversion or erosion have no symptoms, although occasionally the conditions may cause a whitish or slightly bloody vaginal discharge.

Other conditions involving the cervix include **cervical stenosis**—partial or total narrowing of the cervix, which can lead to obstruction—and **cervical incompetence,** the premature opening of the cervix during pregnancy, which creates a high risk of miscarriage.

Cysts and polyps can form on the cervix. **Cer-**

vical cysts occur without symptoms and require no treatment. **Cervical polyps** are also usually harmless, although they may cause irregular bleeding and discharge. Because of these discomforts and because they sometimes affect fertility, cervical polyps are often removed surgically.

Genital warts can also infect the cervix, producing flat, benign lesions. These warts are caused by the human papilloma virus, and there are many subtypes, several of which are associated with an increased risk of cervical cancer.

Another potentially serious cervical problem is **dysplasia,** the abnormal development of cervical cells. Dysplasia is considered a precancerous condition because, if untreated, it leads to cervical cancer in 30 to 50 percent of cases. Although cervical dysplasia strikes women of all ages, it most commonly afflicts women aged 25 to 35. Dysplasia produces no obvious symptoms. The only way to detect the condition is with a test known as a Pap smear *(see Diagnostic and Test Procedures, page 246).*

CERVICAL POLYPS

UTERUS

CERVIX

VAGINA

ENDOCERVICAL POLYP

ECTOCERVICAL POLYP

Cervical polyps are benign growths on the cervix, the lower portion of the uterus that connects to the vagina. Two common types of polyps are endocervical polyps *(above, left),* found within the cervix itself, and ectocervical polyps *(above, right),* found outside the mouth of the cervix. The polyps are usually harmless, but in some cases they may be removed in a minor surgical procedure.

CAUSES

The causes of cervical problems vary. **Cervicitis** is usually associated with other infections of the vaginal cavity caused by sexually transmitted diseases, such as genital herpes, chlamydia, trichomoniasis, and gonorrhea. In some instances lacerations or tears to the cervix during childbirth may also lead to an infection.

What causes **cervical eversion** and **erosion** is not always clear; however, about 20 percent of women are born with eversions, and the friction of intercourse appears to be a factor in erosions. Some doctors believe that the hormones in birth-control pills and the strings of intrauterine devices (IUDs) may cause cervical eversion and erosion, as well as cervicitis. It is estimated that 95 percent of women have an erosion on their cervix at some point during their lives, although often without any symptoms.

Cervical stenosis has a variety of causes. Some women are born with the blockage; others develop it as the result of infections or abnormal growths, such as **polyps** or **uterine fibroids**

(see Uterine Problems). Surgical procedures involving the cervix, such as biopsies and curettage (or scraping) of the cervical canal, can also lead to blockages.

The cause of **cervical incompetence,** which can result in loss of a pregnancy, is unknown, although it has been associated with surgical procedures, such as therapeutic abortions and dilation and curettage (D and C). Abnormal development of the cervix can also lead to cervical incompetence. Women whose mothers took the synthetic estrogen hormone diethylstilbestrol (DES), which was once given in an effort to prevent miscarriage during pregnancy, are at greater risk for cervical and vaginal abnormalities.

A nabothian **cyst,** the most common type of cyst that forms on the cervix, occurs when a mucus gland on the cervix becomes obstructed. Endometriosis, the growth of endometrial tissue outside the uterine cavity, can also cause cysts, known as endometriomas, to form on the cervix.

Cervical polyps often develop after an infection as the body tries to heal itself by growing

CERVICAL PROBLEMS CONTINUED

new cells to cover the old, inflamed ones. Polyps also form during pregnancy and in women who take birth-control pills, as a result of hormonal changes that stimulate the overgrowth of tissue.

Cervical warts are caused by the human papilloma virus (HPV), which is transmitted by sexual contact.

Cervical dysplasia is caused by a subtype of the human papilloma virus, which also causes cervical cancer, but not everyone who is exposed to the virus develops dysplasia or cancer, indicating that other factors are also at work.

DIAGNOSTIC AND TEST PROCEDURES

The first test used to diagnose cervical problems is the Pap smear, a simple procedure in which cells are collected from the cervix with a brush or wooden spatula and examined under a microscope. If the Pap smear indicates a precancerous or cancerous condition, a cervical biopsy—removal of tissue from the cervix for examination—will also be done. The biopsy is performed with a colposcope, a special magnifying instrument. In cases where the area of abnormal tissue extends into the cervical canal, a procedure known as a conization, which removes a cone-shaped piece of tissue from the center of the cervix for analysis, may also be needed. Conizations are done in a hospital under a general anesthetic.

TREATMENT

Some harmless and symptomless cervical problems, such as erosion and nabothian cysts, often require no treatment. Other conditions can be treated with both alternative and conventional methods. For serious cervical problems, such as dysplasia or cancer, however, you should always seek conventional treatment.

CONVENTIONAL MEDICINE

Conventional medical treatments for cervical problems depend on the condition.

Cervicitis is usually treated with an antibiotic or sulfa drug. Your doctor will probably rec-

ommend that you refrain from intercourse until the infection has cleared up to keep it from spreading. In chronic cases of cervicitis antibiotics are not always effective. Your doctor may recommend that the infected tissue be destroyed by either electric cauterization or cryosurgery,

ACUPRESSURE

1 Pressing Small Intestine 3 may help provide relief from back stiffness that sometimes accompanies cervical problems. Place your thumb on the side of the hand, just below the knuckle of the little finger, between the bone and the muscle. Apply pressure for one minute.

2 To reduce neck-muscle stress that may be associated with cervical problems, try pressing Gall Bladder 20. Place the tips of both middle fingers in the hollows at the base of your skull, about two inches apart, on either side of the spine. Press firmly for one minute.

3 Applying pressure to Bladder 10 may provide relief from the stress and tension associated with cervical problems. Press on the ropy muscles a half inch below the base of the skull for one minute.

4 To relieve nervousness and irritability, try pressing Gall Bladder 21. For one minute, use your middle finger to press on the highest point of the shoulders, one or two inches out from the base of the neck. Pregnant women should press lightly on this point.

246

which removes the tissue by freezing it with liquid nitrogen. These procedures, which cause only minor cramping and require no anesthetics, can usually be done in a doctor's office.

If necessary, **cervical cysts** and **polyps** can be removed surgically in your doctor's office under local anesthesia. Surgery to remove blockage caused by **cervical stenosis** is usually done in the hospital. If your cervix begins to close after the surgery, a follow-up procedure to keep it open may be necessary.

Pregnant women with **incompetent cervixes** used to be confined to their beds for their entire pregnancy. Today, the condition is more commonly treated with a procedure called cerclage, which involves stitching the cervix closed, usually during the 12th to 16th week of pregnancy. The stitches are removed in the ninth month of pregnancy. Most women who have the procedure are able to deliver their babies vaginally.

Mild cases of **cervical dysplasia** are treated with cauterization, cryosurgery, or laser surgery, which uses a high-energy beam of light to vaporize the affected tissue. In more advanced cases conization is used. Some doctors recommend a hysterectomy for women with severe cervical dysplasia; however, this is almost always unnecessary. If you have recurring dysplasia that fails to respond to treatment, you should be screened for HIV infection *(see AIDS).*

ALTERNATIVE CHOICES

Alternative treatments may help to heal minor cervical problems.

HERBAL THERAPIES

Goldenseal *(Hydrastis canadensis)* douches are recommended for **cervicitis** and **cervical erosion.** Pour 1 cup of boiling water over 1 tbsp of the herb. Steep the liquid for 15 minutes, then strain and use warm. Pour into a douche container and use as directed on the container package. Repeat every day until symptoms are gone.

HYDROTHERAPY

To stimulate the flow of blood to the cervix and help **cervical erosions** heal, try taking alternating hot and cold sitz baths. Fill one bathtub or large bowl with hot water and another with cold water. Sit in the hot water for 3 minutes, followed by 1 minute in the cold water. Repeat three times, ending with the cold bath, then immediately dress in warm clothing. Take the sitz baths every other day until the cervical erosion heals.

AT-HOME REMEDIES

To help treat **cervical eversion,** douche with a vinegar-and-water solution. By changing the pH of the vagina, the douche may help stop the red columnar cells normally found in the uterus from forming on the vaginal side of the cervical os. To make the douche, mix 2 tbsp white vinegar in a quart of warm water. Use daily until symptoms are gone.

PREVENTION

◆ Practice sexual abstinence or use condoms. Studies have shown that the more exposure to semen a woman has, the greater her risk of **dysplasia** and other cervical problems.

◆ Use barrier methods of birth control—condoms, diaphragms, or cervical caps—when having sex. Such methods offer some protection against sexually transmitted diseases, which can lead to cervical problems.

◆ To help prevent **cervicitis,** eat plenty of fresh vegetables and fruits. These foods are rich in vitamin C, beta carotene (vitamin A), folic acid, and other nutrients that strengthen the immune system and help fight off some infections.

◆ If you smoke, quit. Women who smoke have a greater incidence of dysplasia and cervical cancer.

◆ Women with **erosion** or inflammation of the cervix should be screened for conditions that may cause infertility. ■

CHEST PAIN

Read down this column to find your symptoms. Then read across.

SYMPTOMS	AILMENT/PROBLEM
◆ chest pain that may radiate to jaw, neck, left arm, or elsewhere; possibly, sweating, shortness of breath, nausea, vomiting, anxiety.	◆ Heart attack (damage to the heart muscle)
◆ sudden chest pain with shortness of breath; worsening of pain with deep breathing or cough, which may produce blood-streaked sputum; sweating; fainting.	◆ Blood clot in lung (pulmonary embolism)
◆ sudden chest pain with increasing shortness of breath; worsening of pain with breathing; possibly, recent chest injury.	◆ Collapsed lung (pneumothorax)
◆ severe chest pain beginning during exercise and subsiding after a short rest; possibly, radiation of pain to other areas.	◆ Angina
◆ chest pain with shortness of breath or chest rattle; fever and coughing up of phlegm; worsening pain with deep breathing or cough.	◆ Pneumonia
◆ pain and tenderness on one side of chest after recent severe cough, injury, or chest surgery.	◆ Injured muscle or rib
◆ pain and tightening in chest; possibly, frequent deep breaths; rapid heartbeat; tingling and numbness of lips, arms, or legs.	◆ Stress; anxiety; panic attack
◆ burning pain, usually in lower chest, that worsens on reclining; acid or sour taste in mouth; pain relieved by belching or antacids.	◆ Heartburn (a gastrointestinal problem)

WHAT TO DO	OTHER INFO
◆ **Call 911 or your emergency number now.** *(See Heart Attack.)*	◆ Loosen clothing; try to stay calm. If someone with you has a heart attack and stops breathing, use CPR *(see Emergencies/First Aid: Cardiac and Respiratory Arrest).*
◆ **Call 911 or your emergency number now.** You will be treated to dissolve the blockage.	◆ Hospitalization is usually required for extensive diagnostic testing, including a lung scan.
◆ **Call 911 or your emergency number now.** You may require a chest tube to reinflate the lung.	◆ The cause may be injury, or the lung may collapse spontaneously for an unknown reason.
◆ **Call your doctor now** if you are not already under a doctor's care for angina. See also Heart Disease.	◆ Stop smoking, decrease fat in the diet, and increase exercise, but avoid overexertion.
◆ Call your doctor, who will probably prescribe antibiotics (if the cause is bacterial), plus rest, fluids, and analgesics.	◆ You must get a professional diagnosis and treatment plan for pneumonia.
◆ Rest; apply warm compresses. For pain, wrap chest with a pressure bandage and/or take analgesics. If pain persists, call your doctor to check the possibility of a broken rib.	◆ Chest wall movement tends to worsen chest pain caused by injury, but you must breathe deeply enough to keep lungs inflated.
◆ See the related entries.	◆ Persistent stress (which may also be associated with heart disease) may be relieved by relaxation techniques.
◆ Try an antacid, or consult your doctor about taking other or stronger medication, or if additional symptoms occur. See Heartburn, Gas and Gas Pains, Hiatal Hernia, Indigestion.	

SYMPTOMS

◆ a very itchy rash that spreads from the torso to the neck, face, and limbs. The rash, lasting 7 to 10 days, progresses from red spots to fluid-filled blisters (vesicles) that drain and scab over. Vesicles may also appear in the mouth, around the eyes, or on the genitals, and can be very painful. See also the Visual Diagnostic Guide.

CALL YOUR DOCTOR IF:

◆ you think your child has chickenpox; a doctor can confirm your diagnosis.

◆ chickenpox is accompanied by severe skin pain, and the rash produces a greenish discharge and looks inflamed—signs of a secondary bacterial skin infection.

◆ chickenpox is accompanied by a stiff neck, persistent sleepiness, or lethargy—symptoms of acute encephalitis, a serious illness. **Get medical help immediately.**

◆ your child is recovering from chickenpox and begins running a fever, vomiting, has convulsions, or is somnolent; these are signs of Reye's syndrome, a dangerous, potentially fatal disease that sometimes follows viral infections, particularly if aspirin has been used in treatment. **Get medical help immediately.**

◆ an adult family member gets chickenpox; in adults, the illness can lead to complications such as pneumonia. See your doctor without delay.

◆ you are pregnant, have never had chickenpox, and are exposed to the disease; your unborn child may be at risk for birth defects. See your doctor without delay.

Chickenpox, a viral illness characterized by a very itchy red rash, is one of the most common infectious diseases of childhood. It is usually mild in children, but adults run the risk of serious complications, such as bacterial pneumonia.

People who have had chickenpox develop lifetime immunity. But the virus remains dormant in the body, and if you had chickenpox as a child, you may later develop shingles. Because chickenpox can pass from a pregnant woman to her unborn child, possibly causing birth defects, doctors often advise women considering pregnancy to confirm their immunity with a blood test.

CAUSES

Chickenpox is caused by the herpes zoster virus, also known as the varicella zoster virus. It is spread by droplets from a sneeze or cough, or by contact with the clothing, bed linens, or oozing

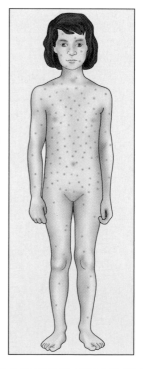

IDENTIFYING THE RASH

Small, red bumps appear on the chest and back and soon form a rash of itchy, fluid-filled blisters that burst and form scabs. Within days the rash spreads to the face, arms, and legs *(right)*. Scabs will dry and drop off about a week after they appear, and the rash should be gone in two weeks. Avoid scratching the scabs; they may become infected and even leave scars if scratched.

vesicles of an infected person. The incubation period is 7 to 21 days; the disease is most contagious a day before the rash appears and up to 7 days after, or until the rash forms scabs.

TREATMENT

Chickenpox is extremely contagious. Keep your child home until most of the vesicles are dry and scabs have fallen off.

CONVENTIONAL MEDICINE

Your pediatrician may prescribe an antihistamine, such as diphenhydramine, to relieve pain and swelling. Antibiotics are called for if a secondary bacterial skin infection arises or if an adult with chickenpox contracts bacterial pneumonia. Acyclovir, an antiviral drug, is sometimes prescribed in severe cases, although some doctors question its effectiveness.

ALTERNATIVE CHOICES

HERBAL THERAPIES

For itching, herbalists recommend the following wash: Add 1 oz each dried rosemary *(Rosmarinus officinalis)* and calendula *(Calendula officinalis)* to 1 qt water. Bring to a boil, then simmer for five minutes. Strain, discard the herbs, and allow the wash to cool. Press a washcloth dampened in the solution to the child's skin after a bath. The wash can be reused for three days if refrigerated.

HOMEOPATHY

Consult a homeopath for appropriate remedies and dosages for children. To relieve itching, your practitioner may prescribe Rhus toxicodendron, especially if itching is worse at night. Sulphur may help when the vesicles are burning.

AT-HOME REMEDIES

- ◆ Trim your child's fingernails or cover her hands with socks or mittens to keep her from scratching, which could lead to infec-

tion as well as to possible scarring.
- ◆ To ease itching, add a handful of oatmeal or baking soda to bathwater; apply cool, wet towels to the skin and allow them to dry.
- ◆ Dab calamine or witch hazel on the lesions to relieve itching. Do not use lotions with diphenhydramine, which may sensitize your child to antihistamines.
- ◆ Leave your baby's diaper off as much as possible to allow the vesicles to dry out and scab.
- ◆ Dissolve ½ tsp salt in a glass of warm water and use as a gargle to ease mouth sores.

PREVENTION

A vaccine to prevent chickenpox received FDA approval in 1995, and many doctors now recommend that children be immunized, usually after the child is a year old, as a protection to vulnerable people such as pregnant women. Consult your pediatrician for advice.

PREGNANCY CONCERNS

If you have not had chickenpox and are exposed to the virus while pregnant, contact your doctor immediately. A varicella zoster immunoglobulin injection, given within 72 hours of exposure, may help lessen the severity of the disease. The virus can still pass to your unborn child through the umbilical cord, but possible complications such as fetal malformation or retarded growth may be less likely to occur. If you give birth while you have chickenpox, the baby should also receive immunoglobulin.

C A U T I O N !

Never give aspirin—even baby aspirin—or other products containing the salt called salicylate to a child who has chickenpox. Aspirin has been linked to Reye's syndrome, a rare but very dangerous illness that causes inflammation of the liver and brain. ■

SYMPTOMS

In men:
- a whitish yellow discharge from the penis.
- a frequent urge to urinate or a burning sensation while urinating.
- redness at the tip of the penis.

In women:
- no symptoms, or mild discomfort that you may mistake for vaginitis or menstrual cramps.

CALL YOUR DOCTOR IF:

- you develop any of the symptoms listed above; chlamydia requires immediate medical treatment to avoid serious complications that can lead to sterility in both men and women.
- you are a woman and you experience high fever and other flulike symptoms, such as chills, backache, weight loss, and diarrhea, along with severe pelvic pain, bleeding after intercourse, severe nausea, or recurring back pain; you may have developed pelvic inflammatory disease, a serious complication of chlamydia that can result in sterility.

Chlamydia, which strikes about three million to five million Americans a year, is the most common bacterial sexually transmitted disease in the United States. Epidemiologists believe it's twice as common as gonorrhea, 6 times as common as genital herpes, and 30 times as common as syphilis.

The good news is that chlamydia is easily cured by antibiotics. The bad news is that 80 percent of women who contract the disease don't know they are infected until they develop serious complications such as pelvic inflammatory disease, which strikes 500,000 women a year and may result in sterility. Men with chlamydia may also develop epididymitis, an inflammation of the scrotal tubes that can cause sterility.

If you're a sexually active woman who is not in a monogamous relationship, ask your doctor to test you for chlamydia during your annual physical. This is especially important if you are pregnant or planning to have a baby. Chlamydia has been linked to ectopic pregnancy and premature birth. Each year in the United States 180,000 babies born to infected mothers suffer conjunctivitis—an inflammation of membranes in the eye—or pneumonia.

CAUSES

Chlamydia is caused by *Chlamydia trachomatis,* a microscopic organism that has the characteristics of both a virus and a bacterium. The disease is spread by vaginal or anal sex, and if you touch your eyes with a contaminated hand, you may also develop conjunctivitis.

CAUTION!

If you're a woman who is pregnant or planning to have a baby, get tested for chlamydia, even if you have no symptoms. Infected infants can develop conjunctivitis, a serious eye disease that could result in blindness.

DIAGNOSTIC AND TEST PROCEDURES

If you suspect you have chlamydia, your doctor may want to test your cervical fluid or penile discharge with a special culture medium, examining the fluids microscopically with a substance that makes bacteria glow. The doctor may draw blood to check for antibodies to the disease.

TREATMENT

In uncomplicated cases of chlamydia, the cure rate is 95 percent. However, because most women don't know they have the disease until it has caused serious complications such as pelvic inflammatory disease, sexually active women should be tested for chlamydia once a year.

CONVENTIONAL MEDICINE

If you are diagnosed with chlamydia, your doctor will prescribe antibiotics such as tetracycline, doxycycline, erythromycin, or sulfa-based drugs such as sulfamethoxazole. If you have pelvic inflammatory disease, you'll need stronger doses of doxycycline, cefoxitin, or penicillin derivatives.

ALTERNATIVE CHOICES

Never attempt to treat chlamydia yourself. You must take the antibiotics your doctor prescribes. However, several alternative remedies may help to reduce symptoms and speed healing.

ACUPRESSURE

Doctors of Chinese medicine believe that sexually transmitted diseases result from the buildup of toxins. They may suggest that you manipulate the chi, or energy flow, of the liver meridian by massaging acupressure points Liver 3, on top of the foot between the big and second toes, and Liver 8, on the inside of the leg above the knee. You may also want to try kneading Kidney 3, on the inside of the leg between the anklebone and the Achilles tendon.

CHINESE HERBS

A doctor of Chinese medicine will prescribe a remedy that is uniquely suited to your symptoms and body chemistry. A typical prescription may include 10 to 20 herbs, such as Chinese foxglove root *(Rehmannia glutinosa)* and dong quai *(Angelica sinensis).*

HERBAL THERAPIES

Saw palmetto *(Serenoa repens),* which contains berberine and stimulates the immune system, is useful in treating genital infections, especially in men. You may drink it as a tea or take capsules.

NUTRITION AND DIET

With any infectious genital disease, it's helpful to cleanse your system and boost its ability to fight off infection. In addition to taking antibiotics prescribed by your physician, you might consider fasting for one to three days. Be sure to ask your physician's advice before beginning a fast.

Juices that may help to rid your body of toxins by stimulating urine flow include pomegranate-cranberry and celery-parsley-cucumber. To increase your body's resistance to chlamydial infection, supplement your daily diet with vitamin E (200 IU) and zinc (15 mg).

To restore healthy intestinal flora after you have taken antibiotics, try eating yogurt with live *Lactobacillus acidophilus* cultures, or take ½ tsp *Lactobacillus acidophilus* powder, 1 tsp *Bifidobacterium* powder, and ½ tsp *Lactobacillus bulgaricus* in a glass of water, three times a day. The preparations are also available in capsules and tablets from health food stores.

PREVENTION

Use a condom to prevent transmission of chlamydia. Women whose partners have symptoms of chlamydia should be tested as well. ∎

SYMPTOMS

A high level of cholesterol in the blood does not have obvious symptoms but can be a risk factor for other conditions that do have recognizable symptoms, including angina, atherosclerosis, heart disease, high blood pressure, stroke, and other circulatory ailments.

- Soft, yellowish skin growths or lesions called xanthomas may indicate a genetic predisposition to the body's inability to process cholesterol and triglycerides normally.
- Obesity and diabetes may be associated with high cholesterol levels.
- In men, impotence may be due to arteries affected by excessive blood cholesterol.

CALL YOUR DOCTOR IF:

- you detect soft, yellowish skin growths on yourself or on your children. You should ask about being tested for a predisposition to high cholesterol.
- you develop symptoms of atherosclerosis, angina, or heart disease, such as pain in the lower legs, kidney failure, dizziness, unsteady gait, or thick speech. Any of these conditions may be associated with high blood cholesterol, and each requires medical intervention.

Cholesterol is a paradox: Everyone needs it, but for some people it's a potential killer. A naturally occurring fat, cholesterol contributes to such vital bodily functions as building new cells, insulating nerves, and producing hormones. The liver makes all the cholesterol the body normally needs, but because this waxy substance is found in all animal products, you ingest it whenever you eat meat and dairy foods. For people genetically predisposed to cholesterol problems, a diet high in saturated fats is the chief cause of high cholesterol levels.

In the bloodstream, cholesterol binds with protein molecules to form various types of so-called lipoproteins. High-density lipoprotein (HDL) is a dense, compact microparticle that transports excess cholesterol to the liver, where it is altered and expelled in the bile. Low-density lipoprotein (LDL) is a larger, less dense particle that tends to remain in the body. Very-low-density lipoproteins (VLDLs) are molecules that transport triglycerides—chemical compounds that store fatty acids, an essential source of energy for the body.

The amount of cholesterol in your bloodstream would not be of such significance were it not for its association with various cardiovascular diseases. The risk of developing these conditions is complex and depends on not only how much cholesterol but also what kind of cholesterol you have in your blood. Generally speaking, LDL—the so-called bad cholesterol—is associated with increased risk of dying from coronary heart disease; HDL—or "good cholesterol"—is associated with decreased risk. However, the risk of cardiovascular ailments posed by high LDL cholesterol varies widely from one person to the next.

Specifically, LDL cholesterol is the type that infiltrates arterial walls, initiating the inflammatory disease known as atherosclerosis; people with atherosclerosis are in turn vulnerable to heart disease, stroke, and other cardiovascular disorders. Even so, most people who have high cholesterol never actually get heart disease, and most heart attack victims do not suffer abnormally high cholesterol levels. Since no one can predict with certainty which people with high cholesterol will develop heart disease, play it safe and keep your cholesterol levels in check.

CAUSES

Having high cholesterol is determined largely by the luck of the genetic draw. Some families are genetically blessed with low total cholesterol or high HDL-cholesterol levels regardless of diet or lifestyle. Other families suffer from various hereditary disorders that significantly increase the risk for high cholesterol; the most prevalent of these disorders are also associated with obesity and diabetes. People with such a genetic predisposition who eat a diet high in saturated fats are very likely to have high blood cholesterol.

On the positive side, vigorous exercisers, such as long-distance runners, tend to have high HDL-cholesterol levels. Before menopause, women tend to have higher HDL cholesterol than men their age. Because some researchers deduce that estrogen may raise HDL, or "good," cholesterol and VLDL while lowering LDL, doctors can weigh the potential benefits when considering hormone replacement therapy for post-menopausal women. *(See Menopausal Problems.)*

DIAGNOSTIC AND TEST PROCEDURES

A laboratory test to determine your blood cholesterol level is now a routine part of most physical checkups. When you have your blood tested you will typically get three readings expressed in milligrams per deciliter: one for total or serum cholesterol, one for HDL cholesterol, and one for triglycerides. Often, a reading for LDL cholesterol will also be included, as well as a figure for the ratio of total cholesterol to HDL cholesterol.

The first concern is your serum cholesterol level: Total cholesterol below 200 is considered normal and safe. Cholesterol levels between 200 and 240 are considered borderline, and a level of 240 or more is definitely high. HDL cholesterol for a man should be above 35, and for a woman it should be above 45. As for LDL cholesterol—the dangerous kind—ideally your level should be below 130; between 130 and 160 is borderline,

and above 160 is high. Your triglyceride level should be below 200. Finally, for the ratio of total cholesterol to HDL cholesterol, the lower the number, the better. For men, 4.2 to 7.3 is average; for women, 3.9 to 5.7 is average. In general, then, any ratio reading below 4 (which means you have more HDL relative to your total cholesterol) is good.

TREATMENT

Advice from your doctor about cholesterol reduction is likely to echo that of nutritionists and most alternative practitioners: Adopt a diet low in fat and cholesterol, lose weight, exercise regularly, and if you smoke, quit.

CONVENTIONAL MEDICINE

For people in the high-normal to borderline serum-cholesterol range—about 40 percent of American men and an even higher percentage of American women—diet and lifestyle changes may reduce cholesterol levels or keep them in a desirable range. If your cholesterol level is close to or above 240, adjusting diet and lifestyle may not be enough. Instead, your doctor may prescribe either a natural cholesterol-reduction plan based on a high-fiber dietary supplement, such as bran or psyllium, or a synthetic cholesterol-reducing drug.

Of the many cholesterol-reducing drugs available, members of the statin family—lovastatin, simvastatin, and pravastatin—are among the more widely prescribed. They operate by blocking an enzyme that the liver uses to manufacture cholesterol. They are tolerated well by most patients, although they are expensive and can sometimes produce unwanted side effects such as liver inflammation. For some people, niacin (vitamin B_3) is an alternative, but to be effective it must be taken in large doses. It is often a poorly tolerated drug and can cause such side effects as skin flushing and stomach irritation. Slow-release or timed-release niacin products may minimize side effects but must always be taken under a doctor's supervision.

A blood-cleansing procedure called LDL apheresis may help people with severe genetic cholesterol disorders. Over several hours, blood is removed from the body, chemically cleansed of LDL cholesterol, then returned to the body. Treatments every two to three weeks can reduce average LDL-cholesterol level by 50 to 80 percent but are costly in terms of both time and money.

ALTERNATIVE CHOICES

Alternative therapists offer a range of natural ways to control your cholesterol levels. All can be pursued independently, many in conjunction with drug therapy. The following list of treatments will let you customize your own program. To be safe, advise your doctor if you are using any alternative therapeutic substances or methods before mixing them with prescription drugs.

AYURVEDIC MEDICINE

Ayurvedic healers have traditionally employed Malabar tamarind, also known as Brindall berry, a yellowish fruit from India used extensively in curries, to treat obesity. Some studies suggest that the fruit may also help reduce total cholesterol and triglyceride levels.

CHINESE MEDICINE

Traditional Chinese healers treat various forms of chronic heart disease, along with factors like high cholesterol, with **acupuncture** and an herbal therapy that employs polygonum (Polygonum multiflorum). Because Chinese herbs almost always work in combinations rather than individually, you should consult a trained herbalist for an appropriate prescription.

HERBAL THERAPIES

A highly touted remedy for fighting high cholesterol is gugulipid (Commiphora mukul), an extract of the mukul myrrh tree of southern India. Gugulipid's ability to control cholesterol and triglyceride levels has been compared to that of some synthetic drugs, with claims that it lowers LDL- and raises HDL-cholesterol levels without side effects.

Other herbs reputed to have cholesterol-

Try the **Corpse** position to promote relaxation. Lie on your back with your feet about 18 inches apart and turned out slightly. Place your hands about 6 inches from your hips, with your palms up. Close your eyes and breathe deeply for 8 to 10 minutes.

lowering properties include alfalfa (Medicago sativa), turmeric (Curcuma longa), Asian ginseng (Panax ginseng), and fenugreek (Trigonella foenum-graecum). You might also consult a nutritionally oriented doctor about the benefits of phytosterol tablets. Phytosterols are plant compounds structurally comparable to cholesterol that effectively block uptake of cholesterol in the liver.

LIFESTYLE

Evidence suggests that even though exercise alone cannot lower total cholesterol, moderate exercise several times a week can help raise HDL-cholesterol levels in many people. Vigorous exercise may raise HDL levels even higher, although at some point athletes apparently reach an "HDL plateau."

MIND/BODY MEDICINE

Stress is believed to contribute to elevated cholesterol, so relaxation techniques that combat stress may help lower cholesterol levels. Progressive relaxation with **guided imagery** is something you can try anywhere, anytime. You might also try **massage** therapy, **yoga** (above), **meditation,** or **biofeedback.**

NUTRITION AND DIET

The basic dietary rules for lowering cholesterol

are simple: Avoid saturated fats and dietary cholesterol. Experts recommend a diet with not more than 30 percent of your daily calories from fat; some say 20 percent. Saturated fats derived from animal products and tropical oils should be kept to a minimum, so avoid eating deep-fried foods and pay attention to nutrition labels on packaged foods. Eat more vegetables, fruits, and grains, which are cholesterol free, virtually fat free, and rich in fiber.

Garlic *(Allium sativum)* and onion *(Allium cepa)* are believed to lower cholesterol, but reports vary on how much you should eat in order to benefit. It's safe to say that the more you eat, preferably raw, the better the effect. For other useful nutritional tips, see **Make Healthy Food Your Ally,** below.

PREVENTION

- Keep your weight in check.
- Eat wisely every day—no more than 300 mg of cholesterol and at the very most 30 percent of calories from fat.
- Exercise several times a week—vigorously if you can, but moderate exercise is better than none at all.
- If you smoke, quit.
- Track your progress. Have your blood cholesterol level tested periodically by your doctor or a reputable lab. At-home test kits, like many consumer health devices, are generally unreliable.

MAKE HEALTHY FOOD YOUR ALLY

People who have a genetic predisposition to cholesterol problems should follow their doctor's dietary recommendations. The rest of us should be able to keep cholesterol levels in check by a self-imposed goal of not more than 30 percent of daily calories from fat.

If you know your foods well, you can distinguish friend from foe. First, cut back on red meat, especially organ meat, because of its high saturated fat and cholesterol content. Eat poultry sparingly and avoid the skin; chicken has less saturated fat than red meat but still contains significant cholesterol. Most fish contains less fat and cholesterol than red meat. Most shellfish is also low in fat, and although it is high in cholesterol, for most people it is preferable to red meat and poultry. Whenever possible, go easy on whole dairy products, mayonnaise, chocolate, tropical oils, and hydrogenated or partially hydrogenated oils or fats such as margarine.

For cooking, replace saturated fats that are solid at room temperature, such as butter and shortening, with liquid monounsaturated fats such as olive, canola, or flax oil. There is evidence that consuming moderate amounts of monounsaturated fat—found in such foods as nuts, seeds, and avocados—may actually lower LDL cholesterol. Avoid tropical oils such as palm and coconut; they contain no cholesterol but are high in saturated fat. Eating grapes may help reduce blood cholesterol, thanks to flavonoid compounds in their skins. Look for grape-seed oil—squeezed from grape seeds after wine pressing—for cooking and for salad dressings.

Limit yourself to three eggs a week: One egg yolk contains almost an entire daily recommended allowance of cholesterol. Vitamins, minerals, and nutrients that have reputed cholesterol-reducing properties include vitamins E, C, and A (beta carotene), L-carnitine, pantethine, chromium, calcium, copper, and zinc. To keep your menus lively, try incorporating rice bran, artichokes, shiitake mushrooms, and chili peppers—all believed to help lower cholesterol.

Finally, select foods that contain water-soluble fiber, which offers an excellent defense against high blood cholesterol. Foods on the high-fiber list are grapefruit, apples, beans and other legumes, psyllium seed, barley, carrots, cabbage, and oatmeal. ■

C

SYMPTOMS

- recent onset of debilitating fatigue.
- fatigue that is not a result of exertion and that is unrelieved by rest.
- persistent low-grade fever.
- muscle soreness and weakness.
- sleep disorders (insomnia or oversleeping).
- swollen, tender lymph nodes.
- migrating joint pain without swelling or redness.
- forgetfulness, confusion, inability to concentrate.
- recurrent sore throat.
- headaches.
- long-lasting malaise following physical exertion.
- symptoms that persist for six months and result in a substantial reduction of activities.

CALL YOUR DOCTOR IF:

- you have overwhelming fatigue and no identifiable, obvious reason for it, such as stress. Your doctor will need to rule out other illnesses that share symptoms with chronic fatigue syndrome, such as depression, thyroid problems, mononucleosis, arthritis, lupus, and cancer.

Chronic fatigue syndrome, or CFS—also known as chronic fatigue and immune dysfunction syndrome (CFIDS), chronic Epstein-Barr virus (CEBV), and myalgic encephalomyelitis (ME)—first came to public attention in the mid-1980s. It primarily strikes young urban professionals, with Caucasian women under the age of 45 accounting for 80 percent of cases; however, all segments of the population, including children, are susceptible.

CFS is characterized by overwhelming fatigue and other flulike symptoms, but it is not contagious. Typically, the onset is sudden and debilitating. The exhaustion felt by CFS sufferers doesn't result from overexertion and isn't alleviated by rest or medications; indeed, it tends to become worse over time.

CFS is not a progressive degenerative or fatal disease, although it may linger one or more years. The symptoms wax and wane and often become disabling before improving, but the vast majority of people do eventually recuperate.

CAUSES

The cause of CFS is not known, but researchers are investigating a variety of possibilities. For example, CFS may be an autoimmune disease that results from a combination of viruses, allergies, and hormonal imbalances. One theory holds that excessive reliance on antibiotics or long-term exposure to pesticides or chemical toxins may be at fault. *(See also Environmental Poisoning.)* Studies also suggest a dysfunction of the immune system. In addition, some scientists are studying enteroviruses such as polio; human herpes viruses; and the recently discovered retroviruses such as HIV, although there is no link between CFS and HIV or AIDS. Others see a link between CFS and chronic yeast infections *(see Yeast Infections).*

Current theory holds that CFS may develop when an opportunistic virus or other agent invades the body at a time when the immune system is already suppressed. Factors that might contribute to this state include physical, emotional, or environmental stress, or a combination of the three.

Although many people, including some physicians, are skeptical and believe that CFS is psychological rather than physiological, research shows that CFS sufferers have disturbances in immunological functioning that make their bodies unable either to eradicate invading viruses or to prevent the reactivation of viruses previously dormant in their systems.

The Epstein-Barr virus, which causes mononucleosis, was once viewed as the cause of CFS but is now known to be an unrelated problem.

DIAGNOSTIC AND TEST PROCEDURES

Your doctor will take your medical history, perform a physical exam, and do a complete blood count to rule out other disorders that share symptoms with CFS, such as HIV, mononucleosis, multiple sclerosis, fibromyalgia (a disease causing muscle pain), Lyme disease, and depression. You may also be given an antinuclear antibody (ANA) test for arthritis, lupus, and other connective tissue diseases. Your thyroid function may be tested to check for an underactive thyroid. An erythrocyte sedimentation rate (ESR) test will show elevated readings if there is any inflammation in your body.

Once other possibilities have been ruled out, your doctor will apply specific guidelines set forth by the Centers for Disease Control and Prevention to determine whether you have CFS. Your symptoms must have been present for at least six months and must meet these guidelines for the diagnosis to be definitive.

TREATMENT

Given that the cause of CFS is unknown, treatment is restricted to relief of symptoms. A number of conventional and alternative therapies can help you weather the course of the disease.

CONVENTIONAL MEDICINE

An often recommended first step with chronic fatigue syndrome is to maintain general good health while avoiding situations that are physically or psychologically stressful, and to balance rest and nonvigorous exercise.

The flulike symptoms of CFS can be temporarily alleviated with a variety of medicines. Your doctor may prescribe a short course of nonsteroidal anti-inflammatory drugs (NSAIDs) or aspirin to counteract your low-grade fever, headaches, and joint or muscle soreness. Low doses of monoamine oxidase (MAO) inhibitors, fluoxetine, or tricyclic antidepressants have improved patients' quality of sleep and helped relieve both fatigue and muscle pain. Studies have shown varying degrees of success in treating other CFS symptoms with intravenous injections of gamma globulin, an age-old blood derivative product. And some doctors are attempting to modulate the immune system with histamine H_2 blockers (a subclass of antiulcer drugs) such as cimetidine and ranitidine, although this form of treatment is still considered experimental.

Sensitivity to a chemical, pesticide, household cleaning product, or another potential environmental toxin may also be contributing to CFS. Try eliminating suspected items, then reintroducing them one by one, to pinpoint what may be causing your symptoms. If you discover that a special sensitivity is your problem, you also might want to consider asking your pharmacist to use preservative-free dilutions in preparing any medications you may be taking.

ALTERNATIVE CHOICES

A number of alternative therapies can help control the various symptoms of CFS. But be sure to check with your doctor for an accurate diagnosis before embarking on a course of treatment.

ACUPRESSURE

Applying gentle pressure to the gallbladder points may help relieve fatigue and depression while strengthening your immune system. See pages 22–23 for help in locating the points on your shoulders and neck known as Gall Bladder 20 and Gall Bladder 21. This sequence can be repeated one or more times a day or whenever CFS symptoms appear. Pregnant women should be careful to press Gall Bladder 21 lightly.

YOGA

1 Stress-reducing exercises may help chronic fatigue. For the **Mountain,** stand with your feet together. Inhale and raise your arms straight out from your sides and join them over your head. Hold for 20 seconds while breathing deeply, then exhale and slowly lower your arms. Do once or twice a day.

2 To do the **Half Moon,** inhale and clasp your hands over your head. Exhale and stretch to the right, pushing out your left hip. Breathe deeply, keeping your shoulders and hips on the same plane. Inhale and return to center. Repeat on the left side. Do once or twice a day.

3 For the **Rag Doll,** stand with your arms at your sides, then exhale and bend forward from the waist. Let the top of your head drop toward the floor (do not force the stretch). Cup your elbows in your palms and relax, breathing deeply. Hold for 20 seconds, then inhale and slowly stand up. Do once or twice a day.

ACUPUNCTURE

An acupuncturist may undertake a series of treatments to attempt to normalize and balance the immune system. In Chinese medicine, enhancing vital energy, nourishing the blood, and strengthening the spirit can be part of therapeutic strategy.

CHINESE HERBS

A commercially prepared mixture called the Astragalus Ten Formula combines Asian ginseng *(Panax ginseng),* licorice *(Glycyrrhiza uralensis),* astragalus *(Astragalus membranaceus),* and other herbs in powder or tablet form. Anecdotal reports describe improvement among CFS patients after taking this formula regularly. Consult an herbalist specializing in Chinese medicine for the proper administration of this herbal remedy.

HERBAL THERAPIES

Goldenseal *(Hydrastis canadensis)* has been shown to increase white blood cell activity in some tests. Echinacea *(Echinacea* spp.) and shiitake *(Lentinus edodes)* mushrooms contain oligosaccharides, known to be extremely potent immune stimulators; take in moderate doses only, as advised by a qualified herbalist. Licorice *(Glycyrrhiza glabra)* is said to have antiviral properties. Silymarin, a component of milk thistle *(Silybum marianum),* may help with the liver problems that sometimes affect people with CFS. German chamomile *(Matricaria recutita),* burdock *(Arctium lappa),* yarrow *(Achillea millefolium),* and Asian ginseng *(Panax ginseng)* are all said to stimulate immune activity and may be beneficial to CFS sufferers if taken regularly. Consult a qualified herbalist for more specific guidelines.

HOMEOPATHY

Some homeopathic practitioners have reported success in treating the symptoms of CFS. As with all chronic ailments, it's best to seek the advice of a homeopathic physician or specialist who can accurately diagnose and treat the specific symptoms of your particular case.

MIND/BODY MEDICINE

Meditation, progressive **relaxation, guided imagery, qigong,** and **yoga** are techniques that may help alleviate CFS symptoms without being tiring. In fact, they may provide you with additional energy because they reduce stress.

NUTRITION AND DIET

One theory holds that a nutritional deficiency may be a contributing factor causing CFS, so it's important to maintain a healthful diet. Avoid caffeine, alcohol, refined sugar, white flour, salt, and fried, preserved, high-fat foods in favor of whole grains, beans, rice, fish, and fresh fruits and vegetables. Add edible seaweeds, shiitake *(Lentinus edodes)* mushrooms, and licorice *(Glycyrrhiza glabra)* to your diet. Eating two cloves of garlic *(Allium sativum)* a day may help boost your immune system's antiviral and antibacterial activity. When garlic is crushed or sliced, a sulfur compound called alliin is converted into allicin, which some people have a difficult time tolerating. If you can't digest fresh garlic, you might want to try one of the commercially prepared aged garlic extract tablets that are available.

Coenzyme Q10 and vitamin B_{12} are nutritional supplements that may lessen symptoms. Some evidence suggests that a combination of malic acid and magnesium may help relieve fatigue and muscle pain. Egg lecithin taken with meals may enhance immunity and promote energy. Other immune system-enhancing vitamins include vitamin C and beta carotene (vitamin A), which is also a natural antioxidant. Vitamins B_5 and B_6, zinc, selenium, manganese, and chromium all play a role in strengthening the immune system as well.

The amino acid tryptophan, found in various foods, may be helpful for some symptoms, and since it helps the body produce serotonin, a natural sedative, it may aid in sleep. However, don't take it in supplement form if you have high blood pressure or are taking antidepressants.

It's not uncommon for people with CFS to have food sensitivities or to have had them as children. These sensitivities may manifest themselves as an allergic reaction or other intolerance to a particular food or several different foods.

When a food that you're allergic to enters your body, your immune system views it as an invader, like a virus or bacterium, and attacks it by flooding your bloodstream with antibodies. The overabundance of these antibodies, in conjunction with the release of histamines and other body chemicals, results in such symptoms as increased mucus production, tissue swelling, headache, sore throat, and sometimes mental confusion.

The simplest way to figure out which food or foods are to blame is to try an elimination diet: For a week or two, stop eating things you think may be causing an allergic reaction. Typical culprits include dairy products, nuts, eggs, shellfish, and preservatives in prepared foods, but other foods can also be the source of your problems. If your symptoms disappear, reintroduce each food, one at a time, and see how your body responds. If your symptoms come back, you will have determined at least one of the foods to which you are sensitive and can then eliminate it in all its variations from your diet.

AT-HOME REMEDIES

Make sure you don't attempt more activity during the day than you can handle. Get plenty of rest, pay close attention to your diet, and exercise lightly on a regular basis.

PREVENTION

Because no one knows what causes CFS, there is no way to prevent it. However, you may be able to avoid any worsening of symptoms by strengthening your immune system with vitamins, a proper diet (including avoiding allergens), mild exercise, avoiding environmental toxins, and keeping any allergies you may have under control. You might also want to consider experimenting with various alternative therapies to determine which ones work best for you. ∎

SYMPTOMS

- cramplike pain, muscle fatigue, and aching in the legs; the blood vessels in your calves, thighs, feet, or hips may be blocked, possibly due to hardening of the arteries *(see Atherosclerosis).*
- bulging, bluish vessels in an aching leg; you may have varicose veins.
- a painful vein; you may have phlebitis.
- a finger, toe, or other body part that feels numb after exposure to cold weather, then becomes red and painful once warmed; you could be suffering from frostbite *(see page 69 in Emergencies/First Aid).*

CALL YOUR DOCTOR IF:

- you experience sudden and severe localized pain, and tissue in the affected area turns pale and cold; you may have a fully blocked blood vessel, which can lead to tissue death.
- you develop skin ulcers, localized skin discoloration, or nonhealing sores; these may be signs of obstructed blood flow.
- you are experiencing pain in leg muscles while walking or resting; your blood flow may be dangerously restricted.

Most of us experience the discomfort of tired, stiff, aching legs every now and then. Many people, however, must cope with this sensation on a daily basis. This condition, called **intermittent claudication**, results from blocked arteries in the pelvis, thighs, or calves and most often is caused by atherosclerosis, commonly known as hardening of the arteries. But circulatory problems come in many other forms as well. Most can be treated effectively at home and in consultation with a doctor. In severe cases, though, a corrective surgical procedure may be appropriate.

Blood circulates through the body via a complex system of vessels. Arteries carry oxygen-rich blood from the heart to the rest of the body; veins return oxygen-depleted blood from distant reaches of the body to the heart. Circulatory problems arise when these vessels become blocked or overly constricted. Such interruptions in normal blood flow can be brought on by a variety of conditions. Weakened arterial walls, for example, can balloon out and form pockets that trap blood. Veins can stretch, causing their internal valves to malfunction, and vascular disease can cause vessels to constrict. Most of the time, the discomfort caused by circulatory irregularities is confined to the buttocks and legs, but it can also affect other parts of the body.

CAUSES

Circulatory problems are rarely linked to a single cause. Rather, they usually come as a consequence of multiple risk factors. The incidence of poor circulation rises with age, as hardening of the arteries becomes more common. Gender also seems to play a role in determining who gets certain circulatory problems. Women, for example, are more likely than men to develop varicose veins. Many circulatory disorders run in families. Lifestyle also wields significant influence. Among the risk factors linked to poor circulation are smoking, obesity, and prolonged periods of sitting or standing. Women taking birth-control pills exhibit a higher incidence of circulatory problems, as do people with diabetes.

TREATMENT

The path to improved circulation usually begins at home. Beyond self-improvement measures, many treatment options are available to those who suffer from circulatory problems. Take the time to learn about your options, then decide which treatment program will work best for you.

CONVENTIONAL MEDICINE

Before suggesting a treatment, your doctor will need to diagnose the underlying cause of your circulatory disorder. You can help in this process by providing information about your lifestyle, family medical history, and personal medical history. If you have diabetes, for example, you stand a greater risk of developing circulatory trouble.

In most cases, a doctor will advise a program of regular aerobic exercise and good nutrition. You may be told to lose weight and to abandon old habits that interfere with circulation. If you are bothered by swelling or inflammation, your doctor may also advise a daily dose of aspirin, which inhibits blood clotting (see Blood Clots).

For more severe cases, treatment options range from drug therapy to surgery. Many doctors prescribe pentoxifylline to improve blood flow to the extremities. In a procedure called angioplasty, doctors insert a small catheter into a blocked blood vessel and inflate a tiny balloon to widen the channel. Another technique is rotational atherectomy, in which a tiny diamond-studded drill is used to break up deposits in peripheral blood vessels. Other, more invasive surgical procedures include revascularization—bypassing blocked vessels with healthy ones taken from elsewhere in the body—and endarterectomy, in which portions of diseased vessels are opened to remove obstructing deposits.

ALTERNATIVE CHOICES

Many nonconventional treatments for poor circulation are attempts to strengthen weak blood vessels or widen their openings, thus allowing greater blood flow to distant parts of the body. Some alternative therapies also help to ease the discomfort or reduce the inflammation and swelling associated with circulatory problems.

BODY WORK

Manipulative techniques such as **massage** and **yoga** can promote blood flow and help to alleviate the discomfort caused by poor circulation.

CHELATION THERAPY

Many people seek relief through chelation therapy, which involves injecting the chemical EDTA into the bloodstream. But this form of treatment is controversial and far from universally accepted. (For more information, see Atherosclerosis.)

CHINESE MEDICINE

A traditional healer may advise a combined program of **acupuncture, herbal therapy,** and **massage.** Chinese herbs are also used in specific combinations to treat circulatory problems. Consult a specialist for the combination that is most appropriate for your condition.

HERBAL THERAPIES

An extract of the small, thorny hawthorn (Crataegus oxyacantha) tree promotes circulation by dilating blood vessels, particularly coronary arteries. And ginkgo (Ginkgo biloba) has a well-documented record of medicinal success. (See "The Medicinal History of Ginkgo," overleaf.) Studies show that concentrated extracts from the leaves of the ginkgo tree may help improve circulation by dilating the arteries. If you have a blood-clotting disorder, consult a doctor before using ginkgo, since the plant contains a substance thought to suppress the blood's clotting ability. Ginkgo has also been shown to cause mild side effects, including excitability and digestive problems.

Taken orally, an Asian herb called gotu kola (Centella asiatica) appears to benefit circulation by strengthening and toning blood vessel walls. Cayenne (Capsicum frutescens) and ginger (Zingiber officinale) may stimulate circulation by dilating arterioles and capillaries near the skin's surface. Butcher's-broom (Ruscus aculeatus) is believed to alleviate swelling and inflammation caused by many circulatory disorders. Butcher's-broom can be prepared and eaten much like its cousin, asparagus, or brewed into a tea.

HYDROTHERAPY
A long soak in a warm bath, followed by a brisk rub with a towel dipped in cold water, can ease general discomfort caused by poor circulation. You might add a decoction of thyme leaves or larch needles (larch is a type of pine) to the bathwater for a stimulating effect. Soak cold feet in a warm footbath for 15 minutes. To promote circulation in the legs, alternate hot and cold footbaths (1 to 2 minutes in hot water, 30 seconds in cold water) for 15 minutes.

MAGNETIC FIELD THERAPY
This controversial technique is based on the assumption that magnetic fields have an influence on the functioning of the body. Practitioners use magnets and electromagnetic equipment—including magnetic blankets and beds—in treatment sessions that can last from just a few minutes to overnight. Most often used to promote bone healing, magnetic field therapy may also be useful in the treatment of circulatory problems. WARNING: Do not use this technique if you are pregnant.

NEURAL THERAPY
Intended to restore electrical conductivity within the body through injections of anesthetics, neural therapy is an especially popular treatment option in Germany for a range of painful conditions, including some circulatory problems. WARNING: Neural therapy should be used only as a complement to orthodox medical treatment, not as a substitute. This technique is not recommended for patients who have cancer, diabetes, or renal failure, or for people who are allergic to local anesthetics.

NUTRITION AND DIET
As a general rule, your diet should be low in fat and high in fiber. Emphasize whole grains and fresh fruits and vegetables. Avoid caffeinated drinks, since caffeine causes blood vessels to constrict. And if you suffer from cold hands and feet,

THE MEDICINAL HISTORY OF GINKGO

The ginkgo, which first took root in northern China about 200 million years ago, is the oldest living tree species on Earth. Almost all of these plants were wiped out during the last ice age. But the few that survived became forebears of an ancient medicinal legacy. Approximately 4,000 years ago, Asian herbalists began investigating the healing properties of ginkgo. Earliest mention of the plant appears in a major Chinese herbal text dating to 1436 and the Ming Dynasty. Ever since, the ginkgo has been prized throughout China for its medicinal properties, particularly as a treatment for asthma.

In 1730 the ginkgo was exported to Europe, where it became popular not for its medicinal properties but for its value as an ornamental tree. Only recently did the plant, also known as the maidenhair-tree, begin to excite scientific curiosity in the West. Over the past two decades, hundreds of scientific studies have been published extolling the benefits of ginkgo. A standardized ginkgo extract was developed in Germany to treat a number of conditions, ranging from circulatory problems to poor memory.

Today ginkgos are grown on plantations in the United States, Europe, Japan, and South Korea. After drying and milling, the leaves are converted into a concentrated extract that can be marketed in both solid and liquid form.

don't fall for the "warming" properties of hot toddies. Alcohol can make you feel warmer, but it ultimately impairs your ability to stay warm. Alcohol makes it more difficult for you to maintain your body temperature in cold weather and may even promote hypothermia.

If you suffer from hardened arteries, eat more fish. Not only is fish low in fat and high in nutritional value, but it also boosts levels of high-density lipoprotein (HDL), the "good" cholesterol that purges blood vessels of fatty deposits. For dessert, try pineapple. Studies suggest that an enzyme in pineapple called bromelain enhances circulation while reducing inflammation.

Healthful doses of certain vitamins and minerals may also improve your circulation. Vitamin C, vitamin E, and niacin, all of which are believed to have a dilating effect on blood vessels, may help to get the blood flowing and make walking less painful. However, consult a doctor or nutritionist before using niacin, as it can cause uncomfortable flushing. Magnesium supplements also may help dilate the vessels and alleviate arterial spasms. Note: Carbonated beverages usually contain large amounts of phosphate, which robs the body of magnesium.

REFLEXOLOGY
Stimulating reflexology areas on the feet for the adrenal glands, in addition to reflexology areas analogous to the localized problem area, may enhance circulation. (See illustration below, left.)

AT-HOME REMEDIES
◆ Take regular walks or bike rides to enhance circulation in your legs. Do simple exercises, such as arm windmills, to get the blood flowing elsewhere.
◆ If you are taking birth-control pills, switch to another form of contraception. Stay away from over-the-counter decongestants; most of these drugs are vasoconstrictors, which can increase heart rate and blood pressure as well as constrict blood vessels.
◆ If you smoke, quit.
◆ Dress appropriately for cold weather. Layer your clothing and wear a warm hat, wool mittens (rather than gloves), and socks made of polypropylene or a polyester blend rather than all cotton.
◆ Take especially good care of your feet, keeping them warm, dry, and comfortable, as even minor problems can turn to major infections in cases of poor circulation.

PREVENTION
◆ Make sure that the food you eat is high in fiber and low in fat and includes plenty of whole grains, fresh fruits, vegetables, and fish. If necessary, supplement your diet with vitamin C, vitamin E, niacin, and magnesium.
◆ If your job requires long hours of sitting, schedule regular breaks into your daily routine; stand up and walk around for a few minutes every hour or so to get blood circulating in your legs and feet.
◆ If you smoke, now's the time to stop. And if you are overweight, try trimming down. ■

REFLEXOLOGY

ADRENALS
WAISTLINE

Improve poor circulation in an area by working its corresponding reflexology area. To enhance overall circulation, also work the adrenal area: Push back your big toe and walk the thumb of your other hand along the extended tendon from the waistline to the adrenals.

SYMPTOMS

Often no symptoms appear until the disease has entered the late stages. When they occur, symptoms can include:

- nausea, vomiting, and loss of appetite.
- unusual gain or loss of weight.
- yellow coloration of the skin and eyes (*see Jaundice*).
- dark urine.
- bloody, black stools, or unusually light-colored stools.
- vomiting of blood.
- abdominal swelling.
- prolonged generalized itching.
- swollen feet or legs.
- red palms.
- sleep disturbances and confusion.
- fatigue or loss of stamina.
- enlarged breasts in men.
- loss of sex drive.
- menstrual disturbances in women.
- spiderlike blood vessels on chest and shoulders.

CALL YOUR DOCTOR IF:

- you notice any of the above symptoms; without proper treatment, cirrhosis can be fatal.

Cirrhosis is a serious degenerative disease that occurs when healthy cells in the liver are damaged—usually as a result of alcohol abuse or hepatitis—and replaced by scar tissue. As liver cells give way to tough scar tissue, the organ loses its ability to function properly. Severe damage can lead to liver failure and possibly death. Cirrhosis poses another danger as well: Dense scarring slows the normal flow of blood through the liver, causing pressure to build up in supplying blood vessels. In some cases this pressure becomes so great that the vessels in the esophagus rupture.

Every year about 26,000 people in the United States die from cirrhosis. The disease cannot be reversed or cured except, in some cases, through a liver transplant. It can often be slowed or halted, however, especially if the disease is detected in the early stages of development. Patients who think they might have cirrhosis should see a physician without delay.

Cirrhosis is serious because of the importance of the organ it affects. The liver, weighing about three pounds and roughly the size of a football, is the largest of the body's internal organs. Among its many functions, the liver serves as an essential part of the digestive system by producing bile, which is stored in the gallbladder, then released into the small intestine, where it helps break down fatty food. The liver also helps maintain the proper composition of the blood by regulating the amounts of fat, protein, and sugar that enter the bloodstream. As the body's primary blood filter, the liver works to detoxify alcohol, drugs, and other potentially harmful chemicals. Along with the spleen, the liver traps and disposes of worn-out red blood cells. And because it aids in the removal of bacteria and viruses from the blood, the liver is a vital component of the immune system. If your liver is not functioning properly, you are more susceptible to infection.

The liver is remarkably tolerant of disease and injury. Even after 70 percent of its mass has been destroyed or removed, the organ can still function, albeit with decreased effectiveness. If the conditions that caused the destruction have been removed or corrected, the liver usually can bounce back. Although function can never be restored to parts of your liver that have turned to scar tissue, you can live a healthy life with the remaining portion if the disease is caught in time. However, there is a point of no return with cirrhosis. As more cells are replaced by scar tissue, fewer healthy cells are left to handle the liver's many tasks. Eventually function problems arise and may remain. This is why it's important to identify the underlying causes as soon as possible and begin taking steps to eliminate them.

CAUSES

Cirrhosis occurs as the result of long-term injury to the liver. Possible causes include viruses, genetic deficiencies, prolonged obstruction of bile flow, and long periods of exposure to drugs and other toxic substances. In the majority of cases, however, the culprit is excessive consumption of alcohol *(see Alcohol Abuse)*.

The link between alcohol and cirrhosis is well documented. Studies show that while moderate drinking may actually help prevent strokes and heart disease, heavy drinking has a clearly harmful effect on the liver. For example, the French—famous for their wine consumption—have a relatively low incidence of heart disease, but the rate of cirrhosis in France is very high. Many physicians believe that more drinkers die from cirrhosis than are protected from heart disease.

Simply put, the more alcohol you drink—and the greater the frequency of drinks—the more likely you are to develop cirrhosis. Because the bodies of men and women process alcohol differently, the amount that you can safely imbibe depends largely on your sex. In general, men can have two or three alcoholic drinks a day without suffering liver damage. Women, on the other hand, can safely consume only one or two drinks daily.

These guidelines notwithstanding, it's important to note that alcohol tolerance may vary from one person to the next. For some people, one drink per day is enough to leave permanent scars in the liver. If you drink—especially if you do so heavily and often—have a physician examine you for signs of cirrhosis. This is necessary even if you feel healthy, since the symptoms of cirrhosis often do not appear until it is too late to arrest the development of the disease or slow its progress.

Excessive drinking almost inevitably causes some liver damage, but it does not always lead to cirrhosis. Some people who drink heavily develop **alcoholic hepatitis,** an inflammation of the liver that can last a week or two, producing symptoms of nausea, fever, loss of appetite, jaundice, and confusion. Over time, the condition can also lead to cirrhosis. Even light drinkers who go on a bender for several days can develop a condition known as **fatty liver,** caused when cells of the liver become swollen with accumulated fat and water. This condition can cause pain or tenderness in the liver, temporary jaundice, and abnormalities in other liver functions. (Fatty liver can also result from diabetes, obesity, and severe malnutrition.)

After alcoholism, the most frequent cause of cirrhosis is hepatitis, a general term meaning inflammation of the liver. Of the various forms of this disease, only two—hepatitis B and hepatitis C—are likely to result in cirrhosis. Scarring usually occurs after hepatitis has become chronic (lasting six months or more). The symptoms may be so mild at first that patients with chronic hepatitis do not even realize their livers are scarring. Meanwhile, the damage continues, perhaps resulting in a serious case of cirrhosis later in life. Therefore, it is important for people with hepatitis to have regular medical checkups. And because hepatitis is contagious, family members of an infected person should also be tested.

Cirrhosis sometimes, though rarely, occurs because of an inherited liver disorder. In **Wilson's disease,** for example, a genetic deficiency inhibits the body's ability to metabolize copper. As a result, excessive amounts of the metal accumulate in various body organs, particularly the liver, where it destroys tissue. Similarly, in **hemochromatosis** the body absorbs excess amounts of iron, which damages the liver and causes scarring. This disorder mostly strikes men between the ages of 40 and 60; women are usually not affected because their bodies lose iron during menstruation.

Children born with **galactosemia** lack an enzyme needed to digest milk sugar. Normally, milk sugar passes harmlessly through the digestive system and out of the body. But in people with galactosemia, the substance accumulates in the liver at levels that become toxic and potentially fatal without proper treatment. Infants with this disorder should be taken off milk and given a substitute formula.

Some babies are born with no bile ducts, or with ducts that are malformed. Because bile is unable to drain out of the body, it accumulates in the liver and eventually poisons it. Although the problem can sometimes be corrected through surgery, most children with this disorder die from cirrhosis before they reach the age of two.

Cirrhosis can result when gallstones block the flow of bile and cause it to back up into the liver for long periods of time. The disease may also come as a consequence of long-term exposure to certain drugs, including methotrexate and isoniazid, and to toxic substances in the environment, such as pesticides and arsenic-based compounds.

DIAGNOSTIC AND TEST PROCEDURES

A patient's history and symptoms, along with the results of a physical examination, are usually enough to determine a case of cirrhosis. Once the diagnosis has been made, the physician may order one or more liver function tests, which use blood samples to identify specific liver diseases and assess the organ's overall health. The doctor may also require a liver biopsy, or tissue sample, to ascertain the cause of the cirrhosis. In this procedure, a needle is inserted into the liver to draw out a fragment of tissue, which is then sent to a lab for analysis.

TREATMENT

The best way to treat cirrhosis is to correct the underlying cause. This could involve giving up alcohol, seeking treatment for hepatitis or an inherited disorder, or eliminating certain substances from your diet or environment.

CONVENTIONAL MEDICINE

Specific remedies for cirrhosis depend on the underlying cause and its stage of development. Besides halting the progress of the disease, conven-

tional treatment also aims at correcting any complications, such as internal bleeding, which in themselves can be disabling or life-threatening.

If your cirrhosis is caused by alcoholism, you simply must stop drinking—immediately and completely. If you continue to drink after you have been diagnosed with cirrhosis, you have less than a 40 percent chance of living longer than five more years. If you stop drinking, however, those chances increase to 60 to 70 percent.

Corking the bottle is also the best way to remedy **alcoholic hepatitis** and alcohol-induced **fatty liver.** Both of these conditions usually clear up when the patient stops drinking long enough for the liver to heal. Conventional treatment of cirrhosis caused by chronic hepatitis emphasizes rest, proper nutrition, and possibly the use of the drug interferon. Some types of hepatitis, however, cannot be cured.

For **Wilson's disease,** doctors generally prescribe medications that rid the body of accumulated copper. It may be necessary to continue these medications for life. In the case of **hemochromatosis,** the best way to dispose of excess iron is to draw blood from the patient once or twice a week. This should be kept up for as long as two years, or until the iron level reaches its normal range. Treatment then continues every two to four months.

Severe cirrhosis may require a liver transplant—a serious procedure usually regarded as a last resort. Transplants are not appropriate for

CAUTION!

Because the liver plays a key role in processing drugs, alcohol, and toxins in the body, people with cirrhosis must avoid anything that will cause further damage to the organ. If you have cirrhosis, your liver may not be able to process drugs properly. Be sure to consult your doctor before taking any medication, including birth-control pills, antibiotics, and over-the-counter drugs such as acetaminophen.

everyone: Some patients are too old, too young, or too sick for the procedure. And people whose cirrhosis is due to alcohol abuse must demonstrate a prolonged period of abstinence before the operation. Doctors generally are hesitant to transplant a liver if the patient is just going to abuse it.

As with any form of major surgery, liver transplants can be risky. The new liver may not function properly, or the body may reject the transplanted organ. There's also the danger that infection will set in after surgery. Still, the procedure has a promising success rate overall. In the United States, 60 percent to 75 percent of adult patients and 90 percent of children survive the operation. Transplant patients live an average of five years after surgery.

ALTERNATIVE CHOICES

Alternative therapies for cirrhosis generally attempt to support the functioning of healthy liver cells as well as relieve some of the discomfort and disability associated with the disease.

CHINESE MEDICINE

Various Chinese herbs, used in combination, may promote healthy liver function. However, self-medication can be dangerous; remedies should be prescribed only by a licensed practitioner.

HERBAL THERAPY

Milk thistle *(Silybum marianum)* is believed to promote healthy liver function. However, consult a licensed practitioner before using this remedy.

HOMEOPATHY

Certain homeopathic remedies, including Taraxacum officinale and Chelidonium majus, may help improve the efficiency of healthy liver cells in cases of cirrhosis. Consult a licensed practitioner for their proper use.

NUTRITION AND DIET

Good nutrition often plays a vital role in the treatment of cirrhosis. Although parts of the liver that have given way to scar tissue can't be restored, a balanced diet—including plenty of fruits, vegetables, grains, milk, and protein—can help promote regeneration among cells in the intact portion. Adults with the disease need to monitor their intake of protein. Too little protein can slow cell regeneration, and too much can raise the amount of ammonia in your bloodstream, possibly leading to mental impairment. Check with a doctor or nutritionist for the amount of protein that's right for you.

Because the liver must filter and refine substances that are introduced into the body, patients with cirrhosis are often told to seek medical advice before taking large doses of vitamins or other dietary supplements. Cirrhosis patients should also avoid eating uncooked shellfish, which are sometimes harvested in polluted estuaries and may carry organisms that cause hepatitis or other diseases.

PREVENTION

◆ If you drink, know your limits and do not exceed them. Generally speaking, men can have two or three drinks a day without suffering liver damage. The safe limit for women is one or two drinks daily. Keep in mind, though, that alcohol tolerance can vary greatly from one person to the next. Doctors often advise people to set a daily limit of one or two drinks and to avoid drinking every day.

◆ Avoid uncooked shellfish.

◆ Never mix alcohol and drugs. Some medications, including acetaminophen, react with alcohol and can damage the liver.

◆ Avoid exposure to industrial chemicals, which can enter the bloodstream and cause liver damage.

◆ Maintain a healthy, balanced diet.

◆ Take precautions to avoid contracting hepatitis. Practice safe sex and—if you use intravenous drugs—be especially careful to avoid dirty needles. Before traveling to countries where the disease is prevalent, ask your doctor about hepatitis vaccinations and immune serum globulin shots. (Immune serum globulin shots provide ready-made defender proteins called antibodies, whereas vaccinations prompt the body to produce its own.) ■

SYMPTOMS

- fluid-filled blisters or red, painful sores on or near the mouth, or on fingers.
- swollen, sensitive gums of a deep red color.
- a fever, flulike symptoms, and swollen lymph nodes in the neck often accompanying the first attack; recurrent sores usually don't produce these symptoms.

CALL YOUR DOCTOR IF:

- you develop a high fever and/or chills; high fevers can be dangerous.
- your sores are very painful; you may be able to get prescription relief.

Cold sores, also called fever blisters, are a painful infection caused by the herpes simplex virus. They may show up anywhere on your body but are most likely to appear on your gums, the outside of your mouth and lips, your nose, cheeks, or fingers. Blisters form, then break and ooze; a yellow crust develops and eventually sloughs off, revealing new skin underneath. The sores usually last 7 to 10 days.

Ninety percent of all people get at least one cold sore in their lives. This first occurrence is often the worst. Some children who are affected may become seriously ill. After the first infection, many people develop antibodies and never have another cold sore. About 40 percent of American adults, however, have repeated cold sores.

Although cold sores generally are not serious, the infection may be life-threatening for anyone who has AIDS or whose immune system is depressed by other disorders or medications. In infants, who usually contract the virus during birth, the infection may spread to other organs, causing serious complications or even death.

The infection from a cold sore may cause blindness if it spreads to the eye; herpes is a frequent cause of infectious blindness.

CAUSES

Cold sores are caused by the herpes simplex virus, which is transmitted by such forms of contact as kissing an infected person or sharing eating utensils, towels, or razors. A person with a cold sore who performs oral sex on another person can give that person genital herpes.

Sores may develop as late as 20 days after exposure to the virus. Once the virus enters your body, it may emerge years later at or near the original site of entry. Before an attack you may experience itching or sensitivity at the site. The virus may be triggered by certain foods, stress, fever, colds, allergies, sunburn, and menstruation.

DIAGNOSTIC AND TEST PROCEDURES

Your doctor may take a culture from your sore or simply examine it to see if you have the virus.

TREATMENT

You can't cure a cold sore, but you can alleviate the pain it causes by avoiding spicy or acidic foods, applying ice, and using over-the-counter remedies. Look for medicines that contain numbing agents such as phenol, and emollients to reduce cracking and soften scabs. To speed healing, apply a water-based zinc ointment as soon as you feel the tingling that precedes a sore.

CONVENTIONAL MEDICINE

If your cold sore is especially painful or irritating, your doctor may prescribe an anesthetic gel to alleviate pain.

ALTERNATIVE CHOICES

Several alternative therapies may help to speed healing and prevent sores from coming back.

AROMATHERAPY

Applying geranium *(Pelargonium odoratissimum)* or eucalyptus *(Eucalyptus globulus)* oils to cold sores every hour may help reduce pain and speed healing of the sores. Aromatherapists believe that tea tree oil *(Melaleuca* spp.) has antiseptic properties.

HERBAL THERAPIES

To dry up a cold sore, herbalists recommend applying witch hazel *(Hamamelis virginiana).*

C A U T I O N !

Cold sore infections can spread to other organs in infants and cause serious illnesses. If your infant develops a sore with a fever, call the doctor. If you have AIDS or a depressed immune system, or are on medication following an organ transplant, guard against developing cold sores. If you touch a cold sore and then touch your eye, you could develop a serious corneal ulcer, a manifestation of herpes.

Herbalists also recommend applying extracts of echinacea *(Echinacea* spp.), nettle *(Urtica dioica)*, goldenseal *(Hydrastis canadensis),* and myrrh *(Commiphora molmol)* to speed healing.

MIND/BODY MEDICINE

Cold sores often are triggered by stress. Try deep muscle **relaxation, biofeedback, guided imagery,** and **meditation.** Don't forget to exercise; activity bolsters your immune system so you can defend yourself against the virus.

NUTRITION AND DIET

The herpesvirus thrives on the amino acid arginine. Stay away from nuts, chocolate, and seeds. Instead, eat foods high in lysine, such as kidney beans, split peas, and corn.

If you have more than three cold sores a year, take 500-mg lysine supplements every day. Double the dosage when you feel yourself developing another sore.

AT-HOME REMEDIES

◆ Apply ice for 15 minutes to relieve pain.
◆ Apply vitamin E oil to help sores heal.
◆ Use Number 15 lip balm sunscreen.
◆ Cover your cold sore with petroleum jelly.

PREVENTION

◆ Don't kiss someone who has a cold sore or use the same utensils, towels, or razors.
◆ Wash your hands after touching a cold sore.
◆ Don't rub your eyes after touching your cold sore; you could develop corneal herpes, which may lead to blindness if left untreated.
◆ Don't touch your genitals after touching your cold sore; you could develop genital herpes.
◆ Replace your toothbrush.
◆ Avoid foods that contain arginine.
◆ Eat foods high in lysine, or take supplments. ■

SYMPTOMS

Colic is not a disease but a pattern of persistent, prolonged crying. Doctors consider it colic if an otherwise healthy infant up to three months old exhibits the following behavior:

- loud crying lasting three hours or more for three or more days a week, over a period of more than three weeks.
- prolonged crying between 6:00 p.m. and midnight in a baby that has been fed.
- while crying, the baby draws his legs to his abdomen and clenches his hands and curls his toes; his face alternately flushes and pales with the effort of crying.
- episodes of crying that sometimes begin or end with a bowel movement or the passing of gas.

CALL YOUR DOCTOR IF:

- ◆ your baby has not had colic before and you suspect he is colicky; your physician will want to rule out other causes.
- ◆ bouts of colic are accompanied by fever, diarrhea, vomiting, or constipation—all possible signs of illness.
- ◆ your baby's crying sounds painful, not fussy—indicating injury or illness is causing the distress.
- ◆ your baby is older than three months and still acting colicky; behavioral problems or illness may be the cause.
- ◆ your colicky child fails to gain weight and is not hungry, which suggests illness.
- ◆ you're exhausted or fear stress might lead you to hurt your baby.

About 20 percent of all infants suffer from colic—spates of crying that go on for hours for no apparent reason. Although distressing for the child and exhausting and emotionally draining for parents, the condition itself is benign and usually ends by the time a child is four months old.

CAUSES

The cause of colic is not known. Experts attribute it to any number of things, including an infant's immature digestive system, allergies, hormones in breast milk, and overfeeding.

TREATMENT

There is no cure for colic, although many at-home remedies have proved helpful in soothing colicky babies. Any of those listed on page 273 may work for your child. It is important to remain calm; communication of your own anxiety or frustration to a colicky child will probably result in more crying. Above all, never punish a colicky baby. If you feel yourself near the breaking point, ask someone else to stay with your child while you rest or get away to compose yourself.

CONVENTIONAL MEDICINE

If you suspect your child has colic, call your pediatrician. After ruling out possible medical causes

COMFORT FOR QUICK RELIEF

Fearing that catering to a colicky baby would spoil the child, doctors used to counsel parents to ignore their baby's cries or to delay in responding to them. Physicians now encourage early, sympathetic response to colic.

of prolonged crying, such as otitis media or respiratory problems, most doctors recommend simple home-management techniques. Some encourage parents to talk with other parents for support. If you have gone through colic with an older child, you may decide to call the doctor only if you think your colicky infant is sick.

ALTERNATIVE CHOICES

ACUPRESSURE

Manipulating certain acupressure points may soothe a crying child. See pages 22–23 for help in locating these points. Apply pressure to the webbed area between your child's thumb and index finger (Large Intestine 4) on either hand. Gently massage Conception Vessel 12, above your child's navel, and the corresponding points near the spine (Bladder 20, 21). Applying pressure to Stomach 36 may also quiet your child.

HERBAL THERAPIES

Teas made with herbs containing carminative oils, which reduce inflammation in the bowels and lessen gas production, may help a colicky child. Try teas made of chamomile (Matricaria recutita), lemon balm (Melissa officinalis), peppermint (Mentha piperita), or dill (Anethum graveolens).

HOMEOPATHY

Homeopathic medicine offers several over-the-counter colic remedies that are considered safe to use without prior consultation with a homeopath. Seek help from a professional if your child does not respond to a remedy within 24 hours.

AT-HOME REMEDIES

Maintain a consistent pattern of comfort. Consistency will help you avoid getting locked into a behavioral problem with your child later. If one of these methods brings the child relief, stick with it.
◆ Give your baby a pacifier.
◆ Motion can relieve colic. Walk with the baby; rock him in your arms or in a swing; go for a car ride; or put him in an infant seat near a clothes dryer, where the vibration can be felt.

COMFORTING A COLICKY BABY

Holding a colicky baby in a secure, restful position can have a calming effect. Hold the baby, stomach down, along your forearm, with head facing outward on your palm and legs on either side of your elbow. You can gently pat the baby on the back with your free hand. This technique may be more effective if you rock in a rocking chair or walk quietly until the baby falls asleep.

◆ White noise may soothe your child. Try running a vacuum cleaner or hair dryer where your infant can hear it.
◆ Wrap the child snugly in a blanket to provide a sense of security and comfort.
◆ Place the baby, stomach down, on a warm water bottle in your lap. Test the temperature of the bottle against your inner wrist.
◆ Ask a relative or friend to take over when you feel yourself getting frustrated or exhausted.

PREVENTION

You can't prevent colic, but if the distress is related to feeding, you may lessen the frequency of episodes by trying the following: Hold your baby upright when feeding; burp often. Feed smaller amounts more frequently. To prevent him from swallowing air, feed your baby slowly. If you are breast-feeding, try eliminating from your own diet cow's milk, caffeinated drinks, and broccoli and other cabbage family vegetables, all of which can promote gas pains in your child. If you are bottle-feeding, try a formula free of cow's milk. ■

SYMPTOMS

- persistent or recurrent diarrhea with blood or pus in the stool.
- abdominal pain.
- bowel movements or diarrhea during the night.
- fever, fatigue, weakness, weight loss, pains or soreness in joints.

CALL YOUR DOCTOR IF:

- you are having heavy, persistent diarrhea; you may be at risk of dehydration.
- you have rectal bleeding, with clots of blood in your stool; your colitis has reached a severe stage.
- you have constant pain and a high fever; you might have **toxic mega-colon,** a severely dilated and inflamed colon. **Get medical help immediately.**

Colitis is a general term for inflammatory ailments of the lower intestine, which include Crohn's disease and chronic ulcerative proctitis. **Ischemic colitis** is an intestinal disorder that affects mainly the elderly. One of the most serious forms of colitis is **ulcerative colitis,** a chronic disease that requires close medical attention.

In **ulcerative colitis,** the colon develops tiny ulcers and other inflammations that flare up periodically and cause attacks of bloody stools or diarrhea that may be painful. It is usually diagnosed in young adults but can occur at any age, and may be associated with various other disorders ranging from eye problems to arthritis in the arm and leg joints. Attacks of ulcerative colitis tend to recur, and the risk of colorectal cancer increases rapidly 8 to 10 years after onset. With regular medical treatment, however, the disease is rarely fatal, and most sufferers can lead fairly normal lives. Doctors recognize several levels of severity:

- With a mild case you will have up to four loose, possibly bloody, bowel movements a day, which may temporarily relieve abdominal pain.
- With a moderate case you will have abdominal pain and four to eight bloody stools daily, as well as a low fever and weight loss.
- With a severe case you will have six or more bloody stools or diarrhea daily and during the night, with fever of 100°F or higher, as well as symptoms of anemia.

CAUSES

Although several theories have been put forward about the causes of colitis, none has been proved conclusively. Colitis-like symptoms can also occur in conjunction with bacterial and parasitic infections, such as salmonella poisoning. Temporary colitis-like symptoms strike some people after they take certain antibiotics, such as amoxicillin, ampicillin, cephalosporins, chloramphenicol, clindamycin, lincomycin, penicillin, tetracycline, or trimethoprim. When the drugs are discontinued, the symptoms tend to disappear.

DIAGNOSTIC AND TEST PROCEDURES

Doctors look for signs of **ulcerative colitis** by examining the inside of the colon with a sigmoidoscope, a flexible tube inserted through the rectum. A diagnosis is often made by taking a biopsy, removing a tiny sample of the colon lining for testing under the microscope.

TREATMENT

Ulcerative colitis is among the most serious systemic illnesses. If left untreated, it can lead to complications in other body systems and is potentially fatal. Prompt diagnosis and appropriate medical treatment are essential. Diarrhea in infants and young children is always a serious matter and must be diagnosed and treated as quickly as possible.

CONVENTIONAL MEDICINE

Doctors focus first on controlling inflammation and stopping diarrhea, and eventually on improving nutrition. If you have intense diarrhea and bleeding, your doctor will probably recommend immediate hospitalization, intravenous feeding, and treatment with appropriate drugs—probably intravenous methylprednisolone or hydrocortisone. Azathioprine, an immunosuppressant, is an option for those who do not tolerate steroids well. When the disease is stable but diarrhea is still a problem, you may need an antidiarrheal remedy such as a loperamide and codeine compound. Because diarrhea tends to dehydrate the body, you need to replace the water you are losing. In severe cases, surgery to remove the colon may be necessary. After the immediate symptoms of colitis are under control, your doctor will probably recommend a high-fiber, lactose-free diet and will encourage you to get regular exercise and to stop smoking.

ALTERNATIVE CHOICES

Because **ulcerative colitis** is a serious, potentially life-threatening illness, you should see a doctor at the first sign of diarrhea with bloody stools. If the medical diagnosis rules out ulcerative or other infectious forms of colitis, however, you may find that alternative therapies are helpful in relieving your symptoms.

ACUPUNCTURE

To provide relief from diarrhea and colitis-like symptoms, your acupuncturist will ask you specific questions about your condition to determine which points to stimulate. The likely points are along the foot-stomach and conception meridians, near the navel and left knee. *(See pages 22–23 for point locations.)*

HERBAL THERAPIES

For soothing an irritated intestine and stimulating antibacterial action, many herbalists recommend a supplemental regimen of garlic, typically one 300 mg capsule of dried garlic, three times a day with meals. *(See also Celiac Disease.)*

HOMEOPATHY

Homeopathy is considered appropriate for relief of colitis and colitis-like symptoms, not only in adults but in infants and children as well. Consult a homeopath for specific treatments; among the commonly prescribed homeopathic remedies for colitis are Arsenicum album and Nux vomica.

NUTRITION AND DIET

Omega-3 fatty acids, found naturally in fish oil and flaxseed oil and available in capsule form at health food stores, may help reduce intestinal inflammation. Consult a knowledgeable health-care practitioner for the dosage appropriate to your condition.

REFLEXOLOGY

In order to relieve the discomfort of intestinal problems, massage the colon, liver, adrenal, lower spine, diaphragm, and gallbladder areas on the bottom of your foot. *(See page 25 for area locations.)* ∎

SYMPTOMS

In its early stage, colorectal cancer usually produces no symptoms. The most likely warning signs include:

- changes in bowel movements, including persistent constipation or diarrhea, a feeling of not being able to empty the bowel completely, or rectal bleeding.
- dark patches of blood in or on stool; or long, thin, "pencil stools."
- stomach discomfort, intermittent cramps, frequent gas pains, heartburn, nausea, vomiting, bloating, or difficulty swallowing.
- unexplained fatigue, or loss of appetite or weight.

CALL YOUR DOCTOR IF:

- you notice a change in your bowel movements, experience bleeding from the rectum, or notice blood in or on your stool. Don't assume you have hemorrhoids; schedule a rectal examination and possibly a sigmoidoscopy.
- you experience persistent abdominal pain, unusual weight loss, or fatigue. These symptoms may be due to other causes, but they could also be linked to cancer.
- you are diagnosed with anemia. In determining its cause, your doctor should check for bleeding from the digestive tract because of colorectal cancer.

Coiled inside your abdominal cavity is a long, tubular digestive tract. The muscular second half of this tube—the large intestine, or bowel—is composed of the colon, which stretches several feet, and the rectum, which is only a few inches long. Together, the colon and rectum act as a waste processor: Digested food moves into the colon, the body absorbs any remaining water, and the solid waste is pushed through the rectum and out of the anus in the form of stool.

The inner lining of the colorectal tube can be a fertile breeding ground for small tumors called **polyps.** About half of all adults over the age of 40 grow at least one colorectal polyp. Most polyps are benign, but at least one type is known to be precancerous. Nine out of ten malignant colorectal tumors develop from polyps in glandular tissue of the intestinal lining, although a few rare types of colorectal cancer arise from nonglandular tissue.

If colorectal cancer is diagnosed and treated while the tumor is still localized, the disease is highly curable, with five-year survival rates of about 90 percent. If the tumor continues to grow, cancer can spread directly through the bowel wall to surrounding tissues and organs, as well as into the bloodstream or lymphatic system. Once the cancer spreads to lymph nodes or other organs, successful treatment becomes more difficult. Depending on how advanced the disease is, five-year survival rates range anywhere from 70 percent to 5 percent.

Cancers of the colon and rectum are jointly responsible for about 12 percent of cancers in the United States, with approximately 150,000 cases diagnosed each year. Like many cancers, colorectal cancer is a particular concern for the elderly. Although detection is often possible at an early stage, many people delay seeking medical care because they are embarrassed or fearful of symptoms related to their bowels. Risk increases significantly after 50 and continues to increase with age. Colorectal cancer is characteristically an urban disease, affecting city dwellers more often than rural dwellers, and Caucasians more than African Americans.

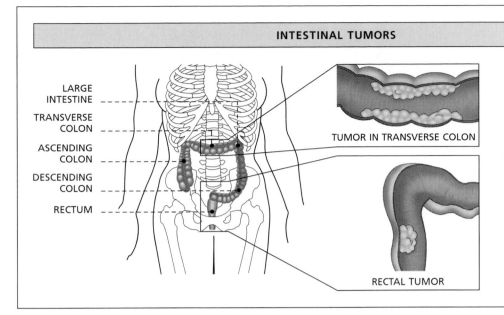

INTESTINAL TUMORS

LARGE INTESTINE

TRANSVERSE COLON

ASCENDING COLON

DESCENDING COLON

RECTUM

TUMOR IN TRANSVERSE COLON

RECTAL TUMOR

The lower digestive tract, or large intestine *(far left)*, includes the colon and the rectum. The large intestine has three main parts: the ascending, transverse, and descending colons. A tumor in the transverse colon *(inset, top left)* can result in abdominal pain, irregular bowel movements, and occult blood in the stool. With a rectal tumor *(inset, bottom left)* blood may be visible in bowel movements.

CAUSES

Colorectal cancer is strongly associated with certain other diseases. Those people considered at high risk include anyone with a personal or family history of colon polyps, inflammatory disease of the colon such as ulcerative colitis or Crohn's disease, and cancers of the pancreas, breast, ovaries, colon, or rectum—especially in a parent or sibling. If you develop ulcerative colitis, the risk of getting colorectal cancer is 20 times greater than average. As with any cancer, potential susceptibility to colorectal cancer is at least partly determined by genetic makeup. A few people inherit a condition called familial polyposis, in which colon polyps develop at an early age; unless treated, these people are almost certain to develop colorectal cancer. *(See box, overleaf.)*

Diet also seems to contribute to the risk, although the cause-and-effect relationship is still unclear. People whose diets are low in fiber because they do not eat enough fruits, vegetables, and grains are known to be at increased risk. Many studies implicate animal fat and protein as promoters of colorectal cancer, although researchers are cautious about drawing any definite conclusions. Some studies show that regularly eating red meat, which is rich in saturated fat and protein, increases risk, while others find no connection. Some scientists think that fat is the main culprit, while others suspect protein. Others contend that it's not the fat and protein themselves, but the way they are cooked. They note that fats and protein cooked at high temperatures—especially when broiled and barbecued—can produce a host of potentially carcinogenic substances linked to colorectal cancer.

Heavy exposure to certain chemicals, including chlorine—which in small amounts is commonly used to purify drinking water—may increase the risk of colorectal cancer. Exposure to asbestos is thought to be potentially harmful, because it has been implicated in causing formation of polyps in the colon.

DIAGNOSTIC AND TEST PROCEDURES

Beginning about the age of 50, everyone should be screened regularly for colorectal cancer. Once a year, your doctor should perform a digital rectal examination and check your abdomen and lymph nodes for signs of swelling or a mass. As part of your annual checkup, a stool sample should be analyzed for occult blood—microscopic traces that could signal bleeding in the digestive tract. Every three to five years, you should

THE GENETIC LINK

Researchers have found that many colorectal cancer patients share certain genetic defects. Having one of these defects means that you are predisposed—but not necessarily bound—to get the disease. For example, scientists have identified a specific gene for hereditary nonpolyposis colorectal cancer (HNPCC), or Lynch syndrome. Presence of the gene—which is extremely rare—predisposes a person to colorectal, stomach, uterine, and certain other cancers of the abdominal organs. Scientists can now test people with a family history of these cancers to find out if an individual carries the flawed gene. Those individuals can then be screened regularly to ensure early cancer detection.

have a sigmoidoscopy, an examination of your rectum and lower, or sigmoid, colon using a flexible, lighted tube called a sigmoidoscope. While this screening technique may not be altogether pleasant, it is extremely valuable for detecting early cancer and other gastrointestinal disorders. *(See also Colitis and Crohn's Disease.)* A noninvasive screening procedure called virtual colonoscopy does away with the tube, instead using spiral computed tomography, which produces a three-dimensional image of the colon after it has been emptied and partially inflated with air.

Any suspicious symptoms or abnormalities will alert your doctor to perform a colonoscopy, a procedure much like sigmoidoscopy that allows a closer view of the inner lining of the bowel. If your doctor finds a polyp or tumor, a biopsy will determine whether or not it is malignant. You may also have x-rays taken of the colon and rectum to view potential masses, along with blood

and urine studies to check for characteristic chemical abnormalities. Should a biopsy confirm cancer, other tests are run to find out whether it has spread to likely sites such as the liver, using x-ray, ultrasound, or CT scans. Further blood tests might be ordered to find out how well the liver is functioning and to measure the blood level of a substance called carcinoembryonic antigen (CEA), often found in higher-than-normal concentration in the presence of colorectal cancer, especially if it has spread.

TREATMENT

Cancer treatment involves not only specific therapies for curing or controlling the disease, but also strategies for meeting a patient's emotional and physical needs. Restoring and maintaining quality of life is a central issue for physicians, as it should be for family members and friends as well. Many complementary cancer therapies can be valuable adjuncts when pursued along with standard medical treatment to help make the stresses of cancer and its treatment more tolerable. However, complementary therapies should never replace standard care.

CONVENTIONAL MEDICINE

Surgery is the most effective treatment for local colorectal tumors. Very small tumors can be removed through a colonoscope, but even with small tumors the surgeon usually prefers to do a laparotomy—removing a significant portion of the bowel and nearby lymph nodes. Often, the surgeon can reconnect the healthy sections of the colon and rectum; when this is not possible, the surgeon forms an opening—known as a stoma—in the abdomen and reroutes the severed colon to it. Waste is collected in a bag worn over the stoma. This procedure, known as a colostomy, often is only temporary; once the bowel has had time to heal, a second operation reconnects the colon and rectum. The need for permanent colostomy is more common with rectal cancer, since retaining the rectum may be difficult. *(See Crohn's Disease.)*

In the treatment of rectal cancer, preoperative radiation or chemotherapy may be advised to shrink the tumor. Radiation and chemotherapy may also be recommended to prevent local tumor recurrence and to lengthen survival time. Radiation is rarely recommended after colon cancer. Instead, doctors have found that chemotherapy combined with immunotherapy can improve the period of survival in patients whose cancer has spread from the colon to surrounding lymph nodes. Chemotherapy may be helpful for patients with rectal or colon cancer that has metastasized to organs in other parts of the body, even though it is not likely to offer a cure. *(See Cancer for more information on therapies.)*

In the immediate postoperative period, the patient can expect to receive painkillers and other medication to ease temporary diarrhea or constipation. Postop patients will be encouraged to eat nutritious foods, rich in calories and proteins, in order to foster strength and healing.

Once cancer of either the colon or rectum achieves remission, follow-up exams to check for recurrence are essential indefinitely. But hundreds of thousands of people are living comfortable, normal lives even after colorectal surgery and a colostomy. Although adjusting to life after a colostomy requires time, support, and understanding, people with stomata have discovered for the most part they can eat, play, and work as well as they did before.

COMPLEMENTARY THERAPIES

Studies published since the 1970s have essentially confirmed that a high-fiber diet substantially reduces the risk for colorectal cancer. Dietary fiber seems to protect the bowel from prolonged exposure to carcinogens by moving waste quickly and by inhibiting formation of some carcinogens. Major studies also show that a diet high in fruit and vegetables reduces risk for colorectal cancer, largely because of the fiber and other nutrients they provide.

While some studies indicate that folic acid, calcium, vitamin D, and the antioxidant vitamins C, E, and A (beta carotene) offer protection against developing colorectal cancer, other studies have failed to confirm these findings and in some cases have flatly contradicted them. For now, the best advice regarding colorectal cancer and nutrition is to include in your daily diet whole grains and at least five fresh fruits and vegetables—especially cruciferous vegetables like cauliflower and broccoli—to ensure that you get ample fiber and many nutrients that may be protective.

PREVENTION

Eat plenty of fresh fruits, vegetables, and whole grains; cut back on red meat and other high-fat foods such as eggs and most dairy products. You can get the protein you need from low-fat dairy products, nuts, beans, lentils, and soybean products. Avoid overcooking or barbecuing meats and fish. To get more fiber, you can add bran or wheat germ to your breakfast cereal.

Speak with your doctor about the latest evidence on aspirin and colorectal cancer. Some studies show that people who regularly take aspirin significantly reduce their risk for colorectal cancer, although other studies find no correlation. In any event, don't start taking aspirin on your own; it is a drug and can cause health problems if taken without a doctor's advice.

If you are over 50, make sure that you are being properly screened for colorectal cancer, especially if you are at high risk for the disease. Home test kits that check for blood in the stool are available at many drugstores. If such a test is positive, see your doctor. If your doctor finds a polyp, have it removed. ∎

SYMPTOMS

- head and chest congestion, perhaps with a runny nose and difficulty breathing.
- sore throat.
- sneezing.
- dry cough that may occur only at night.
- chills.
- burning, watery eyes.
- allover, vague achiness.
- headache.
- constant fatigue.

CALL YOUR DOCTOR IF:

- your newborn (two months or younger) has cold symptoms. For infants, the common cold can be a serious illness.
- congestion makes it hard to breathe, or your chest makes a whistling sound (a wheeze) when you breathe. You may have asthma.
- your throat hurts and your temperature is 101°F or higher; or your cold symptoms worsen after the third day. You may have a bacterial infection (such as strep throat), sinusitis, or bronchitis.
- your temperature is 103°F or higher. You may have pneumonia. **Seek medical care immediately.**
- your cold symptoms occur suddenly with exposure to certain triggers—such as pollen, cats, or perfume—and/or the symptoms continue for weeks. You probably have an allergy.

The aptly named common cold is the most frequent infection in all age groups in the United States. Cold symptoms are triggered when a virus attaches itself to the lining of your nasal passages or throat. Your immune system responds by attacking the germ with white blood cells called neutrophils. If your immune system cannot recognize the virus, the response is "nonspecific," meaning your body produces as many neutrophils as possible (usually more than are needed) and circulates them to the infected sites. This all-out attack kills many viruses, but it doesn't affect the 200 or so viruses that cause colds. Extra neutrophils clumping together at infection sites is what causes the achiness and inflammation of a cold, complete with vast amounts of mucus in the nose and throat.

Cold symptoms settle in between one and four days after you are infected by a cold virus and typically last for about three days. At that point the worst is over, but you may feel congested for a week or more. During the first three days that you have symptoms, you are contagious (meaning you can pass the cold to others), so take preventive measures. *(See Prevention, page 283.)*

Although everyone catches colds, children have them more often than adults. Cold infections are most common during "cold season," which in the United States begins in late fall and runs through spring. During this time of the year people are more likely to congregate indoors, usually with some form of centralized heating on. Closer contact with others, which increases your chances of being exposed to contagious viruses, and hot, dry air, which dries the nose and throat tissues, help create a perfect environment for a viral infection.

Except in newborns, colds themselves are not dangerous. They usually go away in a week or so without any special medicine. Unfortunately, colds do wear down your body's resistance, making you more susceptible to bacterial infections.

CAUSES

More than 200 viruses can infect your nose and throat and cause the common cold. Unfortunately, there is no absolute cure for any of them, so determining which one is causing your cold won't help you recover any quicker. You "catch" a cold virus by breathing minute, airborne droplets from a cold sufferer's cough or sneeze, or by touching a virus-infected surface—such as a doorknob or telephone—and then transferring the germs to your nose or mouth.

DIAGNOSTIC AND TEST PROCEDURES

If your cold is nasty enough to send you to the doctor, your physician will likely examine your throat and ears and may take a throat culture (brushing your throat with a long cotton-tipped swab) to determine if you have a bacterial infection, which requires treatment with antibiotics.

TREATMENT

Conventional and alternative medicine seek the same ends: to make it as easy as possible for your body to fight the cold virus while alleviating the aches and congestion as much as possible. Adequate rest is key to cold recovery; you may find you need 12 hours or more of sleep per night while you're fighting the cold. Drinking water is also important. Mucus flows freely in a well-hydrated body, helping you avoid or recover from infection; and healthy, moist tissues are harder for a virus to infect than dry tissues. If you have a fever, your body is using heat to help kill the cold virus. Giving medication to lower a fever can actually undermine your body's defense efforts. A temperature of 103°F or higher warrants a call to your physician, however.

Pregnant or nursing mothers should check with their doctor before using any type of cold therapy whatsoever, including over-the-counter drugs and herbal remedies.

CONVENTIONAL MEDICINE

No specific treatment exists for the virus that is causing your cold, but in treating your symptoms you can find relief. Ibuprofen can relieve achiness, but acetaminophen and aspirin may make congestion worse. Never give aspirin to a child with a fever; give acetaminophen instead (see Caution below). If your throat is sore, gargle as often as you like with salt water (½ tsp salt in 1 cup water).

It's tempting to acquiesce to an advertiser's claims and try one of the many over-the-counter "cold and flu" preparations, but think twice. These multisymptom drugs likely contain medications for symptoms you don't have, and therefore may result in needless overtreatment. Avoid them entirely for children under 13; even those cold preparations marketed especially for children don't seem to work for this age group, and the drugs commonly induce drowsiness, making everything worse. Over-the-counter decongestants (such as those containing pseudoephedrine) can help break up nasal congestion, but only temporarily: If these drugs are taken regularly for more than five days, your body may "rebound" from them and produce even more mucus—and worse congestion. Pseudoephedrine increases blood pressure and heart rate; do not take it without first checking with your doctor if you have heart disease, high blood pressure, prostate problems, diabetes, or thyroid problems.

Over-the-counter cough suppressants, such as those containing dextromethorphan, can be helpful if your cough is so severe that it interferes

---

CAUTION!

Never give aspirin to a child with a fever; give acetaminophen instead. Reye's syndrome, a neurological disease that can cause coma, brain damage, and death, has been linked to aspirin use in children aged 4 to 15. Reye's syndrome is rare, but typically follows a viral infection: One to three days after the virus has set in, the child becomes extremely tired, vomits heavily, and may be agitated, delirious, and/or confused. Reye's syndrome is an emergency that requires urgent intravenous fluid replacement.

with sleeping or talking. Otherwise, allow yourself to cough as you need to (always covering your mouth as you do), because coughing removes mucus and germs from your throat and lungs. Over-the-counter antihistamines can temporarily make breathing easier, but at a cost: They clear the nose by drying it up, making nasal mucus thicker and harder to drain.

ALTERNATIVE CHOICES

Time is of the essence: Begin to treat your cold as soon as you feel the first symptom. Especially with herbal remedies, an early response often results in a faster and more comfortable recovery.

AROMATHERAPY

Herbal steam can reduce congestion, and if the vapor temperature is 110°F or higher, it will also kill cold germs on contact. Choose eucalyptus (*Eucalyptus globulus*), wintergreen (*Gaultheria procumbens*), or peppermint (*Mentha piperita*). Place either fresh leaves or a few drops of the herb's oil in a bowl and pour in boiling water. Place a towel over your head, lean over the bowl to create a steam tent, and breathe the vapors.

HERBAL THERAPIES

Taken at the first sign of symptoms, echinacea (*Echinacea* spp.) can reduce a cold's intensity and duration, often even preventing it from becoming a full-fledged infection. Echinacea apparently stimulates the immune response, enhancing resistance to all infection. It's available in capsules or tea: Add 2 tsp echinacea root to 1 cup water; simmer for 15 minutes and drink three cups daily. Goldenseal (*Hydrastis canadensis*) helps clear mucus from the throat. It also contains the natural antibiotic berberine, which can help prevent bacterial infections that often follow colds. Steep ½ to 1 tsp goldenseal in 1 cup boiling water for 10 to 15 minutes; drink three cups daily.

For a good "cold tea," combine equal parts of elder (*Sambucus nigra*), peppermint (*Mentha piperita*), and yarrow (*Achillea millefolium*) and steep 1 to 2 tsp of the mixture in 1 cup hot water. This blend can help the body handle fever and reduce achiness, congestion, and inflammation.

Garlic (*Allium sativum*) appears to shorten a cold's duration and severity. Any form seems to work: capsules or tablets, oil rubbed on the skin, or whole garlic roasted or cooked in other foods. If you elect capsules, take 3, three times daily, until the cold is over.

HOMEOPATHY

Cold symptoms often respond well to homeopathic remedies. The dosage is 12c, taken every two hours for a maximum of four doses. Gelsemium may help if you have chills, aching arms and legs, and fatigue, or if your throat hurts. When your runny nose feels as though it burns, your eyes water constantly, and you sneeze often, try Allium cepa. If you feel irritable and have a runny nose that becomes congested at night, take Nux vomica. For a barking cough, a burning sore throat, and a bitter taste that lingers in your mouth, try Aconite.

LIFESTYLE

Refrain from smoking, especially when you have a cold. Smoking assaults the mucous membranes and lungs, increasing your susceptibility to all sorts of respiratory infections, including colds. Once you have a cold, smoke irritates the already-inflamed tissues, making healing and recovery more difficult.

NUTRITION AND DIET

Good nutrition is essential for resisting and recovering from a cold. Eat a balanced diet. Take supplements as needed to ensure you are receiving the recommended dietary allowances for vitamin A, the vitamin B complex (vitamins B_1, B_2, B_5, B_6, folic acid), and vitamin C, as well as the minerals zinc and copper. If your diet is deficient in zinc, your body is low in neutrophils, and you're an easy mark for all types of infections, including colds. Zinc is available as a tablet or throat lozenge.

While you have a cold, avoid dairy products, which tend to make mucus thicker.

The last 20 years have witnessed much research into whether or not taking megadoses (1 gram or more each day) of vitamin C will prevent colds. The jury is still out. Results have varied, but it doesn't appear that megadoses of vitamin C can prevent colds. However, this dosage may lessen the duration and the severity of cold symptoms, possibly because vitamin C is essential for healthy neutrophils.

"Jewish penicillin," also known as chicken soup, has been heralded as a cold therapy since the 12th century. Recent scientific evidence supports the notion that chicken soup reduces cold symptoms, especially congestion. Something (yet to be determined) in the chicken soup keeps neutrophils from clumping together and causing inflammation.

Any food spicy enough to make your eyes water will have the same effect on your nose, promoting drainage. If you feel like eating, a hot, spicy choice will help your body fight your cold.

AT-HOME REMEDIES

◆ Eat hard candies or cough drops to soothe your sore throat, but stay away from minty ones; they can be drying.

◆ Dab petroleum jelly in and around your nostrils to protect against chafing.
◆ Keep your body hydrated by drinking at least 10 glasses of water each day; this will replace the fluids lost through perspiration and your runny nose and minimize nasal and chest congestion. Keep a glass of water on your bedside table to sip during the night.
◆ Humidify your room (especially during the colder months when central heating dries the air) to keep your nose and throat tissues moist.

PREVENTION

A strong immune system is the best defense against all infections, colds included. Boost your body's natural resistance by eating well, not smoking, and drinking plenty of water every day. Minimize contact with people who have colds, or at the very least don't share towels, silverware, or beverages with them. Cold viruses often survive for hours in the open, on doorknobs, money, and other surfaces, so wash your hands frequently.

When you have a cold, do your best to keep it to yourself. A hearty sneeze can carry your cold virus up to 12 feet away, so always cover your mouth when you sneeze (or cough).

Regular, moderate exercise (such as walking for 45 minutes, five times a week) appears to strengthen the immune system and make you less likely to get colds and other infections. Saunas may also help: Swedish researchers have evidence that taking at least two saunas each week can keep you from succumbing to a cold. The reason is unclear, although the sauna's heat may prevent cold germs from reproducing. ■

CONGESTION

Read down this column to find your symptoms. Then read across.

SYMPTOMS	AILMENT/PROBLEM
◆ runny or stuffed nose; scratchy or sore throat; sneezing; head, muscle, and bone aches; thin, clear nasal discharge that turns thick and greenish yellow.	◆ Common Cold
◆ stuffed nose; headache; increasing pressure and pain in the face behind or over the eyebrows, between or over the eyes, on the bridge of the nose, or in the cheeks, upper jaw, or teeth; possible puslike nasal discharge.	◆ Sinus infection
◆ high fever; sometimes, sudden chills, headache, muscle and joint aches, and exhaustion; may be followed by a runny or stuffed nose, nosebleeds, hoarseness, dry cough, and watery eyes.	◆ Flu
◆ stuffed nose with watery discharge; frequent sneezing; itchy eyes and roof of mouth; headache, irritability, exhaustion, possible insomnia.	◆ Hay Fever
◆ a deep, hacking cough that, a day or two later, produces phlegm; tightness or soreness in the chest; possible pain beneath the breastbone when breathing deeply; slight fever, chills, and fatigue.	◆ Acute Bronchitis
◆ difficulty in breathing caused by excess mucus in the lungs; persistent, long-lasting cough with white, yellow, or green phlegm; some wheezing.	◆ Chronic Bronchitis
◆ labored breathing caused by inflamed lung tissue; fever, chills, chest pain, muscle aches, sore throat, cough, and enlarged lymph glands in the neck.	◆ Pneumonia
◆ cough with up to ½ cup of thick, puslike, greenish or blood-streaked, foul-smelling sputum; fever of 101°F or above; sweating, chills, bad breath, and loss of appetite.	◆ Lung abscess

WHAT TO DO	OTHER INFO
◆ See Common Cold. In some people, vitamin C may alleviate symptoms. Colds usually last a week or so; call your doctor if symptoms persist.	◆ Sometimes the first signs of a cold are irritability and restlessness.
◆ See Sinusitis.	◆ Sinus pain may be even worse if you bend forward. Tapping, jolting, or jarring the tender area will hurt. Other symptoms include bad breath, high fever, and a feeling of the "blahs." A sinus infection may occasionally be caused by an abscessed or badly decayed tooth.
◆ See Flu. Call your doctor if symptoms worsen or new symptoms develop.	◆ Different strains of the flu produce different symptoms, including diarrhea, vomiting, and upset stomach. Children may develop swollen neck glands and respiratory problems such as choking and harsh breathing.
◆ See Hay Fever. Try to avoid, eliminate, and protect yourself from airborne substances, such as pollen, dust, mold, and pet dander, that might induce an allergic reaction.	◆ Many medications can relieve the symptoms of hay fever. Be aware of possible side effects, such as drowsiness.
◆ See Bronchitis, especially those sections dealing with the acute form. Call your doctor if your phlegm is blood streaked, your symptoms last more than a week, or your cough interferes with your normal activities and sleep.	◆ Repeated attacks of acute bronchitis may be caused by your environment. The combination of polluted air and cold and damp may increase your susceptibility. Recurrent attacks of acute bronchitis may lead to chronic bronchitis.
◆ See Bronchitis. Call your doctor now if you have symptoms of chronic bronchitis. Stop smoking and avoid irritants.	◆ Chronic bronchitis is a serious form of chronic obstructive pulmonary disease (COPD).
◆ See Pneumonia. There are several types of pneumonia (all serious). Call your doctor now for proper diagnosis and treatment.	◆ Although most people recover completely, pneumonia can be deadly for infants and the very old.
◆ Lung abscesses result from dental disease, pneumonia, or other infection and can be treated with antibiotics. Call your doctor for appropriate diagnosis and treatment.	◆ When treated appropriately, an acute lung abscess can be completely cured without surgery. If it is not treated correctly, an acute lung abscess can become chronic.

SYMPTOMS

◆ Burning itchy eyes that discharge a heavy, sticky mucus may indicate **bacterial conjunctivitis.**

◆ Copious tears, a swollen lymph node, and a light discharge of mucus from one eye are signs of **viral conjunctivitis.**

◆ Redness, intense itching, and tears in the eyes may indicate **allergic conjunctivitis.**

See also Eye Problems and the Visual Diagnostic Guide.

CALL YOUR DOCTOR IF:

◆ you physically injure your eye. Eye injuries can become infected and lead to corneal ulcers, which can endanger your eyesight.

◆ your eyes become red when you wear contact lenses. Remove the lenses immediately and see your ophthalmologist; you may have a corneal infection.

◆ the redness in your eye is affecting your vision and is accompanied by severe pain or excessive yellow or green discharge. You may have a staph infection or a streptococcal infection *(see Strep Throat).*

◆ your conjunctivitis frequently recurs or appears to be getting worse after a week of home treatment; you may have a bacterial or viral infection.

◆ your newborn baby's eyes are inflamed and are not producing tears; this may indicate **ophthalmia neonatorum,** which must be treated immediately to prevent permanent eye damage.

The conjunctiva—the transparent membrane that lines your eyeball and your eyelid—can become inflamed for various reasons. Most cases of conjunctivitis run a predictable course, and the inflammation usually clears up in a few days. Although conjunctivitis can be highly contagious, it is rarely serious and will not damage your vision if detected and treated promptly.

Bacterial conjunctivitis, commonly known as **pinkeye,** usually infects both eyes and produces a heavy discharge of mucus.

Viral conjunctivitis is usually limited to one eye, causing copious tears and a light discharge.

Allergic conjunctivitis produces tears, itching, and redness in the eyes, and sometimes an itchy, runny nose.

Ophthalmia neonatorum is an acute form of **inclusion conjunctivitis** in newborn babies. It must be treated immediately by a physician to prevent permanent eye damage or blindness.

CAUSES

Conjunctivitis is caused by a bacterial or viral infection or by an allergic reaction to pollen, smoke, or other material that irritates your eyes. Children sometimes contract conjunctivitis after a cold or sore throat. Redness and inflammation of the conjunctiva can also be brought on by eyestrain, stress, and poor nutrient levels.

Ophthalmia neonatorum may occur if the baby's tear ducts are not completely opened or if the infant is exposed to bacteria when passing through the birth canal of a mother infected with chlamydia or gonorrhea. The herpesvirus may also be associated with conjunctivitis and corneal infection.

TREATMENT

Traditionally, at-home remedies have been sufficient for soothing conjunctivitis associated with uncomplicated colds, minor infections, or allergies. Treatment consists primarily of cleansing the eyes and preventing the condition from spreading.

A PROTECTIVE LAYER

The conjunctiva is a thin, protective membrane that covers the exposed white of the eye and the inside of the eyelid. Bacterial conjunctivitis—sometimes called pinkeye—is the result of an infection that makes the conjunctiva red, teary, and itchy, with a thick, greenish yellow discharge. When conjunctivitis is caused by an allergy, the discharge is clear and watery.

CONVENTIONAL MEDICINE

If your conjunctivitis symptoms do not appear to be associated with a cold or allergy, you may want to see your doctor or an ophthalmologist for a medical diagnosis. For **bacterial conjunctivitis,** the treatment will probably call for antibiotic eye drops or ointment. **Allergic conjunctivitis** may respond to antihistamine or steroid eye drops, but you should not use steroid drops for either **bacterial** or **viral conjunctivitis.**

ALTERNATIVE CHOICES

Alternative therapies rely on natural remedies to soothe your irritated eyes and ease the itching and inflammation.

HERBAL THERAPIES

Using an eyecup, wash the eye several times a day with one of the following solutions. In each case, cool and strain the eyewash before using.
◆ 1 tsp dried eyebright (*Euphrasia officinalis*) steeped in 1 pt boiling water.

◆ 2 to 3 tsp chamomile (*Matricaria recutita*) in 1 pt boiling water.

HOMEOPATHY

Depending on your symptoms, take the following remedies four times daily for one or two days:
◆ for stinging eyes and red, puffy eyelids, Apis 12x.
◆ for bloodshot eyes and a gritty feeling, Argentum nitricum 12x.
◆ for itchy eyes with a sticky, yellow discharge, Pulsatilla 12x.

AT-HOME REMEDIES

You can cleanse and soothe irritated eyes with a prepared boric acid eyewash, or try the herbal eyewashes above. To relieve discomfort of **bacterial** or **viral conjunctivitis,** apply a warm compress for 5 to 10 minutes, three to four times a day. For **allergic conjunctivitis,** place a cool compress or a cool, moist tea bag on your closed eye. If the condition does not improve in five days, consult an ophthalmologist.

PREVENTION

Bacterial and **viral conjunctivitis** are highly contagious. Unless you take preventive measures, the condition may spread to your other eye or to other people.
◆ Wash your hands often and well.
◆ Keep your hands away from the infected eye.
◆ Do not share washcloths, towels, pillowcases, or handkerchiefs with other family members.
◆ Change your washcloth, towel, and pillowcase after each use, and wash them thoroughly.
◆ Do not use other people's eye cosmetics, particularly eye pencils and mascara.
If your child gets **pinkeye,** keep him or her out of school for a few days. Once one student comes down with conjunctivitis, it is not uncommon for it to spread to an entire class. ■

SYMPTOMS

- hard, compacted stools that are difficult or painful to pass.
- no bowel movements in three days for adults, four days for children.

CALL YOUR DOCTOR IF:

- your constipation is associated with fever and lower abdominal pain, and your stools are thin or loose; these symptoms may be an indication of diverticulitis.
- you have blood in your stools; this may be from a fissure or hemorrhoid but could also be a sign of colorectal cancer; changes in your bowel movement pattern, such as passing pencil-thin stools, may also signal colorectal cancer.
- your constipation develops after you start a new prescription drug or take vitamin or mineral supplements; you may need to discontinue or change dosage.
- you or your child has been constipated for two weeks, with recurrent abdominal pain; this could be a sign of lead poisoning or other serious ailment (see Environmental Poisoning).
- you are elderly or disabled and have been constipated for a week or more; you may have an impacted stool.

Your digestive system is remarkably efficient: In the space of a few hours it extracts nutrients from the foods you eat and drink, processes them into the bloodstream, and prepares leftover material for disposal. That material passes through 20 or more feet of intestine before being stored temporarily in the colon, where water is removed. The residue is excreted through the bowels, normally within a day or two.

Some people—including many alternative therapists—say we should move our bowels one to three times a day to remain healthy, but this opinion is not backed by scientific studies. Depending on your diet, your age, and your daily activity, regularity can mean anything from three bowel movements a day to one every three days. Nonetheless, the longer fecal material sits in the colon, the harder the stool becomes and the more difficult it is to pass. A normal stool should not be either unusually hard or soft, and you shouldn't have to strain unreasonably to pass it.

CAUSES

Our busy, modern lifestyles may be responsible for most cases of constipation: not eating enough fiber or drinking enough water, not getting enough exercise, and not taking the time to respond to an unmistakable urge to defecate. Emotional and psychological problems can contribute to the problem. Persistent, chronic constipation may also be a symptom of more serious disorders, including irritable bowel syndrome, diverticulosis (see Diverticulitis), colorectal cancer, diabetes, Parkinson's disease, multiple sclerosis, and depression.

Bowel habits tend to vary with age and circumstances. Bottle-fed babies, for example, tend to have firmer stools and more bouts of constipation than breast-fed babies. Some children become constipated when they start school or other activities because they are embarrassed to ask permission to use the toilet. Being sensitive to pain, children may avoid the toilet if they have minor splits or tears in the anus from straining or other irritations.

For various reasons, constipation tends to be more common among women, especially during pregnancy. Constipation in the elderly usually occurs for lack of dietary fiber and lack of exercise. Some drugs and vitamin supplements can cause constipation: opiates such as morphine and codeine; aluminum salts in antacids; some dietary iron and calcium supplements; and certain antihistamines, diuretics, antidepressants, antipsychotics, and blood-pressure medications. If you are susceptible to constipation, pay particular attention to the potential side effects of recommended or prescribed medications, and ask your doctor or pharmacist about alternatives if constipation strikes.

DIAGNOSTIC AND TEST PROCEDURES

Occasional constipation does not justify visiting a doctor, but you should seek professional advice for a persistent problem. The doctor will first examine your abdomen for any sign of a hardened mass and may conduct a rectal exam. To check for systemic problems, your doctor may take blood samples. The doctor may examine your colon with a sigmoidoscope, a flexible tube with a magnifying viewer, which is inserted into the rectum. You might also need a barium enema, which coats the intestinal lining so it can be seen on an x-ray.

TREATMENT

Most cases of constipation respond to conservative treatment, such as dietary changes or mild laxatives. Severe or chronic cases will prompt your physician to test for systemic causes and other diseases.

CONVENTIONAL MEDICINE

Your doctor will probably start treatment by getting more fiber or bulk into your diet. For stubborn constipation in older children or adults, the doctor may recommend a nondigestible sugar called lactulose or specially formulated electrolyte solutions. Except for fiber or bulking agents, over-the-counter laxatives should be avoided. Your doctor will also encourage you to take adequate time for moving your bowels and not to suppress the urge to have a bowel movement.

Fecal impaction is a more serious form of constipation that sometimes affects the elderly and disabled. To release hardened material in the rectum, a doctor inserts a gloved finger and manually breaks up the solidified stool. A gentle enema using warm water or mineral oil may also be helpful.

ALTERNATIVE CHOICES

Like many conventional doctors, most practitioners of alternative medicine approach constipation as a lifestyle problem. Corrective measures include increasing fiber consumption, exercising regularly, and setting a routine time to move your bowels.

EXERCISE

Walking for 20 to 30 minutes at a pace fast enough to "get the heart pumping," or a good session at some other exercise, helps stimulate the bowels. Doctors say regular exercise, besides offering cardiac benefits, is an excellent way to correct chronic constipation. People should become accustomed to regular exercise when they are young, so it becomes a healthy, lifelong habit.

HERBAL THERAPIES

Your health food store will have a selection of potentially useful herbal remedies. Try small amounts to test the effect they have on you or take them as recommended by a naturopath. Avoid herbal laxatives containing senna (Cassia senna) or buckthorn (Rhamnus purshiana); they can damage the lining and injure the nerves of the colon, and you can become dependent on them.

HOMEOPATHY

For relief of mild constipation, you can find prepared remedies at a health food store. If your stools are soft but you have to strain to pass them, try remedies containing Bryonia.

LIFESTYLE

Simply recognizing the need to move the bowels solves many cases of constipation. Children respond to praise for sitting on the toilet and having regular bowel movements, and they can be trained at an early age.

For people who are convinced that regular bowel habits are important, the treatment is easy: Sit on the toilet every day at the same time for about 10 minutes, even if you don't have an urge to move your bowels. The best time is after a meal, because food in the stomach stimulates the colon to move. Be patient: It may take a couple of months before this new habit begins to work for you. Remember, however, to heed your body's own signals and never resist the urge to move your bowels at other times.

NUTRITION AND DIET

Almost all Americans should eat more fiber. The American Dietetic Association recommends 30 grams of fiber a day, yet many people consume less than half that amount. Increasing your fiber intake is easy: Eat more raw fruits and vegetables—especially peas, beans, and broccoli—bran cereals, whole-wheat bread, and dried fruits such as raisins, figs, and prunes. A bonus is that most of these foods are rich in vitamins and minerals, yet lower in calories than most processed foods.

It is never too early to start a healthy diet. Children as young as six months can be fed whole-grain cereals, which have more fiber and more nutrients than processed cereals. Even fast-food addicts can be tempted into snacking on fruit and raw vegetables. Otherwise, try a soluble or insoluble fiber supplement like psyllium *(Plantago psyllium)*, which becomes gelatinous when combined with water and adds bulk to the stool. Drink 1 to 2 rounded tsp of powdered psyllium a day, stirred into a glass of cold water or juice, or include an equal amount of powdered flaxseed *(Linum usitatissimum)*, available in many health food stores. Psyllium generally works within two days, but you can take it every day and not become dependent on it.

Insoluble fibers include wheat bran and oat bran. They work as well as psyllium but may give you gas for a few weeks until your system adjusts

---

ACUPRESSURE

1 Digestion may be improved by steady finger pressure on Stomach 36, four finger widths below the kneecap just outside the shinbone. Maintain pressure for one minute, then switch legs. To verify the location, flex your foot; you should feel a muscle bulge at the point site.

2 As an aid to relieving constipation, try applying pressure to Large Intestine 11, on the outer edge of the inside elbow crease. With the arm bent, press deeply into the point with your thumb for one minute, then repeat on the other arm.

3 Pressing Large Intestine 4 in the web between your thumb and index finger may help relieve constipation. Use the thumb and index finger of your right hand to squeeze the web of your left hand for one minute. Repeat on the right hand. Do not use this point if you are pregnant.

4 Pressure on Conception Vessel 6 may help ease abdominal pains from constipation. The point is about three finger widths below the navel. Using the index finger of one hand, press inward as far as you can, then inhale slowly and deeply. Relax and exhale.

to the change. You can mix bran with fruit juice, canned fruit or cereal, or sprinkle it into sandwiches. Start by taking 1 tbsp a day, and gradually increase it to 3 or 4 spoonfuls.

Finally, an old folk remedy for stimulating the bowels is drinking a glass of warm water with the juice of a whole lemon in it after waking up in the morning.

YOGA

The Cobra position is considered one of the best for toning the abdominal organs. Lie on your stomach, with the side of your head resting on the ground and your legs together. Place your hands, palms down, just beneath your shoulders, keeping your elbows close to your body. Inhale and lift your head and chest off the floor with your face forward. Only the upper part of your body should be raised; your navel should touch the floor. Look upward as high as you can and hold this position for three to six seconds. Exhale and slowly bring your head and chest back down. Do this up to four times a day.

The knee-to-chest pose is intended to activate the abdominal organs and relieve gas. Stand straight with your arms at your sides. Lift your right knee up toward the chest. Grasp your right ankle with your right hand and your right knee with your left hand, and pull your leg in as close to your chest as you can. Keep standing straight, and hold for six to eight seconds. Repeat with the other leg. Do this up to three times a day.

AT-HOME REMEDIES

◆ Eat 30 grams of dietary fiber a day. Some good sources are bran and other whole-grain cereals, raw or cooked dried fruits like raisins and prunes, cooked dried beans, popcorn, and nuts.

◆ Drink six to eight glasses of water daily, in addition to your regular beverages with meals.

◆ Go to the toilet at the same time every day—preferably after a meal—and take enough time to let your bowels move fully. If you need to move your bowels at other times, don't resist the urge.

BREAK THE LAXATIVE HABIT

Constipation—real or imagined—is one of the most common medical complaints. In the United States alone, people spend hundreds of millions of dollars a year on laxatives. In many cases, it's not money well spent.

If you take laxative products regularly, your body may become dependent on them, and your constipation is likely to get worse. If you must take laxatives, however, the best ones are fiber-based. They may take a bit longer to work than patent purgatives, but they don't abuse your digestive system.

In any case, don't take over-the-counter laxatives for more than a few days at any one time, and never take a laxative if you have abdominal pain or nausea, if you are vomiting, or if you are pregnant.

PREVENTION

The key to preventing constipation is simple enough: Drink adequate amounts of water—six to eight glasses a day is a good rule—and get sufficient fiber by eating fruits, vegetables, and grains. Fiber is critical because most of our stool is actually made up of bacteria, and fiber gives bacteria a good foundation to grow on. Ample bacterial action results in a larger volume of stool and better bowel function. ■

SYMPTOMS

- A **hard corn** is a compact patch of hard skin with a dense core, located on the top of a toe, the outside of the little toe, or the sole of the foot.
- A **soft corn** is a reddened area of skin up to one-half inch in diameter, with a thin, smooth center, on the side of a toe.
- A **seed corn** is a pluglike circle of dead skin on the heel or ball of the foot.
- A **callus** is a patch of compact, dead skin up to an inch wide on the soles of the feet, the palms of the hands, or any area subject to friction.
- A **plantar callus** is compact dead skin up to an inch wide on the sole of the foot, with a distinctive white center.
- A **hereditary callus** is an area of dead skin up to an inch wide occurring where there is no apparent friction or pressure, such as on the sole of the foot or palm of the hand. This condition runs in families and is usually seen in children.

See also the Visual Diagnostic Guide.

CALL YOUR DOCTOR IF:

- you cut a corn or callus; the break in the skin invites infection.
- a corn discharges pus or clear fluid; it is infected or ulcerated. Either condition requires medical attention.
- you develop a corn and you suffer from diabetes, atherosclerosis, or other circulatory problems. You run the risk of developing a secondary infection.

As annoying as corns and calluses can be, the reason your body forms them is to protect sensitive skin that presses or rubs against underlying bone. Corns generally occur on the toes and balls of the feet, while calluses can develop on hands, feet, or anywhere there is repeated friction—even on a violinist's chin.

A **hard corn** is a small patch of thickened, dead skin with a packed nucleus; a **soft corn** has a much thinner surface and usually occurs between the toes. A **seed corn,** the least common type, is a patch of stiff skin around a tiny plug of cholesterol; a seed corn occurs only on the sole of the foot and often accompanies anhidrosis, or lack of perspiration.

Like corns, calluses have several variants. Besides the **common callus,** usually caused by friction on the hands or feet, there's the **plantar callus** on the sole of the foot and the **hereditary callus,** found on the soles or palms. All are larger than corns—up to an inch in diameter—and lack the corn's telltale center.

CAUSES

Although some corns and calluses on the feet develop from improper walking motion, most are caused by ill-fitting shoes. High-heeled shoes are the worst offenders, putting pressure on the toes and making women four times as likely as men to experience foot problems. **Soft corns** and **plantar calluses** may be caused by either friction or pressure. If your child develops a callus that has no clear source of pressure, it is probably a genetically determined **hereditary callus.** Feet spend most of their time in a closed, moist environment ideal for breeding bacteria; staph infections can start when bacteria enter corns through breaks in the skin and cause the infected corn to give off fluid or pus.

To find out whether a hard patch of skin is a callus or a wart, your doctor will scrape some skin off the affected area. Warts bleed, but calluses just reveal more dead skin. The distinction is useful, because warts are viral and resist treatment, while most calluses (except the hereditary kind) are easily correctable.

TREATMENT

Most corns and calluses gradually disappear when the friction or pressure is removed. To keep corns and calluses on the feet away, wear correctly fitted shoes.

CONVENTIONAL MEDICINE

Most podiatrists discourage the use of over-the-counter salicylic-acid corn remedies; applied improperly, corn plasters can kill healthy tissue around the corn. Properly positioned moleskin pads can help relieve pressure on a corn. Oral antibiotics generally clear up infected corns, but sometimes pus has to be drained through an incision; over-the-counter antibacterial ointments are not effective against infected corns, because most staph bacteria are resistant to them.

Hydrocortisone creams may help remove cracked calluses. Apply the cream and cover the area overnight with a plastic bag or a sock. In the morning, rub off as much of the callus as you can with a coarse towel or brush. Using a pumice to rub the dead skin from a callus after showering, then applying urea-based cream, can also be effective. Do not try this with corns; rubbing will just make them more tender and painful.

You can consider surgery to remove a **plantar callus,** but it is likely to come back anyway. A better approach is to keep your feet dry and friction free. Wear properly fitted shoes and cotton socks, not wool or synthetic fibers that might irritate the skin. If a podiatrist or orthopedist thinks your corn or callus is caused by abnormal foot placement or hip rotation, orthopedic shoe inserts may help correct the problem.

ALTERNATIVE CHOICES

BODY WORK

Some practitioners of alternative medicine work to correct your body imbalance when standing and walking. Types of body work that might help people who suffer from chronic corns and calluses include **Rolfing, Aston-Patterning,** and the **Feldenkrais method**.

HERBAL THERAPIES

Apply a calendula (*Calendula officinalis*) salve two or three times a day to corns or calluses to soften tissue and prevent inflammation.

HYDROTHERAPY

To soothe irritated feet, try a good soak in warm water with Epsom salt. To soften tender corns, rub them with lemon juice.

AT-HOME REMEDIES

The best therapy for corns and calluses is to find the cause of the friction and remove it. In the meantime, be kind to your feet:

◆ Soak your feet in an Epsom salt footbath every day to soothe and soften the skin.
◆ Apply hydrocortisone cream or a calendula-based ointment to a cracked callus. Aloe (*Aloe barbadensis*) cream is also good for soothing and healing the skin.
◆ Elevate your feet and expose them to fresh air whenever possible.
◆ Use pumice or a callus file to gently rub dead skin off a callus, but never rub a corn.
◆ Don't cut or pare away dead skin yourself. Cutting a corn or callus may lead to infection.

PREVENTION

When it comes to corns and calluses, prevention is better than cure. Have both feet professionally measured and buy only properly fitting shoes. Be sure the width is correct and allow up to half an inch between your longest toe and the front of the shoe. Avoid pointed shoes and high heels. Women who wear stylish shoes at work can take some of the pressure off their feet by walking to and from the office in correctly fitted athletic shoes.

Have your shoes repaired regularly. Worn soles give little protection from the shock of walking on hard surfaces, and worn linings can chafe the skin and harbor bacteria. Worn heels increase uneven pressure on the heel bone, which supports 25 percent of your weight. If the soles or heels of your shoes tend to wear unevenly, see an orthopedist about corrective shoes or insoles. ■

SYMPTOMS

More important than the cough itself are aspects of it that provide clues to its cause:

- frequency and duration of the cough.
- length of the coughing spell.
- type of material being coughed up (mucus or phlegm, blood).
- color of the sputum (white, clear, green, yellow, pink, blood-specked).
- consistency of the material coughed up (thick, thin, frothy).
- presence or absence of accompanying pain.

CALL YOUR DOCTOR IF:

- your cough lasts for more than 7 to 10 days; it may be a sign of a serious disease.
- your cough produces yellow, green, pink, or rust-colored sputum.
- your cough is exhausting, persistent, and accompanied by any of the following signs: hoarseness, sore throat, shortness of breath, wheezing, chest pains or tightness, fever of 101°F or higher, headache, back and leg aches, fatigue, rashes, or weight loss. A cough combined with one or more of these symptoms indicates an underlying ailment.

Although it is usually unwelcome and involuntary, a cough is not itself an illness, but rather a protective reflex. Generally, the reflex kicks in when the membranes lining the respiratory tract secrete excessive mucus or phlegm. These secretions help to protect your airways from infections and irritants by trapping and flushing out viruses, bacteria, and foreign particles. Coughing is your body's way of getting rid of this accumulation. The sudden burst of air in a cough not only helps to keep the breathing passages open, but also may prevent infectious mucus from falling into your lungs and bronchial tubes, where it could lead to such serious infections as pneumonia or bronchitis. *(See also Respiratory Problems.)*

Although coughs have many different patterns, they may be categorized according to two characteristics—duration and productivity. Duration refers to how long the person needs to cough. A cough can come and go quickly, as when you cough up something stuck in your throat; it can last for several days if you have a cold; or it can be persistent and chronic, as when you have chronic bronchitis.

A productive cough is one that produces some of the sputum (mucus or phlegm) that protects the lungs and other parts of the lower respiratory tract. A nonproductive, or dry, cough is often the result of irritation caused by mucus running from the nasal passages to the throat.

Although coughing is usually an involuntary act, it can also be voluntary—the result of a conscious decision. In addition, some people cough more often than others because individuals vary in the amount of irritation they can tolerate.

CAUSES

A cough can be caused by anything that irritates the respiratory airways enough to elicit the protective cough reflex. The most common cause is an acute respiratory tract infection, such as the common cold, flu, and sinusitis. In these cases the excessive mucus produced in response to the infection triggers the cough.

Coughs can also be triggered when you accidentally inhale small objects, such as pieces of food, or breathe in irritants such as dust, cigarette smoke, and noxious fumes.

A harsh or forceful cough can itself be an irritant. Coughing causes the airways to contract; repeated contractions lead to irritation of the upper airways, and this prolongs the cough in a sort of vicious cycle.

A dry, nonproductive cough can be a side effect of drugs prescribed for other ailments. There are, for example, five types of angiotensin-converting enzyme (ACE) inhibitors, used in the treatment of high blood pressure and heart disease, that sometimes cause a dry cough. If you are taking one of these drugs and find you are coughing, ask your doctor to prescribe another. A persistent nonproductive cough that interferes with your sleep may indicate a condition called esophageal reflux, in which you involuntarily bring the acidic contents of your stomach back up into the esophagus and then inhale this material.

A chronic, persistent cough should always be considered abnormal. The cough may be caused by smoking, allergies, asthma, or chronic bronchitis, but it may also be an indication of emphysema, tuberculosis, or lung cancer.

DIAGNOSTIC AND TEST PROCEDURES

Any persistent cough may be a symptom of an underlying illness. Your doctor will make the diagnosis based on the frequency, duration, and severity of the cough; breathing difficulties; the type of material being coughed up (the color and consistency of the mucus, phlegm, or blood); and the presence and location of any accompanying pain, swelling, or rash. The doctor may wish to obtain a chest x-ray and a sputum specimen to test for infection.

Although some of the chronic obstructive lung diseases in which coughing may be a symptom are incurable (emphysema, some types of lung cancer, and occupation-related lung diseases, for example), most are treatable. If you have a dry cough along with leg and back aches, fever above 101°F, headache, and a sore throat, you may be diagnosed with flu. A productive cough in which the color of the sputum changes from white (which is normal) to yellow or green may signal infection, possibly bronchitis or sinusitis. If your cough is accompanied by difficulty in breathing, wheezing, and tightness in the chest, you may be diagnosed with bronchial asthma. A cough that produces blood, or pink, yellow, or rust-colored mucus, accompanied by chest pains, headache, fever, and difficulty in breathing, may be diagnosed as pneumonia. And if you have a hacking cough along with a pink rash, muscle aches, fever, and red eyes, you may be diagnosed with measles or German measles.

TREATMENT

Most coughs are not dangerous. Therefore, if you have a nonproductive (dry) cough, along with a runny or stuffed-up nose, sore throat, and sneezing, you have all the classic symptoms of a com-

---

ATTENTION!

COUGHING UP BLOOD

Any cough that produces blood should be evaluated immediately. The underlying cause may or may not be serious, but you should have it checked. Be sure, however, that you are not confusing coughing up blood with blood in your mouth from bleeding gums or a nosebleed.

Hemoptysis (the medical term for coughing up blood) is caused by the rupturing of a blood vessel in the nose, throat, breathing passages, or lungs. The most common cause of a rupture is an infection such as bronchitis, tuberculosis, or pneumonia. Other causes include ailments that produce persistent coughing; blood clots in the lungs; lung cancer; and bleeding disorders such as hemophilia, a hereditary ailment characterized by spontaneous, excessive bleeding.

mon cold, and you should let it run its course.

Since coughing is a protective response by the body, suppressing it with cough medicine, particularly if it is a productive cough, not only reduces the protective clearing action but may serve to mask a more serious underlying problem. Use conventional or alternative cough remedies for no longer than 7 to 10 days and preferably only for temporary relief from nighttime coughing.

CONVENTIONAL MEDICINE

An antibiotic might be prescribed for an underlying bacterial infection. Antibiotics would not be prescribed for a viral infection such as the common cold, however. In that case, your doctor would just prescribe bed rest, aspirin or acetaminophen, plenty of fluids, and moist air (from a humidifier, vaporizer, or teakettle). If your cold or flu produces thick, sticky sputum, an expectorant may help to clear your lungs.

A nonproductive cough can be treated by one or more common therapies: throat soothers and cough suppressants, or antihistamines if your cough is caused by allergies. To relieve a cough's irritation, try cough drops, lozenges, and syrups. Your doctor might recommend a cough suppressant containing the narcotic drug codeine and requiring a physician's prescription, or nonprescription cough drops containing dextromethorphan. Many over-the-counter products contain topical anesthetics that will slightly numb your irritated throat and may provide temporary relief.

Ultimately, for any cough that persists for more than 7 to 10 days, seek medical advice. Based on the diagnosis, your doctor will prescribe the appropriate treatment for the underlying illness or problem.

ALTERNATIVE CHOICES

The following alternative therapies may ease the discomfort of acute or chronic respiratory infections. They do not treat the infection itself, but they may complement conventional care.

ACUPRESSURE

Sometimes a coughing fit can make the muscles in the upper back contract or go into spasm. To relieve the pain this causes, apply pressure to Lung 5 *(above, right)*.

CHINESE HERBS

Sang ju yin, a decoction of mulberry leaf *(Folium mori albae)* and chrysanthemum *(Flos chrysanthemi morifolii),* is a classic cough treatment. It contains a number of other ingredients as well and is available in prepared form. Drink as directed for two to three days. If your cough does not improve, see a practitioner.

HERBAL THERAPIES

A wide variety of herbs act as stimulating or relaxing expectorants that help the body remove

---

COUGH MEDICATIONS

Because coughing is a normal, protective attempt to clear your breathing passages of secretions, irritants, foreign objects, and blockages, it seldom should be stopped. Indeed, unless a physician so orders, children under the age of two should never be given any type of cough medicine. Coughing protects their sensitive lungs (see Croup and Whooping Cough).

If your cough is productive, use a cough suppressant only for temporary relief. An expectorant cough medication may help to loosen the mucus or phlegm and clear your throat, but consuming large quantities of water will have the same effect. Dry, irritating coughs can be controlled by prescribed antitussives and some over-the-counter products. If your throat is dry and sore from coughing, you can try the various throat soothers, such as honey, lozenges, and cough drops.

ACUPRESSURE

Pressing Lung 5 may help ease coughing spasms. Bend your left elbow and make a fist; place your right thumb on the outside crease of the elbow alongside the taut tendon. Press firmly for one minute, and repeat on the other arm. Do three times.

excess mucus from the airways. Stimulating expectorants increase the quantity and then liquefy viscous sputum so it can be cleared out by coughing. Relaxing expectorants loosen the sputum and are soothing if you have a dry, irritating cough.

Since most herbal traditions have remedies for specific types of coughs, you might want to check the many possibilities with an herbalist. However, a basic herbal cough tea that can be taken several times a day for three days consists of 2 parts coltsfoot (Tussilago farfara), 2 parts marsh mallow (Althaea officinalis), 2 parts hyssop (Hyssopus officinalis), 1 part aniseed (Pimpinella anisum), and 1 part licorice (Glycyrrhiza glabra). Add to 1 cup boiling water, steep for 20 minutes, and drink while hot.

HOMEOPATHY

Homeopaths recommend different remedies and dosage schedules for the beginning and later stages of various types of coughs. For relief of early symptoms, take one dose four times a day; for relief of persistent symptoms, take two doses a day for four days. If you are often thirsty and have painful bouts of dry coughs that intensify with the slightest movement, try Bryonia (12c). If your cough is accompanied by hoarseness, difficulty in breathing, and considerable rattling in the chest, take Antimonium tartaricum (12c). If your throat tickles and you get violent coughing fits whenever you lie down, try Drosera (12c). If the slightest draft of cool air initiates a tickling

cough, take Rumex crispus (12c). If you happen to get chilled and develop a fever and a barking cough, try Aconite (12c).

NUTRITION AND DIET

The best thing to do for a cough is to drink plenty of liquids, four to six large glasses a day. A large intake of fluids will loosen the mucus and make coughing it up easier. Warm liquids, or just plain water, are best for this purpose. Try to avoid caffeinated or alcoholic beverages, which are diuretics that cause you to lose more liquid than you take in.

Conventional and alternative practitioners agree that you might speed recovery by drinking fresh fruit and vegetable juices. Some physicians recommend vitamin C supplements; others consider a well-balanced diet just as effective.

AT-HOME REMEDIES

Most of the treatments referred to above can be used at home. In addition to drinking plenty of liquids, including herbal teas, you may find relief by rubbing your throat and chest with essential oil of eucalyptus (Eucalyptus globulus) or myrrh (Commiphora molmol). A simple rub might help you breathe more easily, cough less, and get a good night's sleep.

Another way to reduce persistent night coughing is to sleep with the head of your bed raised six to eight inches. This prevents the pooling of secretions and the return of the irritating acidic contents from your stomach to your esophagus, which you may be breathing in (see Sore Throat). Try to avoid caffeine and peppermint.

You can make an effective expectorant with a large onion and organic honey. Slice the onion into rings, place in a deep bowl, cover with honey, and let stand 10 to 12 hours. Strain and take a tablespoon of this mixture four or five times a day. ■

SYMPTOMS

- severe abdominal pain and diarrhea.
- cramps or pain after eating, especially in the lower right side of the abdomen.
- chronic low-grade fever, loss of appetite, fatigue, or weight loss, especially if accompanied by persistent nausea and vomiting.
- arthritis, with the symptoms above.
- in young children, any of the symptoms above, plus failure to thrive; in older children, failure to grow at a normal rate.

CALL YOUR DOCTOR IF:

- you have a sudden attack of abdominal pain, fever, and the urge to pass gas or have a bowel movement; you may be in the initial stage of appendicitis or colitis.
- you experience prolonged diarrhea, especially if you have had an ileostomy; you may become dangerously dehydrated.
- you have any of the symptoms above accompanied by vomiting; these may signal partial or complete intestinal blockage.

In Crohn's disease, a chronic disorder of the intestines, the gastrointestinal tract becomes inflamed and weak, making digestion difficult and leading to general physical debility. The symptoms are similar to ulcerative colitis; to distinguish between them, your doctor may need to examine a sample of intestinal tissue. The inflammation of Crohn's disease can occur anywhere in the intestinal tract, although it usually strikes the end of the small intestine or the colon.

Crohn's disease is typically diagnosed among people in their twenties and thirties, but the disease can also occur in infants and children. It is more common in women than in men, and it is rare in people of Asian or African descent. The disease is a lifelong ailment that can be controlled but not cured: Crohn's patients usually experience a roller-coaster ride of attacks of abdominal pain and diarrhea followed by weeks or months of remission.

A common complication of Crohn's disease is the development of fistulas that channel through the intestine or the skin itself, often near the anus. Surgery may be required to close the fistulas. Some Crohn's patients show a tendency toward nonintestinal disorders, such as inflammation of the eye, skin eruptions, kidney stones, or arthritis in the knees, ankles, and wrists. People who have had Crohn's for 20 years or more are at risk of developing colorectal cancer, so if you have Crohn's disease and are over 30, you should get regular checkups.

CAUSES

The actual cause of Crohn's disease is unknown, but it may be an autoimmune disorder. The inflammation apparently occurs when the body's own immune system—for reasons not yet understood—attacks a part of the intestine. (See Immune Problems.) Some scientists are studying whether a virus causes Crohn's, but no specific viral agent has been identified. Less likely suspects include food additives such as silica, a chalky substance added to toothpaste and some dietary supplements, and carrageenan, a seaweed derivative widely used as a thickening agent in ice cream and many other dairy products. It is clear, however, that smokers have a greater risk of developing Crohn's than nonsmokers and a poorer prognosis if they continue smoking after developing the disease.

Some antibiotics can cause fever, abdominal pain, and diarrhea—symptoms similar to those of Crohn's disease. Parasitic illnesses such as giardiasis, which can be contracted by drinking water from springs and streams, also cause Crohn's-like symptoms.

DIAGNOSTIC AND TEST PROCEDURES

Crohn's disease can usually be diagnosed from x-rays of the large and small intestines. Your physician may also do a sigmoidoscopy to view the intestines and may take a tiny sample of tissue from the intestinal lining for examination under the microscope.

TREATMENT

At present, Crohn's disease is not curable. Medical treatment typically involves a three-stage approach to controlling the disease—depending on the severity of the symptoms—beginning with drug therapy and a restricted diet, then hospital treatment, and if necessary, surgery.

CONVENTIONAL MEDICINE

You and your doctor will work together to minimize attacks by finding the combination of medications and dosages that works best for you. Some doctors believe Crohn's patients remain free from attacks longer if they take maintenance doses of drugs even when the symptoms are not present; others wait until the patient has recognizable symptoms before prescribing anything. Children with Crohn's disease may need high-protein, high-calorie liquid supplements to keep their growth on track.

Sulfasalazine, an intestinal anti-inflammatory agent, is the cornerstone of conventional medical treatment. It may be prescribed for years at a stretch and is given in varying dosages depending on the severity of the symptoms. Steroids such as prednisone are often prescribed with sulfasalazine to reduce the inflammation of the intestines. Most doctors are wary of prescribing steroids for longer than a few months, however, because of the potentially severe side effects. To reduce the need for steroids, an immunosuppressant such as azathioprine may be substituted. Your doctor may also prescribe an antidiarrheal agent containing codeine for mild bouts of diarrhea. You will probably be put on a bland, well-balanced diet.

If you become severely ill with diarrhea and are losing weight, your doctor may want you to be hospitalized while you receive steroids intravenously. Your doctor may also recommend intravenous (IV) feedings, which allow the intestines to rest. After stabilization, some patients may need IV feedings at home with the help of a visiting nurse.

If the disease does not respond to drugs and diet, your doctor may recommend surgery. A partial colectomy removes the damaged section of the colon but preserves the bowel if possible. In

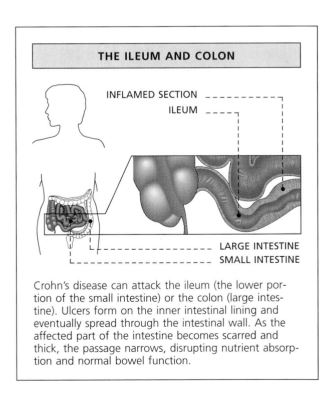

THE ILEUM AND COLON

INFLAMED SECTION

ILEUM

LARGE INTESTINE
SMALL INTESTINE

Crohn's disease can attack the ileum (the lower portion of the small intestine) or the colon (large intestine). Ulcers form on the inner intestinal lining and eventually spread through the intestinal wall. As the affected part of the intestine becomes scarred and thick, the passage narrows, disrupting nutrient absorption and normal bowel function.

a total colectomy, the entire colon is removed and the end of the small intestine is brought to the surface with an ostomy bag for evacuation. (This part of the procedure is known as an ileostomy.) Although the disease may recur after surgery, the symptoms are likely to be less severe and less debilitating than before.

To help you cope with the stresses of having Crohn's disease, your doctor may suggest group therapy, sponsored by the Crohn's and Colitis Foundation or by a local hospital. If you have undergone an ileostomy, you can receive support and tips from your local chapter of the United Ostomy Association.

ALTERNATIVE CHOICES

While Crohn's disease is not curable, many people with mild forms of the disease or Crohn's-like symptoms have found ways to relieve intestinal distress short of drugs or surgery.

ACUPUNCTURE

A trained acupuncturist will ask detailed questions about you and your symptoms of pain and diarrhea. Points near the navel along the foot-stomach meridian are used to treat acute diarrhea. To treat chronic intestinal discomfort, the practitioner may choose points along the liver, spleen, or kidney meridians. *(See pages 22-23 for more information.)*

HERBAL THERAPIES

Powdered slippery elm *(Ulmus fulva)* bark is soothing to the intestines. Dissolve ¼ tsp in a glass of warm water and drink four times a day. Tea made with chamomile *(Matricaria recutita)*, marsh mallow *(Althaea officinalis)* root, or bay-berry *(Myrica cerifera)* is also soothing. Steep 1 tsp of the herb in a cup of boiling water and drink three times a day.

HOMEOPATHY

A homeopath will try to determine the origin of the disease and may want to assess your constitutional makeup before prescribing remedies. For symptomatic relief of diarrhea, try the following remedies every 30 minutes, up to four doses a day:

- Mercurius corrosivus 6c if your stool contains blood and mucus and you have a feeling that the bowel has not emptied.
- Arsenicum album 6c if you have profuse diarrhea with a burning or colicky stomach, anxiety, and chills.
- Podophyllum 6c if you have greenish, painless diarrhea with gurgling and stomach cramps that are worst in the morning.

NUTRITION AND DIET

When the disease is active, you may speed the healing process by drinking juice squeezed from green, leafy vegetables such as cabbage, which are loaded with chlorophyll, or by taking tablets of chlorella, a freshwater alga. Drinking broth made from seaweeds such as kelp *(Fucus* spp.) may also be helpful.

Some doctors recommend a high-protein, high-fiber, low-fat diet to speed healing, with extra B vitamins, vitamin A, magnesium, calcium, zinc, and copper. Be sure to check with your doctor or a licensed nutritionist before taking vitamin and mineral supplements, however, because some have laxative or constipating effects.

Omega-3 fatty acids from fish and flaxseed oils are said to help reduce inflammation. Flavonoids such as quercetin may also reduce inflammation. You can find omega-3 oil and flavonoid supplements in health food stores. Follow the directions on the label or ask your doctor about dosage. Your doctor may also recommend powdered psyllium *(Plantago psyllium)* seed, a soluble fiber, to give your stools more bulk. Mix powdered psyllium in cold water, drink it quickly, and drink another glass of water to increase its effectiveness.

REFLEXOLOGY

To soothe a troubled digestive tract, massage the colon, liver, adrenal, lower spine, diaphragm, and gall bladder areas on the foot *(see pages 24-25 for information and area locations).*

YOGA

The Cobra position is considered one of the best for toning the stomach and bowels. Lie on your stomach, with the side of your head resting on the ground and your legs together. Place your hands, palms down, just beneath your shoulders, keeping your elbows close to your body. Inhale, and lift your head and chest off the floor. With your face forward, look up as high as you can and hold this position for three to six seconds. Exhale and slowly bring your head and chest down. Do up to four times a day.

The Knee-to-Chest pose is intended to activate the abdominal organs and relieve gas. Stand straight with your arms at your sides. Lift your right knee toward your chest. Grasp your right ankle with your right hand and your right knee with your left hand, and pull your leg in as close to your chest as you can. Keep standing straight, and hold for six to eight seconds. Repeat with the other leg. Do up to three times a day.

AT-HOME REMEDIES

Use a juicer to squeeze your own cabbage and other green, leafy vegetable juices, and drink at least one glass every day. A snack of celery sticks is another quick way to get an extra measure of fiber. When the occasional bout of diarrhea strikes, take time to sit down with a cup of chamomile or marsh mallow root tea.

LIVING WITH AN ILEOSTOMY

After surgery to remove the diseased part of the colon, or large intestine, the cut end of the small intestine—the ileum—is led through an opening in the lower abdomen and surgically reconstructed to form a new opening—a stoma—for waste matter. A small plastic bag fastens against the opening to catch waste from the remaining intestine. Because the waste is only partially digested, it is liquid and has a mild acidic odor. A nurse will teach you how to wear and care for the ileostomy bag. Some people change the bag every day; others can go for about a week.

Your body will quickly adapt to having a shorter intestine, and the waste matter will eventually resemble more normal feces. To counteract any unpleasant odors, you can add an aspirin tablet or a little baking soda to each new bag. The stoma eventually shrinks to about the size of a nickel, but the skin around it may remain sensitive and require attention to prevent it from becoming irritated.

People with ileostomies are surprised that the bag hardly interferes with their normal lives. After recovery from an ileostomy, you will probably be able to do everything you could before, even swimming and having normal sexual relations. You can also enjoy a normal diet, although you may have to cut out certain foods, such as popcorn and very fibrous vegetables, that may tend to clog the stoma.

PREVENTION

There is no evidence that food allergies cause Crohn's, but food sensitivities may add to the irritation of the colon. To check for sensitivities, avoid a suspected food for 10 to 30 days, then try it. If a reaction occurs, eliminate the food from your diet. Common allergens are dairy products, eggs, and wheat.

C A U T I O N !

THE DANGER OF DEHYDRATION

If you ever have repeated bouts of diarrhea, be very careful not to let yourself get dehydrated. Taking fluids may not seem sensible after a liquid bowel movement, but it's precisely what you need. A quick antidehydration remedy is drinking several glasses of water mixed with either ½ tsp salt or with baking soda.

Infants and small children with diarrhea should be checked by a doctor as soon as possible after more than two runny bowel movements. Young children tend to become dehydrated quickly and can suffer serious damage to the digestive tract, and in extreme cases, death. In elderly people, severe dehydration has been known to bring on temporary dementia. ■

SYMPTOMS

- a sharp, barking cough, usually accompanied by trouble inhaling and sometimes by a hoarse voice caused by inflamed vocal cords.
- labored breathing that seems to put strain on the neck muscles, ribs, or breastbone, making these areas retract noticeably with each breath.

CALL YOUR DOCTOR IF:

- your child has croup accompanied by a high fever (103°F or more).
- home remedies are not working and the croup symptoms seem to be worsening; hospitalization may be required.
- your child has croup and his respiratory rate exceeds 50, he is having extreme difficulty breathing, he cannot talk, or he is turning pale or blue. These are all symptoms of severe respiratory distress. **Call 911 or your emergency number for immediate emergency help.**
- your child is younger than the age of five and has noisy, rapid breathing; a foreign object may be stuck in his throat.
- your child suddenly begins drooling or can't swallow, has a high fever but no cough, and is leaning forward but can't bend his neck and can't talk. Your child may have a dangerous bacterial infection called epiglottitis, which causes a blocked airway. Do not open the mouth to look inside; doing so can completely close the throat and shut down the child's breathing. **Call 911 or your emergency number for immediate emergency help.**

Croup, a viral infection of the voice box (larynx) associated with signs of a respiratory infection, such as a runny nose or cough, is a relatively common ailment of childhood. Usually the first indication is a cough that sounds like the bark of a seal. Your child may have trouble breathing because the tissue around the larynx is inflamed, constricting the windpipe, and because the bronchial passages are blocked with mucus. The sound of air being forced through the narrowed airways may produce hollow raspy noises, or stridor, with each inhaled breath.

Croup lasts for five or six days and is highly contagious. It usually affects children between three months and six years old (the average age is two), whose small windpipes and bronchial passages are vulnerable to blockage. Most cases are mild and can be managed at home. In severe cases or in the case of epiglottitis—an unrelated bacterial infection of the epiglottis (the flap covering the trachea), whose symptoms mimic croup—your child may need to be hospitalized.

CAUSES

Most croup cases are caused by a parainfluenza virus. The disease is transmitted by airborne droplets from an infected child's cough.

TREATMENT

You and your child may be panicked by the apparent sudden onset of a croup attack. Try to

W A R N I N G !

If your child can't breathe, cough, or speak and he is leaning forward with his neck thrust out, do not open his mouth or tilt his head back to look inside. His throat could close completely, causing respiratory arrest. Call 911 or your emergency number. If your child stops breathing, begin CPR immediately (see pages 50-53).

ACUPRESSURE

1 Gentle pressure on Conception Vessel 17 may help to calm a baby suffering from croup. Place your finger in the center of the child's chest, midway between the nipples, and press lightly. Hold for one minute and release.

2 Coughing spasms may be eased by pressure on Lung 1. Place one finger of each hand about ½ inch below the large hollow under the collarbone, on the outer part of the chest near the shoulder. Apply pressure gently for one minute.

keep your child calm; crying will only make breathing more difficult. Croup usually can be managed with mist or steam therapy, which dissolves sticky or dried mucus in the child's breathing passages. Because the condition commonly worsens at night, many doctors recommend that you sleep in the same room with your child or use a baby-monitoring device to listen for any change in the child's condition. Be ready to get medical help if your child doesn't improve.

CONVENTIONAL MEDICINE

Doctors recommend home care for all but the most serious cases of croup. If the symptoms are severe enough, your pediatrician may take x-rays to check for epiglottitis—which would be treated with antibiotics during a short hospital stay. Severe cases of croup may also require hospitalization; the child will be given inhaled medications such as racemic epinephrine or oral corticosteroids to counter swelling.

ALTERNATIVE CHOICES

ACUPRESSURE
Practitioners suggest pressing at least four of the following points in succession: Large Intestine 4; Triple Warmer 5; Bladder 12, 13; Lung 1, 2; Conception Vessel 17; and Governing Vessel 24. *(See pages 22–23 for information on point locations.)*

HERBAL THERAPIES
To alleviate a persistent cough, herbalists use aniseed *(Pimpinella anisum)*, sundew *(Drosera rotundifolia)*, thyme *(Thymus vulgaris)*, or wild cherry *(Prunus serotina)* bark, which are said to act as mild cough suppressants.

HOMEOPATHY
Aconite, favored by homeopaths for croup, can be given in the 12x or 30c dosage at the beginning of an attack and then every 30 minutes until the child can sleep. If Aconite doesn't work or if the child's breathing sounds like wood being sawed, try Spongia in the same dosage and intervals. For a more mucus-filled bronchial cough, Hepar sulphuris is the third choice for acute croup.

AT-HOME REMEDIES
◆ A cool-mist humidifier may help your child breathe. Direct the mist away from the face and don't put medications in the water; they can irritate your child's throat.
◆ Steam may help loosen phlegm and relax the throat. Turn on the shower and let steam accumulate in your bathroom. Carry your child around in the room (but not under the shower) until the child's breathing becomes easier.
◆ Cold air sometimes offsets croup. If the night is cool, take your child for a ride in the car with the windows down.
◆ Acetaminophen will bring down a fever and lower your child's respiratory rate.
◆ Offer plenty of noncitric liquids to restore fluids and to loosen phlegm.
◆ Keep your child away from cigarette smoke. ■

SYMPTOMS

With most cuts and scratches, the primary danger is infection, particularly if the wound is caused by an animal or a human bite, or if it is deep or ragged, or if it cannot be cleaned completely. Signs of infection include:

- increased pain, redness, or swelling, or discharge from the wound.
- fever, swollen lymph nodes.
- red streaks spreading from the wound site toward the heart.

CALL YOUR DOCTOR IF:

- the bleeding cannot be stopped with pressure. The wound should be stitched or taped within a few hours.
- you suspect **internal bleeding.** Signs include weakness, perspiration, and pain out of proportion to the injury. See Emergencies/First Aid, page 70.
- you believe the victim has suffered a broken bone or a penetrating blow to the body, particularly to the abdomen.
- the victim has a head injury.
- the injury affects a joint or the functioning of the fingers.
- the site of the wound is the face or some other area where scarring would be a concern.
- the victim has not been immunized against tetanus during the last five years.
- signs of infection (swelling, increased pain, increased or smelly discharge) appear.

Cuts, scratches, and minor wounds are an inescapable part of life. Fortunately, the damage usually heals quickly, but two steps should be taken immediately: You must clean the wound and stop the bleeding. *(For severe, persistent bleeding, see Emergencies/First Aid, page 48.)*
Injuries can occur in several forms:

A **cut,** or **incision,** typically caused by a knife, has clean edges. If deep, it can bleed profusely and damage muscles, tendons, and nerves beneath the skin. If contaminated, it may become infected. If spread open, there is a risk of scarring.

A **laceration,** perhaps caused by broken glass or sharp metal, has jagged edges and is likely to involve more damage to deeper tissue than a cut. The risks of infection and scarring are greater.

A **scrape,** or **abrasion,** occurs when skin is rubbed against a hard surface; small blood vessels in the skin are torn and ooze blood. Because of their large surface area, scrapes are easily contaminated by dirt and bacteria.

A **puncture** wound is a narrow, deep hole produced by a nail, tooth, or other penetrating object. Punctures seldom bleed heavily, but they may cause internal injury and carry a risk of tetanus or other infections.

TREATMENT

Before treating yourself or someone else, wash your hands with soap and warm water; even clean-looking skin carries bacteria that can infect.

Commercial healing agents are seldom needed. Antibiotic ointments may help for wounds such as abrasions, but many over-the-counter remedies—including iodine—actually delay healing.

CONVENTIONAL MEDICINE

Cuts and **lacerations:** Let the wound bleed a little; the flowing blood will carry dirt out of the wound. Wash the wound with mild soap and a washcloth under running water. Then use antiseptic wipes, stroking from the wound outward, using a clean section of the wipe for each stroke.

After the wound is clean, blot it dry with sterile gauze or a clean cloth. Put a sterile, absorbent

REMOVING A FISHHOOK

A fishhook embedded just under the surface of the skin (1) can usually be removed without the aid of a doctor. Loop a string around the curve of the hook and grasp the string with one hand. With the other hand, gently press down on the hook's shaft (2) to free the barb from surrounding tissue. Once the barb is disengaged, yank quickly on the string to pull the hook from the wound (3).

dressing or cloth directly on the cut and apply gentle pressure. Once bleeding has stopped, apply a bandage or tape to hold the dressing in place. In addition to protecting the wound from contaminants, the dressing will minimize drying; cells regenerate more rapidly and produce less scarring when kept moist.

Abrasions: Follow the same steps, but because infection is so common, pay extra attention to cleaning the wound; scrub gently but thoroughly. Antibiotic ointment may be helpful.

Punctures: Wash the wound thoroughly with soap and a strong stream of water, apply an antiseptic solution, and bandage the hole with a sterile gauze pad. Do not tape the hole closed and do not apply antibiotic ointment; sealing the wound can increase the likelihood of infection.

For more serious wounds, your most important job is to stop the flow of blood. Pressure is the surest method. Follow these steps:

◆ Wash your hands if possible, and use sterile gloves; or put a few layers of dressing or a layer of plastic wrap between your hands and the wound.

◆ Try to calm and reassure the victim. Lay the person flat, head slightly lower than the torso, or with legs elevated, to reduce the chance of fainting.

◆ Elevate the site of bleeding above heart level if possible; this will slow the flow of blood.

◆ Apply sterile gauze or a cloth dressing (or a piece of clean clothing) and maintain pressure until the bleeding stops. Your goal is to compress the bleeding vessels enough to allow clots to form. When the bleeding has stopped, bind the dressing firmly with adhesive or other tape.

ALTERNATIVE CHOICES

Honey or granulated sugar applied to minor cuts may assist healing. They both inhibit the growth of bacteria and thus retard infection.

AROMATHERAPY

Tea tree oil (*Melaleuca* spp.) provides topical therapy as an antiseptic, similar to hydrogen peroxide. Add a few drops to water when washing a wound.

HERBAL THERAPIES

Topical aloe (*Aloe barbadensis*) soothes the skin and may assist healing of superficial **abrasions** and tissue that is healing or scarred. *Sentilla asiatica* can increase recovery and healing; it should be used under medical supervision.

HOMEOPATHY

Calendula is antiseptic and can be applied as a lotion or ointment. Ledum is effective at reducing pain in **puncture** wounds and may help ward off infection. Staphysagria has been reported of value for lacerations, and Hypericum for cuts in painful areas, such as the lips. Aconite (30c) every 30 minutes for three to five doses may help calm a frightened individual.

NUTRITION

For small wounds, or after healing has begun, vitamin E taken orally (or the oil applied topically) may speed healing. Vitamins A, C, and B complex and the amino acids arginine and glycine (between meals) may also help; bromelain (from pineapple) may reduce inflammation. ■

SYMPTOMS

◆ flakes of skin that range from small and white to large, greasy, and yellow.
◆ itchy flaking that appears on the scalp or eyebrows, or around the hairline, ears, or nose.

CALL YOUR DOCTOR IF:

◆ scaling is greasy and yellow, and does not respond to over-the-counter dandruff shampoos and lotions; you may have seborrheic dermatitis and need more aggressive treatment to relieve the itching and flaking.
◆ your dandruff is localized in a few patches and is very itchy; you may have a fungal infection, which requires treatment with prescription medication.

Dandruff—those dry, white flakes of skin you constantly find yourself brushing off your collar or shoulders—typically poses no health risk whatsoever. But it can be a source of embarrassment, and the itchiness that may come with it is a genuine nuisance. Many people incorrectly assume that the problem has something to do with hygiene and how often you wash your hair. Although it's true that shampooing infrequently can aggravate an existing case of dandruff, it will not bring one on. What actually lies behind dandruff is a simple difference between people in a natural process we all undergo every day: shedding skin cells. The difference is that some of us shed more than others.

CAUSES

Skin cells that grow and die off too fast are the cause of dandruff, but doctors do not know why this happens. Some people with severe flaking have overactive sebaceous glands (whose task is to lubricate the skin with oils); others have an elevated level of the fungus *Pityrosporum ovale,* which is present in most people but to excess in dandruff sufferers. Other causative factors include family history, food allergies, excessive sweating, use of alkaline soaps, yeast infections, and stress. Even the season of the year can contribute to the problem: Cold, dry winters are notorious for bringing on dandruff or making it worse.

If dandruff flakes are greasy and yellow, the probable cause is the skin condition known as seborrheic dermatitis; dry, thick lesions consisting of large, silvery scales may be traced to the less common psoriasis of the scalp. These forms of dandruff—as well as the run-of-the-mill variety—become a hazard only if you scratch to the point of causing breaks in the skin, which can place you at greater risk for infections, particularly from staph and strep bacteria.

TREATMENT

Many over-the-counter shampoos can keep moderate dandruff in check, but consult your doctor about more stubborn forms such as seborrheic dermatitis. Some herbal remedies may relieve the itching and dryness, but it usually takes a tar-based product to subdue the greasy scales.

The U.S. Food and Drug Administration (FDA) has approved only five active ingredients as safe and effective for treating dandruff: coal-tar preparations, pyrithione zinc, salicylic acid, selenium sulfide, and sulfur (the FDA also recognizes a combination of salicylic acid and sulfur as an effective preparation). All other substances have been banned as active ingredients in dandruff shampoos, so read the label.

CONVENTIONAL MEDICINE

If you find that you are still scratching and shedding after trying over-the-counter preparations, see your doctor. You may be using the wrong shampoo for your condition. For really stubborn dandruff cases you may need to use a prescription steroid lotion.

Most doctors recommend that dandruff sufferers use a medicated shampoo daily, leaving the lather on for at least 10 minutes. Be sure to rinse thoroughly; shampoo and soap residue can actually aggravate skin problems. After your dandruff has cleared up, use the medicated shampoo no more than once or twice a week, because it is too harsh for daily use. When possible, let your hair dry naturally instead of blowing it dry.

Brushing your hair with a natural-bristle brush can also prove beneficial. Brush your hair from your scalp outward with steady, firm strokes. This will carry oil from your scalp, where it can cause dandruff, along the hair strands, which need the oil to stay shiny and healthy.

ALTERNATIVE CHOICES

In addition to herbal preparations, other alternative options—including a careful diet, stress-reducing **mind/body** exercises, and **massage**—may prove to be of some benefit in treating dandruff.

HERBAL THERAPIES

To prevent flaking and protect against infection, try massaging tea tree oil (*Melaleuca* spp.) into your scalp. Some practitioners believe it is as effective as prescription steroid creams.

Dried thyme *(Thymus vulgaris),* rosemary *(Rosmarinus officinalis),* or sage *(Salvia officinalis)* may make an effective rinse. Boil 2 heaping tbsp of one of these herbs in 1 cup of water for 10 minutes. Strain and cool. Pour the liquid on damp, clean hair and massage it into your scalp. Do not rinse.

MIND/BODY MEDICINE

Stress may aggravate dandruff. Regular exercise is not only good for your overall health but is also one of the most effective ways to relieve stress. You might also consider adding a relaxation technique such as **yoga** to your weekly routine.

NUTRITION AND DIET

Dandruff is a common symptom of food allergies, often resulting from a cumulative effect that can make it somewhat difficult to identify the source of the allergic reaction. For example, you drink milk every day and never think to associate that with the thickening scales on your head.

If standard dandruff treatments don't seem to be working for you, try cutting fatty foods (such as nuts and chocolate), dairy products, excessive sugar, and seafood out of your diet. Supplements of vitamins, such as biotin, thiamine (vitamin B_1), niacin (vitamin B_3), and cobalamin (vitamin B_{12}), may help eliminate dandruff by improving your body's ability to break down fatty acids.

AT-HOME REMEDIES

◆ Briskly massaging your scalp—either when you shampoo or when you use an herbal preparation such as tea tree oil—will improve the circulation in your scalp; the improved blood flow will help prevent the skin from drying and cracking.

◆ Watch your diet. Dairy products, fatty foods, seafood, and excessive sugar have all been shown to make dandruff worse.

◆ Wash your hair and scalp at least once a week with a medicated dandruff shampoo to prevent recurrences. ■

SYMPTOMS

For **major depression,** you may experience four or more of the following:
- persistent sadness, pessimism.
- feelings of guilt, worthlessness, helplessness, or hopelessness.
- loss of interest or pleasure in usual activities, including sex.
- difficulty concentrating.
- insomnia or oversleeping.
- weight gain or loss.
- fatigue, lack of energy.
- anxiety, agitation, irritability.
- thoughts of suicide or death.
- slow speech; slow movements.

In children and adolescents:
- insomnia, fatigue, headache, stomachache, dizziness.
- apathy, social withdrawal, weight loss.
- drug or alcohol abuse, a drop in school performance, difficulty concentrating.
- isolation from family and friends.

For **dysthymia** (minor but chronic depression), your symptoms will be less intense, fewer in number, but longer-lasting.

CALL YOUR DOCTOR IF:

- you or your child has suicidal thoughts, or has other signs of either **major depression** or **dysthymia;** help is available.

Note: There is a distinct difference between feeling "depressed" and having a depressive illness. If you have low spirits for a while, don't be concerned. However, if you feel you can't lift yourself out of your misery, seek help.

Almost all of us feel low sometimes, usually because of a disturbing event in our lives. But ongoing depression—suffering a period of what is known as **major depression**—is another matter. Depression in some form affects 25 percent of all women, 10 percent of all men, and 5 percent of all adolescents worldwide. It is the most common psychological problem in the United States, afflicting some 17.6 million people each year.

Depressive reaction (minor and often temporary depression) encompasses the normal depressed feelings that arise because of a specific life situation. The symptoms can be severe, but they usually do not need treatment and abate over time—anywhere from two weeks to six months.

Dysthymia (minor, chronic depression), similar to depressive reaction in its symptoms and degree of suffering, lasts longer—at least two years.

Major depression, or depressive illness, is a serious condition that can lead to an inability to function or even to suicide. Sufferers experience not only a depressed mood but also more harmful symptoms, including disinterest in their usual activities, extreme fatigue, sleep problems, or feelings of guilt and helplessness. They are more likely to lose touch with reality, sometimes having delusions or hallucinations. Depressive illness can be treated but often goes undiagnosed because it is confused with depressive reaction. It is a cyclical illness, so though most patients recover from their first depressive episode, the recurrence rate is high—perhaps as high as 60 percent within 2 years and 75 percent within 10 years. Major depression often appears spontaneously, is seemingly unprovoked, and often disappears spontaneously as well, usually in 6 to 12 months. Because of its disabling effects or the possibility of suicide, major depression needs treatment.

Depression can strike at any age, including in childhood. Studies in the United States show that 1.8 percent of prepubertal children and 4.7 percent of 14- to 17-year-olds have some form of depression. However, the common time of onset is early middle age, and depression is particularly rife among the elderly, as a reaction to the facts of growing older—the death of a spouse or friends, the physical limitations of age, and the impending confrontation with death. Elderly widowers are particularly susceptible to suicide.

CAUSES

Depression is an illness that seems to have different causes. **Depressive reaction,** or "normal depression," occurs as a result of a particular event. Depressed moods can also be a side effect of medication, hormonal changes (such as before menstrual periods or after childbirth), or a physical illness, such as the flu or a viral infection.

Although the exact causes of **major depression** and **dysthymia** are unknown, researchers currently believe that both forms are caused by a malfunction of the brain's neurotransmitters, chemicals (particularly serotonin) that modulate moods. This malfunction seems to have a large genetic component: In one study, 27 percent of depressed children had close relatives who suffered from mood disorders.

DIAGNOSTIC AND TEST PROCEDURES

Although very common, depression is often ignored or misdiagnosed and left untreated. Such inattention can be life-threatening; **major depression** in particular has a high suicide rate.

Studies show that 74 percent of people seeking help for depression go to their primary care physician, and that 50 percent of these cases are misdiagnosed. Of the cases that are correctly diagnosed by a general practitioner, 80 percent are given too little medication for too short a time. Some of this mishandling may occur because patients seek a doctor's help with—and physicians prescribe for—physical symptoms, such as sleep problems, fatigue, or weight loss, without considering depression as a possible root cause. Tests should also be made to rule out any organic factors—such as nutrient deficiencies, hypothyroidism *(see Thyroid Problems)*, reactions to drugs (either prescription or recreational)—that can produce similar symptoms.

The elderly are at greatest risk of being overlooked or misdiagnosed. Frequently, primary care physicians, and the elderly themselves, dismiss symptoms of depression as a part of growing old or categorize it as senile dementia—an irreversible condition that causes loss of memory and concentration. This is unfortunate because depression, unlike dementia, is reversible and can be treated successfully.

For all of these reasons, you should consult a psychiatrist or psychopharmacologist (a psychiatrist who specializes in drug therapies for mental illness) for diagnosis and treatment.

TREATMENT

Many therapies—both conventional and alternative—are available for depression. Treatments may vary according to the cause of the depression and its severity. Conventional methods include psychotherapy, antidepressant drugs, and electroconvulsive therapy (ECT).

CONVENTIONAL MEDICINE

Major depression and **dysthymia** are usually treated with a combination of psychotherapy and antidepressants. Psychotherapy aims to teach patients how to overcome negative attitudes and feelings and to encourage them to return to normal activities. Drug therapy is intended to moderate or correct neurochemical imbalances that affect moods.

The group of antidepressants most frequently prescribed today are drugs that regulate the neurochemical serotonin. Known as selective serotonin reuptake inhibitors (SSRIs), the group

---

IMPORTANT!

Depression is not a sign of emotional weakness. It is an illness with physiological as well as psychological causes. Most depression goes undiagnosed and untreated, often because people report only some of their symptoms and primary care doctors fail to consider it as a possibility. If you are suffering from persistent symptoms, do not hesitate to seek help from a psychiatrist or psychopharmacologist who can diagnose and treat your problem correctly.

includes fluoxetine, paroxetine, and sertraline. Bupropion, a drug from another class, is also used to regulate neurotransmitters. For children and adolescents, paroxetine is the drug of choice.

The tricyclics, which have been used to treat depression since the 1950s, are another option, although they are apt to have more unpleasant side effects than the SSRIs. Because adolescents do not tolerate side effects well and tend to stop taking their medication, tricyclics are not recommended for them. Tricyclics include imipramine and amitriptyline, as well as nortriptyline, doxepin, and desipramine.

The third group of antidepressants, the monoamine oxidase (MAO) inhibitors, have also proved effective. MAO inhibitors work more quickly than the tricyclics, but they have more severe side effects and require a change in diet; severe hypertension can occur if patients on MAO inhibitors eat foods containing tyramine—such as cheese, many beans, and various alcoholic beverages. MAO inhibitors are usually prescribed only if the SSRIs and the tricyclics fail to bring improvement.

Lithium carbonate, which is the drug commonly used for manic-depression, is used to treat depression as well.

Electroconvulsive therapy (ECT) involves the application of an electric shock of about 80 volts through electrodes on the head. The shock is not felt by the patient, who is anesthetized. Although doctors are still uncertain exactly how ECT works, its controversial techniques have been refined in the past 20 years and it is thought to be as safe as drugs—and in some cases more effective. Still, ECT should be used only after all other options have been considered—because it requires hospitalization and general anesthesia—or when rapid results are vital, as with suicidal patients or those who refuse to eat or drink. Usually given three times a week for two weeks, treatments generally don't extend beyond 6 to 10 sessions.

ALTERNATIVE CHOICES

Many alternative therapies are effective, particularly for minor depression. For more serious depressions, though, they should be considered as

ACUPRESSURE

Pressing Liver 8 may help relieve the effects of depression. Bending your right knee, place your thumb above the inside knee crease, just below the joint of the knee (swing your leg a few times to find it). Press for one minute, two or three times, then repeat on your left leg.

complementary treatments, not replacements for conventional methods; major or chronic depression should be treated by a psychiatrist.

In addition to the remedies mentioned below, you may want to consider **acupressure** or **acupuncture,** which may be helpful in relieving some symptoms; see a qualified, experienced practitioner. **Massage,** which is both soothing and energizing and enlivens the body, may also help. Try it once a week, if possible.

AROMATHERAPY

Aromatherapy may ease mental fatigue and help with sleep. The essential oils that may benefit depression are basil, clary, jasmine, rose, and chamomile *(Matricaria recutita).* The oil may be placed in a bowl of steaming water (2 or 3 drops), in a bath (5 or 6 drops), or on the edge of your pillow (1 or 2 drops).

BIOFEEDBACK

Anecdotal evidence suggests that EEG (brain-wave) biofeedback (also known as neurotherapy) is effective in reducing the intensity of all types of depression. Neurotherapy attempts to change brain-wave patterns through training—thus doing what drugs do chemically. The number of training sessions depends on the severity of the depression. **Depressive reaction** may need only 6 sessions, **dysthymia** may average 20, and **major depression** may need 30 to 60. Because it is, in effect, self-training, biofeedback has the advantage of putting the depressed person in charge of his own therapy; he can use it at will whenever it is needed.

CHINESE HERBS

"Aspiration" is a combination of several Chinese and Western herbs believed to help lift depression. The formula addresses physical symptoms as well as psychological ones, including loss of appetite, chest constriction, and constipation. It is most effective when taken in conjunction with regular aerobic exercise, daily practice of a **relaxation** technique, and a good diet *(see Nutrition and Diet, right)*. Another Chinese herbal formula, "Gather Vitality," may help with insomnia or oversleeping, aching limbs, and fatigue.

EXERCISE

Exercise should be a part of any therapy for depression; it improves blood flow to the brain, elevates mood, and relieves stress. Even if used alone, it can often bring startling results. Studies show that jogging for 30 minutes three times a week can be as effective as psychotherapy in treating depression. Pick an exercise you like and do it daily, if possible. Any exercise is fine; the more energetic and aerobic, the better.

HERBAL THERAPIES

An experienced herbalist will recommend a particular combination of herbs tailored to your specific symptoms. For a general prescription for depression, one suggestion is: 2 parts St.-John's-wort *(Hypericum perforatum)*, 1 part oat *(Avena sativa)* straw, 1 part lavender *(Lavandula officinalis)*, and 1 part mugwort *(Artemisia vulgaris)*. Take 5 ml of the tincture three times a day for at least one month. St.-John's-wort, taken in any of its forms, is a traditional depression remedy in Europe. However, some herbalists report that its effects are unpredictable: Sometimes the herb gets remarkable results, other times it has no effect at all.

MIND/BODY MEDICINE

Many mind/body practices are helpful with depression. Music and dance can lift the spirits and energize the body. **Meditation** and relaxation techniques, such as progressive muscle relaxation, both stimulate and relax. Other choices include transcendental **meditation** and the Asian exercise techniques of **yoga, t'ai chi,** and **qigong.** Choose one or two that suit you and practice daily.

NUTRITION AND DIET

Because depressive symptoms are exacerbated by nutritional deficiencies, good nutrition is important. Increase your intake of healthful foods such as whole-grain cereals, lean meats, fruits and vegetables, fish, and low-fat dairy products. It's very important to avoid alcohol, but also stay away from junk food, sugar, aspartame, and caffeine, which give you a sudden spurt of energy or a high feeling but then let you down.

Recent clinical studies strongly suggest that vitamin B complex, folic acid (400 mcg daily), and S-adenosylmethionine (two doses of 800 mg daily) are useful in treating depression. The antioxidant selenium (100 mcg daily) was shown to have a mood-elevating effect in regions where food is deficient in selenium.

Many European studies show that the amino acid supplement L-tryptophan, known to increase the synthesis of serotonin, is of value in relieving depression. However, because of the trace contamination of one manufacturer's product, tryptophan in its synthetic form is no longer available in the United States. You can find tryptophan in certain foods, such as turkey, chicken, fish, cooked dried beans and peas, brewer's yeast, peanut butter, nuts, and soybeans. Eat plenty of these foods together with a carbohydrate (potatoes, pasta, rice), which will ease the brain's uptake of tryptophan.

PREVENTION

Some forms of depression may not be preventable since current theory suggests that they may be triggered by neurochemical malfunctioning in the brain. However, there is good evidence that depression may often be alleviated or prevented with good health habits. Proper diet, exercise, vacations, no overwork, and saving time to do things you enjoy all help keep the blues at bay. ■

D

Dry, reddish, itchy skin indicates some type of dermatitis, or skin inflammation, of which there are many types.

- A red rash that is limited to the area of skin exposed to an irritant is probably **contact dermatitis,** an allergic reaction.
- Red, itchy, circular patches of weeping, scaly, or encrusted skin signal **nummular dermatitis,** common in older people who have dry skin or live in dry environments.
- Greasy, yellowish scales on the scalp and eyebrows, behind the ears, and around the nose indicate **seborrheic dermatitis;** in infants it is called **cradle cap.**
- Scaling, greasy-looking, sometimes ulcerated skin appearing inside the lower legs and around the ankles may indicate **stasis dermatitis.**
- Extreme, persistent itchiness may signal **atopic dermatitis,** or eczema.

See also the Visual Diagnostic Guide.

CALL YOUR DOCTOR IF:

- your skin has oozing sores or other signs of infection. You may need treatment with antibiotics or other drugs.
- the affected skin does not respond to treatment with over-the-counter creams or medicated shampoos. You should have a medical diagnosis and treatment.
- during a flareup of eczema you are exposed to anyone with a viral skin disease such as cold sores or warts. You are at increased risk of contracting the viral disorder.

Dermatitis simply means skin inflammation, but it embraces a range of ailments. In most cases the early stages are characterized by dry, red, itchy skin, although acute attacks may result in crusty scales or blisters that ooze fluid. Since many agents can irritate the skin, a doctor will try to narrow the diagnosis to a specific category of dermatitis, even though treatment is similar for most types of skin irritation and inflammation.

CAUSES

The following are the most common general types of dermatitis and their typical causes:

Contact dermatitis typically causes the skin to develop a pink or red rash, which may or may not itch. Pinpointing the exact cause of contact dermatitis can be difficult. Among plants, the leading culprits are poison ivy, poison oak, and poison sumac, although contact with certain flowers, herbs, fruits, and vegetables irritates some people. Common chemical irritants include detergents, soaps, chlorine, some synthetic fibers, nail polish remover, antiperspirants, and formaldehyde (found in permanent-press fabrics, polishes, artificial-fingernail adhesive, particle board, and foam insulation). Wearing rubber gloves, unwashed new clothes, or plated jewelry can also cause contact dermatitis. The inflammation is frequently caused by cosmetics and skin-care products.

Nummular dermatitis consists of distinctive coin-shaped red patches that are most commonly seen on the legs, buttocks, hands, and arms of people 55 or older. Living in a dry environment or taking very hot showers can cause this condition, as can stress and other skin disorders.

Seborrheic dermatitis consists of greasy, yellowish scaling on the scalp and other hairy areas, as well as on the face or genitals, and in skin creases along the nose, under the breasts, and elsewhere. This ailment can be associated with a biotin deficiency in infants—where it is known as **cradle cap**—or with overproduction and blockage of oil glands in adults. It may be aggravated by stress and is common in AIDS patients.

Stasis dermatitis is caused by poor circulation. Veins in the lower legs fail to return blood efficiently, causing pooling of blood and fluid buildup. This leads to unhealthy skin growth and irritation, especially around the ankles.

Atopic dermatitis, or eczema, causes the skin to itch, scale, swell, and sometimes blister. Eczema usually runs in families and is often associated with allergies, asthma, and stress.

For information about other types of skin disorders, see also Diaper Rash, Hives, Impetigo, Psoriasis, Rashes, Scabies, and Shingles.

DIAGNOSTIC AND TEST PROCEDURES

Most types of dermatitis can be diagnosed by a doctor's observation of the irritation and its location on the body. Sometimes a skin scraping will be taken for microscopic analysis. To identify causes of **contact dermatitis,** a doctor may try patch tests, applying suspected irritants to areas of skin on the back. If no inflammation develops after two to four days, the doctor applies other potential irritants until the cause is clear.

TREATMENT

The first step in treating dermatitis is identifying and eliminating the cause. Most mild skin inflammations respond well to warm baths followed by application of petroleum jelly or over-the-counter hydrocortisone cream. **Seborrheic dermatitis** may respond to coal-tar-based shampoo; avoid sunlight for the first few hours after using it, since it increases the risk of sunburn on the scalp. Once irritants causing **contact dermatitis** are identified, treatment will be based on avoidance, allergy relief, or other coping mechanisms. To help dry the sores of **nummular dermatitis,** soak the area in salt water, then apply a corticosteroid cream. If you suffer from **stasis dermatitis,** wear support stockings and rest frequently with your legs elevated to help improve circulation.

CONVENTIONAL MEDICINE

To reduce inflammation and heal the irritation of most types of dermatitis, a doctor usually recom- mends over-the-counter or prescription corticosteroid cream, and might prescribe an oral antihistamine to relieve severe itching and an antibiotic if a secondary infection develops. Severe cases of **seborrheic dermatitis** may call for corticosteroid injections. **Stasis dermatitis** may involve treatment with tar or zinc paste, which must stay on the sores for up to two weeks; this technique requires bandaging by a trained professional.

ALTERNATIVE CHOICES

Because many forms of dermatitis are chronic, most alternative therapies seek only to relieve the symptoms—itchiness, burning, and swelling.

HERBAL THERAPIES

Over the centuries, countless herbs have been used to treat skin ailments. Picking out what's right for your condition can be difficult, so seek help from a trained practitioner. Here are some

C A U T I O N !

THE COSMETIC CONNECTION

If a rash develops on your face, neck, lips, scalp, or hairline, the prime suspects could be among your cosmetics or other skin-care aids, including perfume, deodorants, antiperspirants, shampoos, toothpaste, mouthwash, and aftershave lotion. The irritating ingredient in makeup and skin products is usually a scent or a preservative, but be wary of "unscented" products, too; they may contain chemicals that neutralize natural odors but that can also irritate your skin.

The claim that a cosmetic or skin-care product is "hypoallergenic," "organic," or "nonallergic" can be similarly misleading, since no product can be risk free for everyone. If you have sensitive skin, keep your cosmetics and skin-care aids simple and rely on unscented products.

substances herbalists consistently recommend:

Burdock (Arctium lappa) boosts the immune system and helps reduce inflammation. Brew tea using 1 to 3 tsp of dried root per cup of boiling water, or take up to 1½ tsp of tincture daily.

Some practitioners believe evening primrose oil (Oenothera biennis) works as well as corticosteroids for itchy skin and has fewer potential side effects, but the recommended dose of 500 mg three times a day can be costly. People with liver disease or high cholesterol should use it only under medical supervision; pregnant women should not use this treatment because it can affect their estrogen and progesterone levels.

Topical ointments made with calendula (Calendula officinalis) or chamomile (Matricaria recutita) are effective for treating many types of dermatitis. You can make another herbal remedy by mixing tinctures of nettle (Urtica dioica), cleavers (Galium spp.), and either goldenseal (Hydrastis canadensis) or myrrh (Commiphora molmol) in equal parts; take up to 1½ tsp a day. You can also make a tea from fresh nettles or fresh cleavers—1 tbsp of the herb steeped in a cup of boiling water—and drink three or four cups a day. WARNING: In some cases an allergy to nettle will worsen **atopic dermatitis** (eczema).

HOMEOPATHY

For benign, short-term skin problems, an over-the-counter Calendula cream may soothe the inflammation. Taking Rhus toxicodendron (12x) three or four times a day may relieve the itching of **contact dermatitis**. If you have a chronic form of dermatitis, a homeopath will investigate everything from your sleep patterns to your family history before recommending a remedy.

LIGHT THERAPY

When certain chronic types of dermatitis do not respond to conventional corticosteroid or coal-tar treatment, many doctors recommend using ultraviolet (UV) rays from an artificial light source. In light-therapy treatments, patients expose the affected areas under a sunlamp, which emits UV radiation, for a prescribed period of time. In nearly all cases, the skin clears considerably in a matter of weeks.

MEN JUST DON'T GET SOME TYPES OF RASHES

Paradoxically, unisex fashion trends have uncovered an unsuspected difference between the sexes. Men who wear pierced earrings or other forms of jewelry are far less likely than women to develop contact dermatitis from the nickel in plated jewelry. A team of scientists found that 12 percent of the 15-year-old girls in their study were sensitive to nickel, while less than 2 percent of the young men in a later study had a similar problem. Differences in the types of jewelry the two groups wear may account for some of the disparity, but the researchers also suspect that male and female hormones may play a real but undetermined role.

Despite its apparent effectiveness, light therapy has its drawbacks. At four to eight sittings a month, treatment can be time-consuming for the patient and relatively expensive. Light therapy may cause premature aging of the skin and increase a person's risk of developing skin cancer. In some instances, the dermatitis can recur within a year.

In severe or persistent cases, the treatment can be supported with drug therapy. Light therapy supported with an oral medication called psoralen has good long-term results but carries additional risks. Treatment with psoralen can cause liver problems in some patients; close monitoring by a physician is necessary. Pregnant women should avoid drug-supported light therapy altogether, since psoralen can cause fetal deformities. Women undergoing such therapy should wait several months after stopping treatment before trying to become pregnant.

Some people try to avoid the doctor's office or

hospital by using a tanning salon as their source of UV radiation. They won't find the healing rays they seek, however. Because of concerns about the risks of skin cancer, tanning salons must filter out the type of UV rays used in light therapy. Even patients who own a sunlamp or who can find UV radiation commercially should rely on a doctor's care. Only a qualified physician can tell you how much UV radiation you can tolerate without risking long-term damage to your skin.

MIND/BODY MEDICINE
Since some cases of dermatitis may be stress related, relaxation techniques such as **yoga** may be effective, particularly for **atopic** and **seborrheic dermatitis**. **Guided imagery** can also help: You create and control an image opposite to the physical manifestation of the ailment. For example, if you have a red, dry rash, imagine applying a soothing blue ointment to the affected area. This technique works best if you close your eyes and ears to outside stimuli and concentrate all your senses on the image in your mind; you need to smell the ointment, see the healing, and feel the relief.

NUTRITION AND DIET
Because some patients with **seborrheic dermatitis** are believed to have difficulty metabolizing fatty acids necessary for promoting the body's anti-inflammatory response, a doctor may suggest 50 mg of vitamin B complex twice daily. Vitamin A (25,000 IU a day) and zinc (50 to 100 mg a day) may aid in skin healing, while vitamin E ointment or capsules (200 to 400 IU a day) can help relieve itching and dryness. To avoid the risk of overdose, particularly of fat-soluble vitamins, have your doctor check dosages carefully and monitor your progress; a pediatrician must assess any vitamin supplements given to a child.

AT-HOME REMEDIES
- Over-the-counter oatmeal or cornstarch preparations mixed into a warm bath may soothe the skin and relieve itching. Take care not to stay in the bath too long, because lengthy immersion can strip sensitive skin of essential oils.
- For dryness, rub petroleum jelly or vegetable shortening on affected areas after a bath, or use a topical ointment containing aloe (*Aloe barbadensis*) or zinc.
- Avoid eating potential allergens, such as milk, eggs, and wheat. You may get help from supplemental vitamins A, B complex, and E, as well as zinc.
- If you suspect an allergy to a chemical or cosmetic, try an at-home patch test. Apply a small amount of the suspected irritant to a spot on your arm or back for seven days. If you have a reaction, you know it is a potential irritant.

PREVENTION

The best way to prevent a rash caused by contact with toxic plants like poison ivy is to wash the exposed skin with soap and water as soon as possible after contact. Most other cases of dermatitis develop in people with sensitive skin and can be prevented only by avoiding the irritant. If you have **atopic** or **seborrheic dermatitis,** for example, you have a higher-than-average chance of being allergic to nickel in jewelry or to getting dry skin during the winter. Fair-skinned people seem especially prone to skin problems. If you feel you are at risk, consider these preventive steps:
- Use a humidifier at home and at work to keep the air from getting too dry.
- Wear loose-fitting, natural-fiber clothing; untreated cotton is ideal.
- Avoid plated jewelry, especially in your ears, to prevent nickel-related rashes. Surgical steel or 14-karat gold earring posts are safer choices.
- Don't wear a watchband that presses against your skin for long periods; the friction and sweat buildup can cause rashes.
- Supplement your diet with vitamins A, B complex, and E, and zinc.
- Lubricate your skin after a bath using an unscented, preservative-free lotion or ointment.■

SYMPTOMS

- excessive thirst and appetite.
- increased urination (sometimes as often as every hour).
- weight loss.
- fatigue.
- nausea, perhaps vomiting.
- blurred vision.
- in women, frequent vaginal infections and perhaps the cessation of menstruation.
- in men, impotence.
- in men and women, yeast infections.

CALL YOUR DOCTOR IF:

- you feel nauseated, weak, and excessively thirsty; are urinating very frequently; have abdominal pain; and are breathing more deeply and rapidly than normal—perhaps with sweet breath that smells like nail polish remover. You may need immediate medical attention for ketoacidosis.
- you feel weak or faint; are experiencing a rapid heartbeat, trembling, and excessive sweating; and feel irritable, hungry, or suddenly drowsy. You could be developing hypoglycemia, and may need to eat or drink something quickly to avoid more serious complications.

Diabetes mellitus, the most common disorder of the endocrine system, affects between 10 million and 20 million people in the United States alone. The disease is brought on by disorders in blood levels of insulin, a pancreatic hormone that helps your system convert blood glucose, or blood sugar, into energy. **Type 1 diabetes**—sometimes called insulin-dependent diabetes mellitus (IDDM) or juvenile or juvenile-onset diabetes—results from a shortage of insulin. **Type 2 diabetes**—also known as non-insulin-dependent diabetes mellitus (NIDDM) or adult-onset or stable diabetes—results from the body's inability to process the hormone effectively. About 90 percent of all diabetics have this form.

Regardless of what type of diabetes you have, you need to work closely with your doctor to manage your diet, medication, and activity on a day-to-day basis. Your ability to oversee your own care will make a huge difference in whether you can control the condition and avoid its potentially serious effects.

The many short- and long-term complications of diabetes can demand as much attention as the disease itself. Most important, you need to watch your blood sugar levels every day to prevent an attack of hypoglycemia, in which available levels of blood sugar are too low to fulfill your body's energy needs. Hypoglycemia can easily be remedied, however, once you recognize its symptoms.

Hyperglycemia, or high blood sugar, can bring on a serious diabetic condition known as ketoacidosis, in which the blood becomes increasingly acidic from the accumulation of toxic by-products called ketones that are produced as the body breaks down fat for energy. Ketoacidosis occurs in Type 1 diabetics if they do not receive adequate supplementary insulin and their bodies are starved for energy sources. Ketoacidosis can also occur in diabetics if glucose and insulin levels are not properly balanced, or if the body comes under sudden physical stress, perhaps from an accident or illness. (Any sort of illness increases the body's need for insulin to process blood glucose into the energy required to fight illness or infection.)

If you are diabetic, be especially alert for the warning signs of ketoacidosis: nausea, excessive thirst, frequent urination, extreme weakness, abdominal pain, and rapid deep breathing. Failure to respond immediately with injections of insulin and intravenous salt solutions (to replenish lost body fluids) can result in coma or death.

Long-term complications of diabetes can damage the eyes, nervous system, kidneys, and cardiovascular and circulatory systems, as well as hinder the body's overall resistance to infections. Cuts and sores heal more slowly for people with diabetes, and diabetics are also prone to gum problems, urinary tract infections, and mouth infections such as thrush, caused by an overgrowth of yeast organisms. *(See also Urinary Problems and Yeast Infections.)*

Complications from diabetes are the primary cause of adult blindness in the United States. Within 10 years after their condition is diagnosed, about half of all diabetics develop an eye disorder called diabetic retinopathy, which can weaken the capillaries that supply blood to the retina, and eventually affect vision. Almost all of those who have had the disease for at least 30 years experience some degree of diabetic retinopathy. Diabetics are also more likely to develop cataracts and glaucoma.

People with diabetes stand a higher than normal chance of developing heart disease and circulatory problems such as high blood pressure, hardening of the arteries *(see Atherosclerosis),* heart attacks, and strokes. Poor circulation also makes diabetics more susceptible to skin ulcers, cramps, and gangrenous (tissue-destroying) infections. Damage to the blood vessels in the kidneys from diabetes may lead to kidney failure.

A number of people with diabetes suffer from a condition known as diabetic neuropathy, which causes a gradual deterioration of the nervous system. The condition appears to begin early in both types of diabetes mellitus and affects motor nerves as well as sensory nerves. As a result, diabetics commonly experience a variety of aches and pains. Some develop slowed reflexes, loss of sensation, numbness and tingling in the legs, impotence, and circulatory problems.

ATTENTION!

LURKING DANGERS

Some over-the-counter remedies that are safe for nondiabetics contain ingredients that can cause problems for diabetics. For example, aspirin taken in large amounts can alter blood glucose levels. Diabetics seeking relief from respiratory ailments must be careful when using phenylephrine, epinephrine, or ephedrine, all of which can raise blood sugar levels. Type 2 diabetics tempted to use appetite suppressants to control their weight need to know that these drugs usually contain caffeine, which boosts blood sugar. Fish oil, commonly taken as a way to improve cholesterol levels, also raises blood sugar. To learn about potential hazards lurking in non-prescription medications, talk to your doctor and your pharmacist, and read labels carefully.

CAUSES

In **Type 1 diabetes,** the pancreas secretes little or no insulin. Unable to use glucose in the blood, the body tries to produce energy by burning fat and muscle. Type 1 diabetes develops fairly quickly, usually striking people under age 30. Recent research suggests that many Type 1 diabetics may have had a genetic predisposition to the disease that was triggered by a viral infection.

Type 2 diabetes usually develops in people over age 40, and there appears to be a strong link between obesity and the development of Type 2 diabetes. Although this particular group of diabetics may have sufficient or even excessive amounts of insulin in their systems, their bodies are unable to use the hormone effectively. Excessive food intake boosts blood glucose levels, and the pancreas cannot produce enough insulin to convert the extra sugar into energy. Sometimes a similar form of this disease, called gestational diabetes, occurs as a temporary condition in women who are pregnant.

D

FIRST AID FOR DIABETICS

You can take steps to help someone who is experiencing a diabetic emergency. First, check to see if the victim is wearing or carrying a Medic Alert tag. If the person has diabetes, the tag should indicate this, and possibly the type of diabetes as well. Hyperglycemia (high blood sugar) can occur in either Type 1 or Type 2 diabetics. Hypoglycemia (low blood sugar) can also strike all diabetics and, in some cases, people who don't have the disease.

Hyperglycemia symptoms include rapid, heavy breathing; abdominal pain; sweet-smelling breath; frequent urination; vomiting; drowsiness; and possibly unconsciousness. What you should do: If the person is conscious and can swallow, give him something to drink that contains no sugar (to prevent dehydration), then take him to the hospital. **If the victim is unconscious, call 911 immediately.**

Hypoglycemia symptoms include pale, clammy skin; excessive hunger; disorientation; aggressive behavior; and possibly unconsciousness. What you should do: If the victim is conscious and can swallow, give him something to eat or drink that contains sugar—such as fruit juice, candy, a soft drink, or plain sugar— then take him to the hospital. **If the victim is unconscious, call 911 immediately.**

If the victim is conscious and you are unsure whether he is hyper- or hypoglycemic, give him something to eat or drink that contains sugar, such as fruit juice, candy, a soft drink, or even plain sugar, then take him to the hospital. (Even if the person has hyperglycemia, the additional sugar will do no harm.) **If the victim is unconscious, call 911.**

DIAGNOSTIC AND TEST PROCEDURES

Your doctor may suspect that you have diabetes if a routine physical examination indicates that excess sugar in your body is being flushed out in your urine. Actual diagnosis begins with an examination of your glucose levels, which the doctor does by taking a blood sample in the morning before you have had anything to eat; if your pancreas is producing little or no insulin (Type 1), or if the body is not producing enough insulin to process blood sugar (Type 2), your glucose levels will be elevated. Additional tests for diabetes include a glucose tolerance test, which measures the body's ability to convert glucose into energy. After fasting for a period, you drink a very sweet beverage containing glucose, then have your blood glucose levels checked.

TREATMENT

Treatment for both forms of diabetes mellitus requires adjustment of insulin levels in the body and strict management of diet and exercise. By paying close attention to the content and timing of your meals, you can minimize or avoid the "seesaw effect" of rapidly changing blood sugar levels, which can require quick changes in insulin dosages.

CONVENTIONAL MEDICINE

If you have **Type 1 diabetes,** it is essential that you receive supplementary insulin every day, at least twice a day, to promote your body's use of blood glucose. Since insulin is a protein and is destroyed by digestive enzymes, it cannot be taken orally. Rather, it must be injected directly into the body at set intervals. While some diabetics use a computerized pump that administers insulin on a set basis, most doctors advise direct injections. Learning to give injections to yourself or to your infant or child may at first seem the most daunting part of managing Type 1 diabetes, but the process quickly becomes routine.

Most insulin in use today is processed synthetically, although some is still derived from animal hormone. The medication comes in three varieties: short-acting (taking effect within 30 or 40 minutes and lasting for 6 hours); intermediate-acting (taking effect in 2 to 4 hours and lasting up to 24 hours); and long-acting (taking effect in 6 to 8 hours and lasting up to 32 hours). Each injection plan is tailored for the individual diabetic and adjusted to accommodate events such as periods of stress, adolescent growth, and the pre-menstrual period of a woman's monthly cycle.

By monitoring your own blood glucose levels, you can track your body's fluctuating insulin demand and help your doctor calculate the most appropriate insulin dosage. One self-monitoring technique involves a special meter that reads glucose levels in a sample of your blood dabbed on a strip of treated paper. Another method uses paper strips that change color when exposed to a drop of blood to indicate glucose levels.

For some **Type 2 diabetics,** diet and exercise are sufficient to keep the disease under control; others require drug therapy, which may include insulin or an oral hypoglycemia medication such as tolbutamide, acetohexamide, glipizide, glyburide, or chlorpropamide. If you take any of these drugs for Type 2 diabetes, ask your doctor about possible interactions with other prescription drugs, including chloramphenicol, phenylbutazone, oxyphenbutazone, and clofibrate.

Maintaining a balanced diet is vital in both Type 1 and Type 2 diabetes, so work with your doctor to set up a menu plan. If you have Type 1 diabetes, and the timing of your insulin dosage is determined by activity and diet, when you eat and how much you eat are just as important as what you eat. Usually, doctors recommend three small meals and three to four snacks every day to maintain the proper balance between glucose and insulin in the blood. Carbohydrates—especially some starches and other complex carbohydrates, which release glucose relatively slowly into the bloodstream—should make up 50 to 60 percent of your total caloric intake; proteins should compose from 20 to 25 percent; and fats, from 20 to 30 percent.

Recommended proportions of carbohydrates, proteins, and fats for Type 2 diabetics are essentially the same, although patients who are overweight are encouraged to lower their intake of fat and eat more complex carbohydrates and fiber. Since Type 2 diabetics are usually not concerned with scheduled doses of insulin, they do not need to time their meals so carefully.

Another crucial element in a diabetic's daily program is exercise, which can help Type 2 diabetics in particular lose excess weight. For people with either type, exercise can also help mitigate cardiovascular complications of the disease, and it may offer stress relief as well. Type 1 diabetics need to remember, however, that exercise lowers blood glucose levels. To prevent an attack of hypoglycemia, plan to eat a carbohydrate snack approximately half an hour before you begin exercising, and make sure you have something to eat or drink if you start to feel hypoglycemic symptoms. With either type, check with your doctor before starting an exercise program.

It is also a good idea to wear a Medic Alert bracelet or tag indicating that you have diabetes; this will make others aware of your condition in case you have a severe hypoglycemic attack and are not able to make yourself understood, or if you are in an accident or another situation and need emergency medical care. Identifying yourself as a diabetic is important because hypoglycemic attacks can be mistaken for drunkenness, and victims often aren't able to care for themselves. Without prompt treatment, hypoglycemia can result in a coma or seizures. And since your body is under increased stress when you are ill or injured, your glucose levels will need to be monitored by any medical personnel who give you emergency care.

ALTERNATIVE CHOICES

Since diabetes that is incorrectly treated can be life-threatening, you should never try to treat the disease without the help of a doctor, and you should always discuss any possible treatments thoroughly. Some alternative remedies offer variations of diabetic diets. Others emphasize supplemental vitamins and minerals, prescribe herbs to restore blood sugar levels, or treat secondary effects. Stress-reduction practices may also help lower blood glucose levels.

D

ACUPUNCTURE

Stimulation of certain points may relieve pain associated with diabetic neuropathy, boost the immune system, and minimize circulatory system complications. Consult a licensed practitioner.

CHINESE HERBS

Chinese herbal medicines, including ginseng root *(Panax ginseng),* are frequently used to alleviate some symptoms of diabetes; consult a practitioner for a comprehensive treatment plan.

HERBAL THERAPIES

Check with a practitioner to make sure herbs are appropriate for your condition. Remember: If you need insulin to manage your diabetes, there is no herbal substitute for the hormone.

Blueberry *(Vaccinium myrtillus)* leaves in a decoction may lower blood glucose levels and help maintain the vascular system. This remedy may also help to keep the blood vessels of the eye from hemorrhaging if you develop diabetic retinopathy. Diabetics in one study who ate crackers made from the powdered form of burdock *(Arctium lappa)* after a starchy meal had a lowered incidence of hyperglycemia. A cream made with cayenne *(Capsicum frutescens)* may relieve pain associated with peripheral neuropathy, a type of diabetic neuropathy.

Supplementing the diet with fenugreek *(Trigonella foenum-graecum)* seeds has been shown in clinical and experimental studies to reduce blood glucose and insulin levels while lowering blood cholesterol. Garlic *(Allium sativum)* may lower blood pressure as well as levels of blood sugar and cholesterol.

Ginkgo *(Ginkgo biloba)* extracts have been used to stem deteriorating vision in patients by maintaining adequate blood flow to the retina. Other reported benefits of ginkgo include reducing the risk of heart disease, hypertension, and elevated cholesterol levels.

Onion *(Allium cepa)* may free up insulin to help metabolize glucose in the blood, thus lowering blood glucose levels. Both raw and boiled onion extracts have been found to have this effect. Onion is also considered beneficial in maintaining a healthy cardiovascular system.

LIFESTYLE

In laboratory tests, exercise has been shown to increase the tissue levels of chromium, which the body uses to regulate blood glucose and cholesterol levels. For **Type 1 diabetics,** exercise has also been found to increase the body's ability to use available insulin so that fewer insulin injections are needed. WARNING: If you have Type 1 diabetes, keep in mind that exercise lowers your blood glucose; eat a carbohydrate snack before exercising, and eat or drink again if you feel the warning symptoms of a hypoglycemic attack.

Type 2 diabetics who need to lose weight can benefit from moderate exercise. However, if you are a Type 2 diabetic, you should avoid weight-lifting or other forms of exertion that involve pushing or pulling heavy objects; these activities raise blood pressure and may aggravate any eye problems that stem from diabetes.

If you are diabetic, be sure to take good care of your teeth and floss regularly; diabetes can exacerbate gum disease.

MIND/BODY MEDICINE

Any sort of practice that will lower your stress level, such as **biofeedback, meditation, hypnotherapy,** or other relaxation techniques, may help lessen your insulin requirements.

NUTRITION AND DIET

Some practitioners claim that diabetes is a disorder of Western lifestyles, pointing out that when people in other cultures abandon native foods for a diet of refined and processed foods, diabetes rates begin to rise. The high-carbohydrate high-plant-fiber diet (HCF diet) is an alternative to the conventional diet plan for diabetics.

The HCF diet calls for diabetics to follow these daily guidelines in planning their meals: Eat 70 to 75 percent complex carbohydrates, 15 to 20 percent proteins, and only 5 to 10 percent fats. The HCF diet is said to boost insulin's ability to promote blood glucose as an energy source, improve cholesterol levels, reduce the incidence of hyperglycemia and hypoglycemia, and help with weight loss for Type 2 diabetics.

A modified version of the HCF diet further restricts what foods may be eaten but increases the

ESSENTIAL FOOT CARE

If you are diabetic, your foot is your Achilles heel, so to speak. This is because nerve damage from diabetic neuropathy can deaden your perception of pain and allow small injuries such as blisters to develop into major infections before you notice anything is wrong. Diabetics need to examine their feet closely every day, looking for red spots, bruises, cuts, blisters, swelling, or any sign of infection. Watch out for dry skin, which can crack and allow bacteria and fungi to invade. Cut toenails straight across to avoid ingrown toenails. Wear comfortable shoes, and don't risk injuring your feet by walking barefoot or wearing sandals.

allowable amount of complex carbohydrates. One university study indicated that a high-carbohydrate, high-fiber diet could reduce the insulin demands of Type 1 diabetics by 30 to 40 percent, and of Type 2 diabetics by 75 to 100 percent.

Diabetics should avoid sugar, as it can lower the body's glucose tolerance and worsen circulatory problems. Nutritionists also emphasize the importance of certain foods, vitamins, and minerals, including the following:

Chromium supplements can be very helpful for people with diabetes. Chromium not only lowers blood glucose levels and improves glucose tolerance but it also lowers insulin levels and helps hold down blood cholesterol levels.

Inositol, a B-complex vitamin, has been shown to help protect diabetics from peripheral neuropathy by relieving numbness and tingling in the hands and feet. However, since inositol might alter blood sugar levels, make sure to check with your practitioner before starting supplements. Biotin, also called vitamin H, may improve glucose metabolism in diabetics.

Vitamin B_6 may help decrease the severity of diabetic neuropathy and reduce insulin demands in Type 2 diabetics. Vitamin B_{12} may help treat diabetic neuropathy; injections may prove more beneficial than oral doses.

Diabetics may need supplements of vitamin C to make up for low blood levels of insulin, which normally works to help cells absorb the vitamin. Proper amounts of vitamin C help the body maintain good cholesterol levels, fight off infection by bolstering the immune system, and prevent cataracts. Although some practitioners recommend supplementing your diet with up to 1 gram of vitamin C per day, you should consult your practitioner to make sure this is a safe dosage for you to take. Vitamin E may help limit damage to the vascular system and improve blood cholesterol levels.

Manganese helps the body metabolize glucose; diabetics often have a serious manganese deficiency. Magnesium supplements may help control diabetic retinopathy and reduce the possibility of cardiovascular damage.

Zinc may help increase glucose tolerance, and potassium may improve a diabetic's ability to utilize insulin. Copper supplements may help improve cardiovascular fitness.

Okra and peas can help stabilize blood sugar levels and provide fiber in a high-complex-carbohydrate diet. Some research suggests that cinnamon can lower insulin requirements in Type 2 diabetics; seasoning your food with as much as $1/4$ tsp at every meal may help regulate blood sugar levels.

PREVENTION

Because of the apparent link between obesity and Type 2 diabetes, you can do a great deal to help reduce your chances of developing the disease by slimming down if you are overweight. This is especially true if diabetes runs in your family.

A good exercise program and a nutritionally balanced diet can greatly limit the effects of both Type 1 and Type 2 diabetes. If you smoke, quit; smoking can significantly increase the risk of heart disease, particularly for diabetics. ∎

SYMPTOMS

- redness over the diaper area—around the genitals, buttocks, and thighs, but not on the abdomen.
- tight, papery skin, or skin that is shiny and bright red.
- a strong smell of ammonia.
- in boys, an inflamed penis.

See also the Visual Diagnostic Guide.

CALL YOUR DOCTOR IF:

- you see no improvement after four days of home treatment, or you also see white patches inside the mouth that appear red after being wiped with a clean cloth; your child may have a yeast infection called candidiasis, or sometimes thrush.
- the rash is scaly and has a yellowish hue and appears not only in the diaper area, but elsewhere on the body, such as behind the ears or under the arms; your child may have seborrheic dermatitis.
- the diaper rash does not go away within a few days or worsens; your child may have developed a strep or staph infection or a local reaction to a particular lotion, soap, or laundry detergent.
- the diaper area is covered with blisters that leave shallow red sores; your child may have impetigo, which requires treatment with antibiotics.
- your son's penis is swollen and red and you can't retract the foreskin, or you notice a greenish discharge from the penis; your child may have a painful condition called balanitis, which requires antibiotics.

Almost all babies develop a diaper rash—an inflammation of the skin on the buttocks, genitals, and thighs—at some time in their young lives. Although a diaper rash may cause a baby discomfort and even some pain, it is rarely serious. Most cases are of short duration, lasting only three or four days. But sometimes a rash will persist, an indication that a secondary skin condition or infection has developed.

Your baby can get diaper rash whether you use disposable or cloth diapers; moisture, not the diaper itself, is the culprit. Keeping your child clean and changing a diaper soon after it is soiled is the key to battling diaper rash.

CAUSES

Diaper rash can be caused by anything that irritates your baby's sensitive skin. The most common source of the problem is urine and stool left in contact with the skin for too long, but a rash can also be caused by inadequate drying of the baby's skin after a bath or by an allergic reaction to lotions or soaps used directly on the baby's skin or to chemicals in the laundry detergent used to clean fabric diapers. Seborrhea, an inflammatory skin condition that affects the oil glands, can trigger a diaper rash as can thrush, a type of yeast infection. Babies receiving antibiotics for other illnesses are particularly susceptible to thrush-related diaper rash because the drugs allow fun-

C A U T I O N !

When baby powder or talc comes in contact with broken skin, it may cause an inflammatory reaction called granulation. If inhaled, the fine powder may cause lung damage. To help keep diapered areas dry, most pediatricians now recommend barrier creams or cornstarch, which is coarser and heavier than powder. Do not use cornstarch if your baby has a yeast infection, however: Yeast thrives on cornstarch.

gal growth. Eczema, an allergic skin condition, can also occur as a diaper rash in reaction to foods or other allergens.

TREATMENT

Most diaper rashes respond well to home treatments and require no medical care. If your baby's rash fails to improve after three or four days, see a pediatrician. The rash should be diagnosed to rule out the presence of a more serious infection.

CONVENTIONAL MEDICINE

For an ordinary rash, the doctor may recommend an over-the-counter ointment containing zinc oxide to protect the skin. If your child has developed a bacterial infection, a topical or oral antibiotic may be prescribed. For thrush, your pediatrician will prescribe an antifungal cream for the rash and possibly an oral antifungal liquid to clear up patches of thrush in your baby's mouth. For diaper rashes involving seborrheic dermatitis or eczema, doctors sometimes prescribe hydrocortisone cream. Over-the-counter antifungal and hydrocortisone creams are also available; however, you should check with your child's pediatrician before using them instead of prescription creams.

ALTERNATIVE CHOICES

Alternative remedies can be very effective in treating and preventing common diaper rashes. Seek professional medical care, however, if your child's rash does not improve within several days.

AROMATHERAPY

Mix 2 drops each of essential oils of sandalwood, peppermint *(Mentha piperita)*, and lavender *(Lavandula officinalis)* in 4 tbsp of a carrier lotion or oil such as sweet almond oil; gently apply the lotion to the reddened area of skin.

HERBAL THERAPIES

Calendula *(Calendula officinalis)* cream may relieve diaper rash. Herbalists also recommend the following ointment, which you can make at home:

- 1 tbsp each: dried chickweed *(Stellaria media)* leaves, powdered marsh mallow *(Althaea officinalis)* root, and powdered comfrey *(Symphytum officinale)* root.
- ⅛ tsp goldenseal *(Hydrastis canadensis)* root powder.
- 1 cup sweet almond oil.
- ¼ cup beeswax.

In a cast-iron pan, heat the herbs in the oil for 5 to 10 minutes. Don't let them burn. Add beeswax and let it melt. Strain the mixture through cheesecloth into a jar with a tight-fitting lid. Refrigerate until solid. Apply when you diaper your baby. The rash should improve after three or four applications. Discard after two months.

AT-HOME REMEDIES

- ◆ At the first sign of redness, wash your baby's bottom with warm water, and dry it thoroughly. Then apply an antiseptic cream and a barrier ointment, such as zinc oxide, to protect the skin.
- ◆ Change your baby's diaper as soon as it becomes soiled. Let your baby go without diapers as often as possible.
- ◆ Use disposable diaper liners, which allow urine to pass through to the diaper while keeping the baby's skin dry.
- ◆ Until the rash clears up, avoid plastic pants or diaper covers, which trap moisture.

PREVENTION

You can't prevent diaper rash, but you can limit its duration or severity by keeping your baby dry and clean and by changing the baby's diaper as soon as it becomes soiled. Wash cloth diapers in hot water, use bleach or vinegar in the rinse water, and add extra rinse cycles to help kill bacteria and remove traces of soap. If the entire diaper area is red and irritated, the child may be allergic to your detergent. Try another brand to see if the rash clears. The best preventive measure is to let your baby go without diapers as much as possible. ■

DIARRHEA

Read down this column to find your symptoms. Then read across.

SYMPTOMS	AILMENT/PROBLEM
◆ frequent or watery stools; possible abdominal cramping after eating or drinking coffee.	◆ Overeating fiber-rich foods such as whole grains, vegetables, and/or fruit, or drinking too much coffee
◆ frequent or watery bowel movements after beginning a new medication.	◆ Side effect of drugs such as antibiotics, antacids, cimetidine, quinine, and others
◆ frequent or watery stools during times of stress or depression.	◆ Emotion-induced diarrhea
◆ recurrent stools with mucus; lower abdominal pain that worsens with eating or stress.	◆ Irritable bowel syndrome
◆ recurrent, foul-smelling, watery stools that are pale or yellowish; flatulence; stomach cramps; weakness.	◆ Malabsorption, a digestive disorder in which fats and nutrients are not properly absorbed by the intestines
◆ relentless watery bowel movements; nervousness; insomnia; excessive sweating.	◆ An overactive thyroid gland, diabetes, or an underactive adrenal gland
◆ loose stools, possibly with visible blood.	◆ Many possibilities, including colorectal cancer
◆ sudden attack of watery, frequent stools that may be bloody; nausea; fever; abdominal cramping.	◆ Gastroenteritis, such as intestinal flu, traveler's diarrhea, food poisoning; or gastritis
◆ frequent, watery stools (perhaps with blood or pus); abdominal pain; weakness; lack of appetite; possible vomiting, mild fever, joint pain.	◆ Colitis or Crohn's disease
◆ episodes of frequent, watery stools; coughing; wheezing; flushed face.	◆ A carcinoid tumor (a growth in the intestine that may be benign or malignant)
◆ watery stools that may be black; center or left abdominal pain; possible bright red anal bleeding.	◆ Diverticulitis

WHAT TO DO	OTHER INFO
◆ Drink plenty of water, continue to eat a normal diet, avoid coffee.	◆ Diarrhea should resolve itself in less than 48 hours.
◆ Ask your doctor about changing or stopping your medication.	
◆ Experiment with stress-reducing techniques until you find one that works and fits into your daily life. Seek treatment for depression.	
◆ Anything that reduces stress, such as regular meditation or moderate exercise, often relieves this diarrhea.	◆ Taken 3 times daily, peppermint (*Mentha piperita*) or chamomile (*Matricaria recutita*) tea may ease intestinal spasms and cramps.
◆ Call your doctor today; see Anemia, Celiac Disease, Lactose Intolerance, Pancreatic Problems.	◆ Malabsorption is common after bowel surgery. Dietary changes alone can often relieve symptoms.
◆ See your doctor for treatment. See Diabetes, Thyroid Problems.	
◆ Call your doctor today. The many causes of anal bleeding range from harmless to dangerous.	◆ Any anal bleeding should be examined by a doctor. If you are over age 50, get a routine check every three years for hidden anal bleeding (and colorectal cancer).
◆ Keep your body well hydrated by drinking plenty of water, fruit juice, and/or prepared electrolyte solutions (available at the drugstore).	◆ Most gastroenteritis resolves itself in a day or two.
◆ Avoid stressful situations and foods that disagree with you.	◆ Avoid spicy and high-fat foods, as they worsen colitis-induced diarrhea.
◆ See your doctor for diagnosis and treatment, which may include anticancer drugs and/or surgery.	◆ Carcinoid tumors spread very rapidly and should not be ignored.
◆ Call your doctor today to get a proper diagnosis.	

D

SYMPTOMS

Many cases of damaged spinal disks have no physical symptoms. However, if your disk problem directly affects spinal nerves, you may have one or more of the following symptoms:

- sharp pain in the back, sometimes going down the back of one or both legs, immediately upon or shortly after exertion or injury.
- inability to bend or straighten your back, accompanied by severe pain.
- gradual development of neck or lower-back pain, possibly intense on arising or when sneezing or coughing.
- numbness or tingling in an arm or leg, and possibly a progressive loss of strength in one or both legs.

CALL YOUR DOCTOR IF:

- you experience persistent pain in the upper or lower back; you may be suffering from ankylosing spondylitis or a form of arthritis.
- back pain is accompanied by fever; you may have a viral or bacterial infection.
- you have sudden loss of feeling or weakness in your extremities; you may have an injury to your spinal cord.

Only a person who has experienced it understands the agony and helplessness that come with a damaged spinal disk. The pain is excruciating, and every movement makes it worse. Like most kinds of pain, however, it is actually a valuable warning signal. If you heed the warning and take proper action—or, more appropriately, inaction—the discomfort usually stops and the problem can be corrected. If you ignore the warning, you could suffer permanent physical and neurological damage.

As children, some of us may have heard parents or relatives grumble about the pain of a slipped disk. We may have pictured a wobbly stack of pennies with one sticking out enough to tip the rest over. As with other myths and mysteries of childhood, there was a little truth in the image, but not much. Intervertebral disks are actually flexible pads tightly fixed between the vertebrae—the specialized bones that make up the spinal column (see Back Problems). Each is a flat, circular capsule roughly an inch in diameter and perhaps one-quarter-inch thick, made of a tough, fibrous outer membrane called the annulus fibrosus, surrounding an elastic core called the nucleus pulposus.

The disks are firmly embedded between the vertebrae and are held in place by the ligaments connecting the spinal bones and by the surrounding sheaths of muscle. There is really little if any room for them to slip or move. The points on which the vertebrae actually turn are called facet joints, which stick out like arched wings on either side of the vertebrae and keep the vertebrae from bending and twisting far enough to damage the spinal cord, the vital network of nerves that runs through the center of each bone.

The disk is sometimes described as a shock absorber for the spine, which makes it sound more flexible or pliable than it really is. While the disks separate the vertebrae and keep them from rubbing together, they are far from pneumatic or springlike. In children they are actually gel- or fluid-filled sacs, but they begin to solidify as part of the normal aging process. By early adulthood, the blood supply to the disk has stopped, the soft inner material has begun to harden, and the disk is less elastic. In middle-aged adults the disks are tough and quite unyielding, with a consistency similar to that of a piece of hard rubber.

Under stress, it is possible for the inner material to swell and herniate, pushing through the tough outer membrane of the disk. The entire disk becomes distorted, and all or part of the core material actually protrudes through the outer casing at a weak spot, causing pressure against surrounding nerves. If further activity or injury causes the membrane to rupture or tear, the disk material can injure the spinal cord or the nerves that radiate from it, producing extreme, debilitating pain—an unmistakable signal to stop all movement immediately. Such damage to a disk can be irreversible.

By far the majority of disk injuries occur in the lumbar region of the lower back, with less than 10 percent affecting the neck and shoulders. Not all herniated disks press on nerves, however, and it is entirely possible for a person to have deformed disks without any pain or discomfort. For that reason, an x-ray or MRI scan showing a distorted disk can sometimes misdiagnose pain that has an entirely different cause.

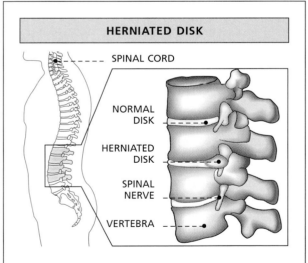

HERNIATED DISK

SPINAL CORD

NORMAL DISK

HERNIATED DISK

SPINAL NERVE

VERTEBRA

A normal intervertebral disk acts as a cushion between the bones in the spinal column. A disk is said to be herniated or prolapsed when the soft inner core pushes through the weakened or ruptured outer layer. If it touches a nerve, the result is immediate, excruciating pain.

Herniated disks are most common in men under 50, although they can occur in active children and young adults. Older people, whose disks no longer have fluid cores, are much less likely to encounter the problem. People who do regular, moderate exercise are much less likely to suffer from disk problems than their sedentary counterparts. They also tend to stay flexible considerably longer, without the annoying stiffness that many people take for granted as they grow older.

CAUSES

Although a violent injury can damage a disk, problems with disks are often brought on by everyday activities—lifting heavy objects the wrong way, stretching too hard during a tennis volley, or slipping on an icy sidewalk. Any such event can cause the fibrous outer covering of the disk to break or distort to the point that it impinges on a spinal nerve. Sometimes, however, a disk swells, tears, or degenerates without any apparent cause.

Disk problems are sometimes lumped together under the term **degenerative disk disease.** Change in the condition of the disk is a natural result of aging, and it contributes to a gradual loss of flexibility as we grow older. But disk degeneration is far more serious in some people than in others. Severe cases may be the result of a deficiency in collagen, the material that makes up cartilage. Poor muscle tone and obesity also put excessive strain on the spine and the ligaments that hold the disks in place.

DIAGNOSTIC AND TEST PROCEDURES

The classic procedure for identifying a herniated disk is the straight-leg-raising test. The patient lies on his or her back while the doctor holds the ankle and slowly raises the leg; pain in the back of the leg often—though not always—indicates a herniated disk in the lower back. The doctor will also look for weakness and loss of reflexes in legs and feet. Locating the site of the pain may be enough to identify the herniated disk.

A spinal x-ray may eliminate other potential

causes, but because x-rays do not show soft tissue clearly, magnetic resonance imaging (MRI), computed tomography (CT) scans, or myelography—a radiological technique for viewing the spinal cord—may be used to identify and determine the extent of a herniated disk.

TREATMENT

Both conventional and alternative therapies call for pain relief, rest, steps to reduce inflammation, and measures to restore strength and normal activity. Except in severe cases of disk degeneration's affecting nerves that control muscle movement, herniated disks generally heal themselves, and surgery is rarely necessary.

CONVENTIONAL MEDICINE

Doctors usually prescribe bed rest and pain-killing medication such as aspirin, ibuprofen or another nonsteroidal anti-inflammatory drug (NSAID), and in some cases corticosteroids and muscle relaxants. With a herniated disk, any movement of the back can heighten the pain and potentially aggravate the injury, so full bed rest is a must, at least for the first few days after the onset. Once the patient is well enough to move, the doctor may call for a back brace or neck collar to limit movement and ease the pressure on sensitive nerves while the disk heals. In severe cases, full or partial traction may be needed.

If the disk is just temporarily distorted, the potential for complete recovery is excellent. If the outer membrane actually breaks or ruptures and loses some of its gelatinous center, however, the damage may be permanent unless more aggressive steps are taken.

When the herniated disk causes weakness or paralysis of the nerves that control muscles of the back and limbs, the doctor may recommend epidural injections or surgery. Epidural injection consists of a combination of an anesthetic and corticosteroids injected through a long needle into the space between the affected disk and the covering of the nerve and spinal cord. Surgery may be performed to remove some of the soft core of a swollen disk with a hollow needle so that the disk no longer impinges on a nerve. Other microsurgical procedures can remove fragments of core material that have broken through the fibrous outer wall. Discectomy is the surgical removal of part of a herniated disk, and is done to relieve pressure on the nerve. In this procedure, the core of the disk is removed, leaving the tough outer casing in place between the vertebrae. Like epidural injection, it sometimes brings long-term relief, but there is no guarantee of permanent recovery. Because any invasive therapy near the spinal cord is potentially dangerous, surgery should be undertaken only in extreme cases, when the herniated disk is causing weakness or paralysis of nerves going to muscles.

Injections of the drug colchicine may be helpful in relieving acute pain and inflammation of a ruptured disk. A somewhat controversial treatment, now largely out of favor, is chemonucleolysis, which is said to dissolve material in a herniated disk by an injection of the enzyme chymopapain.

Just as artificial replacements for damaged or worn parts are being surgically implanted in other parts of the body, intervertebral disk replacement has passed the experimental stage and is being performed in other countries. The safety and long-term success of disk replacement remain to be seen, but like stainless-steel hip joints and plastic heart valves, synthetic versions of intervertebral disks may offer yet another medical option in the not-so-distant future.

ALTERNATIVE CHOICES

Besides pain relief and rest immediately following an episode of a herniated disk, alternative therapies tend to focus on relaxation and gentle exercise to restore full movement.

ACUPRESSURE

While acupressure can be highly effective for treating lower-back pain, acupressure therapists exercise caution when dealing with pain from spinal disks. Rather than applying pressure to the spine or to points on meridians next to the spinal column, an acupressure therapist may recom-

1 The **Knee Down Twist** stretches lower-back muscles. Lie on your back with arms out, inhale, and put your right foot on your left knee. Exhale, turn your head to the right, and bring your right knee toward the floor to your left. Hold 15 to 20 seconds. Repeat on the other side.

2 The **Rag Doll** restores flexibility. From a standing position, slowly bend forward from your hips, head down, as far as you can go without straining your back or bending your legs. Hold 15 to 20 seconds as you breathe slowly. Inhale and come back to an upright position.

3 The **Child** stretches low-back muscles. Sit on your heels, knees together. Exhale and bend from the hips. Extend your upper body over your knees with arms at your sides, palms up. Move your forehead toward the floor. Breathe slowly, hold 15 to 20 seconds, then sit up again.

mend preventive treatment to relax the back muscles before a problem occurs. One such recommendation is sleeping in the shrimp position, lying on your side with the back curled, and using warm compresses or moist heat to improve circulation.

ACUPUNCTURE

An acupuncturist will determine the precise location of the nerve or nerves affected by a herniated disk and will most likely treat points along the governing vessel meridian. *(See pages 22–23 for more information.)*

BODY WORK

Alternative therapists focus on the body mechanics that have led to stress on the disk. **Reflexology** manipulates certain areas in the hands and feet. For pain and tension relief in the lower back, advocates of reflexology cite positive results from applying firm pressure behind the anklebone and at the outer edge of the instep.

After initial symptoms are under control, a practitioner trained in the **Alexander technique** or the **Feldenkrais method** may help people with chronic problems reestablish good posture and body control, which in turn can help prevent the recurrence of disk problems.

CHIROPRACTIC

Today's chiropractic treatment for chronic disk problems is likely to include manual examination or x-ray diagnosis to determine the location of the affected vertebra. Hands-on procedures to correct muscle and joint malfunction—with due caution not to exacerbate the disk strain—are likely to be followed by a regimen of massage and exercise that will soothe and strengthen the surrounding muscles.

PREVENTION

Yoga is a well-established, long-term approach to relaxing and conditioning both the body and the mind. The exercises at left are recommended for strengthening the back and neck as well as for relieving overall bodily stress. ∎

D

SYMPTOMS

- severe, cramping abdominal pain that is usually more severe on the left side.
- nausea.
- fever.
- constipation, thin stools, diarrhea.
- pain in the lower left quadrant of the abdomen that increases when the sore spot is touched.

CALL YOUR DOCTOR IF:

- you have fever, chills, and abdominal swelling, or are vomiting; you could have peritonitis, an infection of the membrane that lines the abdominal cavity. **Get medical help immediately.**
- blood appears in stools; this indicates **internal bleeding.** *(See also page 70 in Emergencies/First Aid.)*
- you have a fever; you may have an infection that requires medication.
- severe pain continues despite treatment; you may have another abdominal disorder.

Diverticulitis is the inflammation or infection of small pouches, called diverticula, that develop along the walls of your intestines. The formation of the pouches themselves is a relatively benign condition known as diverticulosis. The pouches can develop anywhere on the digestive tract, but they most commonly form at the end of the descending and sigmoid colons, and they also frequently occur on the first section of the small intestine (although they rarely cause problems there). If you have diverticulosis, you may not even be aware of it, because the diverticula are usually painless and cause few, if any, symptoms. You may experience some cramping on your left side that disappears when you pass gas or move your bowels. And because diverticula sometimes bleed, bright red blood may appear in your stool.

The more serious disease, diverticulitis, may involve anything from a small abscess in one or more of the pouches to a massive infection or perforation of the bowel. The symptoms are similar to those of appendicitis, except that the pain is located in the lower left side rather than the lower right side.

Diverticulitis may be acute or chronic. The acute form can manifest itself with one or more severe attacks of infection and inflammation. In chronic diverticulitis, inflammation and infection may subside, but they may never clear up completely. The inflammation of diverticulitis can eventually result in a bowel obstruction, which is indicated by constipation, thin stools, diarrhea, abdominal distention, and abdominal pain. If the obstruction persists, abdominal pain and tenderness will increase, and you may experience nausea and vomiting.

If it is left untreated, diverticulitis can lead to serious complications requiring extensive surgery. Abscesses may form around the infected diverticula, and if these go through the intestinal wall, you may develop peritonitis, a potentially fatal infection that requires immediate treatment. An infected diverticulum can also reach an adjoining organ and form a connection, or fistula, between them. This most frequently occurs between the large intestine and the bladder, and it can lead to an infection of the neighboring kidneys. Another potential complication is severe internal and colonic bleeding.

CAUSES

Aging and heredity are primary factors in the development of diverticulosis and diverticulitis, but diet also plays a role; eating a lot of low-fiber, refined foods can greatly increase the risk. Indeed, in Western societies, an estimated 20 to 50 percent of people over 50 eventually develop diverticular disorders; the figure may be higher than 50 percent in the United States.

If you are often constipated and usually strain at bowel movements, you may create enough pressure in the intestinal walls to begin the development of diverticular pouches. If the diverticula then become filled with fecal material or with undigested food, they are vulnerable to bacterial infection, leading to the inflammation of diverticulitis.

THE DIVERTICULA

— COLON
— DIVERTICULUM
— ABSCESS

If the lining of the colon is weakened for some reason, internal pressure can force small pockets of the lining to bulge through the muscle wall. Undigested food or fecal matter lodged in the bulges—or diverticula—can become infected. If the condition is not treated, the resulting inflammation—called diverticulitis—may cause abscesses that can break through the intestinal wall into the abdominal cavity.

DIAGNOSTIC AND TEST PROCEDURES

If you think you have either diverticulosis or diverticulitis, your doctor will probably have tests done on both your blood and stool to help diagnose possible infection. Because cancer, irritable bowel syndrome, and diverticulitis can share the same symptoms, your doctor will need to thoroughly examine your intestines. A barium enema, which fills the colon with barium and allows an x-ray to show an outline of the inside of the intestines, can help confirm a diagnosis of diverticulitis. You may also have the insides of your intestines examined with a flexible lighted tube in a procedure called a sigmoidoscopy. Sometimes a bit of tissue may also be removed for a biopsy, to test for cancerous growth. If you have an acute case of diverticulitis, both barium enemas and biopsies can injure your intestine, so your doctor may choose instead a CT scan, which shows the bowel wall and the outside of the colon and can also confirm the diagnosis.

TREATMENT

Diverticulosis can be treated at home, but if you have diverticulitis, you need to see a physician to make sure you fully recover and to avoid possibly life-threatening complications. Conventional medicine treats diverticulitis using diet modifications, antibiotics, and possibly surgery. Alternative treatments for diverticulitis may be used in conjunction with conventional treatment to help ease the symptoms and bolster the digestive tract.

CONVENTIONAL MEDICINE

If you have a mild case of diverticulosis, your doctor may have you eat a high-fiber diet to make sure your bowels move regularly and to reduce your odds of getting diverticulitis. If you do go on to develop diverticulitis but have only a mild infection, you may need just bed rest, stool softeners, a liquid diet, antibiotics to fight the inflammation, and possibly antispasmodic drugs.

However, if you have had a perforation or develop a more severe infection, you will probably

D

be put in the hospital for intravenous antibiotic therapy. You may also be fed intravenously to give your colon time to recuperate. In some cases, your doctor may want to drain infected abscesses and give your intestinal tract a rest by performing a temporary colostomy. A colostomy creates an opening so your intestine will empty into a bag that is attached to the front of your abdomen. Depending on the success of your recovery, this procedure may be reversed during a second operation. (See also Colorectal Cancer.)

If you have several attacks of acute diverticulitis, your doctor may want to remove the infected section of the intestine when you are free of symptoms. You may also need surgery if intravenous therapy does not effectively treat your acute attack of diverticulitis. Whatever your treatment, your chances for a full recovery are very good if you receive prompt medical attention.

ALTERNATIVE CHOICES

Alternative practitioners may treat some mild cases of diverticulitis, but more serious cases require conventional treatment in order to prevent dangerous health complications.

ACUPUNCTURE

To treat diverticulitis, an acupuncturist will target points intended to relieve pain and distention, reduce inflammation, regulate intestinal peristalsis, and improve the tone of the intestinal wall. Treatments are performed once or twice a week depending on the severity of the condition, with a full course of treatment requiring about 10 visits. It's very important to observe good dietary habits while undergoing acupuncture therapy.

AROMATHERAPY

Inhaling two drops of hyssop (Hyssopus officinalis) three times daily may serve as an abdominal relaxant.

CHINESE HERBS

Some Chinese herbs that are used to treat systemic disorders may prove helpful for diverticulitis. See a practitioner of Chinese medicine for recommendations and treatment.

HERBAL THERAPIES

Slippery elm (Ulmus fulva) may be soothing to infected diverticula: Put 1 tsp powder into ½ cup water, bring to a boil, and simmer 15 minutes. Drink three times daily.

Always check with a practitioner first to see if using this herb is appropriate for your particular illness.

HOMEOPATHY

Many homeopathic remedies, such as Belladonna, Bryonia, and Colocynthis, may be used to treat diverticulitis. Check with a homeopathic physician to see which medicines and dosages might be appropriate for you.

MASSAGE

Use a light vegetable oil to massage your lower abdomen with circular clockwise strokes for five minutes while you are lying down each morning. Follow the massage by drinking an herbal tea such as chamomile (Matricaria recutita), which may help promote relaxation.

MIND/BODY MEDICINE

Relaxation techniques may help you deal with the stress and pain of diverticulitis.

NUTRITION AND DIET

Drink at least six glasses of water daily to prevent constipation. If you do become constipated, prunes, prune juice, or herbal teas specifically formulated for constipation may serve as natural laxatives. Keep to a low-fat diet; fat slows down passage of food through the intestine. Get yourself tested for food allergies to identify foods that irritate your system and that you should avoid.

During acute attacks of diverticulitis, try a one- to three-day water or vegetable-juice fast. Eat low-bulk foods (broths and low-fiber breads) while diverticula are still inflamed and sensitive. During an attack of acute diverticulitis, make the following foods a significant part of your diet: cooked vegetables, cooked fruits, and apples—all of which will be soothing to the inflamed intestine. Avoid milk and milk products (yogurts and cheeses), which could worsen your illness, especially if you have diarrhea.

REFLEXOLOGY

To stimulate secretion of norepinephrine and hydrocortisone (which help your body deal with stress and reduce infection) and maintain intestinal muscle tone, a practitioner will massage adrenal gland areas on the foot. Stimulating intestine areas helps intestines contract regularly and remove wastes as will stimulating areas corresponding to the location of the inflamed diverticula in the intestine (the descending colon area). Stimulating the diaphragm/solar plexus area may help with stress and tension.

AT-HOME REMEDIES

◆ Use a heating pad to treat mild pain and spasms in your abdomen. However, do not use high settings for prolonged periods, and never sleep on a heating pad; you could burn yourself.

◆ To promote regularity, try to move your bowels at the same time every day (after meals is usually easier).

◆ Stay in bed if you are feverish or having a great deal of pain, and get medical help soon.

PREVENTION

The best preventive action you can take against diverticulitis, of course, is to keep from developing the small intestinal sacs called diverticula. You have a good chance of doing that simply by modifying your diet and lifestyle. Eat whole-grain breads, oatmeal, bran cereals, fibrous fresh fruits, and vegetables, or try an over-the-counter preparation containing psyllium *(Plantago psyllium)* to increase the bulk in your diet. You can also try ground psyllium seed: Add 1 tsp over any cold liquid, and drink once a day—within a few minutes of preparing, before the mixture gels. Make sure you drink plenty of fluids if you increase your intake of fiber, and take care to add fiber gradually; a sudden switch to a high-fiber diet can cause your abdomen to become distended and create an uncomfortable amount of intestinal gas. Adjust your diet to remove foods that are difficult for you to digest.

Avoid refined foods such as white flour, white rice, and other processed foods. Contrary to popular wisdom, however, it is not necessary to avoid nuts and seeds; they are no more likely than other foods to become caught in diverticula.

Try over-the-counter stool softeners to fight constipation. If you have the urge to move your bowels, don't delay or ignore it. Regular exercise can help the muscles in your intestine retain their tone, which encourages regular bowel movements. Don't use suppositories for constipation, because your system may become addicted to them. Prunes, prune juice, and psyllium seed are all good natural laxatives. Specially formulated teas to fight constipation are available in health food stores, but some may be very strong, so use them only as directed; avoid products containing senna *(Cassia senna),* which is an especially strong herbal laxative. ■

DIZZINESS

Read down this column to find your symptoms. Then read across.

D

SYMPTOMS	AILMENT/PROBLEM
◆ dizziness (your head or everything around you seems to spin) with no obvious associated symptoms.	◆ Dizziness (general)
◆ dizziness with weakness, paralysis, or numbness in arms or legs; possibly, blurred or temporary loss of vision or difficulty speaking.	◆ Stroke or transient ischemic attack
◆ dizziness with persistent or recurrent headache; less commonly, nausea, vomiting, seizures, personality change, vision loss, speech problems, weakness or paralysis, memory impairment, or coordination or balance problems.	◆ Brain tumor or bleeding
◆ dizziness when turning the head, with pain and stiffness in joints, in a person older than 50.	◆ Cervical osteoarthritis
◆ continuous severe dizziness that worsens with movement; loss of hearing, ringing in ears; possibly, nausea, vomiting; previous viral infection.	◆ Inflamed inner ear and/or nerve (labyrinthitis)
◆ attacks of intermittent dizziness; loss of hearing, ringing in ears; possibly, headache, nausea and vomiting, pallor, or exhaustion.	◆ Ménière's disease
◆ dizziness when changing the position of your head.	◆ Postural dizziness (benign positional vertigo)

WHAT TO DO	OTHER INFO
◆ Sit, close your eyes, bow your head, and breathe deeply. If attacks are severe, call your doctor to check on possible causes that could be treated; you may need to change a medication you're taking.	◆ Many drugs can cause dizziness, such as nonsteroidal anti-inflammatory drugs (NSAIDs), antibiotics, and antihypertensives.
◆ **Call 911 or your emergency number now.** The usual procedure is hospitalization for tests, medication to prevent further strokes, and possibly surgery. See Stroke.	◆ A stroke is a sudden loss of brain function caused by blockage of or damage to a blood vessel to the brain. In transient ischemic attack, the disruption of blood supply is temporary and the symptoms subside.
◆ **Call your doctor, 911, or your emergency number now.** A brain tumor may require surgical removal, radiation therapy, and/or chemotherapy. Bleeding within the skull is an emergency and may require surgery. See Brain Cancer.	◆ A tumor develops slowly over a period of time, whereas bleeding may begin suddenly as the result of trauma or abnormalities of the blood vessels.
◆ Call your doctor, who may prescribe a neck collar or anti-inflammatory drugs to relieve pain. See Arthritis.	◆ Dizziness may be caused by bony outgrowths and inflammation of neck joints, which put pressure on nerves and blood vessels.
◆ The usual treatment is bed rest, the antihistamine meclizine, and possibly, anti-anxiety drugs.	◆ With or without treatment, recovery usually takes several days to three weeks. The cause of this inflammation is believed to be viral.
◆ Call your doctor. The usual treatment is bed rest and the antihistamine meclizine for relief of vertigo.	◆ Sometimes a tube is inserted to equalize air pressure on both sides of the eardrum. Vitamin B_6 (50 mg, three times a day) may be helpful.
◆ Call your doctor if the symptoms are troublesome. Head-tilting exercises may help to bring on and then blunt the vertigo.	◆ Postural dizziness usually subsides in a few seconds without treatment.

DRUG ABUSE

SYMPTOMS

◆ changes in appearance and behavior that affect relationships and work performance.

◆ in children, abrupt changes in mood or attitude, poor school performance, temper flareups, or increased secrecy.

Specific symptoms depend on the drug:

◆ Extreme energy, weight loss, dilated pupils, insomnia, and trembling may indicate abuse of **stimulants,** or "uppers."

◆ Lethargy, slurred or confused speech, lack of balance, constricted pupils, or excessive sleep may point to abuse of **sedatives,** or "downers."

◆ Mood swings, red eyes, dilated pupils, slowed time sense and reflexes, dizziness, and lethargy may indicate **marijuana** use.

◆ Ulcerated nostrils are typical of **cocaine** sniffing; a runny nose or sniffles are typical of smoking crack cocaine; needle marks on the arms may indicate intravenous cocaine abuse.

◆ Weight loss, lethargy, mood swings, excessive sweating, slurred speech, constricted pupils, and poor appetite suggest **opiate** abuse.

◆ Hallucinations, dilated pupils, trembling, and sweating indicate abuse of **psychedelic** drugs.

CALL YOUR DOCTOR IF:

◆ you detect any of the above symptoms in a family member—especially a child or teenager—and suspect drug abuse. The abuser will often deny the problem; you will need professional guidance to deal with the situation.

Drug abuse is the use of a psychoactive drug—legal or illegal—enough to cause the abuser physical, mental, emotional, or social harm. Addiction or dependence is the compulsive, continued use of a drug. *(See also Alcohol Abuse and Nicotine Withdrawal.)* While the term "drug abuse" conjures up violent images of the illegal drug trade, abuse of legal drugs is an even larger health problem. Between two and three million Americans are addicted to prescription drugs, and hospitals report as many emergencies from abuse of legal drugs as from illegal drugs. Like alcohol abusers, drug abusers commonly deny their problem by playing down the extent of drug use or blaming external factors, such as job or family stress. Families may join in denial in a misguided effort to defend the abuser, creating a powerful barrier to treatment and recovery.

Commonly abused drugs fall into several broad categories:

Central nervous system (CNS) depressants. Sleeping pills and antianxiety drugs are among the most prescribed medications in the United States; about seven million people take some form of CNS depressant at least once a week. Barbiturates bring on effects like those of alcohol: Small doses are relaxing, but large amounts can damage both mind and body. Taken with alcohol, barbiturates can be fatal. The risks of addiction and overdose are so well known that doctors prescribe barbiturates with extreme caution.

Benzodiazepines are safer than barbiturates but can cause dependence as patients develop tolerance to them after a few weeks of use. This class includes the popular antianxiety agents diazepam, alprazolam, and triazolam. Their abuse brings on drowsiness, slurred speech, and lack of coordination, which may progress to memory impairment, tremors, and paranoia. A drug abuser being treated with benzodiazepines for anxiety during withdrawal is quite likely to start abusing a benzodiazepine.

Stimulants. Addictive stimulants cause rapid speech, agitation, and a debilitating pattern of highs followed by crashes. People addicted to amphetamines, or uppers, often try to calm themselves down with CNS depressants, or downers, and become caught in an up-and-down cycle. A more powerful and more habit-forming stimulant is cocaine; the smoked version called crack is highly addictive. There are an estimated two million cocaine addicts in the U.S.

Opiates. About half a million people in the U.S. are addicted to opium, morphine, or heroin. The addiction typically causes depression, anxiety, low self-esteem, and reduced coping ability. Intravenous injection of these drugs carries the additional risk of hepatitis, AIDS, and other transmissible diseases.

Cannabis. Smoking marijuana can depress short-term memory, motivation, and energy levels. Chronic use brings increased heart rate, vision problems, poor lung function, changes in sex hormones, and increased risk of lung cancer. Marijuana and other forms of cannabis such as "hash" are not highly addictive but are considered entry drugs: Marijuana users are significantly more likely to use cocaine than are nonusers.

Other commonly abused substances range from **tobacco** and **alcohol** to **psychedelic drugs** like LSD. Athletes who use **anabolic steroids** to add muscle face the possibility of violent behavior, heart disease, and severe liver and hormone damage. Babies of pregnant women who abuse either legal or illegal drugs face special dangers, ranging from premature birth and malnutrition to life-threatening birth defects. Many adolescents are tempted to experiment with drugs and are highly vulnerable to peer pressure—especially those in poverty or with nonsupportive families.

CAUSES

There is little agreement on the underlying cause of substance abuse, but experts are more likely to regard it as a disease than a lack of will power. Chronic alcohol and drug abusers may have a genetic predisposition to addiction, but environmental and social factors such as poverty, family dysfunction, and peer pressure are also significant. Certainly the social context can be crucial: One cannot become addicted to drugs without starting to use them in the first place.

Many people consider that drug dependence comes from a natural desire to alter a person's

Misuse of legal drugs

Millions of Americans abuse legal prescription and nonprescription drugs. Even mild, "everyday" drugs such as cough medicines and diet pills can be abused to the point of dependence and physical harm. Aspirin and ibuprofen can cause bleeding stomach ulcers, long-term use of laxatives can damage the bowels, and nasal sprays can produce a dependence that actually increases congestion. All medications should be taken only as directed; if a drug is not achieving the desired effect, consult your doctor before taking more.

consciousness or an effort to achieve wholeness. One reason addictive drugs are so dangerous is that most people who use them believe they are immune to addiction. Once drug dependence is established, the pattern is hard to break—whether or not the abuser is aware of the problem. Tolerance to opiates and stimulants increases with use, so chronic abusers have to take more to get the same effect. For the most addictive drugs, such as heroin and cocaine, continued use is often reinforced by the desire to avoid the pain of withdrawal.

TREATMENT

Treatment is a two-step process. **Withdrawal** from drug use may require only days or weeks, but can be unpleasant and even dangerous without professional supervision. **Recovery** is the extended stage of remaining drug free.

CONVENTIONAL MEDICINE

The first step in treating drug abuse is awareness. Some addicts may not know they are drug dependent; others deny it. At this stage, family, friends, or a trusted professional must make the case for abstinence and treatment.

No single treatment fits all abusers; appropriate treatment depends on the type and severity of the addiction. Approaches range from outpatient maintenance programs, psychotherapy, and self-help groups like Narcotics Anonymous to residential programs lasting weeks or months. An addicted person may need not just drug treatment but also medical care, welfare support, and psychiatric or social counseling. Successful recovery programs strive to establish social support, raise self-esteem and a sense of spirituality, and help the addict avoid situations that can trigger relapse. For many abusers, the key to success may involve finding regular employment, drug-free housing, and friendships with people who do not use drugs.

Withdrawal from **CNS depressants,** or downers, can be painful and even life-threatening. Stopping the chronic use of barbiturates and some benzodiazepines can produce delirium tremens, rapid pulse, weakness, convulsions, and hallucinations. Because of the danger of seizures, withdrawal should be done under a doctor's care if the drugs have been used for more than four to six weeks.

Breaking away from **stimulants,** or uppers, can produce lethargy, anxiety, fatigue, hallucinations, and depression. Because most stimulants do not produce physical addiction as strong as that of barbiturates or heroin, withdrawal symptoms may not be as severe. The exception is cocaine, which is very difficult to relinquish. Post-withdrawal treatment of chronic cocaine abuse often requires extensive counseling, along with group and family support. Therapy and group support are equally essential for abusers of amphetamines; patients may become depressed and even suicidal after withdrawal.

Withdrawal from an addiction to **opiates**—with shakes, sweats, tremors, and acute craving for the drug—has been widely dramatized. As disagreeable as the symptoms are, they are not as dangerous to the addict as those of alcohol or barbiturate withdrawal. While opiate addiction was once thought almost impossible to break, the experience of many Vietnam War veterans who voluntarily quit their drug habits on returning

DRUGS AND THE ELDERLY

Older people often suffer adverse drug effects or become unwitting abusers for several reasons. We metabolize and excrete drugs more slowly as we age, so it is easier to take an overdose. Many people do not even realize that cough medicines, sleeping aids, diet pills, and laxatives are drugs. Older people often increase the risk of dangerous interactions and side effects by simultaneously taking several prescription drugs for different ailments or combining prescription and nonprescription drugs without their physicians' knowledge.

In older people, symptoms of drug intoxication are easily mistaken for mental illness or other ailments. Complications of drug abuse are more common in the elderly, and detoxification is more complex. Certain drugs are of special concern. Diuretics, commonly used to lower blood pressure, can deplete the body's store of potassium and other minerals, causing weakness and appetite loss. Some antihypertensive drugs may bring depression, fatigue, or fainting. Antianxiety drugs may cause drowsiness, shakiness, confusion, and amnesia if taken to excess. While anyone taking medication should follow dosages meticulously, it is especially important for older people to do so and to tell their physicians about all the medications they take. Supervising or helping an older person with medications is not just a kindness—it may be a lifesaver.

home has shown that self-initiated cure is possible. After withdrawal from heroin or morphine, some users are "maintained" on prescribed doses of methadone, a less addictive narcotic, under a doctor's care. While controversial, methadone maintenance is still customary because stress or depression can easily trigger a return to more harmful drugs even after years of nonuse.

Recovery is the stage after withdrawal when the individual must strive to remain drug free. This stage is often very difficult because it requires the addicted person to change habits and lifestyle, and to control the use of potentially addicting substances throughout life. The backing of family, friends, employers, and drug-support groups can be a powerful—often vital—part of an addict's recovery. For adolescents, group treatment is often more successful than individual therapy. Since a child's addiction is often part of a family problem, treatment should involve all family members. Because of the power of peer pressure, an adolescent may need more reinforcement than an adult to stay with a recovery regimen.

ALTERNATIVE CHOICES

Many alternative therapies can help reduce the stress that accompanies or underlies drug abuse, strengthen the body, and reduce cravings.

ACUPUNCTURE

Acupuncturists report success in treating addicts of heroin, cocaine, and other drugs. In particular, acupuncture on several points of the ear is reported to reduce withdrawal symptoms and cravings, prevent relapse, and raise recovery rates.

HERBAL THERAPIES

Cleansing the body of toxins is an important step in healing. Silymarin, found in milk thistle *(Silybum marianum)*, is taken to strengthen the liver. Wild oat extract, burdock *(Arctium lappa)* root, echinacea *(Echinacea* spp.), and licorice *(Glycyrrhiza glabra)* are said to cleanse the blood, while skullcap *(Scutellaria lateriflora),* valerian *(Valeriana officinalis),* and vervain reduce anxiety. See a professional herbalist for dosages.

HYDROTHERAPY

Some therapists believe that cleansing the body of drugs takes months. A daily 10- to 20-minute bath containing half a cup of baking soda or sea salt can be a powerful aid to detoxification.

MIND/BODY MEDICINE

Biofeedback, meditation, relaxation response, and **guided imagery** techniques can help reduce stress and bring about behavioral changes as aids to recovery. For specific techniques, see Stress.

NUTRITION AND DIET

Drug abusers tend to eat poorly and may overuse sugar. For lasting recovery, eat at least three regular meals a day with a good balance of protein, vegetables, and complex carbohydrates. If you have an irresistible craving for sweets, use barley malt or rice syrup instead of sugar, and take a 250 mcg capsule of chromium picolinate daily to help stabilize erratic blood sugar levels. Ask your doctor about the potential benefits of supplemental vitamins C and E, pantothenic acid (vitamin B_5), adrenal extract, magnesium, calcium, potassium, choline, and folic acid.

PREVENTION

While efforts to eradicate illegal drugs have shown little success, both treatment and public education make a difference. One study found that a dollar spent on treatment of cocaine users was seven times as effective in cutting cocaine consumption as a dollar spent on law enforcement.

Parent groups, community efforts, public education and prevention programs, drug-free workplaces, and strong national leadership have all played a role in discouraging illegal drug use. Parents may not be able to stop their children from experimenting with drugs, but they can give them accurate information about drug abuse—especially the genetic risk to their own unborn children. Lectures and scare tactics are rarely successful, but adolescents should understand the internal and external pressures that make people start using drugs, hear rebuttals to pro-drug arguments, and learn techniques for resisting peer pressure. But if you don't want your children to abuse drugs—including alcohol and tobacco—the best first step is to set the right example. ■

EARACHE

Read down this column to find your symptoms. Then read across.

SYMPTOMS	AILMENT/PROBLEM
See Otitis Media or the Atlas of the Body for an illustration of the anatomy of the ear.	
◆ earache that gets worse over weeks or months; blocked feeling and ringing in the ears; partial hearing loss.	◆ Excess earwax that has hardened in the outer ear canal, blocking the eardrum
◆ following air travel or scuba diving, ear pain that may radiate into the cheeks and forehead; dizziness; ringing in the ears; ears feel blocked.	◆ Barotrauma (strained or damaged eardrum, due to large changes in atmospheric pressure)
◆ feeling that something is in your ear; hearing loss; ear pain.	◆ Presence of a foreign object, such as a bug, a seed, or an earplug, in the ear
◆ itching in the ear, later becoming sharp or dull ear pain; pain worsens if you pull on your earlobe; yellowish discharge; possibly, fever and temporary hearing loss.	◆ Swimmer's ear
◆ ear pain that is either sharp and sudden or dull and throbbing; fever; nasal congestion; muffled hearing.	◆ Otitis media
◆ pressure in the ear; a lump outside or inside the ear canal; excessive earwax; possibly, hearing loss and infection (fever, ear pain, and swelling).	◆ A benign (noncancerous) cyst or tumor in or just outside the ear canal
◆ earache; persistent tooth or jaw pain.	◆ Tooth or gum trouble, such as tooth decay or abscess; temporomandibular joint syndrome
◆ dull pain, redness, and swelling both within and behind the ear; mild fever; thick pus discharge from ear; possibly, partial hearing loss.	◆ Mastoiditis (infection of the mastoid process, the honeycomb-like bone behind the ear)
◆ sudden ear pain, usually after an injury or an infection; bleeding or pus discharge from the ear; dizziness; ringing in the ear; partial hearing loss.	◆ Ruptured eardrum

◆ For three days, place a few drops of warm baby oil or mineral oil in the ear twice daily to soften wax. Then use a bulb syringe to flush out the wax with warm water.

◆ Flushing the ear may cause dizziness. Never try to remove wax by inserting an object—even a cotton-tipped swab—in your ear; you could damage your eardrum.

◆ Symptoms should dissipate within a few hours without treatment. If they don't, consult your doctor.

◆ During flight, hold your nose and gently blow air into it, or constantly suck hard candy or chew gum; this may help equalize the pressure on either side of your eardrum.

◆ See Emergencies/First Aid: Ear Emergencies.

◆ Never try to remove an object that is lodged in your ear; you risk perforating your eardrum. See your doctor.

◆ Take acetaminophen for pain. Your doctor may also prescribe ear drops containing an antibiotic, an antifungal drug, or cortisone (to reduce inflammation).

◆ Keep water out of your ears (when swimming and showering) for at least three weeks after symptoms have subsided. Don't use earplugs; they can be harmful.

◆ Place a warm compress over the ear and take acetaminophen. Call your doctor; you may need prescription antibiotics.

◆ A few drops of warm mineral or olive oil in your ear may lessen pain.

◆ Often no treatment is needed. If the cyst or tumor becomes extremely large or infected, your doctor will remove it.

◆ Call your dentist today. An abscessed tooth is an emergency. See also Gum Problems; Toothache.

◆ Relaxation techniques may ease mild cases of temporomandibular joint syndrome.

◆ Call your doctor today. You need aggressive antibiotic therapy, perhaps for several weeks. Persistent infection may call for surgical removal of the mastoid process.

◆ Without treatment, mastoiditis can cause serious problems, such as meningitis and facial paralysis.

◆ Take acetaminophen for pain until you can see a doctor. You may need a patch for the eardrum (to speed healing) and antibiotics. Large tears can be surgically repaired.

◆ Don't blow your nose or allow water in your ear until the rupture has healed (which should take two months or so).

SYMPTOMS

◆ patches of chronically itchy, dry, thickened skin, usually on wrists, face, and inner creases of the knees and elbows.

◆ skin lesions, patches of redness, scaling, and—in dark-skinned people—changes in skin color; sometimes small bumps or blisters that may ooze fluid.

See also the Visual Diagnostic Guide.

CALL YOUR DOCTOR IF:

◆ you develop an otherwise unexplained rash and have a family history of eczema or asthma. You should have a medical diagnosis of the condition.

◆ the inflammation does not respond within a week to treatment with over-the-counter coal-tar preparations or steroid-based creams. A physician may suggest more aggressive forms of treatment.

◆ you develop yellowish to light brown crust or pus-filled blisters over existing patches of eczema. This may indicate a staph or other bacterial infection that should be treated with an antibiotic.

◆ during a flareup of eczema you are exposed to anyone with a viral skin disease such as cold sores, genital warts, or genital herpes. Having eczema puts you at increased risk of contracting the viral disorder.

◆ you develop numerous small, pus-filled blisters. You may have **eczema herpeticum,** a rare but potentially serious complication caused by the herpes simplex II virus.

Strictly speaking, eczema is a form of dermatitis characterized by chronically itchy, inflamed skin. The affected area typically becomes dry, the skin flakes off, and occasionally blisters develop. When eczema appears on fair-skinned people, the affected areas typically turn a brownish gray color; on people with dark skin, it generally alters their natural pigmentation, making the affected area either lighter or darker. Eczema appears most frequently on the face, wrists, elbows, and knees but is not limited to those areas.

Eczema—also known as **atopic dermatitis**—afflicts between 3 and 7 percent of the population to some degree, and in more than 70 percent of patients, it runs in the family. It is most common among infants, many of whom grow out of it before their second birthday. If it persists, the child is likely to be a chronic sufferer and may develop distinctive thickened, brownish gray skin in the areas that break out most frequently. Eczema is often associated with asthma, so children with that disorder may be at greater risk of skin problems. Since eczema may be in part an internal response to some sort of external stress, initial treatment focuses on identifying and reducing the possible cause.

CAUSES

Many cases of eczema are allergy related. In susceptible people, outbreaks can be caused by ingesting certain foods, such as cow's milk, eggs, wheat, and nuts—as well as by inhaling airborne irritants like dust mites and pollen. Eczema is also caused by contact with irritants in common substances, such as woolen and synthetic fabrics, latex rubber, certain detergents, chlorine-based products, the mineral nickel used in plated earrings and other jewelry, and chemicals like formaldehyde, found in permanent-press fabrics, polishes, rugs, foam insulation, and particle board.

In people predisposed to eczema, doctors think outbreaks may be caused by a change in the way a person's immune system reacts to certain kinds of physically, chemically, or emotionally induced stress. Besides contact with potential allergens, any emotionally charged event—from a move to a new job—may trigger a flareup of the disorder. *(See Immune Problems and Stress.)*

DIAGNOSTIC AND TEST PROCEDURES

To determine whether an allergy is the underlying cause of the inflammation, ask your doctor about taking a radioallergosorbent test (RAST).

TREATMENT

Because eczema is generally a benign disorder, and because the underlying causes differ from person to person, primary treatment is directed at alleviating symptoms. At-home remedies and over-the-counter medications are usually sufficient. For chronic eczema, a doctor will focus on identifying allergens, building up the immune system, or relaxing the patient. For information on light therapy for eczema, see Dermatitis.

CONVENTIONAL MEDICINE

To relieve itchiness, most doctors will start patients on such basic therapies as a warm bath to remove crusted skin followed by immediate application of petroleum jelly or vegetable shortening, which helps conserve the skin's natural moisture. Topical coal-tar preparations also work, but they can be messy and smelly; they should not be used by pregnant women, and their prolonged use may increase the risk of skin cancer.

If symptoms persist, the doctor may recommend application of an over-the-counter steroid-based hydrocortisone cream. Doxepin cream may also be effective at relieving itchiness associated with eczema. Apply the ointment as a thin film four times a day for up to eight days. Most patients report no side effects, but the cream may cause a burning sensation in some cases.

If the eczema is allergy related, taking oral antihistamines may help. In severe cases, the doctor may prescribe oral corticosteroid medication; steroids should always be taken with caution and never without medical supervision.

For extreme cases of eczema, particularly in children, a wet body wrap can be effective in get-

ting moisture back into the skin. The patient sleeps in wet pajamas covered with dry clothes or a nylon sweat suit; some doctors suggest covering the face with wet gauze wrapped with an elastic bandage, and covering the hands and feet with a pair of wet, then a pair of dry, tube socks. The patient's room must be kept warm.

ALTERNATIVE CHOICES

Alternative therapies are available to address both the symptoms of eczema and some of the underlying causes. Patients should be aware, however, that some herbal therapies can cause allergic reactions and that certain Chinese herbs can be toxic to the liver and immune system. Long-term treatment with herbs should be undertaken only with thorough knowledge of the potential effects and under the guidance of trained therapists. Use extreme caution when giving herbs to children, pregnant women, and the elderly.

ACUPRESSURE

Acupressure is not intended to cure eczema, but applying deep pressure several times a week to Liver 3, on top of the foot, and Stomach 36, be-

---

CAUTION!

Although steroid creams or steroids may be appropriate for acute outbreaks or severe episodes of eczema, long-term use is not advisable because of the considerable risk of side effects. Topical steroid creams can cause thinning and spotting of the skin, acne, and permanent stretch marks. If used around the eyes, topical steroid medications can, in rare cases, lead to glaucoma. Eczema patients who take oral steroids for longer than the usual two-week cycle and then stop using the drug face the additional risk of severe relapse. For these reasons, steroid therapy is advised only under a doctor's supervision.

low the knee, may relieve the tension that can bring on episodes of inflammation. *(See pages 22-23 for more information on point locations.)*

AROMATHERAPY

Essential oils of lavender *(Lavandula officinalis)*, thyme *(Thymus vulgaris)*, jasmine *(Jasminum officinale)*, and chamomile *(Matricaria recutita)* may be effective in soothing allergy-related eczema. Add a few drops of one of these oils to a bowl of hot water to scent a room.

BODY WORK

Among the many forms of alternative therapy that relieve tension, **shiatsu** and **reflexology** are the most widely used body work techniques. Consult licensed practitioners about appropriate treatment for your condition.

CHINESE HERBS

Studies suggest that a particular traditional Chinese herbal tea mixture can be beneficial to certain eczema patients. The herbs include siler *(Ledebouriella divaricata)* root, Chinese foxglove *(Rehmannia glutinosa)*, and licorice *(Glycyrrhiza uralensis)*, which are said to be anti-inflammatories, and peony *(Paeonia lactiflora)*, which is said to affect the immune system. The researchers caution against long-term use of such mixtures, however, because of potential liver toxicity and because the skin condition may return after patients stop drinking the tea. Because of the wide range of Chinese herbal products, a licensed professional should monitor your use of any long-term treatment.

HERBAL THERAPIES

Evidence suggests that evening primrose oil *(Oenothera biennis)* may effectively treat itching associated with eczema. Some practitioners consider it as effective as corticosteroids without their potential side effects. However, people with liver disease or high cholesterol should use this treatment only under medical supervision, and pregnant women should not use it at all because of its effect on estrogen and progesterone levels.

Burdock *(Arctium lappa)* root and dandelion *(Taraxacum officinale)* root may also be effective in treating some forms of eczema. Take up to 1½ tsp of the fluidextract a day. You can also brew teas from either of these roots: Simmer 1 tbsp of the dried root in a cup of boiling water for 10 minutes, strain, and drink up to three cups a day. Chamomile *(Matricaria recutita)* ointment soothes dry, flaky skin and helps to combat inflammation and itching. Do not take any of these herbs for longer than one month without supervision by a medical herbalist or other trained practitioner.

HOMEOPATHY

A homeopathic remedy to soothe inflamed skin that patients can apply safely at home is topical Calendula ointment. Do not attempt to treat eczema with other homeopathic remedies, however, without consulting a licensed homeopath. Because eczema is a chronic, systemic problem, a homeopath will make a complete examination of all your symptoms—including sleep patterns, food cravings, body temperature, moods, and family history—before deciding on a plan of action. During homeopathic treatment, eczema may actually get worse before it gets better, so professional supervision is important.

NUTRITION AND DIET

Since many eczema patients have allergy problems, they should pay particular attention to their diets. In addition to avoiding the traditional suspects—cow's milk, eggs, wheat flour, and nuts—patients should be wary of eating too much red meat, because animal fats contain fatty acids that promote the body's inflammatory response.

The oils of mackerel, herring, and salmon are high in eicosapentaenoic acid (EPA), shown to reduce skin inflammation and itchiness. Since you would have to eat up to two pounds of fresh fish a day to get the necessary amount of EPA, it's more convenient to take 1 tbsp cod-liver oil or four 1,000-mg fish-oil capsules a day.

Patients may benefit from a daily 50-mg zinc supplement; many eczema sufferers have a zinc deficiency, and zinc helps the body metabolize fatty acids. Your doctor may recommend taking vitamin A, also found in cod-liver oil, which is essential for the repair and renewal of skin. You can take doses of up to 25,000 IU a day. To avoid the

BEWARE OF SECONDARY INFECTIONS

Eczema sores can create tiny openings in the skin through which moisture is lost and bacteria and viruses can enter the body. Scratching the skin affected by eczema creates more openings. This is a particular problem with babies, who tend to develop eczema on the cheeks and forehead. If your baby has eczema, keep her nails cut short and—if she tends to scratch the sores—put mittens on her hands inside out, especially at bedtime.

Open eczema sores make a person more susceptible than normal to highly contagious viral skin diseases. Anyone with eczema must be careful to avoid exposure to people with cold sores, warts, and other diseases caused by viruses. In particular, the herpes simplex II virus causes eczema herpeticum, a rare but potentially serious complication of adult or infant eczema. It is recognizable by numerous small, pus-filled blisters, which require immediate medical attention.

risk of overdose, particularly with fat-soluble vitamins, ask your doctor to monitor your progress.

MIND/BODY MEDICINE

With all the possible causes of eczema, many patients overlook the key element of emotional or physical stress. A Swedish study of adult eczema patients found that those who used relaxation techniques along with their regular regimen of topical preparations improved much faster than those who received topical medication alone.

AT-HOME REMEDIES

◆ To soothe itchiness and help the skin retain moisture in mild forms of eczema, try a

warm bath followed by an application of topical ointment. Use simple, nonmedicated salves like petroleum jelly or vegetable shortening, or ointments made with zinc oxide, chamomile, or calendula—and no additives, preservatives, oils, or perfumes.

◆ Relax. To relieve stress and improve circulation, take a brisk walk or exercise on a regular basis. Come home to a warm bath sprinkled with a few drops of essential oil of lavender.

◆ Soothe and rehydrate your skin by sleeping overnight in wet pajamas, covered with a nylon sweat suit or rain gear. Be sure to keep the room warm.

◆ Eat little or no red meat. Be wary of highly allergenic foods such as cow's milk, wheat, and eggs. Take daily supplements of fish oil, vitamin A, and zinc.

◆ If your baby has eczema, keep her from scratching by putting mittens on her hands when she goes to bed. To avoid the possibility of loose threads wrapping around the baby's wrists or fingers and cutting off circulation, always put the mittens on inside out.

PREVENTION

Since eczema often runs in families, parents may have a good idea whether their own children may be at risk. But even if your baby inherits the predisposition, you may be able to lower her chances of being a chronic sufferer. One study suggests that children weaned from breast milk before the age of four months were nearly three times as likely to develop recurrent eczema as children who were weaned later. If possible, babies should live on their mothers' milk exclusively for the first three months, and doctors advise continuing breast milk for at least up to six months as you introduce your baby to solid food. To avoid triggering food allergies that might bring on eczema, do not offer any eggs or fish until the child is at least a year old. Babies should also be protected from such potential allergens as tobacco smoke and pet hairs, and from airborne irritants such as mites and molds. ■

SYMPTOMS

Emphysema progresses slowly over time and is often mistaken for other ailments, ranging from asthma to heart disease. Typical symptoms of emphysema include:

- shortness of breath, worsening over the years.
- a chronic, mild cough, sometimes accompanied by a small amount of phlegm.
- a distended, "barrel-shaped" chest.

CALL YOUR DOCTOR IF:

- your cough produces unusual amounts of phlegm, especially if the phlegm is dark in color and thick. This is a symptom of bronchitis and an accompanying upper respiratory infection that may require antibiotics.
- you have a lingering, mild cough (sometimes dismissed as "smoker's cough") that does not go away after several months. This symptom points to emphysema, but it could also signal the early stages of lung cancer.
- you begin to lose weight inexplicably. This symptom is associated with emphysema, but it is also characteristic of cancer.
- you regularly become breathless after simple activities, such as climbing a flight of stairs. Again, breathlessness is associated with emphysema, but it could also be a sign of cancer or heart disease.

Emphysema, a potentially fatal lung disease characterized by increasing loss of elasticity in the lungs, typically causes chronic, mild coughing and shortness of breath. Although a number of factors—including heredity, pollution, and a preexisting chronic lung disease such as asthma—can play a role in its development, emphysema is most often caused by long-term, heavy smoking. In many cases, emphysema patients also suffer from chronic bronchitis, which accounts for some of the overlapping symptoms.

More people in the United States die from emphysema than from any other respiratory disease. To date, no cure has been found and no treatment can reverse its effects. However, by seeking professional medical help in the beginning stages of the disease, you can substantially slow its advance.

Emphysema results when the alveoli—tiny, thin-walled air sacs clustered at the ends of the airways deep within the lungs—become damaged or enlarged. Healthy lungs contain about 300 million of these spongy sacs, which are responsible for delivering oxygen into the bloodstream and drawing out carbon dioxide waste. But when the lungs' airways become constricted or damaged, usually from smoking, breathing becomes more forced and difficult. Long periods of labored breathing put pressure on the lungs that eventually stretches the alveoli beyond their normal limits. Over time they lose their natural elasticity and sometimes they burst. Such damage not only prevents the alveoli from working efficiently; it also significantly reduces the surface area and overall elasticity of the lungs. As emphysema develops, sufferers are often unable to carry out even the simplest forms of exercise, such as walking up a flight of stairs, without becoming breathless.

Emphysema is most common in men between the ages of 50 and 70 who have smoked heavily for years, but the disease is becoming more common in women as they join the ranks of heavy smokers. People with emphysema are particularly vulnerable to pneumonia, bronchitis, and other lung infections, as well as to cardiovascular problems such as heart failure. Although emphysema patients need to be monitored by a medical professional, they can make changes in their lifestyle, learn breathing techniques, and supplement their doctor's care with a number of other therapies to make their lives more comfortable.

CAUSES

By far the most common cause of emphysema is heavy, long-term smoking. Cigarette smoke is thought to break down the elastic fibers in the walls of the alveoli, making the air sacs more susceptible to rupture. Smoking also has the effect of weakening the walls of the lungs' branching airways, causing them to collapse on exhalation, trapping stale air. Besides its role in the development of emphysema, smoking also makes people with the disease more vulnerable to lung infections and other serious disorders, such as chronic bronchitis.

Even one puff on a cigarette is enough to cause temporary paralysis in the tiny, hairlike cells known as cilia that are responsible for brushing debris and excess mucus from the lungs.

ALVEOLI

HEALTHY ALVEOLI

STRETCHED AND DAMAGED ALVEOLI

LUNG

Deep in the lungs, the job of delivering oxygen to the bloodstream and removing carbon dioxide is carried out by tiny, thin-walled air sacs called alveoli. When airways become constricted, usually because of smoking, the lungs are forced to work harder, and this puts tremendous pressure on the fragile alveoli. Over time, the sacs may swell or even burst, hampering the vital exchange of gases.

Cilia damaged by continued smoking function only poorly and eventually may stop working altogether. Clogged with mucus, the lungs are then vulnerable to viral and bacterial infections, which over time distort and permanently damage the lungs' airways.

Any lung disease that causes the narrowing of the respiratory airways—such as chronic bronchitis or asthma—may contribute to the development of emphysema, since the resulting pressure on the lungs may exhaust and ultimately damage the alveoli. In rare cases, emphysema can also be caused by the lack of a cellular enzyme that helps to maintain the elasticity of fibers in the walls of the alveoli. People who have inherited this enzyme deficiency have an increased chance of coming down with emphysema sometime in their thirties or forties, even if they don't smoke.

DIAGNOSTIC AND TEST PROCEDURES

A doctor can diagnose emphysema by simply tapping on your chest and listening with a stethoscope. If the tapping produces a hollow sound, more than likely the lungs' air sacs are enlarged or ruptured—the telltale signs of emphysema. After diagnosis, the doctor will probably take an x-ray of your chest to help gauge the extent of the lung damage.

TREATMENT

No treatment will restore your lungs to a healthy state, but there are things you can do to keep your emphysema from getting worse. The first important step is to see a doctor if you develop any of the symptoms listed on page 346. Never dismiss a "smoker's cough" as harmless or merely bothersome; if you smoke, and if you have coughed steadily for more than a month or have suffered chronic breathlessness, chances are your lungs are already damaged. You must stop smoking immediately. If you don't, your condition will almost certainly deteriorate. Breathing techniques, aromatherapy, and oxygen therapy (usually necessary in advanced emphysema) may help you cope with the disease.

CONVENTIONAL MEDICINE

It is important to see a physician regularly if you have emphysema. Your doctor can teach you how to do breathing exercises correctly and how to practice controlled coughing as a way to remove excess mucus from your lungs. Mild physical exercise is also recommended for people with emphysema. A doctor may also prescribe bronchodilators to help ease breathing.

In severe cases of emphysema, at-home oxygen therapy may be necessary; oxygen-delivering devices are widely available for at-home use in both stationary and mobile tanks. In some cases, surgery may be an option. One procedure—in which damaged portions of the lungs are removed—has been shown to alleviate some of the symptoms of emphysema.

ALTERNATIVE CHOICES

If you have emphysema, you should think of alternative choices only as supplements to supervised medical care. The following remedies may provide some relief from the discomfort associated with the disease.

AROMATHERAPY

Essential oils such as eucalyptus *(Eucalyptus globulus)*, hyssop *(Hyssopus officinalis)*, aniseed *(Pimpinella anisum)*, lavender *(Lavandula officinalis)*, pine *(Pinus sylvestris)*, and rosemary *(Rosmarinus officinalis)* may help ease breathing and relieve nasal congestion. Inhale through your nose directly from the bottle, or from a tissue dabbed with a few drops of one or more essential oils. You might also try massaging your chest with 2 tsp of light vegetable oil mixed with 2 drops of essential oil.

CHINESE HERBS

The Chinese herb ephedra *(Ephedra sinica),* also called *ma huang,* is a potent bronchodilator. Note, however, that large quantities of ephedra have the same effect as large quantities of epinephrine; do not use this herb if you have high blood pressure or heart disease. Prepare an infusion by combining 5 grams ephedra, 4 grams cinnamon *(Cinnamo-*

mum cassia) sticks, 1.5 grams licorice *(Glycyrrhiza uralensis),* and 5 grams apricot seeds *(Prunus armeniaca).* Let the mixture steep in cold water, then bring it to a boil. Drink it hot.

HERBAL THERAPIES

A number of herbs act as soothing expectorants and may be appropriate in the treatment of emphysema. Elecampane *(Inula helenium),* for example, is believed to help clear excess mucus from the lungs. To prepare an infusion, shred the root to yield 1 tsp and add a full cup of cold water. Let the infusion stand for 10 hours, then strain and drink it hot three times daily.

Mullein *(Verbascum thapsus)* tea is recommended for soothing the mucous membranes, especially during episodes of nighttime breathlessness. Other herbs that may help relieve shortness of breath include grindelia *(Grindelia* spp.), *Euphorbia pilulifera,* lobelia *(Lobelia inflata),* wild black cherry *(Prunus serotina)* bark, licorice *(Glycyrrhiza glabra),* motherwort *(Leonurus cardiaca),* and aniseed *(Pimpinella anisum).*

HOMEOPATHY

To treat emphysema, a homeopath might recommend the following substances, taken twice a day for a week or as needed. For wheezing and congestion, Antimonium tartaricum (6c). For symptoms that worsen on damp days, in stuffy rooms, or early in the morning, Ammonium carbonicum (6c). For symptoms that grow worse at night or in cold air and drafts, Hepar sulphuris (6c).

NUTRITION AND DIET

Some nutritionists recommend avoiding foods that cause excess mucus production, such as dairy products, processed foods, and white flour products.

REFLEXOLOGY

Toes outstretched, massage the upper surface of both feet, just below the second and fourth toes; this area corresponds to the lungs and chest.

YOGA

The following **yoga** exercises can help you learn to breathe more efficiently.

- With your fingertips on your shoulders, breathe in and join your elbows together in front of you. Lift your elbows as high as you can, then lower them, creating a circle with your arms as you exhale. Repeat.
- While sitting on a stool or standing, make a breaststroke motion with your arms; slowly stretch them behind you. Clasp your hands, lowering your arms below your buttocks, and pull your shoulders back. Then, still clasping your hands behind you, breathe in and lift your arms up as far as you can. Breathe out, lower your arms, and unclasp your hands. Repeat.

AT-HOME REMEDIES

Inhaling steam can help loosen phlegm in your lungs. First, fill a sink with boiling water. Keeping your eyes closed, drape a towel over your head and inhale the steam for two to five minutes. To further ease breathing and help relieve nasal congestion, try adding a few drops of one or more essential oils to the hot water. *(For a list of suggested oils, see Aromatherapy.)*

The warm steam distributed by vaporizers can also help clear the lungs. However, in an average-sized room, most vaporizers aren't powerful enough to generate the density of steam necessary to be truly helpful. If you want to use a vaporizer, place it in a smaller space, such as a bathroom. Don't use cold humidifiers: They must be scrubbed daily with bleach; otherwise, they can spread germs and encourage mold or mildew growth, increasing your chances of developing lung infections.

PREVENTION

If you smoke, the best way to prevent emphysema is to stop right away. Organizations such as Smokenders and the American Lung Association offer programs that will help you kick the habit. There are also a number of alternative smoking-cessation techniques available *(see Nicotine Withdrawal).*

LEARNING TO BREATHE EASIER

Although there is no cure for emphysema, you can practice some simple exercises and breathing techniques that will help you cope with the disease. *(See Yoga for more breathing exercises.)*

Take a walk. Physical fitness is very important for people with emphysema, and daily walking is one of the best means to that end. Begin with a short walk and increase your distance every day. Try to avoid highly polluted areas, or do your walking indoors, perhaps at a local shopping mall.

Arm lift. From a standing position, lift both arms high over your head while breathing deeply. When your lungs are completely filled, slowly lower your arms and exhale. Repeat the exercise three times at first, then increase the number of repetitions each day.

Leg lift. Lie comfortably on your back with knees bent and feet on the floor. Inhale deeply. Slowly raise one knee toward your chest as you exhale; lower your leg as you breathe in. Repeat three times with the same leg, then switch.

Sitting stretch. While seated in a chair, lean back, breathe deeply, and raise your arms high over your head. With your chin tucked into your chest, breathe out as you slowly slump forward; bring your head to your knees and let your arms hang loosely by your sides. Repeat three times.

Diaphragmatic breathing. (This exercise can help increase the efficiency of your lungs and strengthen the muscles that control breathing.) While lying on your back, put the fingertips of one hand over your diaphragm, which lies immediately below your rib cage in the center of your abdomen. Inhale deeply through your nose and concentrate on pushing your diaphragm against your fingers while keeping your chest motionless. Count slowly to three, then exhale to the count of six. When you can take about a dozen breaths this way without tiring, try diaphragmatic breathing while sitting, then while walking, and eventually while climbing stairs. ■

SYMPTOMS

- sharp abdominal pains before, during, or just after menstrual periods.
- sharp abdominal pain during intercourse.
- menstrual periods that are abnormally heavy, especially if they produce large clots and last more than seven days.
- infertility.

CALL YOUR DOCTOR IF:

- you suspect you are suffering from endometriosis; a proper diagnosis is essential to treatment.

Normally, the tissue that lines a woman's uterus, known as the endometrium, is found only in the uterus. However, in a woman suffering from endometriosis, microscopic bits of this tissue migrate outside the uterus, become implanted on other organs and tissues, and grow there. These lesions, or areas of abnormal tissue, usually develop within the abdominal cavity—often involving other portions of the reproductive system, such as the ovaries or the muscular wall of the uterus—but in rare cases they can affect other organs, such as the lungs.

Like the endometrium itself, the transplanted tissue responds to the hormones estrogen and progesterone by thickening and then bleeding every month. But because the transplanted tissue is embedded in other tissue, the blood it produces cannot escape and ends up irritating the surrounding tissue, causing cysts, scars, and adhesions to form. These can eventually bind the reproductive organs together so that they move as one mass when manipulated by a physician.

Cases of endometriosis are classified as minimal, mild, moderate, or severe, depending on

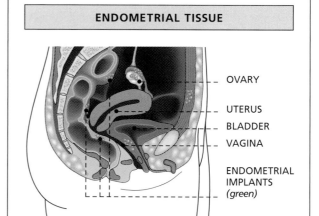

ENDOMETRIAL TISSUE

OVARY

UTERUS

BLADDER

VAGINA

ENDOMETRIAL IMPLANTS *(green)*

Special tissue called endometrium is flushed out of the uterus as part of the natural menstrual process. If fragments of endometrial tissue become implanted in other organs in the pelvic cavity, they can grow, become irritated, and cause pain and abnormal bleeding. Left untreated, the tissue growths can eventually form cysts that disrupt the function of the reproductive organs.

the size of the lesions and how deeply they reach into host organs. Symptoms vary, and about 10 percent of patients have no noticeable symptoms at all. Others experience abnormally heavy and painful periods and sharp, deep abdominal pain during intercourse. Endometriosis accounts for 30 to 40 percent of female infertility. In women who are able to conceive, symptoms may diminish or disappear during pregnancy, but they may return a year or two later.

Endometriosis is most likely to strike women in their thirties and forties; it usually stops at menopause with the marked decline in the production of estrogen.

CAUSES

Researchers do not know definitively how endometrial tissue reaches other parts of the body. One likely possibility involves a condition known as retrograde, or backward, menstruation. Normally during menstruation, portions of the sloughed-off uterine lining exit the uterus through the cervix and the vagina. But in retrograde menstruation, fragments of the endometrium flow back into the fallopian tubes and may then be carried into the abdominal cavity, giving rise to endometriosis. Indeed, doctors have found that endometriosis occurs more often in women with physical conditions that increase retrograde menstruation, such as obstructions in the vagina and cervix.

There is some controversy as to whether tampon use can cause retrograde flow. Evidence seems to suggest that it does not, but some women who have endometriosis avoid tampons, just to be on the safe side. *(See also Toxic Shock Syndrome for guidelines on tampon use.)*

In the rare cases of endometriosis affecting the lungs or other tissue far from the uterus, researchers speculate that the stray endometrial fragments travel through the bloodstream or the lymphatic system, although no one knows just how this happens.

Another theory suggests that endometrial tissue migrates outside the uterus on a fairly routine basis but develops into endometriosis only in women who have an immune system problem that prevents the body from destroying the displaced fragments.

Despite uncertainty about the specific mechanisms behind endometriosis, researchers can point to correlations. The fact that the condition tends to run in families suggests that genetic influences may play a role. Studies have also shown that endometriosis occurs more often in women who have a shorter-than-normal menstrual cycle or a longer-than-normal flow: Women who have fewer than 25 days between periods or who menstruate for more than 7 days are twice as likely to develop endometriosis. Recent evidence also points to exposure to dioxin, an industrial chemical, as a possible cause.

There seems to be no direct relationship between the size of lesions and the severity of pelvic pain. Some women with small lesions report debilitating pain, while others with extensive lesions have no symptoms. Pain probably comes from the scarring and irritation caused by bleeding, or from endometrial tissue invading or growing on a nerve.

How the disease causes infertility is also unclear, but it doesn't appear to be related to the severity of the case; many women with tiny lesions are infertile. Some investigators think the endometrial implants upset the process of ovulation. The implants may also hinder passage of the egg through the fallopian tubes by interfering with the cilia responsible for moving the egg. Other research suggests that endometrial implants secrete chemicals that create an environment hostile to fertilization.

TREATMENT

Endometriosis may respond to both conventional and alternative treatments, ranging from hormonal drugs and surgery to herbal remedies. However, the condition is managed, not cured; symptoms often return when treatment is stopped. Menopause usually ends the symptoms, but in women who take estrogen during and after menopause, symptoms may continue.

Since endometriosis often recurs and often

causes infertility, you may wish to join an endometriosis support group to get help in coping with the uncertainties of the condition. Many hospitals can refer you to a support group.

CONVENTIONAL MEDICINE

Your doctor will usually perform a pelvic examination in order to rule out other potential causes of your symptoms. However, diagnosis can be made only by laparoscopy—visual examination with a slim, lighted instrument that the doctor inserts into the abdominal cavity through a small incision. This procedure is usually done under general anesthesia; many doctors also do a biopsy to confirm the diagnosis.

For women who can conceive and want a child, pregnancy is thought by many doctors to be a good treatment. Pregnancy alleviates symptoms, probably because it temporarily stops menstrual cycles. In some women endometriosis does not return after they have given birth. Alternatively, your doctor may have you take birth-control pills continuously for nine months or more, producing a pseudopregnancy that halts the menstrual cycle and stops the bleeding of the endometrial lesions. This treatment can be effective, but it does not work as well as actual pregnancy; symptoms frequently return.

If a continuous course of birth-control pills fails to bring relief, your doctor may advise treatment with androgens—male hormones. Drugs with hormonal effects such as danazol and nafarelin work by stopping the menstrual cycle, thus keeping uterine tissue from bleeding. Danazol, however, has masculinizing side effects that may not be reversible, such as increased body hair growth and—rarely—deepening of the voice, and it cannot be taken for long periods of time. Indeed, with all such drug therapies, complete cure is uncommon, since the implants remain attached to organs and may resume monthly bleeding when therapy ends.

Analgesics such as ibuprofen and naproxen may relieve the discomfort of cramps but will not affect the implants' cyclic changes, so again they address the symptoms without addressing the underlying cause.

YOGA

1 The **Boat** strengthens the spine and conditions the pelvic area. Lying on your stomach, inhale and lift your head, chest, arms, and legs off the floor. Stretch your arms behind you and hold the position for 15 to 20 seconds, then exhale and relax back onto the floor. Do once or twice a day.

2 The **Bow** increases the elasticity of the spine. Lie on your stomach and grasp both ankles. While inhaling, squeeze your buttocks and slowly raise your head, chest, and thighs off the floor. Hold for 15 seconds, breathing slowly. Exhale, then release. Do once or twice a day.

3 The **Locust** tones the muscles in the pelvic area. Lie on your stomach with your arms at your sides. Squeeze your buttocks as you press down with your arms. While inhaling, raise your legs, keeping them straight as you press outward through the toes and heels. Hold for 15 seconds, then exhale and release. Do once or twice a day.

If tissue growth is rampant and drug treatment is ineffective, your doctor may advise surgery. If all the implanted tissue is removed, your symptoms should disappear. However, some tissue fragments may remain and regrow, and your symptoms may recur, even after a hysterectomy. Your doctor may thus combine surgery with continued drug therapy.

ALTERNATIVE CHOICES

Most alternative remedies aim at relieving symptoms; but since they tend not to affect lesions directly, they are often less effective than comparable conventional treatment.

ACUPRESSURE
You may be able to alleviate cramping by applying pressure to Spleen 6, located on the inside of the leg two inches above the ankle. Do not use this point if you are pregnant. (See pages 22–23 for more information on point locations.)

HERBAL THERAPIES
Some herbal formulas may relieve pain. Skullcap (Scutellaria lateriflora), black cohosh (Cimicifuga racemosa), and wild yam (Dioscorea villosa) may address underlying hormonal problems. Valerian (Valeriana officinalis) may help you relax, but do not take it for longer than a month unless directed by your healthcare practitioner. Life root (Senecio aureus) and black cohosh enhance the health of pelvic organs. Consult a medical herbalist for specific formulas.

NUTRITION AND DIET
The body contains hormonelike substances called prostaglandins that, among other things, play a role in muscle contractions and thus contribute to menstrual cramping. Eating foods rich in natural antiprostaglandins—including mackerel, sardines, salmon, and tuna—may therefore help reduce symptoms. You may choose to take these nutrients in the form of fish-oil supplements and cod-liver oil.

A daily multivitamin-multimineral supplement containing vitamin B complex (50 to 100 mg), vitamin E (400 to 600 IU), calcium (1,000 mg), and magnesium (400 to 600 mg) may help balance estrogen and prostaglandin levels and reduce menstrual cramps.

AT-HOME REMEDIES
◆ In addition to taking an analgesic for pain relief, apply a heating pad or moist heat, and drink warm beverages to help relax cramping muscles. Exercise moderately to increase endorphins, your body's natural painkillers.
◆ To reduce tension, drink soothing herbal teas made with herbs such as hops (Humulus lupulus) and valerian (Valeriana officinalis).

PREVENTION
◆ Avoid exposure to dioxin, which recent evidence has shown may play a role in causing some instances of endometriosis.
◆ If you use tampons, change them frequently, especially when your flow is heavy, and consider alternating tampons with sanitary napkins; these measures may help prevent menstrual flow from backing up—which is one theory for the cause of endometriosis.

RISK FACTORS!
Several factors correlate with increased risk of endometriosis. Be aware of the greater likelihood that you will get this disease if:
◆ you have a close relative with endometriosis, especially a mother or a sister.
◆ your menstrual cycle is consistently short— fewer than 25 days.
◆ your menstrual flow during each period is long—more than a week.
◆ you experience heavy flow during periods.
◆ you use tampons and change them less often than every eight hours.
◆ you use an IUD.
◆ you have a medical condition that blocks or constricts your cervix or vagina.
◆ you have a congenital anomaly of the uterus, such as a double uterus or a double cervix.
◆ you have been exposed to dioxin. ■

SYMPTOMS

For **acute environmental poisoning,** see Emergencies/First Aid: Poisoning.

The symptoms of **chronic environmental poisoning** are wide ranging and often vague. Among the most common:

- cough, headache, nose and eye irritation, diarrhea, dizziness, blurred vision, anxiety, lightheadedness, memory loss, drowsiness, tingling in extremities, aching in muscles and joints, difficulty concentrating, fatigue.
- in severe cases, depression, an overwhelming feeling of weakness, and difficulty breathing.
- disappearance of symptoms when you are not around the possible toxic agent (for example, during the weekend when you are not at your workplace).

CALL YOUR DOCTOR IF:

- your symptoms are persistent, and you can think of no obvious explanation for them but have reason to believe you've been exposed to a toxic substance; you need to be checked and tested to see whether you are indeed suffering from environmental poisoning.

NOTE: **Acute environmental poisoning,** which usually occurs as a result of a catastrophic accident or a one-time event such as a child ingesting a toxic chemical, requires immediate help. **Call 911 or a poison control center now.**

The human body is remarkable for its ability to handle the onslaughts of what can at times be a hostile environment. It is capable of neutralizing or expelling many potentially harmful agents, whether they are organic microbes or industrial chemicals or minerals. However, if your body absorbs low levels of some chemicals or minerals over a period of months or even years, you may develop **chronic environmental poisoning.** (Another form of environmental poisoning is **acute environmental poisoning,** which results from exposure to or ingestion of dangerous amounts of a toxic substance; for information on how to deal with acute poisoning, see Emergencies/First Aid: Poisoning.) Symptoms of chronic environmental poisoning are often vague and can vary in severity; the condition is thus sometimes mistaken for another ailment or remains undetected altogether.

Some people cannot tolerate even minimal exposure to certain chemicals because a genetic malfunction interferes with the production of enzymes that would normally metabolize the toxins and neutralize their damaging effects. Other people are just more sensitive to toxins in the environment: This increased sensitivity can be due to age (both the very young and the elderly being more susceptible to environmental poisoning) and health factors (including smoking, drinking, diet, exercise, and existing chronic disease).

Many conditions fall into the category of environmental poisoning. In some people, for example, environmental poisoning may take the form of an allergy, a physical reaction to a substance that most people are able to tolerate. People who work in poorly ventilated buildings with unhealthy levels of airborne toxins may develop what is known popularly as **sick building syndrome,** while agricultural workers who use pesticides day after day are at risk for **pesticide poisoning.** Although not universally accepted in the medical community as a physical illness, **multiple chemical sensitivity**—in which the body reacts adversely to a wide range of substances, from plastics to perfumes, that do not normally trouble most people—is yet another condition attributed to chronic exposure to potential environmental toxins.

Studies suggest that, once lodged in the body, toxic substances are a factor in the development of many other diseases and conditions that may not at first glance seem directly related to environmental poisoning. Among these are birth defects, endometriosis, infertility, other reproductive and developmental problems, coronary heart disease, respiratory illness, and many types of cancer, especially of the lung, skin, and breast.

Because we encounter low levels of so many environmental toxins in daily life, identifying the toxin or toxins that may be responsible for environmental poisoning can be difficult. Some of the most common and hazardous toxins are lead, asbestos, gasoline and other petroleum distillates, radon, carbon monoxide, organophosphates, formaldehyde, and drinking-water contaminants.

Benzene is one hazardous substance that is found in many forms. It is used in the production of deodorant, oven cleaner, soap, and perfume, and it is a component of paints, pesticides, asphalt, and gasoline and jet fuel. It can contaminate ground-water and surface-water supplies and pollute the air via auto exhaust, manufacturing processes, and cigarette smoke. Yet despite its widespread presence in the environment and its classification as a cancer-causing agent (carcinogen) in the United States, benzene is generally considered a hazard only for the two million or so industrial workers who are exposed to elevated benzene levels at their jobs.

Another common industrial chemical is formaldehyde, which is found in a wide variety of products, including plastics, paper, cosmetics, and carpets. Construction materials, such as particle board, building insulation, and plywood, can emit formaldehyde gas for several years after their manufacture and installation. Several studies since the 1980s have indicated that long-term exposure to formaldehyde is a health risk. The Environmental Protection Agency (EPA) classifies the chemical as a probable carcinogen, although only industrial workers are considered at risk. Some researchers claim that much lower levels of exposure can irritate the eyes and respiratory tract, but many people routinely exposed to formaldehyde at such levels do not develop even these milder symptoms of toxicity.

CLEANSING YOUR SYSTEM

To cleanse your body, eat a high-fiber diet, which helps the gastrointestinal tract move out toxins that have not been absorbed into the bloodstream or stored in other parts of the body. Also, to help the kidneys flush toxins from your system, drink at least two quarts of purified water each day.

Two substances that have received public notice as known carcinogens are asbestos and radon. Asbestos is a fine, fiberlike mineral that until recently was used in construction. Radon and its breakdown products, which are present in the Earth's crust, are released naturally into the air via radioactive decay. Both radon and asbestos are indoor air pollutants that have been significantly linked to the development of lung cancer. Not all buildings contain asbestos, however; and only certain areas of the United States emit radon at levels considered health-threatening.

Carbon monoxide is a common, yet poisonous, gas that is released into the air whenever fuel, wood, or tobacco products are burned. Heavy rush-hour traffic can generate high levels of carbon monoxide, and dangerous, sometimes lethal levels can build up in poorly ventilated garages or houses where faulty heating devices emit exhaust fumes that stay trapped indoors. When carbon monoxide enters the bloodstream, it disrupts the body's usual mechanisms for transporting and absorbing oxygen. Mild cases of carbon monoxide poisoning may cause headaches, nausea, or dizziness; severe cases can lead to respiratory failure and death.

The mineral lead is another contaminant of the air, water, soil, and food. Poisonous at even low levels, lead is known to have a damaging effect on the reproductive system, the kidneys, the nervous system, and the production of blood cells. Since the use of lead-free gasoline has become widespread, lead levels in the air have been significantly reduced. The EPA sets permissible limits for lead in drinking water. However, young children are still at risk of developing lead poisoning from ingesting particles of lead-based paint, which was used in most homes and buildings until it was banned in 1978.

Organophosphates are a potential toxic hazard for farm workers, gardeners, veterinarians, and other people who work with pesticides or insecticides. These chemicals, which are usually absorbed by the skin, retain their potency for several days after they have been applied to field crops. Their toxic effects can range from extreme fatigue, skin irritations, and nausea to depression, breathing problems, seizures, or coma. Agricultural workers who are routinely exposed to high levels of pesticides are considered at greatest risk of developing serious side effects, but some researchers believe that homeowners who use these products regularly in their houses or gardens may also be at risk.

Taking preventive actions, from checking your home for radon emissions to wearing protective gear when exposed on the job to hazardous chemicals, is the key to combating any level of environmental poisoning. The more you know about the particular risks involved, the better you can avoid toxic substances before they become a problem.

CAUSES

Toxic chemicals can get into the body through inhalation (for instance, carbon monoxide), penetration of the skin (pesticides), or ingestion (lead). Some substances can affect the human fetus by crossing the placenta; some also contaminate breast milk and thus may be ingested by a nursing infant.

Once inside the body, toxins can act in a number of ways. Despite how or where a toxin enters the body, it may have its greatest effect on certain target organs. The liver and kidneys, which filter impurities from the body, are often the most susceptible to toxins, especially inhaled industrial solvents. Some chemicals and minerals

are stored in the body's fat or bones and may be released later. Lead, for example, is stored in the bones and may be released when a woman becomes pregnant and her body draws on its stores of bone calcium. Some hazardous agents may be effectively broken down by metabolic processes once they are in the body, but others may become even more harmful as a result.

DIAGNOSTIC AND TEST PROCEDURES

A doctor will probably give you a complete physical examination and take a detailed medical history. You may be asked to keep a diary of your diet and other behavior. Your blood, urine, hair, and fatty tissue may be analyzed for chemical content, and you may also have a liver function test to see how it responds to certain chemicals.

Some doctors are currently studying the usefulness of "environmental control units," special chemically sterile chambers in which patients suspected of having **multiple chemical sensitivity** are exposed to various substances until those specifically linked to their illness are identified.

TREATMENT

CONVENTIONAL MEDICINE

The treatment you receive will depend on which toxic substances are identified as causing your illness. For instance, lead poisoning is often treated with chelation therapy, which involves injections of chemicals that bind with lead in the blood; the lead is later eliminated in urine. However, most treatments for environmental poisoning focus on monitoring symptoms and identifying and eliminating offending substances from the patient's immediate environment.

ALTERNATIVE CHOICES

Regular exercise, a balanced diet, and stress-reduction techniques, such as **yoga** and **meditation,** can help strengthen your immune system, enabling your body to be more resilient to environmental toxins.

HERBAL THERAPIES

Milk thistle *(Silybum marianum),* burdock *(Arctium lappa),* and dandelion *(Taraxacum officinale)* may help detoxify the liver. For general immune support try Siberian ginseng *(Eleutherococcus senticosus),* astragalus *(Astragalus membranaceus),* and cleavers *(Galium* spp.). For advice on how best to treat your specific condition, consult an herbal practitioner.

PREVENTION

Be aware of your environment. Ask questions. Pay close attention to what you are eating and breathing. A recent study—the largest ever on the health effects of airborne particles from smokestacks and traffic—found that people in the most polluted U.S. cities are about 15 percent more likely to die prematurely than those living in cities with the cleanest air.

Here are some specific preventive steps that you can take:

◆ Talk to your state environmental office to see if your house is located in an area known for radon contamination; if so, have it tested.

◆ If you are removing paint from your house, have it tested for lead content. Painting over the old paint may be preferable to removing it, because sanding can release lead particles into the air. Some communities have regulations for removing lead paint; check with your local environmental or health department before beginning the job.

◆ When using hazardous products, always follow the instructions, and wear protective clothing and eye gear.

◆ Keep your children and pets off lawns that have recently been treated with pesticides. (Some communities require that homeowners post a notice when chemicals have been applied.) Stay indoors with the windows closed if trees in your neighborhood are being sprayed with chemicals.

◆ Use nontoxic cleaning products and insecticides around your house. Many of these products are now available in stores or through catalogs.

◆ In buildings, be alert to obvious—or overpowering—chemical odors that may be emitted by paints, pesticides, new carpets, office machines, or other offenders. Make sure the ventilation in your office meets or exceeds standards.

◆ Some studies indicate that certain houseplants can help remove impurities from the air. Consult your local horticultural society or garden center.

◆ To help avoid pesticides, thoroughly wash fruits and vegetables, peel produce, and consider buying organic.

◆ Avoid walking or running near streets with heavy automobile traffic; your increased respiration will increase the amount of carbon monoxide and other toxins that you inhale.

◆ Install a carbon monoxide detector in your home. Without a detector, you may remain unaware of a buildup of the gas, which is colorless, tasteless, and odorless and may not cause any physical irritation.

◆ A balanced diet will help your body maintain its ability to fight toxins. Vitamin deficiencies have been linked to increasing the toxic effects of several substances. Your susceptibility to lead poisoning, for example, increases if your body is deficient in calcium, phosphorus, copper, magnesium, iron, vitamin C, or vitamin E. However, because some vitamins and minerals can be toxic in large doses, never exceed the amounts recommended on the label for your daily requirements, without first consulting a nutritionist.

◆ Weight-loss diets, which make your body metabolize existing fat for energy, will also result in the release of any chemicals that have been stored in those fat cells. If you want to lose weight, do so slowly so that your system does not become flooded with a sudden release of these substances. ∎

SYMPTOMS

Seizures—episodes of abnormal mental or muscular activity—are the basic indicator of epilepsy. They vary widely:

- Staring straight ahead and lapsing into complete immobility for a few seconds characterize a **petit mal seizure.**
- Loss of consciousness, rhythmic jerking motions, and incontinence are among the signs of a **grand mal seizure**, which may last up to 30 minutes.
- Repetitive lip smacking, aimless fiddling movements, and a sense of detachment from surroundings may indicate a **temporal lobe seizure.**
- Rhythmic twitching of a hand, a foot, or the face, often followed by a period of weakness or paralysis, indicates a **Jacksonian seizure.**
- Convulsions in an already ill child three months to three years old, resulting from a sudden climb in fever, indicate a **febrile seizure**. See page 74 for guidelines on how to help someone having a seizure.

CALL YOUR DOCTOR IF:

- you or someone without a prior history of epilepsy experiences a seizure for the first time. You need a doctor's diagnosis; the cause could also be poisoning, stroke, or drug overdose. In feverish infants, convulsions could be a sign of meningitis; **get medical help immediately.**
- one seizure follows another without a return to consciousness; the brain could be deprived of oxygen—**call 911 or your emergency number now.**

Epilepsy is an elusive neurological disorder with a broad range of symptoms, widely differing degrees of severity, and much mystery about why it strikes. In all cases, however, it results from electrical storms in the brain—erratic discharging by neurons. The electrical misfiring of brain cells produces epilepsy's characteristic seizures, which may occur infrequently or in rapid succession.

While every case of epilepsy is distinct, a standardized classification scheme has been developed to describe seizures. The attacks are divided into two main types: generalized (involving the entire brain) and partial (misfirings originating in one area of the brain). Within these categories, seizures are further identified according to the pattern of the attack. The two most common forms of seizure are both of the general type: a **petit mal seizure,** which may include such symptoms as swallowing motions or staring, and can recur many times in a day; and a **grand mal seizure,** which may begin with a cry, a loss of consciousness, and a fall, followed by rigidity, then jerking motions, a period of confusion, and sometimes deep sleep. Among the partial types are **temporal lobe seizures,** which may be preceded by a vague feeling of abdominal discomfort, sensory hallucination, and distorted perceptions such as déjà vu; and **Jacksonian seizures,** with localized twitching of muscles that sometimes spreads to the whole body.

The first signs of epilepsy are usually seen in childhood or adolescence. Very young children with high fevers may have convulsions, but this is not true epilepsy, and such seizures generally disappear after the age of three.

CAUSES

Most cases of epilepsy are of unknown origin. Sometimes, however, a genetic basis is indicated, and other cases may be traceable to birth trauma, lead poisoning, congenital brain infection, head injury, alcohol or drug addiction, or the effects of organ disease. Triggers for the attacks also vary widely. Among the factors that can bring on attacks are certain chemicals or foods, sleep deprivation, stress, flashing lights, menstruation, some prescription and over-the-counter medications, and possibly oral contraceptives.

DIAGNOSTIC AND TEST PROCEDURES

An electroencephalogram (EEG) performed on a sleep-deprived individual can reveal abnormal brain waves characteristic of epilepsy, and imaging tests such as an MRI or CT scan can identify physical trauma that may be causing seizures.

TREATMENT

Epilepsy can often be well controlled by medication. A recommended precaution for epileptics is to wear a Medic Alert bracelet so that other people can quickly recognize what is happening during a seizure and lend effective assistance.

CONVENTIONAL MEDICINE

In the great majority of cases, seizures can be reduced in frequency and severity or eliminated altogether with regular medication; side effects vary, but most are mild. Anticonvulsants commonly prescribed include phenytoin, phenobarbital, valproic acid, carbamazepine, and gabapentin.

ALTERNATIVE CHOICES

Self-medication should never be practiced in place of a doctor's care, and your doctor should be aware of all separate treatments to avoid any drug incompatibility. There is no substitute for the benefits of prescribed drug therapy.

HOMEOPATHY

You may want to consider consulting a homeopath if conventional prescription drugs are not completely controlling seizures. Homeopathic remedies can serve as an effective adjunct to conventional drugs, but don't expect results overnight; the homeopath will advise you on how long it will be before treatments begin to work.

MIND/BODY MEDICINE

Electroencephalogram **biofeedback** may be effective in helping epileptics alter their brain waves to prevent seizures. With guidance, they learn to control their own brain waves by watching them on a computer screen.

OSTEOPATHY

When epilepsy appears to have resulted from a physical injury, cranial osteopathy or craniosacral therapy may help; consult an osteopath.

AT-HOME REMEDIES

◆ Regularly practice biofeedback techniques, learned from a trainer, to ward off epileptic attacks.
◆ Make sure you get ample sleep; too little can increase the likelihood of seizures.

PREVENTION

Identify and watch for particular foods, environments, or physical and emotional signs that precede attacks. It's not uncommon, for example, to feel annoyed or elated several hours prior to a **grand mal seizure**, and immediately before the attack, to become aware of a warning "aura"— perhaps a taste or smell; this warning may allow you to lie down in time to avoid falling. In cases where the aura is a smell, some people are able to fight off seizures by sniffing a strong odor, such as garlic or roses. When the preliminary signs include depression, irritability, or headache, an extra dose of medication (with a doctor's approval) may help prevent an attack. In the case of a **Jacksonian seizure**, firmly squeezing the muscles around those that are twitching can sometimes halt the attack. ∎

EYE PROBLEMS

Read down this column to find your symptoms. Then read across.

SYMPTOMS	AILMENT/PROBLEM
For more information about eye problems specifically related to your vision, see Vision Problems.	
◆ eye is red and painful; upper and lower eyelids may be swollen.	◆ Corneal abrasion or other corneal injury
◆ eyes feel tired, may burn and water; usually occurs in older people and contact lens wearers; is more common in women.	◆ Dry eyes
◆ both eyes are turned inward (crossed eyes); one eye is turned outward (walleye); one eye holds the line of sight while the other wanders.	◆ Strabismus (inability of both eyes to be directed at the same object at the same time; usually caused by weakness or defect in one of six muscles controlling eye movement)
◆ inflammation at one point along the edge of the eyelid, usually at the base of an eyelash; the area reddens and may be painful, a pimple may form, and the pimple may discharge pus.	◆ Sty

WHAT TO DO	OTHER INFO
◆ Call your doctor, who may prescribe an antibiotic and a painkiller, remove any foreign matter, and place a patch over the eye. **Call your doctor immediately** if your vision is impaired; these symptoms could indicate a variety of eye problems, some of which can be very serious.	◆ To avoid scratching the cornea, do not rub your eye if you think you have something in it. See Emergencies/First Aid: Eye Emergencies for instructions on how to remove a foreign object from your eye. Always see your doctor if you have suffered an eye injury.
◆ Try using artificial tears, found in over-the-counter eye drops. Avoid those with vasoconstrictors, which constrict blood vessels in tissues overlying the eye. For an herbal therapy, try bathing your eyes in a solution made with eyebright *(Euphrasia officinalis)*.	◆ Use a humidifier in winter to avoid too much dry heat. Protect your eyes from sun and wind with wraparound sunglasses.
◆ Call your doctor or ophthalmologist. Treatment aims to correct unbalanced eye muscles, and may include eye drops or ointment, corrective lenses, or surgery. Eye exercises may help balance the muscles.	◆ Eye muscle problems are usually congenital but may also result from a loss of vision in one eye from any cause. Treatment is most effective in young children.
◆ In most cases a sty will clear up on its own. See your doctor if the inflammation recurs; you may need an antibiotic.	◆ Apply a hot compress to the area periodically to help bring the sty to a head. *(See also the Visual Diagnostic Guide.)*

FACIAL PAIN

Read down this column to find your symptoms. Then read across.

SYMPTOMS	AILMENT/PROBLEM
◆ stabs of intense pain in lip, gum, cheek, or chin, usually triggered by touch, in people over 50.	◆ Trigeminal neuralgia
◆ dull pain around eyes and cheeks that worsens on bending forward; possibly, thick discharge from nose, temporary loss of smell, nasal speech, headache, malaise, sore throat, fever, toothache.	◆ Sinusitis
◆ throbbing forehead pain; the artery crossing your temple may be swollen and painful to the touch; possibly, mild fever, loss of vision.	◆ Inflamed artery (temporal arteritis, giant cell arteritis)
◆ continuous throbbing pain on one side of face when tooth is touched; tooth feels loose; possibly, swollen glands in neck, fever.	◆ Tooth abscess
◆ pain or bruised feeling on one side of face; red, blistery rash on face, ear, or throat; inability to move facial muscles; tingling, itching, prickly sensation of skin; low fever.	◆ Shingles (herpes zoster nerve infection)
◆ throbbing pain around one eye, subsiding and recurring; usually accompanied by nasal congestion; sweating; tearing and reddening of eye.	◆ Cluster headache
◆ clicking or popping around jaw joint and pain on opening mouth; jaw pain; possibly, recurrent headaches and pain radiating through face and around the neck and shoulders.	◆ Temporomandibular joint (TMJ) syndrome

F

WHAT TO DO	OTHER INFO
◆ Call your doctor, who may prescribe analgesics to kill the pain, possibly with low doses of an anticonvulsant or antidepressant drug to maximize pain relief.	◆ This nerve inflammation could be caused by a blood vessel pressing on a nerve. Deep-tissue massage and acupuncture may help relieve pain. Surgery is sometimes required.
◆ The usual treatment is an analgesic, decongestant, or antibiotic (if cause is bacterial); or antihistamines, immunotherapy, or inhaled corticosteroids (if cause is allergy).	◆ Allergies and dental abscesses may predispose you to sinusitis. Acupuncture and homeopathy may be helpful for acute pain or to prevent recurrence.
◆ Call your doctor, who may prescribe corticosteroids to reduce inflammation and prevent loss of vision.	◆ Treatment brings a 75 percent chance of complete recovery.
◆ **Call your dentist now;** treatment is essential. Take an analgesic; rinse mouth hourly with warm salted water. See Toothache.	◆ Emergency dental treatment is essential to prevent damage to the jawbone through spread of infection.
◆ Call your doctor for treatment that may include prescribed pain relievers, an antiviral medication, or rarely, an antibiotic.	◆ High doses of vitamin E (500 IU, three times a day, taken under a doctor's supervision) may be helpful. Shingles is caused by a recurrence of the same virus that causes chickenpox.
◆ Call your doctor if you have not yet been diagnosed. See Headache.	◆ The trigger may be alcohol or medications that dilate blood vessels, such as nitroglycerin. Inner nasal applications of cayenne (Capsicum frutescens) ointment may relieve pain.
◆ Call your dentist for treatment that may include correction of jaw misalignment or of other dental problems.	◆ Treatment may include anti-inflammatory drugs, moist heat, physical therapy, and soft foods. Acupuncture, shiatsu, and relaxation techniques such as biofeedback are especially effective.

FAINTING

Read down this column to find your symptoms. Then read across.

SYMPTOMS	AILMENT/PROBLEM
◆ brief loss of consciousness, possibly preceded by pallor and lightheadedness, usually lasting several minutes.	◆ Fainting (general)
◆ faintness or fainting after exertion or several hours spent in hot (usually humid) air; fatigue; possibly, nausea, vomiting, headache, weakness, rapid heartbeat.	◆ **Heat exhaustion** or **heatstroke**
◆ faintness or fainting in someone who is vomiting blood or passing bloody or black, tarry stool.	◆ Digestive tract bleeding (ulcer, polyps, inflammatory or infectious diseases, cancer)
◆ faintness or fainting when standing abruptly after sitting, lying, or bending, especially in persons taking antihypertensive drugs.	◆ Low blood pressure (hypotension)
◆ faintness or fainting in a person who has diabetes or who has not eaten recently; possibly, weakness, tingling in hands, feet, and lips, trembling, nausea, headache, rapid heartbeat.	◆ Low blood sugar (diabetes, hypoglycemia)
◆ faintness or fainting after an emotional shock or other stressful event or in a person with a panic disorder.	◆ Stress; anxiety
◆ sudden faintness or fainting with numbness and weakness; possibly, blurred vision, confusion, difficulty speaking, or paralysis.	◆ Stroke; transient ischemic attack
◆ sudden fainting in someone with irregular pulse or heart disease.	◆ Heart disease; heart attack

WHAT TO DO	OTHER INFO
◆ **Call 911 or your emergency number** if someone is unconscious for more than five minutes or has no pulse; start CPR (*see Emergencies/First Aid: Loss of Consciousness*). Otherwise, make the person comfortable after consciousness returns.	◆ Brief, infrequent fainting with no other symptoms usually is not a cause for concern.
◆ **Call 911 or your emergency number now.** Move to a cool place; drink water; apply cool compresses. See Emergencies/First Aid: Heatstroke and Heat Exhaustion.	◆ A victim of heatstroke does not sweat, despite a body temperature of 100°F or higher; pulse may be rapid and strong.
◆ Call your doctor without delay; proper diagnosis is essential.	◆ Your doctor will order tests to detect the cause of bleeding.
◆ Rise more slowly. If you frequently faint when standing, call your doctor to check for underlying ailments.	◆ If you take antihypertensive drugs, your doctor may reduce dosage. If fainting recurs, seek evaluation for another condition.
◆ Call your doctor if fainting recurs. Anyone with low blood sugar should carry a sugar or protein snack to eat when feeling faint.	◆ Treatment for diabetes is designed to normalize blood levels of glucose and insulin through diet and sometimes medication.
◆ You may benefit from counseling or psychotherapy. See also Phobias, Panic Attack, Posttraumatic Stress Disorder.	◆ You may benefit from relaxation exercises such as biofeedback, meditation, or yoga. Acupuncture or massage may also reduce anxiety.
◆ **Call 911 or your emergency number now;** immediate medication may prevent further damage.	◆ Stroke rehabilitation may include speech and physical therapy, including gentle aerobic exercise.
◆ **Call your doctor or 911 or your emergency number now** unless you have a chronic, stable, benign heart arrhythmia. See also Heart Disease and Heart Attack.	◆ Fainting can follow pump failure, arrhythmia, valve problems, and other factors that lower blood flow. Smoking cessation, changes in diet, exercise, and stress reduction may help prevent heart disease.

FATIGUE

Read down this column to find your symptoms. Then read across.

SYMPTOMS	AILMENT/PROBLEM
◆ following recent travel, persistent fatigue; sleeplessness; hunger at seemingly odd times.	◆ Jet lag (disruption of your body's normal rhythms for sleeping and eating)
◆ general lethargy that somewhat limits daily activities; possibly, obesity; tendency to feel stressed.	◆ Your lifestyle is working against you and needs change
◆ fatigue that develops after starting a new medication.	◆ Side effect of prescription or over-the-counter medication such as sleeping pills, cough and cold preparations, and blood pressure drugs
◆ fatigue during the day; trouble falling asleep, and/or difficulty sleeping through the night.	◆ Insomnia
◆ persistent sadness, fatigue, and pessimism; sudden change in appetite; difficulty sleeping, or tendency to oversleep; sometimes, thoughts of death or suicide.	◆ Depression
◆ nighttime sleep that is interrupted by sudden awakenings from a choking sensation, followed by drowsiness and more sleep; fatigue during the day.	◆ Sleep apnea (episodes of interrupted breathing—for up to one or two minutes at a time—during sleep)
◆ debilitating fatigue that lasts for six months or more; fatigue is not from exertion and is not relieved by rest; persistent low-grade fever; aching, weak muscles; swollen lymph nodes; joint pain; headache; confusion; sore throat.	◆ Chronic fatigue syndrome
◆ weakness and fatigue; dizziness; faintness; pale skin; heart palpitations; loss of appetite.	◆ Anemia

WHAT TO DO	OTHER INFO
◆ Keep your body well hydrated: Drink water and avoid alcoholic beverages. When you arrive at your destination, force your body to adjust to the local time zone quickly.	◆ The hormone melatonin is believed to help regulate the body's rhythms; melatonin supplements, available in health food stores, may help fight jet lag.
◆ Determine what lifestyle patterns (over-working, not exercising enough) are contributing to your fatigue, and make changes; begin a diet to lose weight, and/or adopt a stress-reduction technique—such as yoga—that you're comfortable with and will do regularly.	◆ Aromatherapy may help reduce stress: Place 2 drops of essential oil of peppermint (Mentha piperita) on a handkerchief, and inhale.
◆ Talk to your doctor or pharmacist about the side effects of any medications you are taking.	
◆ If your insomnia lasts longer than a month, visit your doctor; you may have an underlying problem such as hypothyroidism. Mild insomnia is normal during pregnancy.	◆ Use different strategies to help yourself sleep; before bed, try taking a warm bath, reading a book for pleasure, practicing deep breathing, or having a cup of chamomile (Matricaria recutita) tea.
◆ Depression often responds to both conventional and alternative treatments. Consult your doctor, a psychotherapist, or a counselor such as a member of the clergy.	◆ Regular exercise is a significant aid to recovering from depression.
◆ See your doctor for an accurate diagnosis. Treatments are available for mild cases (see Snoring), but surgery to keep airways open is sometimes necessary.	◆ Other disorders that can mimic sleep apnea include asthma and slight heart failure.
◆ See your doctor; this condition is easily confused with AIDS, mononucleosis, and other ailments.	◆ The cause for this syndrome is not clear; viruses, allergies, and hormonal imbalances have all been implicated.
◆ See your doctor without delay. Anemia can have serious complications.	◆ Treatment will depend on the cause and extent of your anemia, and may include dietary changes, nutritional supplements, and/or surgery.

Read down this column to find your symptoms. Then read across.

SYMPTOMS	AILMENT/PROBLEM
◆ extreme fatigue; fever; sore throat; chills; headache; body aches; nasal congestion; cough.	◆ Flu
◆ severe fatigue, headache, sore throat that may be severe, chills, muscle aches, fever, cough; possibly followed by swollen lymph nodes, yellowish skin, rash that resembles measles, soreness in upper-left abdomen.	◆ Mononucleosis
◆ lack of appetite; fatigue; mild fever; muscle or joint aches; nausea and vomiting; abdominal pain; possibly, dark-colored urine, light-colored stools, yellowish, itching skin.	◆ The liver is either inflamed (hepatitis) or degenerating (cirrhosis)
◆ fatigue, weight loss, cough (occasionally with bloody sputum), slight fever, nighttime perspiration; sometimes, pain in the chest, back, and/or kidneys.	◆ Tuberculosis; possibly, lung cancer
◆ fatigue; weight gain; numbness and tingling in hands; constipation; dry skin and hair; increased sensitivity to cold; persistently low body temperature.	◆ Hypothyroidism (failure of the body to produce enough thyroid hormones)
◆ fatigue; excessive thirst and frequent urination; increased appetite; weight loss; recurring yeast infections.	◆ Diabetes
◆ weakness; fatigue; weight loss; salt cravings; darkening skin; hair loss.	◆ Addison's disease (a potentially fatal illness that occurs when the adrenal glands cannot produce adequate amounts of the hormone cortisone)
◆ frequent waking during the night to urinate; persistent fatigue; weight loss; dry, itching skin; pallor; shortness of breath; swelling of hands and feet; unpleasant taste in mouth.	◆ Kidney disease
◆ shortness of breath; fatigue and weakness; coughing; swelling in abdomen or legs; rapid heartbeat.	◆ Congestive heart failure (heart not pumping at full capacity, causing fluid to accumulate in other areas of the body)

WHAT TO DO	OTHER INFO
◆ Rest as much as possible and drink plenty of water. Take an anti-inflammatory painkiller such as ibuprofen if necessary.	◆ Vaccines for some forms of flu are offered each year and are recommended for anyone over 65, as well as for other groups at high risk for developing serious complications.
◆ See your doctor. Complete bed rest is essential, with a gradual return to normal activity; no other treatment is usually given.	◆ Most people feel better within two or three weeks, but the fatigue may last for months.
◆ See your doctor without delay. Treatment will depend on the type and severity of your illness. See Hepatitis and Cirrhosis.	◆ Cirrhosis may be caused by one of several viruses, by overuse of alcohol or drugs, or by ingesting one of many toxins.
◆ See your doctor today. For tuberculosis, you will need one or several antibiotics. Lung cancer therapy is wholly dependent on the extent of the disease.	◆ Taken as an infusion or in capsule form, echinacea (*Echinacea* spp.) is reputed to stimulate immune system activity, thereby helping to fight infection.
◆ You will likely need hormone replacement therapy; consult your doctor. See Thyroid Problems.	◆ Avoid foods that interfere with thyroid hormone production, including cabbage, peaches, spinach, and peanuts.
◆ See your doctor for a diet and medication regimen to avoid serious (and possibly lethal) complications.	◆ Type 1 diabetes requires insulin injections; Type 2 does not and can be controlled through diet and exercise alone.
◆ **Call your doctor now.** You will need regular cortisone supplements to avoid going into adrenal shock.	◆ Once Addison's disease develops, it is a lifelong condition that requires regular cortisone-like supplements.
◆ **Get medical care immediately.** Kidney disease is a life-threatening condition that often requires emergency care.	◆ Ask your doctor or nutritionist for dietary guidelines for minimizing stress on your kidneys.
◆ **Get emergency medical care.** You may be hospitalized to stabilize your condition; treatment may include surgery, medication, changes in diet, and specific exercises.	

FEET, ACHES AND PAINS

Read down this column to find your symptoms. Then read across.

SYMPTOMS	AILMENT/PROBLEM
◆ pain when putting weight on your foot; hard, flat lump of roughened skin on sole; mild pain when the lump is squeezed; possibly, tiny black dots on the lump's surface.	◆ Plantar wart
◆ pain at the base of your big toe and the ball of your foot; bony protrusion at the side of your foot near your big toe; swelling, redness, tenderness, and limited joint motion.	◆ Bunion
◆ pain under the heel and arch of your foot, especially if you walk or run a lot; possibly, stiffness and numbness in your heel.	◆ Plantar fasciitis (inflammation of connective tissue in the foot)
◆ persistent, shooting pains between your third and fourth toes.	◆ Morton's neuroma (a benign mass of nerve tissue)
◆ sharp pain when you put weight on your foot or heel.	◆ Bone spur
◆ pain, swelling, redness, warmth, and stiffness in joints of your foot and elsewhere.	◆ Rheumatoid arthritis
◆ intense pain in your big toe; swelling, warmth; possibly, alternating chills and fever.	◆ Gout
◆ pain in your foot following an injury or sudden movement; possibly, swelling and the inability to put weight on the foot.	◆ Broken bone or other injury

WHAT TO DO	OTHER INFO
◆ Most warts go away on their own, so you may choose to do nothing. But if the wart is especially troublesome, see your doctor about removal methods.	◆ To prevent the spread of this highly contagious virus on your own feet or to others, do not pick at the warts; wear rubber shoes in the shower.
◆ Wear soft, wide shoes; consider made-to-order shoes. If the pain is severe, your doctor or podiatrist may recommend surgery.	◆ Although you may inherit a tendency to get bunions, the condition is worsened by wearing tight shoes. Bursitis or osteoarthritis may also be present, causing pain and stiffness.
◆ Try an over-the-counter arch support; call your doctor for diagnosis and rehabilitation recommendations.	◆ This so-called overuse injury causes tissues in the sole of your foot to become inflamed.
◆ For quick relief, remove your shoes and massage the area. If the pain persists, your doctor may suggest corticosteroid injections or surgery.	◆ A neuroma is typically caused by an inflamed, pinched nerve. Avoid tight shoes and high heels. Over-the-counter metatarsal arch supports may help.
◆ Avoid tight shoes; try putting a foam rubber pad, with a hole cut out under the spur, in your shoe. Take an anti-inflammatory painkiller such as ibuprofen.	◆ Acupuncture or physical therapy may help to relieve the discomfort.
◆ Try taking an anti-inflammatory painkiller such as ibuprofen. Arthritic joints require a balance of rest and exercise. See Arthritis.	◆ The pain of arthritis may be helped by acupuncture and various relaxation techniques.
◆ The usual treatment is a nonsteroidal anti-inflammatory drug (NSAID) and/or the drug colchicine.	◆ The homeopathic remedy Colchicum, from the plant from which colchicine is extracted, may relieve the pain.
◆ **Call your doctor or get emergency care now** if you cannot walk or move your foot or if you are unsure of the severity of injury. If there is no fracture, rest with the foot raised and apply an ice bag. See Sprains and Strains and Emergencies/First Aid: Fractures and Dislocations.	◆ A fracture may require a firm bandage or plaster cast or, possibly, surgery to reposition bones. Soft-tissue injuries may be massaged with an over-the-counter anti-inflammatory cream or Arnica cream, provided there is no break in the skin.

FEVER AND CHILLS

F

Read down this column to find your symptoms. Then read across.

SYMPTOMS	AILMENT/PROBLEM
◆ fever (a higher-than-normal body temperature, usually above 98.6°F), with or without other symptoms; possibly, chills, especially while fever is climbing.	◆ Fever (general)
◆ fever with severe headache and stiff neck; possibly, nausea, vomiting, light sensitivity, drowsiness, confusion.	◆ Meningitis
◆ fever with convulsions, shaking, and/or blue color to face, usually in a baby or child.	◆ Fever with convulsions
◆ fever in a child under 12, accompanied by earache, rash, swollen jaw , noisy breathing, runny nose, red eyes, or dry cough.	◆ Various illnesses of infancy and childhood, such as ear infection, croup, measles, German measles, chickenpox, mumps
◆ abrupt onset of fever (102°F to 106°F); possibly, chills, headache, malaise, diarrhea, runny nose, dry cough, sore throat, or aches in muscles or joints.	◆ Flu or other viral infection
◆ fever after several hours in heat or strong sun; fever in a baby dressed too warmly.	◆ Overheating or **heat exhaustion**
◆ fever with sore throat; pain in back and painful urination; pelvic pain; nausea, vomiting, and diarrhea; chest pain when taking a breath, cough, and shortness of breath.	◆ Various infections, such as tonsillitis, pharyngitis, or laryngitis; bladder or kidney infection; pelvic inflammatory disease; gastroenteritis; bronchitis or pneumonia; malaria; AIDS
◆ fever after taking medication.	◆ Drug reaction
◆ fever with throbbing face pain, especially when tooth is touched; possibly, swollen glands in neck.	◆ Tooth abscess

WHAT TO DO	OTHER INFO
◆ Call doctor if fever lasts longer than 48 hours or if fever in an infant between three and six months exceeds 100.5°F (rectal). Take fluids and aspirin or acetaminophen (do not give aspirin to a child).	◆ Most fevers are caused by bacterial or viral infections. A baby who won't drink liquids may need intravenous rehydration.
◆ **Call your doctor now.** Unless treated, meningitis can cause permanent neurological damage.	◆ The usual treatment is antibiotics for bacterial infection, or intravenous fluids and analgesics for viral infection.
◆ **Call 911 or your emergency number** if child's skin turns blue or if patient is adult. Sponge with tepid water to lower fever.	◆ Fever convulsions do not represent a seizure disorder, but infants should be examined for an underlying problem.
◆ Call your doctor; treatment depends on the illness. See related entries.	◆ Adults should not be exposed to measles, chickenpox, or mumps if they have not had them. Childhood diseases are more serious in adults.
◆ Rest; increase fluid intake. Call your doctor if you have shortness of breath or if fever lasts more than 48 hours. See Flu.	◆ Flu may lead to secondary infections, such as pneumonia, especially in patients who are elderly, very young, chronically ill, or smokers.
◆ Rest in a cool place. Call your doctor if temperature continues to rise. See Emergencies/First Aid: Heatstroke and Heat Exhaustion.	◆ Vigorous exercise can temporarily raise your temperature well above normal.
◆ Call your doctor for a proper diagnosis. The usual treatment is antibiotics if the infection is bacterial. Otherwise, treatment depends on the disease. See related entries.	◆ Seek treatment for fever with back or pelvic pain (possibly kidney infection or pelvic inflammatory disease) or chest pain with shortness of breath (possibly pneumonia).
◆ Check on changing your prescription.	◆ Penicillin and some antihypertensives may cause fever.
◆ **Call your dentist now** for emergency treatment. See Toothache.	◆ Treatment is needed to prevent spread of infection, possible damage to jaw, and blood poisoning.

SYMPTOMS

- fever—usually between 101°F and 102°F, but occasionally as high as 106°F—sometimes alternating with chills.
- sore throat.
- dry, hacking cough.
- aching muscles.
- general fatigue and weakness.
- nasal congestion, sneezing.
- headache.

CALL YOUR DOCTOR IF:

- you experience any of these symptoms and your immune system is already weakened by cancer, diabetes, AIDS, or other conditions; or if you have a serious illness like chronic heart or kidney disease, impaired breathing, cystic fibrosis, or chronic anemia. You may be at risk of developing serious secondary complications and need to be carefully monitored as long as symptoms last.
- your fever lasts more than three or four days, you become short of breath while resting, or you have chest pain. You may have developed pneumonia.

nfluenza—commonly shortened to "flu"—is an extremely contagious viral disease that appears most frequently in winter and early spring. The infection spreads through your upper respiratory tract and sometimes goes into your lungs. The virus typically sweeps through large groups of people who share indoor space, such as schools, offices, and nursing homes. The global influenza epidemic of 1918—which started in a military training camp in Kansas—eventually killed some 500,000 people throughout the United States.

Although both colds and influenza stem from viruses that infect the upper respiratory tract, the symptoms of influenza are more pronounced and its complications more severe. Influenza occurs most commonly in school-age children, but its most severe effects are felt by infants, the elderly, and people with chronic ailments. Despite advances in prevention and treatment, influenza and its complications are still fatal to about 20,000 people in the U.S. annually. Specific strains of the disease can be prevented by injections of antibodies in a flu vaccine, but after influenza—or any other viral infection, for that matter—has started, there is no cure except to let it run its course.

CAUSES

The flu virus is transmitted by inhaling droplets in the air that contain the virus, or by handling items contaminated by an infected person. The symptoms start to develop from one to four days after infection with the virus.

Researchers divide influenza viruses into three general categories: types A, B, and C. While all three types can mutate, or change into new strains, type A influenza mutates constantly, yielding new strains of the virus every few years. This means that you can never develop a permanent immunity to influenza. Even if you develop antibodies against a flu virus one year, those antibodies are unlikely to protect you against a new strain of the virus the next year. Type A mutations are responsible for major epidemics every several years. Types B and C are less common and result in local outbreaks and milder cases. Type B has also been linked to the development of Reye's syndrome, a potentially fatal complication of influenza and other viral infections—such as chickenpox—that usually affect children.

Most influenza viruses that infect humans seem to originate in parts of Asia where close contact between livestock and people creates a hospitable environment for the mutation and transmission of viruses. Swine, or pigs, can catch both avian (meaning from birds or poultry) and human forms of a virus, and act as hosts for these different viral strains to meet and mutate into new forms. The swine then infect people with the new form of the virus in the same way in which people infect each other—by transmitting viruses through exchange of droplets in the air.

DIAGNOSTIC AND TEST PROCEDURES

All three types of influenza mimic the basic symptoms of the common cold, such as cough and headache. Your doctor may take a throat culture or blood test to rule out the possibility of other ailments such as strep throat or, if public-health officials are gathering statistics on an influenza outbreak, to identify the specific viral strain.

TREATMENT

Influenza will run its course regardless of how you treat it. Because it is a viral disease, it does not respond to antibiotics. If you are in good health, influenza will probably pass with no complications after a week or so of bed rest and self-care at home. If you are over 65, are a diabetic, or have another chronic disease, talk to your physician about being immunized before winter sets in (see Prevention, page 377). If you then come down with flu anyway, make sure your doctor monitors your progress so that any complications can be caught and treated appropriately.

CONVENTIONAL MEDICINE

Doctors have no single treatment that applies to all cases of influenza. You will probably be told to rest in bed, eat nourishing food, and drink lots of liquids. Fluids are especially important to help avoid dehydration from fever and for loosening up respiratory tract secretions.

You can try over-the-counter medicines to ease the discomfort of your cough, nasal congestion, and sore throat. A steam vaporizer in your room puts moisture into the air and may make breathing easier. If you are feverish and have muscle aches, analgesics like aspirin, ibuprofen, or acetaminophen may help you feel better. Because it has been linked to Reye's syndrome, you should not give aspirin to children.

If these remedies don't help a severe bout of flu, your physician may give you amantadine or ri-

A COLD OR THE FLU: WHICH IS IT?

The common cold and influenza are both contagious viral infections of the respiratory tract. Although the symptoms can be similar, influenza is worse: A cold may drag you down a bit, but influenza can make you shudder at the very thought of getting out of bed.

Congestion, sore throat, and sneezing are common with colds, and both ailments bring coughing, headache, and chest discomfort. With influenza you are likely to run a high fever for several days, and your head and body will ache. Usually, complications from colds are relatively minor, but a severe case of influenza can lead to a life-threatening illness like pneumonia.

Over 100 types of cold viruses are known, and new strains of influenza evolve every few years. Since both diseases are viral, neither can be conquered by antibiotics; those drugs are useful only against a secondary bacterial infection that may cause sinusitis or pneumonia.

mantadine, oral antiviral drugs that are active against type A influenza. You need to give yourself time to fully recuperate from influenza and prevent the development of secondary infections that can cause bronchitis, sinusitis, or pneumonia.

ALTERNATIVE CHOICES

Alternative therapies may help strengthen your body's ability to fight the virus and recover from the illness as well as ease temporary flu symptoms.

ACUPRESSURE

Pressure on a number of points can be recommended for various flu symptoms; refer to pages 22–23 for the location of acupressure points. Bladder 36 is recommended for stimulating natural resistance to colds and flu. Bladder 2, Stomach 3, Large Intestine 20, Gall Bladder 20, and Governing Vessels 16 and 24 may be helpful for relieving nasal congestion, headaches, and eyestrain. Large Intestine 11 may help fight fever and strengthen your immune system. Large Intestine 4 may offer general relief from flu symptoms, but do not press it if you are pregnant. Conception Vessel 22 and Kidney 27 may help relieve chest congestion and coughing. Finally, try Bladder 38 to relieve coughing, breathing difficulties, and other respiratory complications.

AROMATHERAPY

In flu season, when those around you are coming down with the virus, protect yourself by gargling daily with one drop each of the essential oils of tea tree (*Melaleuca* spp.) and lemon in a glass of warm water; stir well before each mouthful. If you come down with the flu despite your best preventive measures, 2 drops of tea tree oil in a hot bath may help your immune system fight the viral infection and ease your symptoms. Tea tree oil can be irritating to the skin, however, so don't use more than 2 drops in a full bath.

If you have a congested nose or chest, add a few drops of essential oils of eucalyptus (*Eucalyptus globulus*) or peppermint (*Mentha piperita*) to a steam vaporizer. If you are asthmatic, do not use steam; instead, sprinkle a few drops of these essential oils on a handkerchief and inhale.

HERBAL THERAPIES

For an herbal approach to stimulating your immune system, try taking ½ tsp each of tincture of goldenseal (*Hydrastis canadensis*) and echinacea (*Echinacea* spp.) twice a day. If flu symptoms appear, chew a clove of raw garlic (*Allium sativum*) for its antiviral properties, but do not eat raw garlic on an empty stomach.

An infusion of boneset (*Eupatorium perfoliatum*) may relieve aches and fever and clear congestion: Simmer 1 cup boiling water with 2 tsp of the herb for 10 to 15 minutes; drink a cupful every hour, as hot as you can stand it. To combat chills, try taking 30 drops of yarrow (*Achillea millefolium*) or elder (*Sambucus nigra*) flower tincture every four hours until your chills are gone.

HOMEOPATHY

For homeopathic self-care, try one of the following remedies in 12c dosages every 6 to 8 hours for a day or two. If you don't notice an improvement in your condition after 24 hours, try another homeopathic remedy.

◆ If you feel tired, weak, "heavy," and chilled, with headache and stuffy nose, try Gelsemium.

◆ If you feel general achiness in your muscles, with headache and irritability that are worse when you move around, and if you are thirsty for cold fluids and have a dry hacking cough, try Bryonia.

◆ If you are restless, chilled, and thirsty with a dry mouth, hoarse voice, and aching joints, try Rhus toxicodendron.

◆ If you have a dry cough with achiness, or if your body feels bruised and chilled, and you are thirsty for cold drinks although they upset your stomach, try Eupatorium perfoliatum.

NUTRITION AND DIET

Eat vitamin C-rich fresh fruits and vegetables like citrus fruits, Brussels sprouts, and strawberries; or take 1,000 mg of vitamin C every two to three hours when awake. Increase zinc intake with lean meats, fish, and whole-grain breads and cereals.

REFLEXOLOGY

To support your respiratory system, press your thumb into the solar plexus/diaphragm point for a few seconds, or massage the point with your thumb. *(See page 25 for information about locating this point.)*

AT-HOME REMEDIES

◆ Take two tablets of aspirin, acetaminophen, or ibuprofen every four hours to reduce fever, headache, and body aches: These symptoms are usually worst in the afternoon and evening. Do not give aspirin to anyone under 21, because some people in this age group may be at risk of developing Reye's syndrome.

◆ If you have a sore or scratchy throat, try a salt-water gargle. Dissolve 1 tsp salt in 1 pt warm water. Gargle whenever your throat is uncomfortable, but don't swallow the mixture.

◆ Use a heating pad on body aches.

◆ When you feel like eating, try bland, starchy food like dry toast, bananas, applesauce, cottage cheese, boiled rice, rice pudding, cooked cereal, and baked potatoes. These foods provide a gentle transition for your digestive system when you have not been eating regularly.

◆ Don't drink alcoholic beverages; they leave you dehydrated and can lower your body's ability to fight illness and secondary infection. Avoid over-the-counter flu remedies that contain alcohol.

◆ If you take over-the-counter pain relievers, make sure your symptoms are actually diminishing, not just temporarily suppressed, before you get out of bed. If you don't give yourself enough time to recover fully, you may end up prolonging your illness or developing complications.

PREVENTION

The most effective preventive measure against influenza is to be inoculated every fall against strains that have developed since the previous outbreak. If you are vaccinated against one or more type A and B strains, you may still come down with flu, but your symptoms are likely to be milder than they would have been had you not had a vaccination.

Influenza vaccine is available through physicians and public-health facilities. Because influenza is a serious threat, the U.S. Centers for Disease Control and Prevention recommend vaccination for everyone over 65; nursing home residents and employees; anyone whose immune system is compromised by AIDS, cancer, or other chronic ailments; and people who work in medical facilities. The vaccine is usually given as a single injection, although children may receive two. If you are pregnant, wait until your second trimester and make sure your doctor approves of the vaccination. Some people develop low fever and muscle aches as side effects of the vaccine. Because the vaccine is grown in chicken embryos, it is not recommended for people allergic to eggs.

Amantadine and rimantadine are oral antiviral medications that may lessen your risk of contracting type A flu, but they are most effective if you begin to take them a few weeks before flu season begins or within two days after symptoms appear. Usually these drugs are prescribed for people at high risk for developing complications from flu, such as people with chronic lung disease or the elderly. If the virus has already begun to circulate in your community, a doctor may also prescribe amantadine while you are waiting for a vaccination. If so, continue taking it for two weeks after you are vaccinated to ensure that you are adequately protected while your body builds up its immune response to the vaccine. Other preventive measures you can take during flu season are to:

◆ Give up smoking—which damages your respiratory tract—and alcohol, since both substances lower your resistance to infection in general.

◆ Avoid sleeping in a room with someone who has flu; the virus is easily spread in the air.

◆ Wash your hands often to kill viruses you may have picked up by touching contaminated objects like doorknobs or phone receivers.

◆ Try to avoid crowds, and give people who are coughing or sneezing a wide berth. Airplanes are especially effective at exposing people to flu viruses because cabin air is recirculated.

◆ Stay warm and dry so that your body can fight off infection by flu and other viruses. ■

FLUID RETENTION

Read down this column to find your symptoms. Then read across.

SYMPTOMS	AILMENT/PROBLEM
◆ painless swelling of the ankles and/or feet; no other symptoms.	◆ Edema (fluid accumulating in ankles and/or feet)
◆ prominent dark blue blood vessels in the legs and feet; aching or tender legs that often swell after standing for any length of time; possibly, discolored, peeling skin or skin ulcers.	◆ Varicose veins
◆ in women, bloating; headache; painful breasts, muscle aches, irritability; anxiety; depression; anger; fatigue; insomnia; food cravings.	◆ Premenstrual syndrome (PMS), a group of symptoms related to the hormonal changes of the menstrual cycle
◆ fatigue and nausea followed by swelling in the abdomen and legs; abdominal pain; dark-colored urine; light-colored stools; yellowish, itching skin.	◆ Severe cirrhosis; substantial degeneration of the liver
◆ swelling in the hands and feet; frequent waking during the night to urinate; persistent fatigue; weight loss; elevated blood pressure; pallor; unpleasant taste in mouth.	◆ Kidney disease
◆ swelling in the feet and legs; rapid weight gain; headache; shortness of breath; little or no urination.	◆ Acute renal failure
◆ shortness of breath; fatigue; cough; swollen abdomen, legs, and ankles; rapid or irregular heartbeat; low blood pressure.	◆ Congestive heart failure (heart not pumping at full capacity, causing fluid to accumulate in other parts of the body)
◆ in pregnant women, swelling in hands and face; sudden weight gain; possibly, headache, blurred vision, confusion, irritability, and/or stomach pain.	◆ Preeclampsia, also called toxemia; a form of high blood pressure that occurs in 5 to 10 percent of all pregnancies

WHAT TO DO	OTHER INFO
◆ Elevate your feet to encourage fluids to circulate, and avoid sitting for long periods of time. If swelling is persistent, call your doctor.	◆ Causes may include weak veins in the legs, staying seated for long periods of time, and/or pregnancy.
◆ See your doctor for advice. Your treatment will depend on the severity of your problem, and will likely include over-the-counter aspirin or ibuprofen for pain.	◆ Special elastic support stockings can help minimize discomfort.
◆ See your doctor for an accurate diagnosis. Treat your symptoms as needed. (Try over-the-counter analgesics for achiness; avoid salt, and drink plenty of fluids to minimize bloating.) If PMS is debilitating, your doctor may suggest medication.	◆ If you are deficient in magnesium, zinc, or vitamin B$_6$, supplements may alleviate your symptoms.
◆ **Get emergency medical care.** You may need to stay in the hospital until your condition stabilizes.	◆ A diet of small, frequent meals with low salt, no alcohol, and as few medications as possible will minimize stress on the liver.
◆ **Get medical care immediately.** Kidney disease can be a life-threatening condition that requires emergency care.	◆ Consult your doctor before taking any drugs, including over-the-counter medications such as ibuprofen and acetaminophen, which may contribute to kidney disease.
◆ **Get emergency care immediately.** With proper treatment, the kidneys often become functional again.	◆ Causes may include the worsening of a long-term kidney disease; shock; an infection; or a reaction to drugs.
◆ **Get emergency medical care.** You may be hospitalized to stabilize your condition; treatment may include surgery, medication, changes in diet, and specific exercises. See Heart Disease.	◆ Risk of developing congestive heart failure is highest if you have existing heart disease, you smoke, or you abuse alcohol.
◆ **Get emergency medical care.** Mild cases respond well to treatment, and a full-term delivery is likely; severe situations may require an early delivery to save the baby's and the mother's lives.	◆ The elevated blood pressure of preeclampsia usually drops to normal within 24 hours of the baby's birth. If you did not have chronic high blood pressure before becoming pregnant, you'll most likely not have it after your pregnancy, either.

Read down this column to find your symptoms. Then read across.

SYMPTOMS	AILMENT/PROBLEM
◆ flushed face accompanied by fatigue, nausea, and/or headache.	◆ Most likely a result of excessive alcohol consumption
◆ flushed face; warm, dry skin; excessive thirst and hunger; possibly also frequent urination, rapid breathing, vomiting, confusion.	◆ Diabetes
◆ face flushes easily during emotional stress or during exercise; in the case of exercise, may be accompanied by a headache, possibly a migraine.	◆ A natural propensity to blush; a physiological response to exertion
◆ fatigue, dizziness, nausea, extreme sweating, and headaches followed by flushed face, hot and dry skin, and rapid but weak pulse.	◆ Heatstroke (sunstroke)
◆ flushed face accompanied by gas, belching, possibly nausea, gurgling stomach, and acidic and bitter-tasting regurgitation rising to the throat and mouth.	◆ Indigestion
◆ abnormally flushed cheeks and nose that may progress to pus-filled pimples; aggravated by spicy foods, hot drinks, or alcohol; most common in women over 30.	◆ Rosacea
◆ Flushing of the face often accompanies a high fever (104°F or above); see Fever and Chills for more information. A rosy glow in the cheeks and face is common in pregnant women.	

WHAT TO DO	OTHER INFO
◆ Avoid drinking more than one or two alcohol-based drinks per day. See Alcohol Abuse.	◆ Dilated blood vessels associated with a flushed face cause the body to lose heat more rapidly than normal and during cold weather can put you at risk for hypothermia; drinking alcohol is thus not a good way to try to warm someone up.
◆ See Diabetes.	
◆ Blushing is not a health problem, and it is also normal to flush in the face when exercising. If you are troubled by how easily you flush, consider seeing a specialist in Chinese medicine, who will focus on correcting a presumed energy imbalance between the upper and lower halves of your body. See also Headache.	◆ Some alternative practitioners associate quick flushing of the face with a disturbed physiology that could be a signal of potential health problems; you may want to consider seeing an acupuncturist or homeopath for an evaluation.
◆ Cool down with a cold shower or wet washcloths; **get medical help immediately**. See also Heatstroke in Emergencies/ First Aid.	◆ Homeopaths often suggest Belladonna as a complement to emergency care for heatstroke.
◆ Try an over-the-counter antacid or upset-stomach remedy. See Heartburn and Indigestion.	◆ Ayurvedic, herbal, and homeopathic therapies offer several viable alternatives.
◆ See Acne.	◆ If left untreated, rosacea can develop into sebaceous hyperplasia, in which enlarged oil glands create a bulbous nose. Rosacea responds particularly well to antibiotics, dietary changes, or large doses of B vitamins, especially riboflavin (vitamin B_2).

F

SYMPTOMS

Generally, food poisoning causes some combination of nausea, vomiting, and diarrhea that may or may not be bloody, sometimes with other symptoms.

- Abdominal cramps, diarrhea, and vomiting, starting from one hour to four days after eating tainted food and lasting up to four days, usually indicate **bacterial food poisoning.**
- Vomiting, diarrhea, abdominal cramps, headaches, and fever and chills, beginning from 12 to 48 hours after eating contaminated food—particularly seafood—usually indicate **viral food poisoning.**
- Vomiting, diarrhea, sweating, dizziness, tearing in the eyes, excessive salivation, mental confusion, and stomach pain, beginning about 30 minutes after eating contaminated food, are typical indications of **chemical food poisoning.**
- Partial loss of speech or vision, muscle paralysis from the head down through the body, and vomiting may indicate **botulism,** a severe but very rare type of bacterial food poisoning.

CALL YOUR DOCTOR IF:

- you recognize symptoms of **botulism.** You need immediate medical treatment for a life-threatening illness.
- you recognize symptoms of **chemical food poisoning.** You need immediate medical treatment to avoid potential damage to one or more of your vital organs. *(See also Emergencies/First Aid, page 73.)*
- the vomiting or diarrhea is severe and lasts for more than two days. You are at risk of becoming dehydrated.

You can get food poisoning after eating food contaminated by viral, bacterial, or chemical agents. Food poisoning causes mild to acute discomfort and may leave you temporarily dehydrated. Mild cases last only a few hours and at worst a day or two, but some types—such as **botulism** or certain forms of **chemical poisoning**—are severe and possibly life-threatening unless you get medical treatment.

CAUSES

Many bacteria can cause food poisoning. People who are ill or infected can transmit staph bacteria to food they are preparing. People who eat or drink contaminated food or water can get **travelers' diarrhea,** usually caused by the bacterium *E. coli.* Bacteria can contaminate poultry, eggs, and meat, causing **salmonella** poisoning; though potentially fatal, most cases cause only mild discomfort. Harmful bacteria grow in cooked and raw meat and fish, dairy products, and prepared foods left at room temperature too long; dishes made with mayonnaise are notorious culprits.

Canned goods—especially home-canned produce—can harbor a bacterium that needs no oxygen to multiply and is not destroyed by cooking. This bacterium causes **botulism,** a rare but potentially fatal food poisoning. Infants may develop botulism from eating honey because their immature digestive systems, unlike those of adults, cannot neutralize its naturally occurring bacteria.

Raw seafood—especially contaminated shellfish—may bring on **viral food poisoning.** Certain mushrooms, berries, and other plants are naturally poisonous to humans and should never be eaten; potato sprouts and eyes also contain natural toxins. Toxic mold can form on improperly stored fruit, vegetables, grains, and nuts. **Chemical food poisoning** can be caused by pesticides or by keeping food in unsanitary containers.

DIAGNOSTIC AND TEST PROCEDURES

If your symptoms are mild, you probably don't need a doctor. If symptoms last beyond two days, you may need your stool, blood, or vomited material tested to identify the cause of your illness.

Botulism is diagnosed from a description of symptoms and by tests for the bacteria in samples of blood, stool, or the suspect food. **Chemical food poisoning** can usually be diagnosed by a description of symptoms and by testing food potentially responsible for the poisoning.

TREATMENT

Vomiting and diarrhea are the body's way of flushing poison out of your system, so don't take any antiemetic or antidiarrheal medicine for 24 hours after your symptoms develop. Once you can keep fluid in your stomach, drink clear liquids for about 12 hours. Then eat bland foods like rice, cooked cereals, and clear soups for a full day.

Because repeated vomiting or diarrhea can remove large amounts of water from your system, dehydration is a potentially dangerous complication, especially in children and older adults. You must see that lost fluids are replaced promptly and completely. If you cannot keep liquids down, intravenous fluid replacement may be necessary.

CONVENTIONAL MEDICINE

If symptoms are severe or persistent, your doctor may prescribe antidiarrheal or antiemetic drugs until the condition is under control. Infants, children, elderly people, and anyone with diabetes or other chronic conditions will be monitored for dehydration and other potential complications.

If you have **botulism,** you will be hospitalized immediately. Although botulism can lead to respiratory failure and even death, prompt treatment greatly increases your chance for full recovery. If symptoms indicate **chemical poisoning,** you should have your stomach pumped out as soon as possible, or the poison could affect other organs by the time you receive treatment for the specific toxin. (See Emergencies/First Aid, page 73.)

ALTERNATIVE CHOICES

Try one or more of these alternative remedies while the body rids itself of the poison.

ACUPRESSURE

To relieve general nausea, try pressing Pericardium 6 on your inner forearm, two finger widths from the wrist crease, for one minute.

HERBAL THERAPIES

Ginger (Zingiber officinale) can be an effective remedy for nausea: Take two capsules or a cup of ginger tea every two hours as needed. An infusion of meadowsweet (Filipendula ulmaria), catnip (Nepeta cataria), or slippery elm (Ulmus fulva) may help soothe stomach and intestinal membranes: Steep 2 tsp of the herb in a cup of boiling water for 15 minutes; drink three times daily.

HOMEOPATHY

Try any of the following over-the-counter remedies in 12c potency every three to four hours until symptoms improve: Arsenicum album, Veratrum album, Nux vomica, or Podophyllum.

NUTRITION AND DIET

After symptoms subside, restore strength by eating foods like white rice, bland vegetables, and bananas. To restore essential bacteria to your digestive tract, eat plain yogurt with active Lactobacillus acidophilus cultures, or take Lactobacillus acidophilus capsules. Avoid unfermented milk products, which may be difficult to digest.

PREVENTION

◆ Always wash your hands before preparing any food; wash utensils with hot soapy water after using them to prepare any meat or fish.
◆ Don't thaw frozen meat at room temperature. Let meat thaw gradually in a refrigerator, or thaw it quickly in a microwave oven and cook immediately.
◆ Avoid uncooked marinated food and raw meat, fish, or eggs; cook all such food thoroughly.
◆ Don't eat any food that looks or smells spoiled, or any food from bulging cans or cracked jars.
◆ Set your refrigerator at 37°F; never eat cooked meat or dairy products that have been out of a refrigerator more than two hours. ■

SYMPTOMS

Gallstones most frequently make their presence known when they become lodged in one of the ducts that carry bile, a digestive juice, from the gall-bladder to the small intestine. When such an obstruction occurs, you might experience the following:

- severe and sudden pain in the upper right abdomen and possibly extending to the upper back.
- intermittent or recurring indigestion.
- fever and shivering.
- severe nausea and vomiting.
- jaundice.

CALL YOUR DOCTOR IF:

- your abdominal pain begins quite suddenly, lasts more than three hours, and is followed by a mild aching sensation in the right upper abdomen; you may have gallstones or a bile-duct infection.
- you notice jaundice; gallstones may be obstructing the bile duct, causing bile to back up into the liver and seep into your bloodstream.

Gallstones are crystal-like deposits that develop in the gallbladder—a small, pear-shaped organ that stores bile, a digestive juice produced by the liver. These deposits may be as small as a grain of sand or as large as a golf ball; they may be hard or soft, smooth or jagged. You may have several gallstones or just one.

One out of every 10 people in the United States has gallstones or will develop them at some time in life, yet most of those who have the condition do not realize it. In this case, what you don't know probably won't hurt you; gallstones that are simply floating around inside the gallbladder generally cause no symptoms and no harm. These "silent" stones usually go unnoticed unless they show up in an ultrasound examination conducted for some other reason. However, the longer a stone exists in the gallbladder, the more likely it is to become problematic. It may take as long as 25 years for a gallstone to start causing trouble.

When symptoms do occur, it's usually because the gallstone has moved and become lodged within the cystic duct, a small conduit that connects the gallbladder to another tube called the common bile duct. The typical symptom is abdominal pain, perhaps accompanied by nausea, indigestion, or fever. The pain, caused by the gallbladder's contraction against the lodged stone, generally occurs within an hour of eating a large meal or in the middle of the night. Stones can also clog the common bile duct, which carries bile into the small intestine.

Obstructions in the bile pathway can cause a duct to become inflamed and possibly infected. If the problem continues for a number of years, liver damage and possibly liver failure may result. Blockage of the common bile duct, which merges with the pancreatic duct at the small intestine, can also lead to inflammation of the pancreas (see Pancreatic Problems).

In a rare but dangerous condition that occurs most often in older women, gallstones migrate into the small intestine and block the passageway into the large intestine; symptoms include severe and frequent vomiting. Gallstone problems can also lead to cancer of the gallbladder or bile duct.

DISRUPTION OF BILE FLOW

GALLBLADDER

CYSTIC DUCT

COMMON
BILE DUCT

GALLSTONES

Crystal-like deposits called gallstones often go unnoticed if they remain in the gallbladder, which stores bile produced by the liver. But a stone that exits the gallbladder and becomes lodged in the cystic duct or the common bile duct *(above)* can cause intense pain and inflammation. Prolonged blockage can lead to infection, liver damage, or severe pancreatic problems.

Approximately a million new cases of gallstones are diagnosed in the United States each year. For reasons that are still unclear, women are four times as likely as men to be afflicted. Gallstones are also more common in people over the age of 40, in those who are obese or have lost a lot of weight in a short amount of time, and in women who have had multiple pregnancies.

CAUSES

The primary function of the gallbladder is to store bile, a brown or greenish fluid that helps the body break down fatty food. When you eat a meal, the gallbladder releases its stored bile into the cystic duct. From there the fluid passes through the common bile duct and into the small intestine.

Chief among the ingredients of bile are cholesterol and bile acids. Normally, the concentration of bile acids is high enough to break down the cholesterol in the mixture and keep it in liquid form. However, a diet high in fat can tip this delicate balance, causing the liver to produce more cholesterol than the bile acids are able to handle. As a result, some of this excess cholesterol begins to solidify into crystals, which we call gallstones. About 80 percent of all gallstones are created this way. The remaining 20 percent consist of calcium mixed with the bile pigment bilirubin.

If the liver fails to produce adequate amounts of bile acids, gallstones can form even in people who eat properly. And as researchers have found, a diet extremely low in fat can also contribute to gallstone formation: With little fatty food to digest, the gallbladder is called into play less frequently than usual, so the cholesterol has more time to solidify. Other factors that can reduce activity in the gallbladder, possibly leading to gallstone formation, include cirrhosis, the use of oral contraceptives, and pregnancy.

DIAGNOSTIC AND TEST PROCEDURES

If your symptoms suggest a gallstone-obstructed duct, your doctor might first examine your skin for jaundice, then feel your abdomen to check for tenderness. A blood test may reveal evidence of an obstruction.

Because other digestive problems, such as an infection of the duct, can produce symptoms similar to those of a gallstone attack, the doctor may also run other tests to determine if gallstones are in fact the culprit. The most common technique is an ultrasound examination. This quick, painless procedure uses high-frequency sound waves to create pictures of the gallbladder, bile duct, and their contents.

A more complicated test may be used if the doctor suspects that a gallstone is lodged in the bile duct. Commonly known by the acronym ERCP, this test allows the physician to look at the bile duct through a small flexible tube called an endoscope. The doctor sprays the back of the patient's throat with an anesthetic drug to prevent gagging, then passes the endoscope into the mouth, through the stomach, and into the area of the small intestine where the bile duct enters. Dye is injected through the tube and into the bile duct, then x-rays are taken. The procedure takes about an hour and can be done in the doctor's office.

G

TREATMENT

In most cases, treatment of gallstones is considered necessary only if they are symptomatic. Of the various conventional treatments that are available, surgical removal of the gallbladder is the most widely used. Some alternative treatments have also been found to be effective in alleviating the symptoms of troublesome gallstones.

CONVENTIONAL MEDICINE

When deciding what course of action to take for symptomatic gallstones, doctors usually choose from among three main treatment options: watchful waiting, nonsurgical therapy, and surgical removal of the gallbladder.

Watchful Waiting. While a gallstone episode can be extremely painful or frightening, almost a third of all people who experience an attack never have a recurrence. In some cases, the stone dissolves or becomes dislodged and thereby resumes its "silence." Because the problem may solve itself without intervention, many doctors take a wait-and-see approach following the initial episode.

Even when the patient has had repeated gallstone episodes, the physician may postpone treatment or surgery because of other health concerns. If your surgery has been delayed, you should remain under a doctor's care and report any recurrences of gallstone symptoms immediately.

Nonsurgical Therapy. If you are unable or unwilling to go through surgery for a gallstone problem that requires treatment, your physician may recommend one of several noninvasive techniques. Note: While these methods may destroy symptom-causing gallstones, they can do nothing to prevent others from forming.

Some gallstones can be dissolved through the use of a bile salt, although the procedure can be used only with stones formed from cholesterol and not from bile pigments. Taken as a tablet, the salt dissolves the stone by increasing the level of bile acids in the gallbladder. Depending on its size, the gallstone may take months or even years to go away. Another nonsurgical technique, shock wave therapy, uses high-frequency sound waves to fragment the stones. Bile salt is administered afterward to dissolve the small pieces.

A method called contact dissolution can also be used to dissolve gallstones. Not strictly speaking a nonsurgical therapy because it involves an incision, this procedure is less invasive than direct surgical removal of the gallbladder. The doctor inserts a catheter through the abdomen, then injects a special drug directly into the gallbladder. In many cases, the stone disappears within a few hours.

Surgical Removal of the Gallbladder. While the gallbladder serves an important function, it is not essential for a normal, healthy life. When gallstones are persistently troublesome, doctors often recommend removing the organ entirely. This operation is considered among the safest of all surgical procedures. It is also the only treatment method that eliminates the possibility that other gallstones will develop in the future.

When the gallbladder has been removed, bile flows directly from the liver into the small intestine, and this sometimes leads to digestion problems. Because bile no longer accumulates in the gallbladder, quantities of the digestive fluid cannot be stored up and used to break down an especially fatty meal. This condition is not considered serious, however, and can be corrected by simply limiting fat in the diet.

Until recently, removal of the gallbladder was done through traditional "open" surgery, which requires surgeons to make a large incision in the abdomen. Patients faced a two- or three-day hospital stay plus several weeks of recovery at home.

Today, however, the most commonly used surgical technique is a much simpler approach known as laparoscopic cholecystectomy. The doctor makes a half-inch incision in the abdomen, then uses special pencil-thin instruments to remove the gallbladder. A tiny microscope and video camera, snaked through the incision to the site, allow the physician to view the operation.

Laparoscopic surgery is highly effective and very safe. It has reduced the hospital stay to a day or two. Patients report less pain and are generally able to resume a normal lifestyle in a short period of time. However, people who are obese or who have a severe infection or inflammation in the gallbladder may still be considered candidates for traditional open surgery.

ALTERNATIVE CHOICES

Some alternative therapies, administered by a skilled practitioner, may help alleviate gallstone symptoms. Like most nonsurgical conventional treatments, however, alternative therapies do not necessarily prevent future gallstone problems.

ACUPUNCTURE

Some patients have found that acupuncture, if administered by a licensed practitioner, can relieve the pain associated with gallstones.

CHINESE HERBS

Very small gallstones may be dissolved through the ingestion of Chinese herbs such as pyrrosia leaf (Pyrrosia lingua) and rhubarb (Rheum palmatum). These herbs must be blended carefully by a skilled practitioner.

HOMEOPATHY

A number of homeopathic remedies can be used to treat gallstone-related symptoms. For acute pain, a homeopath might prescribe Dioscorea, Colocynthis, or Belladonna. Inflammation of gallbladder tissue may call for Berberis vulgaris, Hydrastis, or Chelidonium majus. You should consult a professional homeopath for exact medicine and dosages.

NUTRITION AND DIET

Depending on the severity of your condition, an improved diet may help relieve gallstone symptoms. Gallstones occur more frequently in people who are obese than in those at or near their proper weight. Though a reduction in the intake of fat may help prevent gallstones, general weight reduction seems to be the best way to avoid their development and to relieve the painful symptoms once gallstones have formed. If you are overweight, a balanced diet and exercise will help you trim down and reduce your chances of developing gallstones.

PREVENTION

A sensible diet is the best way to prevent gallstones. Seek out good sources of fiber—raw fruits and vegetables, cooked dried beans and peas, whole-grain cereals, and bran, for example—and avoid eating too much fat. A high-fiber, low-fat diet helps keep bile cholesterol in liquid form. However, don't cut out fats abruptly or eliminate them altogether, as too little fat can also result in gallstone formation.

Recent studies have found that moderate consumption of olive oil (about 2 tbsp a day) may actually lower your chances of developing gallstones. An ingredient in olive oil evidently helps reduce cholesterol levels in the blood and gallbladder. Researchers have found that the incidence of gallstones is relatively low among people who live in areas where olive oil consumption is high.

Studies suggest that lecithin—a natural substance used as a thickener in ice cream, mayonnaise, and other foods—may help prevent gallstones by keeping cholesterol from solidifying in the gallbladder. Lecithin is found in a number of foods, including soybeans, oatmeal, eggs, milk, peanuts, cabbage, and chocolate. Even though most people get plenty of lecithin in their normal diet, supplements are available in tablet or liquid form at health food shops and drugstores. Take one tablet or 1 tbsp before each meal, or follow the instructions on the label. WARNING: Over time, large amounts of choline, a chemical in lecithin, could lead to liver problems or other complications. Check with your doctor or nutritionist before taking lecithin supplements. ■

GAS AND GAS PAINS

SYMPTOMS

◆ abdominal bloating and pain.
◆ belching.
◆ flatulence (passing rectal gas).

CALL YOUR DOCTOR IF:

◆ you have persistent, unexplained bloating for more than three days; you may have a more severe abdominal disorder.
◆ you have severe abdominal pain; you may have appendicitis.
◆ you have pain in your upper right abdomen; you might have gallstones or a stomach ulcer.
◆ you are flatulent and have lower abdominal pain that decreases when you pass gas or have a bowel movement; you may have irritable bowel syndrome.
◆ you are flatulent, are losing weight, and have pale, foul bowel movements; you might have a malabsorption disorder, in which your intestines are not able to digest fat.

Gas and gas pains are a normal part of your digestive process. People may typically pass gas more than 10 times a day, but you can greatly exceed that average and still be perfectly healthy. You can usually prevent and treat gas and gas pains without professional care, but if you have other symptoms, you should consult with a doctor to find out if you have a more serious health problem.

CAUSES

When air enters your stomach, you may expel it through belching. You can take in air when you eat or drink, especially if you eat quickly. Drinking through a straw, drinking carbonated beverages, chewing gum, wearing false teeth, or swallowing air from nervous habit may also increase the amount of air that gets into your stomach.

If you eat high-fiber foods such as beans, vegetables, fruit, or grains, the partially digested cell walls of these foods will pass into your intestines, where bacteria begin a fermentation process that produces gas. If you have lactose intolerance, you do not produce enough lactase, a digestive enzyme that breaks down milk sugars, and you are more likely to produce gas after eating dairy foods. A gastrointestinal infection may also produce intestinal gas.

TREATMENT

You can usually treat gas and gas pains without the active involvement of a healthcare professional. Conventional medicine suggests decreasing excessive gas through changes in diet and use of over-the-counter preparations. Alternative medicines offer a wide variety of treatments.

CONVENTIONAL MEDICINE

A doctor will probably suggest you treat gas problems by changing what you eat. Avoid high-fiber foods like beans, milk products, alcohol, and carbonated beverages. Moderate exercise after meals can help move gas through your system more quickly. You may also decide to try over-the-counter preparations for gas pains. Simethicone, the active ingredient in most of these over-the-counter preparations, appears to help break up gas bubbles in the large intestine. Activated charcoal tablets absorb intestinal gas, but check with your doctor before using them, because they also absorb medications. If you are lactose intolerant, lactase supplements can help you to digest milk products more effectively. An over-the-counter product containing alpha-galactosidase may reduce the gas that is produced in digesting beans.

ALTERNATIVE CHOICES

There are many alternative therapies for gas problems. Most of them can be practiced at home, but you should check with a practitioner to make sure a particular therapy is suitable for your needs.

ACUPRESSURE

Pressing the following points may help to alleviate gas pains: Conception Vessel 6, Large Intestine 4, Spleen 6, and Stomach 36. *(See pages 22–23 for information on point locations.)*

ACUPUNCTURE

A practitioner can provide treatment for gas using the same points used in acupressure except for Conception Vessel 8, where heat might be applied instead.

HERBAL THERAPIES

Anise water, made by steeping 1 tsp of aniseeds in 1 cup of water for 10 minutes, may be helpful. Teas made with peppermint *(Mentha piperita),* chamomile *(Matricaria recutita),* or fennel *(Foeniculum vulgare)* may also relieve gas pains.

HOMEOPATHY

Carbo vegetabilis is the most commonly used homeopathic remedy, but Lycopodium is used as well. Nux vomica is used for gas associated with constipation, and Chamomilla is preferred for gas in infants. Talk to a homeopath about which is most suitable for you.

LIFESTYLE

Regular exercise stimulates digestion and promotes the reabsorption and expulsion of gas.

MIND/BODY MEDICINE

Biofeedback and **qigong** can relieve stress and reduce gas production.

NUTRITION AND DIET

Increase your fiber intake slowly and try avoiding beans, peas, and fermented foods such as cheese, soy sauce, and alcohol. Asafetida powder dispels intestinal gas and may be used as a spice with beans. Drink fewer carbonated drinks. Avoid mixing proteins and carbohydrates at the same meal. Do not overeat, and eat fewer different food items at one sitting. For people who are lactose intolerant, replacing cow's milk with soy milk may help.

REFLEXOLOGY

Stimulate stomach areas to encourage stomach digestion, liver area to trigger bile secretion, gallbladder area to trigger release of stored bile, intestine areas to stimulate regular contractions in both intestines, and pancreas area to encourage secretion of digestive enzymes. *(See page 25 for area locations.)*

AT-HOME REMEDIES

Dissolve a teaspoon or two of superfine white, green, or yellow French clay (available at health food stores) in water and drink at least once daily (but not with meals). The clay absorbs impurities and intestinal gas; check with your doctor to make sure it won't absorb medications you may be taking as well.

PREVENTION

One of the main methods of preventing gas and gas pains is also the primary treatment: Avoid foods that generate gas in your system. Try to become more aware of the air that you swallow; you can avoid some gas, for instance, by not gulping your food. ■

SYMPTOMS

Any of a variety of mild-to-severe stomach symptoms may indicate gastritis. The most common are:

- upper abdominal discomfort or pain.
- nausea.
- vomiting.
- diarrhea.
- loss of appetite.

CALL YOUR DOCTOR IF:

- you are vomiting blood or have bloody, black, or tarry stools; you have **internal bleeding** and need immediate medical attention. *(See page 70.)*
- stomach pain becomes severe; you may have a gastric or duodenal ulcer *(see Stomach Ulcers).*
- you have excessive thirst, a dry mouth, or decreased urination; you may be dehydrated and need fluid replacement.

Gastritis is a general medical term for inflammation of the stomach lining. Attacks of **acute gastritis,** marked by discomfort, nausea, vomiting, or diarrhea, usually last only one or two days. The term "acute" means that the attacks are short, not necessarily that the symptoms are severe. People with **chronic gastritis** may have no pain but may experience appetite loss or nausea. Chronic gastritis can lead to pernicious anemia, a deficiency in blood cells caused by a lack of vitamin B_{12}.

Gastritis occurs most often among the elderly, but it can affect anyone at any age. Self-care is often the best treatment for mild gastritis. For more-severe cases the treatment offered by your practitioner will depend on the underlying cause of the inflammation.

CAUSES

Many conditions can irritate your stomach and cause acute or chronic gastritis. Aspirin and other over-the-counter and prescription drugs may cause erosion of the stomach lining. Viral or bacterial infections, as well as ingested substances, may cause stomach inflammation.

DIAGNOSTIC AND TEST PROCEDURES

Your doctor may suspect acute gastritis from your symptoms and order tests to confirm the diagnosis. A barium x-ray, for instance, may show stomach lesions. Another possible procedure is gastroscopy, a visual examination of the stomach's interior. A confirmed diagnosis of chronic gastritis requires a biopsy.

TREATMENT

In both conventional and alternative medical practices, treatment for gastritis depends upon the type of gastritis you have. Conventional medicine uses over-the-counter antacids, prescription drugs, antibiotics, and in rare cases, surgery to treat gastritis. Both conventional and alternative practitioners frequently suggest changes in lifestyle—such as stopping smoking—that reduce your risk of developing gastritis.

CONVENTIONAL MEDICINE

For a mild case of gastritis, over-the-counter antacids are recommended. If you find these are not effective, your doctor may prescribe cimetidine, ranitidine, or famotidine, which reduce production of stomach acid. Gastritis caused by bacteria can be treated with antibiotics and with over-the-counter preparations that contain bismuth subsalicylate. Chronic gastritis can also usually be treated with over-the-counter antacids. If your stomach lining has been seriously eroded by excess stomach acid and you have internal bleeding, you may need blood transfusions and other intravenous fluids. Surgery may be needed to control the bleeding if other treatments don't work or if you have ulcers or perforations through the stomach wall.

ALTERNATIVE CHOICES

Alternative treatments focus on treating gastritis with both physical and mental techniques. Some require a practitioner's care, but you can try some at home as well.

Drugs and Gastritis

Anti-inflammatory drugs, often used for arthritis and other disorders, can irritate your stomach lining to the point that gastritis and other stomach problems develop. Aspirin and many nonsteroidal anti-inflammatory drugs (NSAIDs) like ibuprofen, naproxen, indomethacin, and tolmetin are among the drugs that can be harsh on your stomach. Avoid them if you have been diagnosed with gastritis.

ACUPRESSURE AND ACUPUNCTURE

A practitioner can treat gastritis by using many points, depending on your symptoms, or you can press the points associated with digestive system problems, such as Conception Vessel 6 and 12, Pericardium 6, Spleen 34, and Stomach 36. *(See pages 22–23 for point locations.)*

HERBAL THERAPIES

To soothe your stomach, drink a tea made of 1 tsp chamomile *(Matricaria recutita)* steeped in 1 cup boiling water for 10 minutes. Licorice *(Glycyrrhiza glabra)* extract in capsule or liquid form may also help.

HOMEOPATHY

For acute gastritis, try one of the following remedies every hour for up to four doses; if that one doesn't work, try one of the others, and if the gastritis persists, consult a homeopath for other possibilities.

◆ Burning pains and vomiting that are relieved by cold food and drinks: Phosphorus (12x).
◆ Nausea, tender stomach, and a sensation like a stone in your stomach: Bryonia (12x).
◆ A sensation like a knot in your stomach, acid reflux, hiccups, and increased discomfort after eating and drinking: Nux vomica (12x).
◆ Stomach pain that is better after eating but returns two hours later: Anacardium (12x).

NUTRITION AND DIET

Limit or eliminate alcohol, caffeine, and carbonated drinks from your diet; contrary to popular belief, though, you do not need to avoid spicy foods in particular. Eat more noncitrus fruits, cooked vegetables, and bland foods, and eat fewer refined carbohydrates such as white bread and white rice. Supplements of zinc and vitamin A may help heal the stomach lining.

AT-HOME REMEDIES

Over-the-counter antacids and acetaminophen may offer relief. Don't eat solid food on the first day gastritis develops; drink lots of water and other liquids—but not milk, which increases acid secretion—to prevent dehydration. ∎

SYMPTOMS

Gastroenteritis is also often called stomach flu or intestinal flu. Its symptoms generally last less than 48 hours. They include:
- nausea and vomiting.
- diarrhea.
- abdominal cramps and pain.
- fever.
- weakness.

CALL YOUR DOCTOR IF:

- symptoms last longer than two days, your fever is 102°F or higher, or your symptoms recur after treatment; you may have a more serious gastrointestinal disorder.
- you have mucus or blood in your stool, or are vomiting blood; this indicates internal bleeding *(see also Emergencies/First Aid)*.
- you have excessive thirst, are urinating less frequently, have a dry mouth, and feel confused; you may be dehydrated and need fluid replacement.
- you have severe pain or swelling in the abdomen; you may have appendicitis or another abdominal disorder.

Gastroenteritis is a general term that applies to many types of irritation and infection of the digestive tract. Unless you have a severe case or complications set in, you probably don't need a professional diagnosis or treatment. However, children, the elderly, and people with chronic health conditions need to be watched for complications such as dehydration.

CAUSES

Gastroenteritis may be caused by many things. The most common cause is a virus that can spread quickly through an office, school, or daycare center. Food poisoning, bacteria, and parasites also can cause gastroenteritis. Bacterial infection in the digestive tract is often responsible for travelers' diarrhea. Sometimes taking certain medications or drinking excessive amounts of alcohol can irritate your digestive tract enough to cause gastroenteritis.

DIAGNOSTIC AND TEST PROCEDURES
A doctor can usually diagnose gastroenteritis by your symptoms alone. Lab tests of your stool can show if you have a parasitic or bacterial infection.

TREATMENT

Unless you have a bacterial form of gastroenteritis, or develop complications, you probably don't need professional care. Alternative methods treat nausea, vomiting, diarrhea, and other symptoms.

CONVENTIONAL MEDICINE
If you have a simple case of gastroenteritis, your doctor will probably recommend rest, drinking lots of liquids, and eating bland foods if you can tolerate them. Over-the-counter remedies that contain bismuth subsalicylate or absorbent clays may help control diarrhea. Other drugs may be prescribed to treat severe diarrhea. If your vomiting is severe, your doctor may prescribe prochlorperazine or trimethobenzamide. If your

gastroenteritis is caused by a bacterial agent, antibiotics may also be prescribed; they may make your diarrhea worse but are necessary to kill the harmful bacteria. If you become dehydrated from vomiting and diarrhea, you may be put in the hospital to have the lost fluids replaced intravenously. This happens most frequently to infants, elderly people, and people with chronic diseases such as diabetes.

ALTERNATIVE CHOICES

Like most conventional medical treatment, alternative choices mainly offer self-help treatments for the symptoms of gastroenteritis.

ACUPRESSURE AND ACUPUNCTURE

In addition to using the acupressure techniques illustrated at right, press Pericardium 5 for vomiting and nausea (see pages 22–23 for point locations). See a practitioner for acupuncture treatment to harmonize the digestive organs.

HERBAL THERAPIES

Meadowsweet (Filipendula ulmaria) can reduce nausea and stomach acidity: Pour 1 cup boiling water on 2 tsp dried meadowsweet and steep for 15 minutes; drink three times daily. Slippery elm (Ulmus fulva) may also help calm your digestive tract when the worst symptoms have passed: Mix 1 part powdered slippery elm with 8 parts water and bring to a boil; simmer for 15 minutes, and drink half a cup three times a day.

HOMEOPATHY

If symptoms are severe, take 12x dosages of one of the following homeopathic preparations every two hours until symptoms improve. If you do not feel any better after two or three doses, try another preparation.

◆ Arsenicum album for restlessness, exhaustion, chills, thirst, vomiting, diarrhea, and burning pains.
◆ Ipecac for extreme nausea and vomiting.
◆ Nux vomica for symptoms caused by exhaustion, overeating, or drinking too much alcohol or coffee.

Acupressure on points PE 6 and ST 36 may help relieve nausea, stomach disorders, and indigestion. PE 6 is located between the two bones of the forearm, two finger widths from the center of the inner wrist crease (top). ST 36 is located four finger widths below the bottom of the kneecap on the outside of the large leg bone (bottom). Press your thumb firmly into each point and hold for one minute. Repeat on the other arm and leg; press on each point three to five times.

NUTRITION AND DIET

Drink lots of fluids. After symptoms are gone, eat live-culture yogurt with Lactobacillus acidophilus, bananas, whole-grain foods, and vegetables. These help soothe the stomach and restore protective bacteria in your digestive system. Avoid milk products for two weeks after diarrhea ends; they can cause a recurrence of diarrhea while your system readjusts to absorbing milk.

REFLEXOLOGY

Stimulate the adrenal areas to fight infection and the stomach areas to restore normal function. See page 25 for area locations.

PREVENTION

◆ Wash your hands frequently to avoid picking up or passing along germs that cause gastroenteritis.
◆ See Food Poisoning for important safeguards about preparing and storing food. ∎

SYMPTOMS

◆ numbness, tingling, or burning in the genitals.
◆ burning sensation while urinating or having intercourse.
◆ painful urination or frequent need to urinate.
◆ watery blisters in the genital area.
◆ flulike symptoms.

CALL YOUR DOCTOR IF:

◆ you have any of the symptoms listed above; your condition needs to be properly evaluated and diagnosed.

Herpes is the most common viral sexually transmitted disease in the United States, affecting more than 20 million people. The disease is both highly contagious and incurable, but it is not fatal, and you can learn to live with it.

Usually, herpes spreads only if the infected person is experiencing an outbreak of blisters. However, people can sometimes spread it even if they have no symptoms; it can also be spread through oral sex if one partner has a herpes sore on the mouth or genitals.

The first outbreak is usually the most extensive and painful, and can last from five days to three weeks. As much as 30 percent of those who have one outbreak never have another. Many people experience precursor signals several hours prior to an outbreak of blisters: pain running down the buttocks or in the knees, and/or itching in the genital area.

CAUSES

Genital herpes is caused by a virus that invades the body through tiny breaks in the skin. After symptoms disappear, the virus travels to deep nerve centers at the base of the spinal cord near the buttocks. When reactivated, the virus moves out along the nerves, resulting in a new outbreak.

People who are chronically ill or under severe stress seem to have the most attacks, and many kinds of stimuli or stress may reactivate the virus, including sunburn, sexual intercourse, and menstruation. Outbreaks may also occur in response to certain foods or medications.

TREATMENT

There is no cure for herpes, but there are ways to lessen the discomfort and speed healing.

CONVENTIONAL MEDICINE
A doctor may prescribe acyclovir, either as a pill taken orally or applied as a cream. The drug can prevent recurrences or lessen them in up to 90 percent of people who have herpes. If you are

pregnant, however, the doctor will recommend another medication, because acyclovir may cause fetal damage. Analgesics such as aspirin may lessen the pain, and drying agents such as calamine lotion may help heal the sores.

ALTERNATIVE CHOICES

There are several things you can do yourself to alleviate herpes symptoms and prevent recurrences. For example, because herpes outbreaks are often brought on by stress, the disease responds well to **relaxation** techniques. Changes in diet and vitamin supplements may also help.

ACUPRESSURE

Acupressure massage is said to relieve fatigue and tension, which may trigger outbreaks. Press the highest point of the shoulder muscle midway between the outer tip of the shoulder and the spine. Do this several times a day.

CHINESE HERBS

A doctor of Chinese medicine will prescribe a formula tailored to your needs. It may include herbs such as gentiana *(Gentiana scabra)* and dong quai *(Angelica sinensis)*.

HERBAL THERAPIES

Echinacea *(Echinacea spp.)* and garlic *(Allium sativum)* are thought to strengthen the body's defenses against viral infection. Research also suggests that glycyrrhizic acid, a constituent of licorice *(Glycyrrhiza glabra),* inactivates the herpesvirus. Drink herbal teas or take capsules as directed by your physician or an herbalist.

HOMEOPATHY

A homeopath will prescribe a specific combination of remedies that may include Rhus toxicodendron, Sepia, Natrum muriaticum, Hepar sulphuris, and Thuja occidentalis.

MIND/BODY MEDICINE

By reducing stress, you can prevent outbreaks or lessen their severity. See page 27 for descriptions of various techniques, such as **meditation,** that help relieve stress.

NUTRITION AND DIET

The herpesvirus needs the amino acid arginine to thrive; conversely, the amino acid lysine prevents it from flourishing. Avoid arginine-rich foods such as peanuts, cashews, and chocolate. Lysine-rich foods include beef, lamb, fish, milk, and cheese. You can also take 500 mg of lysine in capsule form daily to help prevent outbreaks; as soon as you notice symptoms, take 1,000 mg every four hours. In addition, vitamin E may decrease pain and speed the healing of lesions.

AT-HOME REMEDIES

◆ Apply diluted lemon juice, vitamin E, or tea tree oil (*Melaleuca* spp.) to dry up sores.
◆ Apply ice 10 minutes on, 5 minutes off to relieve pain.
◆ Use zinc sulfate ointment to heal sores.
◆ Soothe lesions with baking soda compresses.
◆ Add 3 tbsp salt to a warm bath; follow with a cold bath. Soak about 15 minutes in each.

PREVENTION

If an infected partner is having a herpes outbreak, don't have intercourse, even if you use a condom. If the infected person is symptom free, use a condom anyway; he or she may still be contagious. Don't practice oral sex if one of you has a cold sore.

C A U T I O N !

If you are pregnant and have herpes, follow your doctor's advice carefully. If you deliver your child while you're having an outbreak, you could pass the disease to the baby. In such cases, your doctor may recommend that you undergo a Cesarean section. ■

SYMPTOMS

- painless flesh-colored or grayish white growths on the vulva, anus, or penis that may develop a cauliflower-like appearance.
- growths that are itchy or mildly sore.

CALL YOUR DOCTOR IF:

- you develop any of the symptoms listed above; although genital warts are harmless, they are contagious and require medical treatment.

Genital warts (*Condylomata acuminata*) affect an estimated 10 million to 20 million Americans. As many as a million people contract genital warts each year; pregnant women and people with impaired immune systems are more susceptible than is the general population to this infection.

Sometimes what appear to be genital warts are merely accumulations of normal skin that have no medical significance; about 1 in 100 men has these. But because genital warts are contagious, you should see a doctor if you discover any such growths.

Although the warts are harmless in themselves, there appears to be some link between genital warts and cervical cancer. Several studies have shown that 90 percent of women who have cervical cancer also had genital warts. This doesn't mean cancer is inevitable, but if you have genital warts you should probably play it safe and get a Pap smear every six months.

CAUSES

Genital warts are caused by the human papilloma virus, or HPV, the same virus that causes warts on the hands, feet, and face. The virus lives inside your body's cells, where it replicates; eventually the virus breaks out of its original host cell to infect other cells.

DIAGNOSTIC AND TEST PROCEDURES

Your doctor may want to take a culture to determine whether your warts are contagious. If you are a woman and are diagnosed with warts, make sure to be tested for cervical irregularities during your regular gynecological exams. Your doctor may take a Pap smear or insert a colposcope, a device to microscopically inspect the vaginal walls and cervix for abnormal cells.

TREATMENT

Although there is no cure and no vaccine for genital warts, they are easily controlled and should in no way disrupt your life. About one-fifth of all warts disappear spontaneously within six months, and two-thirds go away after two years. Nevertheless, unlike warts on other areas of the body, genital warts should not be left untreated because they are much more contagious. And even though conventional treatments will remove the warts themselves, the virus remains in the body and may cause later outbreaks.

CONVENTIONAL MEDICINE

Don't attempt to get rid of genital warts with over-the-counter remedies. The genital area is too sensitive for these products and you could damage your skin. Instead, let your doctor remove warts with a chemical "paint" called podophyllin. Podophyllin treatment usually is effective within a few weeks. If you're pregnant, your doctor will want to use another treatment, since podophyllin may be absorbed into the bloodstream and cause fetal abnormalities. Warts may also be frozen with liquid nitrogen or solid carbon dioxide (dry ice), burned off with lasers, or surgically removed. Another treatment involves injections of interferon alpha, or Intron A. In some studies, the drug eliminated warts in half the subjects.

ALTERNATIVE CHOICES

Because genital warts are contagious, you should see a physician before exploring alternative methods to help alleviate symptoms and prevent warts from coming back.

CHINESE HERBS

A doctor of Chinese medicine will give you a unique herbal prescription to cleanse your liver and build up your immune system. Ingredients may include Chinese foxglove root *(Rehmannia glutinosa)* and gentiana *(Gentiana scabra)*.

HERBAL THERAPIES

To help heal warts, apply garlic *(Allium sativum)*, or the juice of a sour apple, a dandelion stalk, a fresh pineapple, or fresh green figs. Calendula *(Calendula officinalis)* juice and the sap of a celandine stalk applied to the area may be beneficial as well. All have properties that are therapeutic to skin conditions.

HOMEOPATHY

A homeopathic physician will prescribe a treatment to strengthen your immune system. Some homeopaths may recommend that you apply Thuja occidentalis tincture to the warts. Sabina, taken orally, is another common remedy.

MIND/BODY MEDICINE

Several studies have shown that **hypnotherapy** may be effective in reducing or eliminating warts. Ask your physician if hypnotherapy might help you. Stress may also contribute to outbreaks, so find a relaxation technique that works for you. Many forms of **meditation** and self-hypnosis can be practiced at home.

NUTRITION AND DIET

To prevent HPV infections from recurring, eat plenty of foods that contain vitamins A and C, which help the body fight off infections, and folic acid, which strengthens the immune system. Both broccoli and spinach are good sources of these nutrients.

AT-HOME REMEDIES

◆ Apply tea tree oil *(Melaleuca spp.)* to warts to help them heal.
◆ Eat a balanced diet with plenty of fruits and vegetables.
◆ Meditate regularly. Try listening to guided meditation cassettes.

PREVENTION

The best way to prevent genital warts is to use condoms. If your partner discovers a wart, insist that he or she see a doctor, and if the warts prove to be venereal, get tested yourself—even if you have no symptoms.　■

SYMPTOMS

A child with German measles may not look or act sick, but symptoms may include:

- a low-grade fever and swollen glands behind the ears and at the back and sides of the neck.
- loss of appetite, irritability, loss of interest in personal care.
- in an older child or teenager, joint pain.

A rash appears in only about half the cases of German measles. When it does appear, it starts on the face and torso and spreads to the arms and legs. Over the course of about four days, the rash fades. See also the Visual Diagnostic Guide.

CALL YOUR DOCTOR IF:

- you are pregnant and you think you have been exposed to German measles; the virus can pass from you through the umbilical cord to your unborn child, possibly causing birth defects.
- your child has German measles and is having trouble staying fully awake or is extremely lethargic. This may indicate encephalitis, a rare complication.
- your child has German measles and has abdominal pain accompanied by vomiting; these are possible symptoms of pancreatic or liver inflammation.

German measles, or rubella, is a mild illness, in many cases no more uncomfortable for your child than a cold. People who have had German measles once develop a lifetime immunity.

The danger of German measles is to the unborn child, especially during the first trimester. A pregnant woman who contracts German measles runs a 20 percent to 50 percent risk of bearing a child with birth defects, including blindness, deafness, and congenital heart defects. Before becoming pregnant, a woman should confirm that she is protected *(see Prevention, opposite)*.

Many states require children to be immunized before entering public school *(see page 33)*.

CAUSES

German measles is caused by a virus and transmitted by droplets from a sneeze or cough. The incubation period—when the virus multiplies and the child is not contagious—is 14 to 21 days from exposure. Infected children are contagious from 2 days before to 7 days after any rash is visible.

TREATMENT

Your child should stay at home while sick or up to a week after any rash disappears.

CONVENTIONAL MEDICINE

No medical treatment of a child with German measles is required. If you are pregnant and are exposed to rubella, you should contact your doctor immediately. The risk of birth defects is higher the earlier in your pregnancy the exposure occurs, and in some cases your doctor may advise you to consider a therapeutic termination of your pregnancy. However, after the 20th week of your pregnancy the risk of a defect being caused by exposure to German measles drops to zero.

ALTERNATIVE CHOICES

Many alternative practitioners believe it is better for an otherwise healthy child to contract Ger-

The first signs of German measles are fever and swollen glands in the neck. In about half of all cases, tiny, pinkish spots develop on the face and trunk two or three days later *(right)*. Unlike measles, the spots do not merge into a solid, uniform rash.

After several days the rash on the face subsides, and the spots spread to the arms and legs. They last up to five days and do not itch.

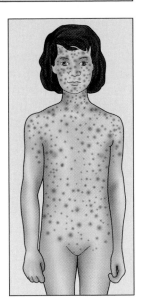

man measles than to be vaccinated, because immunity is then permanent. However, since an infected child can pass the disease to others at risk, especially pregnant women, you should seriously consider immunization.

HOMEOPATHY
Always consult a homeopathic physician for appropriate dosages and remedies for children. Belladonna, Pulsatilla, and Phytolacca are three remedies often prescribed; the choice depends on your child's symptoms and temperament.

OSTEOPATHY
Gentle, rhythmic pressure applied over the spleen, a procedure known as spleen pumping, may enhance the release of white blood cells into the blood. Seek help from an osteopath.

AT-HOME CARE
◆ Keep your child quiet, especially if she has a fever; confinement to bed is not necessary. Children should be kept home while any rash is visible and for a week thereafter.

◆ Cool sponging will help relieve fever and discomfort from a rash. An acetaminophen-based pain reliever may also help.

PREVENTION

Immunization of children as a protection to others is strongly recommended by most healthcare practitioners, but be aware that vaccination does not always provide lifetime immunity. The homeopathic version is not an accepted equivalent and will not provide adequate protection.

The MMR (measles, mumps, and rubella vaccine) is now given at 12 or 15 months, with a booster at the age of 4 to 6 or 10 to 12. If a household member is pregnant and there is any question of her not being immune, your doctor will recommend delaying immunization of your children to prevent exposing the mother-to-be to the live, though weakened, virus in the vaccine.

At least three months before trying to become pregnant, a woman should have a blood test to see if the rubella antibodies are present; if not, she should be immunized or reimmunized.

PREGNANCY CONCERNS
If you are pregnant, are not sure of your immunity to rubella, and suspect you have been exposed, contact your doctor immediately, because the virus can pass to your unborn child. If your child has German measles, notify any at-risk individuals who have had contact with your child during the illness and up to 10 days before symptoms appeared, so they can seek appropriate care.

C A U T I O N !
Never give a child aspirin—even baby aspirin—or other products containing the salt called salicylate to reduce a fever or to relieve pain. Aspirin has been linked to Reye's syndrome, a rare but very dangerous illness that causes inflammation of the liver and brain. ■

SYMPTOMS

- Teary, aching eyes, blurred vision, occasional headaches, and progressive loss of peripheral vision are signs of **chronic glaucoma.**
- A sudden onset of severe throbbing pain, headaches, blurred vision, rainbow halos around lights, redness in the eye, dilated pupils, and sometimes nausea and vomiting are signs of **acute glaucoma.**
- Blurred vision, headaches, and halos around lights following an eye injury are signs of **secondary glaucoma.**
- In infants, teary or cloudy eyes, unusual sensitivity to light, and enlarged corneas are signs of **congenital glaucoma.**

CALL YOUR DOCTOR IF:

- you have symptoms of **acute glaucoma.** You need immediate medical attention to prevent potentially permanent eye damage or blindness.
- you become drowsy, fatigued, or short of breath after using eye drops containing beta-adrenergic blockers such as timolol, betaxolol, or bunolol. The medication may be aggravating a heart or lung problem.
- you are prescribed drugs for other ailments. Many medications, especially those used to treat stomach and intestinal disorders, may aggravate glaucoma.

More than two million adult Americans suffer from glaucoma, making it one of the leading causes of blindness. **Chronic glaucoma,** which accounts for 90 percent of cases in the United States, usually appears in middle age and seems to have a genetic component: 1 out of 5 sufferers has a close relative with the condition. Doctors often refer to **chronic glaucoma** as the "sneak thief in the night" because it comes on gradually to steal your vision. It may be well established before you notice the warning signs: You have headaches, you need new glasses, you start losing side vision, and eventually you develop blank spots where you can't see anything.

Other forms of glaucoma are less common but no less serious. If you have sudden, severe pain in the eyes, blurred vision, and dilated pupils—sometimes with nausea or vomiting—it may be an attack of **acute,** or **narrow-angle, glaucoma.** This type accounts for less than 10 percent of reported cases, but it comes on quickly and requires urgent medical attention. If left untreated, it can irreversibly damage the optic nerve, which carries visual images from the eye to the brain, causing blindness—sometimes in a matter of days.

Secondary glaucoma is usually associated with another eye disease or disorder, such as an enlarged cataract, uveitis (an inner-eye inflammation), an eye tumor, or an eye injury. People suffering from diabetes are also susceptible to **neovascular glaucoma,** a particularly severe form of the disease. **Congenital glaucoma** is an extremely rare, inborn condition affecting babies; 80 percent of cases occur by the age of one.

CAUSES

The eye's lens, iris, and cornea are continuously bathed and nourished by a water-based fluid called aqueous humor. As new fluid is produced by cells inside the eye, excess fluid normally drains out through a complex network of tissue called the drainage angle, where the cornea and iris meet *(illustration above, right).* An imbalance between the rate of production of aqueous humor and the rate of drainage will bring on **chronic,** or **open-angle, glaucoma.** This is the most

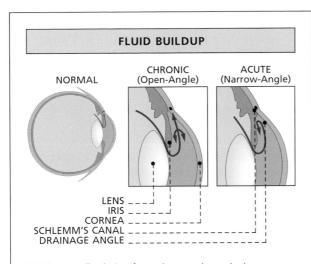

FLUID BUILDUP

NORMAL CHRONIC (Open-Angle) ACUTE (Narrow-Angle)

LENS
IRIS
CORNEA
SCHLEMM'S CANAL
DRAINAGE ANGLE

Fluid normally drains from the eye through the drainage angle—located between the cornea and the iris—and out through the tiny Schlemm's canal. **Chronic,** or **open-angle, glaucoma** *(inset, left)* occurs when fluid is produced faster than it can drain out. **Acute,** or **narrow-angle, glaucoma** *(inset, right)* occurs when the iris blocks the drainage angle.

prevalent form of the ailment and generally develops slowly with age.

Some people apparently inherit a condition of the inner eye in which the iris can block normal drainage channels. When this happens, the fluid does not drain out of the eye fast enough, and the sudden pressure from fluid buildup causes **acute glaucoma.** In newborns, defects in the drainage angle are the cause of **congenital glaucoma.** Both conditions need prompt medical attention to prevent potential loss of sight.

Depending on the individual, the onset of glaucoma may be related to gradual changes in drainage-angle tissue, increased fluid production, or a congenital abnormality. Whatever the specific cause, the effect is the same: The increase in pressure from excess fluid damages the optic nerve, which relays visual messages to the brain. As the optic nerve deteriorates, your field of vision narrows and you have difficulty discerning things at either side. If nerve damage continues, it can affect your central vision and lead ultimately to total blindness.

Researchers are not certain what triggers these abnormalities, but they do know some things that may induce or aggravate them. Using certain antidepressants, antihypertensives, and steroids for a long period may increase pressure within the eye. A change in the body's collagen metabolism may also contribute to glaucoma. Collagen, one of the most abundant proteins in the body, plays an integral role in maintaining the strength and utility of your eye tissue. Corticosteroid eye drops, sometimes prescribed for other eye disorders, are thought to destroy collagen balance in certain situations *(see Eye Problems and Vision Problems).* Stress and allergies may aggravate symptoms of chronic glaucoma.

DIAGNOSTIC AND TEST PROCEDURES

Procedures for glaucoma screening are brief and painless. Your optometrist will routinely measure your inner-eye pressure with an air-puff tonometer; an ophthalmologist may use a more sensitive instrument called an applanation tonometer. But the mere presence of higher-than-normal pressure within the eye does not mean that you have glaucoma: Slight pressure in your eye without evidence of damage to your optic nerve is called **ocular hypertension.** In most cases, this condition calls only for repeat testing at regular intervals to check for early signs of nerve damage.

If glaucoma is suspected, your ophthalmologist may dilate your eyes and examine the optic nerve with a hand-held ophthalmoscope. You should have a visual field test, which measures your peripheral, or side, vision.

Congenital glaucoma is difficult to diagnose because a child under a year old cannot describe the symptoms. If the cornea in your child's eye appears cloudy, a congenital condition may be present. Babies are routinely checked for the disorder at birth, but if you suspect congenital glaucoma, see a pediatric ophthalmologist at once.

TREATMENT

Treatment of glaucoma requires measures to control the flow and drainage of aqueous humor in the eye, restoring the normal balance of inner-eye pressure. **Chronic glaucoma** may not be noticed until it has progressed to a relatively advanced stage, but it can usually be controlled. Both medical and surgical approaches have high rates of success in treating **chronic glaucoma,** but you can help yourself by relieving stress and maintaining collagen production. **Acute glaucoma** is different: If the pressure of excess fluid in the eye is not relieved quickly, the result can be blindness.

CONVENTIONAL MEDICINE

Appropriate therapy depends on the nature and stage of the ailment. Your ophthalmologist may not prescribe any therapy for **ocular hypertension** when the pressure in your eye is minimal; periodic evaluation with close monitoring of your peripheral vision and of the appearance of the optic nerve may be sufficient.

Chronic glaucoma is typically managed with eye drops. Those that contain epinephrine or pilocarpine help increase fluid outflow but may have undesirable side effects: Pilocarpine may cause headaches and blurred vision; epinephrine may cause excessively red, teary eyes and in rare cases may aggravate heart problems. Eye drops containing beta-adrenergic blockers such as timolol, betaxolol, and bunolol may have heart or lung side effects. Oral carbonic anhydrase inhibitors help decrease fluid production but may cause stomach upset or tingling hands and feet. Because of potential drug interactions, your ophthalmologist should know before prescribing eye drops about any other medications you take.

If your chronic glaucoma does not respond to medication, or if you cannot tolerate the side effects, your doctor may recommend one of several surgical techniques:

◆ Trabeculoplasty creates 50 to 100 small laser burns at the drainage angle, where the iris and cornea meet, increasing the outflow rate of aqueous fluid. This relatively brief procedure can be done in an ophthalmologist's office.
◆ Trabeculectomy creates an artificial channel for fluid outflow in advanced cases in which the inner-eye pressure is high and the optic nerve continues to be damaged. Results vary, but generally the success rate is high.

When glaucoma is unresponsive to surgery or when the risks of a surgical procedure are too high, other options are available to destroy the cells that produce too much aqueous fluid: Ultrasound treatment uses high-frequency sound waves, diathermy uses heat, and cryosurgery uses a freezing process.

Many medications, especially those used to treat stomach and intestinal disorders, may aggravate your glaucoma by actually increasing inner-eye pressure. Always make sure your physician and ophthalmologist are each aware of what the other prescribes for you.

ALTERNATIVE CHOICES

Alternative approaches to treating glaucoma emphasize prevention and good eye maintenance. Natural remedies may help keep glaucoma at bay or—if you are already under a doctor's care—may complement conventional treatment. Some therapies seek to relieve stress in order to control inner-eye pressure. Herbal and dietary applications attempt to maintain collagen balance and replenish any nutrient deficiencies.

ACUPUNCTURE
Performed in conjunction with herbal therapy and a nutritious diet, acupuncture may help relieve tension and reduce pressure in the eye. The acupuncturist will concentrate on points along the bladder, gallbladder, liver, and kidney meridians. *(See pages 22–23 for point locations.)*

BODY WORK
According to **reflexology** therapists, the nerve endings where your toes meet the rest of your foot influence the nerves in your visual system. Therapeutic **massage** and manipulation of your foot in this area relieve stress and tension, which may help reduce eye pressure.

HERBAL THERAPIES
A variety of herbs have properties that address the factors contributing to glaucoma.
◆ Bilberry *(Vaccinium myrtillus)*—or its American equivalent, huckleberry—helps maintain collagen balance and prevents the breakdown of vitamin C. Eat 2 to 4 oz three times a day

whenever the fresh berries are available.

◆ *Cannabis sativa,* also known as marijuana, contains the chemical compound tetrahydrocannabinol (THC). Clinical studies have demonstrated that it reduces the inner-eye pressure that causes glaucoma. Though a controlled substance, cannabis can be prescribed by a licensed professional to treat glaucoma.

MIND/BODY MEDICINE

Eye exercises may relieve stress and eyestrain caused by overworked eyes and many eye problems, including glaucoma. *(See Vision Problems.)*

Hydrotherapy may be used to stimulate circulation in the eye. Soak a cloth in hot water, wring it out, and place it on your eyes for up to three minutes. Then do the same with a cold compress, and alternate each compress three times.

NUTRITION AND DIET

Studies suggest that vitamin C lowers inner-eye pressure and restores collagen balance, making it especially useful if you are unresponsive to oral medications or eye drops. Foods high in vitamin C include cauliflower, broccoli, turnip greens, strawberries, grapefruits, and oranges. Alternatively, take up to 3,000 mg of a vitamin C supplement daily. Chromium and zinc may also deter glaucoma, as most people with the disease exhibit deficiencies of these minerals, as well as of thiamine (vitamin B_1).

When used in conjunction with traditional drug therapies, rutin is said to reduce inner-eye pressure and restore collagen balance. It can be found in supplement form in varying strengths at health food stores. See the product label or ask your doctor for appropriate dosages.

It is important to identify and avoid any foods and other substances you may be allergic to, since an allergic reaction may induce excess pressure within the eye.

AT-HOME REMEDIES

Early detection is crucial. Only an ophthalmologist can diagnose the condition, but you must be aware of the warning signs. So if you sense that your vision is deteriorating—especially if you are

▼ RISK FACTORS

The following factors increase the risk of developing glaucoma. If one or more apply to you, have your eyes examined annually.

◆ *Chronic glaucoma usually develops after the age of 40.*

◆ *Diabetics are three times as likely to develop glaucoma as are non-diabetics. Neovascular glaucoma, a severe form of the disease, is linked to diabetes.*

◆ *High blood pressure, migraine headaches, and nearsightedness are associated with the onset of glaucoma.*

◆ *Glaucoma is sometimes inherited, although a person may have a genetic predisposition to the disorder without developing it.*

◆ *African Americans develop glaucoma-induced blindness at a rate several times higher than that of Caucasians. Researchers have yet to find the reason for a greater incidence of glaucoma in certain racial groups.*

over 40—a complete eye examination is a must.

If you are already near- or farsighted, a balanced diet and eye exercises may be effective preventive measures against glaucoma. If you have diabetes or high blood pressure, you should diligently stick to your prescribed treatment to reduce the inherent risk of developing glaucoma. Once you have been diagnosed with glaucoma, however, you can expect to remain under the regular care of your physician or ophthalmologist. Although you may have to use eye drops for the rest of your life, you can use some of the alternative treatments listed above to complement your professional medical care. ■

GOITER

SYMPTOMS

- swelling at the base of the neck, ranging from a small lump to a general enlargement (see illustration opposite).
- If you have **hyperthyroidism** (an overactive thyroid gland), you may also experience weight loss despite an increased appetite, an increased heart rate, elevated blood pressure, nervousness, diarrhea, muscle weakness, and hand tremors.
- If you have **hypothyroidism** (an underactive thyroid gland), you may also experience lethargy, slowed physical and mental functions, depression, a lower heart rate, an intolerance to cold, constipation, easy weight gain, and tingling or numbness in your hands.

CALL YOUR DOCTOR IF:

- you have a large goiter and experience dizziness, hoarseness, or difficulty in swallowing; the goiter may be pressing on your jugular vein, windpipe, esophagus, or the nerve that runs to your larynx. The growth requires treatment and may need to be surgically removed.

Goiters can be any one of several types of growths in the thyroid gland, located at the base of the neck. In the case of Graves' disease, the entire thyroid gland becomes enlarged. Another type, called **nodular goiter,** results when one or more nodules, or adenomas, develop in the thyroid and trigger excess production of thyroid hormone. A goiter may be a temporary problem that will remedy itself over time without medical intervention, or a symptom of another, possibly severe, thyroid condition that requires medical attention (see Thyroid Problems).

CAUSES

Goiters can occur when the thyroid gland produces either too much thyroid hormone **(hyperthyroidism)** or not enough **(hypothyroidism).** The problem may arise when the pituitary gland stimulates thyroid growth to boost production of the hormone. But most goiters are caused by insufficient iodide, a key ingredient in the manufacture of thyroid hormone. To make up for the resulting shortfall of the hormone, the gland begins to grow. Sometimes a slight swelling is enough to correct the problem, but if the goiter interferes with breathing, it must be treated or removed.

Another type of thyroid growth, called a **sporadic goiter,** can form if your diet includes too many goitrogenic (goiter-promoting) foods, such as soybeans, rutabagas, cabbage, peaches, peanuts, and spinach. These foods can suppress the manufacture of thyroid hormone by interfering with your thyroid's ability to process iodide. Drugs such as iodides, propylthiouracil, and phenylbutazone may have the same effect.

DIAGNOSTIC AND TEST PROCEDURES

A goiter may be large enough for you to see or to feel with your hand, or it may remain unnoticed until a physician discovers it, perhaps during a routine exam. In any case, the first step is to determine whether the goiter is a symptom of another thyroid condition. Radioactive iodide uptake tests track how much iodide the thyroid takes in within a certain time period. Higher-than-normal

404

NORMAL THYROID GLAND

ENLARGED THYROID GLAND

cancerous, the entire thyroid gland may have to be surgically removed.

ALTERNATIVE CHOICES

Alternative therapies treat goiters by attempting to boost production of thyroid hormone and correct the body's chemical imbalance.

CHINESE HERBS

Notoginseng root *(Panax notoginseng)* and tang-kuei formula may help reduce the size of a goiter. Consult a practitioner for appropriate dosages.

HERBAL THERAPIES

To improve an underactive-thyroid condition, try bladder wrack *(Fucus vesiculosus)* three times a day. Take it in tablet form or as an infusion, which is prepared by steeping 2 to 3 tsp dried bladder wrack in 1 cup boiling water for 10 minutes.

amounts indicate possible **hyperthyroidism;** low levels indicate **hypothyroidism.** Blood tests also can measure levels of thyroid hormone.

TREATMENT

A goiter may require no treatment, especially if it is small and has succeeded in boosting production of thyroid hormone. However, if the goiter develops because of excessive thyroid hormone production, fails to produce enough hormone, or causes discomfort, you should seek medical help.

CONVENTIONAL MEDICINE

If your goiter requires treatment, supplementary iodide or a synthetic hormone such as levothyroxine may stop the pituitary gland from secreting the excess hormone that is causing the goiter to grow. When the medication takes effect, the thyroid will begin to return to its normal size. However, a large **nodular goiter** with a lot of internal scar tissue will not shrink with hormone treatment. If the goiter is uncomfortable, causes overproduction of thyroid hormone, or becomes

A PINCH OF PREVENTION

Dietary supplements of iodide, which the body uses to make thyroid hormone, have proved to be an effective weapon in the war against goiters. People who live in coastal areas usually get plenty of iodide from their food and drinking water—even from ocean mists. But in mountainous or inland regions, the amount of available iodide is normally very low. In the United States the incidence of goiters dropped dramatically after manufacturers began adding iodide to table salt in 1924. In fact, no cases of iodide deficiency have been reported in the U.S. since 1970. By contrast, in developing countries—such as India—that have not implemented iodide supplements, goiters remain a common medical complaint. ∎

SYMPTOMS

- a puslike urethral discharge that may be yellowish, cloudy, green, white, or bloodstained.
- frequent need to urinate.
- burning sensation while urinating.
- severe pelvic and lower abdominal pain.
- constant urge to move bowels **(anal gonorrhea).**
- nausea, vomiting, fever, chills.
- pain during intercourse.
- reddened, irritated tip of penis.
- severe sore throat, pain on swallowing **(pharyngeal gonorrhea).**

CALL YOUR DOCTOR IF:

- you have any of the above symptoms. Gonorrhea is a serious contagious disease that can lead to severe complications.

Incidents of gonorrhea—a bacterial infection of the genitourinary tract and, occasionally, the rectum, pharynx, and eyes—are on the rise in the United States, especially among teenagers and young adults. Approximately 2.5 million cases of gonorrhea are reported annually.

If you're a woman and you have gonorrhea, there's a good chance you won't know it; women often experience no symptoms until the infection has done serious damage. On the other hand, 95 percent of men develop symptoms within days or weeks. If your partner has symptoms, both of you should see a doctor and seek treatment. Because the disease is so contagious, doctors must report cases of gonorrhea to local public-health officials; you should be prepared to answer questions concerning your recent sexual contacts.

Left untreated, gonorrhea may spread and damage the heart or cause gonococcal arthritis. In men, it can lead to prostatitis, urethritis *(see Prostate Problems and Urinary Problems),* or epididymitis, an inflammation of the scrotal tubes. In women, the infection may spread to the uterus and fallopian tubes, causing pelvic inflammatory disease, which may result in scarring of the tubes and sterility.

Even if you have no symptoms, you should ask your doctor to perform a gonorrhea test once a year. This is especially important for women who are pregnant or plan to be; newborns may be permanently blinded as a result of exposure to the organism during birth.

CAUSES

Gonorrhea is caused by a bacterium called *Neisseria gonorrhoeae,* which is transmitted sexually.

DIAGNOSTIC AND TEST PROCEDURES

Your gynecologist may discover gonorrhea during a routine pelvic exam if your cervix is red or there is a discharge coming from the center of it. The doctor will culture any discharge from the infected area—cervix, urethra, pharynx, or rectum—and may examine the sample under a microscope after it is stained with a special dye.

TREATMENT

Because gonorrhea is a contagious disease with serious consequences, you must seek conventional medical treatment first.

CONVENTIONAL MEDICINE

Your doctor will prescribe analgesics to relieve pain, as well as antibiotics such as ceftriaxone, doxycycline, ampicillin, or erythromycin to kill the bacteria. Because of the advent of newer, drug-resistant strains, the doctor may also treat you with probenecid, a drug that enables antibiotics to remain active longer in your system. If the infection has spread to other organs, you may be treated with amoxicillin.

ALTERNATIVE CHOICES

In addition to conventional treatment, a number of alternative therapies may speed healing.

ACUPRESSURE

In Chinese medicine, a white discharge is said to be due to lack of chi, or energy. To cleanse your system and build up energy, try massaging acupressure points Liver 3, on top of the foot between the big and second toes, and Liver 8, on the inside of the leg above the knee. Also try kneading Kidney 3, on the inside of the leg between the anklebone and the Achilles tendon. *(See pages 22–23 for more information about point locations.)*

CHINESE HERBS

To cleanse your system, a doctor of Chinese medicine may prescribe an herbal formula tailored to your body's needs. This might include gentiana *(Gentiana scabra)*, Chinese foxglove root *(Rehmannia glutinosa)*, dong quai *(Angelica sinensis)*, bupleurum *(Bupleurum chinense)*, and licorice *(Glycyrrhiza uralensis)*. Herbs such as coptis *(Coptis chinensis)* are considered helpful in strengthening the urinary and reproductive systems, especially when pelvic inflammatory disease is a complication.

HERBAL THERAPIES

Calendula *(Calendula officinalis)*, myrrh *(Commiphora molmol)*, and thuja *(Thuja occidentalis)* may reduce the inflammation and discharge that accompany gonorrhea; use these herbs as a tea or douche. Pipsissewa *(Chimaphila umbellata)*, a woodland wildflower once used to flavor soft drinks, may also help, as could uva ursi *(Arctostaphylos uva-ursi)*, goldenseal *(Hydrastis canadensis)*, and burdock *(Arctium lappa)*.

HOMEOPATHY

A homeopathic physician may want to attack the gonorrhea bacteria with antibiotics and then prescribe a remedy to strengthen your immune system and prevent recurrences.

NUTRITION AND DIET

If your doctor approves, try fasting for one to three days to clean out your system. Drink the juices of pomegranate and cranberry or a mixture of celery, parsley, and cucumber to flush out toxins from the urinary tract. Because antibiotics destroy beneficial intestinal bacteria as well as pathogenic kinds, eat yogurt containing live cultures or take acidophilus supplements.

AT-HOME REMEDIES

◆ Take hot baths to help reduce pain and inflammation.
◆ Eat a balanced diet, including live-culture yogurt.
◆ Supplement antibiotic therapy with the herbs listed above.
◆ Use ice packs to reduce abdominal pain.
◆ Apply moist heat to infected joints to ease the pain of gonococcal arthritis.

PREVENTION

Always use a condom. If your partner develops symptoms, both of you should be tested and treated by a doctor. ■

- sudden, intense pain in a joint, typically the big toe or ankle, sometimes the knee.
- swelling, inflammation, and a feeling that the joint is very hot.
- in extreme cases, alternating chills and fever.
- usually strikes unexpectedly and may recur, but the symptoms typically do not last more than a week.

CALL YOUR DOCTOR IF:

- severe pain in a joint recurs or lasts more than a few days, especially if the pain is accompanied by chills or fever; you may be experiencing the early signs of rheumatoid arthritis or, in rare cases, lead poisoning.
- symptoms of gout increase or other side effects occur while you are taking allopurinol to reduce uric acid production or colchicine to relieve pain; these drugs may be interacting adversely with other medication.

Without warning and, for some reason, in the middle of the night, it strikes—an intense pain in a joint, most often the big toe, but sometimes other joints, including knees, elbows, thumbs or fingers. Attacks of gout can be unexpected and excruciatingly painful. With prompt treatment, the pain and inflammation disappear after a few days, but they may recur at any time.

Nine out of ten gout sufferers are middle-aged men, and about half of them have a hereditary predisposition to the ailment. Gout is uncommon in women and very rare in children. Men who are overweight or suffering from high blood pressure are particularly prone to gout—especially if they are taking thiazide diuretics to lower the body's water retention.

Gout is actually a form of arthritis; specifically, it is the body's reaction to irritating crystalline deposits in the space between the bones in a joint. In spite of the extreme pain at onset, gout responds well to prompt treatment; mild cases may be controlled by diet alone. Chronic attacks of gout, however, may require long-term medication to prevent damage to bone and cartilage, as well as deterioration of the kidneys because of excess uric acid production.

Chronic gout sufferers may feel tiny, hard lumps accumulating over time in the soft flesh of the hands, feet, or earlobes. These harmless deposits, called tophi, are concentrations of uric acid crystals that can eventually cause aching, stiffness, and protrusions. If similar deposits form in the kidneys, they can lead to painful and potentially dangerous kidney stones.

CAUSES

Gout is brought on by an excessively high level of uric acid in the blood. Uric acid is essential to the digestive process, and the excess is filtered through the kidneys and eliminated in urine. If the body produces too much uric acid or fails to excrete it, crystals of sodium urate become concentrated in the joints and tendons, causing inflammation, pressure, and severe pain.

Although the precise mechanism that causes

gout to develop is unknown, the disorder is often associated with an injury or surgical procedure, periods of stress, or reactions to alcohol and certain drugs, including antibiotics. Gout may also occur in the presence of some tumors or cancers. Research shows a relation between gout and kidney disorders, enzyme deficiencies, and lead poisoning. Gout may also accompany psoriasis or anemia. Susceptibility to gout can be inherited, and repeat attacks are common if the body's uric acid level is not kept under control.

Pseudogout, or false gout, is a similar but generally less painful condition caused by calcium crystals in the joints. More common after age 60 in both sexes, pseudogout is treated with anti-inflammatory agents or, in severe cases, surgery followed by cortisone injections.

DIAGNOSTIC AND TEST PROCEDURES

Because other diseases may masquerade as gout, it is important to see a physician for an accurate diagnosis of any kind of joint pain.

Blood and urine tests may or may not be useful diagnostic tools, since you can have a high level of uric acid without having gout, or the level may appear normal after an attack. To confirm the presence of uric acid crystals in persistent cases, a specialist may take x-rays or draw fluid from the synovial sac that cushions the joint.

TREATMENT

Anyone who experiences a gout attack quickly realizes that the first order of business is to ease the pain. Clothing or other covering only aggravates the discomfort of the swollen, sensitive joint, so most doctors advise keeping the foot or affected extremity bare, even when sleeping. The next stage of treatment will be an oral pain-killer, typically a nonsteroidal anti-inflammatory drug (NSAID).

After the initial discomfort is relieved, the answer to controlling gout is keeping the body's level of uric acid in balance.

Even without conventional or alternative treatment to relieve pain and inflammation, the

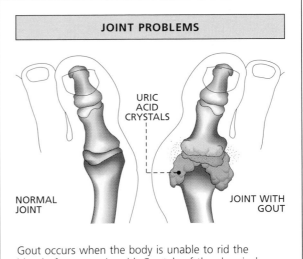

JOINT PROBLEMS

URIC ACID CRYSTALS

NORMAL JOINT

JOINT WITH GOUT

Gout occurs when the body is unable to rid the blood of excess uric acid. Crystals of the chemical accumulate between the bones of certain joints, most commonly in the big toe. The result can be sudden and severe pain, inflammation, and in severe cases, joint deformity.

immediate symptoms of gout will disappear in a few days or a week. Nonetheless, all incidents of suspected gout should be diagnosed and treated by a physician. Left untreated, uric acid deposits can eventually cause irreversible damage to the kidneys and other tissues.

CONVENTIONAL MEDICINE

Many doctors recommend oral doses of ibuprofen, available in both prescription and nonprescription versions, or other anti-inflammatory agents. Low doses of aspirin, which may have been recommended for other conditions, should be discontinued, as it can slow the elimination of uric acid.

Corticosteroid injections in the affected joint may be helpful in reducing pain and inflammation in severe attacks or chronic cases. However, steroids such as hydrocortisone can have undesirable side effects in some patients and must always be administered by a licensed specialist. (See also Bursitis.)

The standard treatment favored by many physicians to treat acute or chronic gout attacks consists of the anti-inflammatory agent col-

G

GOUT ATTACKS

Although gout is most likely to strike the big toe, the disorder can also affect other joints, including the elbows, hands, and knees. Recurrent attacks of gout may affect several areas at once.

chicine, a medication that has been in use for centuries. CAUTION: Colchicine may cause adverse side effects or interact with a number of antidepressants, tranquilizers, or antihistamines; it should not be taken by pregnant women because of the risk of birth defects.

Your physician will probably recommend that you cut out certain protein-rich foods, especially those high in purines, chemicals essential for the body's production of uric acid. These foods include organ meats, shellfish, fatty fish, asparagus, spinach, and most dried beans. Although you should drink plenty of liquids, you should avoid alcohol, which retards the elimination of uric acid. Obese patients may be put on an even stricter regimen.

Keeping the body's level of uric acid in balance can be done through the diet and, if necessary, by one of several drugs, such as allopurinol, that reduce the body's production of uric acid. Allopurinol may cause rashes, drowsiness, and disorientation, and it can have adverse reactions with other medications, particularly anticoagulants and diuretics.

To encourage excretion of excess uric acid in the long term, the drugs of choice are probenecid and sulfinpyrazone. But like other medications used to combat gout, they may cause adverse interactions with other drugs or complications with existing ailments such as blood disorders, ulcers, and kidney problems.

In many cases, prompt treatment with appropriate drugs solves the problem permanently. Since recurring attacks are possible, however, chronic sufferers may have to remain on low-level drug therapy for extended periods, sometimes for life.

ALTERNATIVE CHOICES

Nonconventional approaches to treating gout begin with reducing the immediate pain and inflammation, then continue with therapies to control excessive uric acid production.

ACUPRESSURE

Among recommended acupressure points for relieving the pain of a gouty toe are several locations on the affected foot itself: Spleen 3, at the side of the metatarsal joint just behind the big toe; Stomach 42, at the center of the top of the instep; and Liver 2, just behind the space between the big and second toes. Press each of these points firmly for 60 seconds. If the pain permits, you can also use two other points at the back corners of the big toenail. (See pages 22–23 for more information about point locations.)

ACUPUNCTURE

Because acupuncture can be administered to areas other than the swollen joint, this procedure may be more tolerable than direct treatments, such as **massage,** to patients in the initial stages of gout. See a professional for treatment.

HERBAL THERAPY

Drink an infusion of 2 tsp celery (Apium graveolens) seed or gravelroot (Eupatorium purpureum) in a cup of water, three times a day, to stimulate elimination of uric acid. Do not take herbal teas if colchicine has been prescribed.

HOMEOPATHY

A homeopath may consider predisposition to gout in an overall constitutional treatment. Colchicum, or autumn crocus, the plant from which colchicine is extracted, can be effective in relieving the pain of an attack. Other mixed homeopathic remedies may include dilute doses of Arnica, Ledum, Urtica urens, Benzoicum acidum, Lycopodium, and Pulsatilla.

NUTRITION AND DIET

In general, gout seems more common with diets that include meat and animal fats but is unusual in people following vegetarian diets. Dietary regimens for preventing attacks of gout in people showing a hereditary predisposition to the disease usually eliminate red meat and meat extracts such as bouillon and gravies; yeast and other enzyme-producing products; organ meats such as liver, sweetbreads, and kidneys; shellfish and certain kinds of preserved fish, including sardines, herring, and anchovies.

Foods that appear to suppress the immediate symptoms of gout include complex carbohydrates, particularly from cereals, fruits, and leafy green vegetables. Simple carbohydrates, such as those in refined sugar, are likely to increase uric acid production and should be avoided.

Several authorities report favorable results in treating the pain of chronic gout by having patients eat fresh or canned cherries—up to 8 oz a day—or drink cherry juice. Similar effects are claimed for strawberries, blueberries, and other red-blue berries.

Some practitioners recommend a teaspoon of activated charcoal three times a day to stimulate uric acid elimination in the urine.

Drinking plenty of clear, nonalcoholic fluids—fruit juices, herbal teas, or water—helps to dilute the urine and promote excretion of uric acid through continued flushing of the kidneys.

REFLEXOLOGY

To help restore balance to the kidneys and spleen, the organs responsible for uric acid production, a reflexology practitioner will massage the appropriate area at the center of the sole of the foot. Some advocates of reflexology assert that this direct massage technique serves to break up deposits of uric acid crystals that have become concentrated in the feet.

AT-HOME REMEDIES

The first concern in an attack of gout is to reduce pain and inflammation. If you can stand it, apply a plastic bag containing a few ice cubes or a bag of frozen vegetables to the joint; this will help relieve painful swelling. Wrap the cold bag in a soft cloth or towel and hold it against the painful area for up to five minutes at a time, then repeat as needed.

Because even the pressure of a sheet or blanket can be painful to a gout-afflicted joint, at bedtime rest the gouty foot inside a cardboard box or a plastic laundry basket that has been placed on its side.

PREVENTION

If gouty arthritis runs in the family, men in particular should moderate their intake of alcohol, fats, and high-purine foods, and should keep their weight within recommended ranges. Blood and urine tests during routine checkups will signal potential susceptibility to gout attack.   ∎

THE PRICE OF HIGH LIVING

The old image of the gout sufferer as a rotund, aging aristocrat, surrounded by roast beef and flagons of ale, swollen foot propped on a cushion, wasn't entirely mythical. While gout isn't simply a sign of "high living" and can occur anytime in adulthood, we now know that rich foods and alcohol can contribute to the real cause of gout and will certainly aggravate the disease after the initial attack.

SYMPTOMS

- weight loss despite increased appetite.
- faster heart rate, higher blood pressure, and increased nervousness.
- excessive perspiration.
- increased sensitivity to heat.
- more frequent bowel movements, sometimes with diarrhea.
- muscle weakness, trembling hands.
- development of a goiter (enlargement of the thyroid gland, causing a swelling at the base of the neck).
- bulging eyes.
- in women, change in frequency or total cessation of menstrual periods.

CALL YOUR DOCTOR IF:

- you are feverish, agitated, or delirious, and have a rapid pulse. You could be having a **thyrotoxic crisis,** in which the effects of too much thyroid hormone suddenly become life-threatening.

First described by Sir Robert Graves in the early 19th century, Graves' disease is one of the most common of all thyroid problems. It is also the leading cause of **hyperthyroidism,** a condition marked by excessive production of thyroid hormones. Once the disorder has been correctly diagnosed, it is quite easy to treat. In some cases, Graves' disease goes into remission or disappears completely after several months or years. Left untreated, however, it can lead to serious complications—even death. Although the symptoms can cause discomfort, Graves' disease generally has no long-term adverse health consequences if the patient receives prompt and proper medical care.

CAUSES

Hormones secreted by the thyroid gland control metabolism, or the speed at which the body converts food into energy. The metabolic rate is directly linked to the amount of hormone "fuel" that circulates in the bloodstream. If, for some reason, the thyroid gland secretes an overabundance of this fuel, the body's metabolism goes into high gear, producing the pounding heart, sweating, trembling, and weight loss typically experienced by hyperthyroid people. Normally, the thyroid gets its production orders through another chemical, called thyroid-stimulating hormone (TSH), released by the pituitary gland in the brain. But in Graves' disease, a malfunction in the body's immune system results in the manufacture of abnormal antibodies, or defender proteins, that mimic the pituitary's messenger chemicals. (See Immune Problems.) Spurred by these false signals to produce, the thyroid's hormone factories work overtime and exceed their normal quota.

Exactly why the immune system begins to produce these aberrant antibodies is unclear. Heredity and other characteristics seem to play a role in determining susceptibility. Studies show, for example, that if one identical twin contracts Graves' disease, there is a 50 percent likelihood that the other twin will get it too. Also, women are more likely than men to develop the disease. And smokers who develop Graves' are more prone to eye problems than nonsmokers with the disease.

Eye trouble—usually in the form of inflamed and swollen eye muscles and tissues that can cause the eyeballs to protrude from their sockets—is a distinguishing complication of Graves' disease. However, only a small percentage of all Graves' patients will experience this condition, known as exophthalmos. Even among those who do, the severity of their bout with Graves' has no bearing on the seriousness of the eye problem or how far the eyeballs protrude. In fact, it isn't clear whether such eye complications stem from Graves' disease itself or from a totally separate, yet closely linked, disorder. If you have developed exophthalmos, your eyes may ache and feel dry and irritated. Protruding eyeballs are prone to excessive tearing and redness, partly because the eyelids no longer can shelter them effectively from injury.

In severe cases of exophthalmos, which are rare, swollen eye muscles can put tremendous pressure on the optic nerve, possibly leading to partial color blindness or a decrease in visual acuity. Eye muscles weakened by long periods of inflammation can lose their ability to control movement, resulting in double vision.

DIAGNOSTIC AND TEST PROCEDURES

Although Graves' disease can be diagnosed from the results of one or two tests, your doctor may use several methods to double-check the findings and rule out other disorders. An analysis of your blood will show if the levels of two hormones—thyroxine and triiodothyronine, which are produced or regulated by the thyroid—are higher than normal. If they are, and if levels of thyroid-stimulating hormone in your blood are abnormally low, you are hyperthyroid, and Graves' disease is the likely culprit. Blood analysis can also detect the presence of the abnormal antibody associated with Graves' disease, but this test is somewhat expensive and generally not necessary.

To confirm a diagnosis of Graves' disease, your doctor may conduct a radioactive iodide uptake test, which shows whether large quantities of iodide are collecting in the thyroid. The gland needs iodide to make thyroid hormones, so if it is absorbing unusually large amounts of iodide, it obviously is producing too much hormone.

IMPACT ON THE EYES

Protruding eyeballs are an occasional symptom of Graves' disease. When tissues lining the eye socket become inflamed, they can swell and force the eyeball forward, a condition known as exophthalmos. If the lid cannot close over it, the eye may become dry and irritated. Prolonged inflammation can weaken eye muscles, impairing eyeball movement and causing vision problems.

If exophthalmos is your only symptom, your physician will probably run blood tests to check for hyperthyroidism, since this eye disorder can occur apart from Graves' disease. The doctor may also evaluate your eye muscles using ultrasound, a CT scan, or magnetic resonance imaging (MRI). Signs of swelling in any one of these tests will confirm a diagnosis of Graves' disease.

TREATMENT

If you have Graves' disease, or even suspect that you have it, you should have a professional diagnosis and, if necessary, a treatment plan that suits your particular condition. Although the disorder is rooted in a malfunctioning immune system, the goal of both conventional and alternative approaches is to restore thyroid hormone levels to their correct balance and to relieve discomfort.

CONVENTIONAL MEDICINE

If you have a mild case of Graves' disease, you and your practitioner may simply decide to see how the disease develops before initiating any treatment. Should medical intervention be necessary, the two most frequently used conventional treatments involve disabling the thyroid's ability to produce hormones.

One common approach uses a strong dose of radioactive iodide to destroy certain cells in the thyroid gland. This procedure attempts to halt excess hormone production by thinning the ranks of cells responsible for manufacturing the chemicals. The amount of radioactive iodide you receive depends on the estimated size of your thyroid—determined either through a physical exam or by ultrasound—and on the gland's level of activity, as indicated by the results of an iodide uptake test. Despite its destructive effect on thyroid cells, the iodide used in this procedure will not harm surrounding tissues and organs.

At the beginning of the treatment, you will be given a capsule or liquid containing the radioactive iodide. Either way you take it, you should not feel any effects as the substance enters your system. Most of the iodide will gather and remain in your thyroid; excess amounts will be excreted in your urine. It is a good idea to drink several extra glasses of water per day for about a week after the treatment to help flush the material out of your body as quickly as possible. To be on the safe side, you should also limit contact with infants, children, and pregnant women for at least seven days after you ingest the iodide.

You probably won't notice any changes in your body for several days after taking the radioactive iodide, but if your thyroid gland feels inflamed and sore, acetaminophen, ibuprofen, or aspirin can offer some relief. Over the next several months, the thyroid's hormone secretion should gradually begin to drop. During this time you need to see your doctor for periodic checkups to determine how well the treatment is progressing. Chances are good that a single dose of radioactive iodide will be sufficient to correct your hyperthyroidism. However, if your condition hasn't improved three months or so after your initial treatment, your practitioner may give you a second dose of iodide. Once the doctor has decided that your Graves' disease is effectively under control, you will still need to have routine

checkups to make sure that your thyroid levels remain within the normal range.

Although radioactive iodide treatments are generally safe, they cannot be given to pregnant women because the chemical may destroy the thyroid gland in the fetus. Therefore, you must make sure that you are not pregnant before you take radioactive iodide for Graves' disease. It is best to let several months pass after your last dose of radioactive iodide before you become pregnant; confirm the length of time you should wait with your practitioner. Except during these periods following the treatment, radioactive iodide poses no health risks for women who want to become pregnant, and it will not affect the fertility of either women or men.

Antithyroid drugs such as propylthiouracil and methimazole, which interfere with thyroid hormone production, can be used to treat Graves' disease. After you begin treatment, it may take several months for your hyperthyroid symptoms to subside. This is because the thyroid has already generated and stored enough hormone to keep it circulating at elevated levels. Once the stores are drained, hormone production should drop to its normal level. Although your disease may seem to go away entirely, you might still need drug therapy to keep your thyroid operating properly. Even if your case of Graves' disease does go into remission and your doctor says it's safe to stop taking your medication, you will need to be evaluated every year or so to make sure your hyperthyroidism has not returned.

Beta-adrenergic blockers such as atenolol and propranolol, frequently prescribed to treat heart disease and hypertension, are also used by some patients to alleviate the heart palpitations and muscle tremors that characterize Graves' disease. Before prescribing beta blockers for this condition, however, your doctor needs to know if you are asthmatic or have any kind of heart trouble.

Radioactive iodide treatments and antithyroid drugs are usually effective in slowing down thyroid hormone output, but in some cases surgery is the best approach for Graves' disease. If you develop the disorder before or during pregnancy, for example, or if you are reluctant or unable to undergo radioactive treatment or are allergic to antithyroid medication, your doctor may recommend subtotal thyroidectomy, a relatively safe and simple procedure in which most of the thyroid gland is removed.

Because many conventional remedies severely limit the thyroid's ability to manufacture thyroid hormone, they increase the chances that you will develop **hypothyroidism,** a potentially serious condition marked by insufficient thyroid hormone production (see Thyroid Problems). Therefore, if you have undergone any of the aforementioned treatments for Graves' disease, you must continue to see your doctor for periodic checkups to make sure the problem has not been overcorrected, causing your thyroid hormone levels to drop too low.

Only about 5 percent of people with Graves' disease will develop eye problems severe enough to warrant professional treatment. And almost half of those who develop exophthalmos, the condition that causes the eyeballs to protrude, will have mild cases that can be helped with simple treatments (see At-Home Remedies, right).

Graves' disease patients with eye problems can find temporary relief from the redness, swelling, and pain through a number of drugs, including prednisone, methylprednisolone, and dexamethasone. However, these medications should not be used for long periods of time, as they can lead to bone loss, muscle weakness, and weight gain. Vision problems and severe cases of eye protrusion can often be corrected through radiation therapy and surgery. Make sure to ask your doctor about any possible complications before undergoing surgery.

ALTERNATIVE CHOICES

Alternative treatments generally serve to complement conventional medicine's more direct goal of thyroid hormone suppression. Some of these therapies help alleviate the unpleasant symptoms of Graves' disease, while others seek to improve general thyroid function.

HERBAL THERAPIES

For relief from the symptoms of Graves' disease, try a combination of 4 parts bugleweed (Lycopus

spp.), 2 parts motherwort (Leonurus cardiaca), 2 parts skullcap (Scutellaria lateriflora), and 1 part hawthorn (Crataegus laevigata) in a tincture, three times a day.

LIFESTYLE

After the heart rate has stabilized, aerobic exercise for 15 to 20 minutes a day is thought to be very good for maintaining good thyroid function.

NUTRITION AND DIET

If you are hyperthyroid, eating foods that inhibit the manufacture of thyroid hormones might help lower hormone secretion. These include cabbage, peaches, radishes, peanuts, rutabagas, soybeans, and spinach. Vitamin B complex injections may also prove useful.

YOGA

The Shoulder Stand position, practiced at least once daily for 20 minutes, can help some people with Graves' disease improve overall thyroid function. Lie on your back and lift your legs up so that your hips come off the floor. Supporting your hips with your hands, extend your legs into a vertical position. Slide your hands farther toward your shoulders, with your thumbs at the front of your body and your fingers at the back, making sure that the weight of your body is supported by your shoulders, not your head and neck.

AT-HOME REMEDIES

◆ If your lids cannot close completely over your eyes, use eye patches at night. This will help keep your corneas from drying out.
◆ Use over-the-counter or prescription artificial tears to moisten your eyes whenever they feel dry.
◆ If your eyes are red and swollen in the morning, sleep with your head elevated.
◆ Wear tinted glasses to protect your eyes from bright light, sunlight, and wind. ■

SYMPTOMS

◆ pain and stiffness in one or both sides of the groin when you try to walk or sit; may be accompanied by swelling or black-and-blue discoloration.

CALL YOUR DOCTOR IF:

◆ you detect a swelling or bulge along the crease between your leg and stomach, especially if you are overweight or have been engaging in strenuous activity; you could have a hernia.

◆ you run a high temperature or have chills associated with pain in the groin; these may be symptoms of a bone or kidney infection.

◆ the pain extends to the small of the back, whether or not your temperature is high; you may be suffering from a kidney stone or a prostate problem.

◆ the pain extends to the lower abdomen; you may have a digestive or (if you are a woman) gynecological disorder, or a viral infection. If the pain happens during a menstrual period, discuss the symptoms with your gynecologist.

By definition, the groin is where your torso joins your legs. It's the place where your trunk and your legs can bend forward, backward, and to the sides. Because the groin is the center of a lot of body movement, it is subject to potential strain, particularly in athletes, dancers, and people who do physical labor. Less active people can also suffer groin injury: Ordinary lifting, stretching, running, and weekend sports can put great strain on the bones and muscles of the groin.

The effect of a strain to these key muscles and tendons—sometimes called a groin pull—is immediate and often immobilizing. The pain is intense, and you cannot walk, sit, or put weight on your leg without extreme discomfort. As a protective reflex, you tend to stiffen up and limp, favoring the injured side of the groin. In some cases you may have to be carried to a place where you can lie down, relax, and ease the pain.

CAUSES

The immediate cause of a groin pull is bruising or tearing the muscles that run from the pelvis down the thighs. It may also involve a torn tendon connecting the ends of the muscle to a bone. Groin pulls are usually caused by overexertion, lifting heavy objects improperly, or failing to warm up before a strenuous activity. Sometimes a strained groin muscle comes from external causes, such as falling against a solid object or being struck with great force, as in an accident.

TREATMENT

A minor groin pull will generally heal itself with rest in a matter of hours or a few days. If the muscle tissue is actually torn, the healing process may take a week or more. In severe or recurring cases, surgery may be necessary to repair the damage to muscles and tendons.

CONVENTIONAL MEDICINE

To reduce the swelling and inflammation of your groin strain, apply an ice pack as quickly as pos-

REFLEXOLOGY

GROIN

ADRENAL
WAISTLINE

GROIN

To reduce muscle tension in the groin, work the groin and adrenal areas. Holding your foot straight back, walk your left index finger from one side of the groin area to the other; walk back with your right finger. Repeat several times. Then push the big toe back and walk your thumb along the inside of the main tendon on the bottom of your foot from the waistline area to the adrenal area.

sible after the injury. You might also take aspirin or a nonsteroidal anti-inflammatory drug (NSAID) to relieve pain. Rest the affected muscle until the swelling and inflammation subside. Later you can apply a warm compress to relax the damaged muscle tissue and encourage the body's natural healing processes.

If your groin pull is due to an athletic injury, you may want to see a specialist in sports medicine, not just to relieve the pain but also to advise you on how to prevent a pull from happening again. Among young people who play team or individual sports, groin pulls are fairly common and tend to heal quickly—as long as the victim resists the urge to "play through the pain." Older people with groin strain—especially those who are not athletically inclined—should allow plenty of time to let the natural healing process work.

ALTERNATIVE CHOICES

Like conventional approaches, alternative treatments center on pain relief and rest until the muscles and tendons restore themselves to their normal condition and capability.

ACUPRESSURE

To relieve immediate pain in the thigh and groin, try pressure at the Liver 8 or Spleen 6 point. *(See pages 22–23 for more information on point locations.)*

BODY WORK

After relieving the immediate pain of a minor groin pull with a cold compress and rest, massaging the area using a warm body oil is an excellent way to relax muscles.

A **reflexology** therapist will manipulate the area along the front of the ankle where it joins the foot—a technique intended to stimulate circulation and lymphatic activity and to help relieve muscle tension in the groin.

HOMEOPATHY

Arnica is the homeopath's first-aid remedy for muscle injuries. It can be taken orally and applied as a salve to the painful area. Rhus toxicodendron and Ruta may also be useful for muscle strains.

AT-HOME REMEDIES

If you suffer a groin pull, lie down in a comfortable place and let your body relax. Apply a cold pack—a plastic bag of ice cubes or a packet of frozen vegetables wrapped in a towel—for 10 minutes on and 10 off until the pain recedes. Avoid exertion for several days, until you can use the affected muscles without pain.

PREVENTION

The single most important factor in avoiding muscle strain—in the groin or anywhere else in your body—is to warm up your muscles with moderate exercises before starting any strenuous activity. When a warmup period is not possible, work into the activity gradually, letting your muscles and tendons stretch and become more elastic. ∎

G

G

SYMPTOMS

- swollen, red gums that may bleed easily.
- localized pain, loose teeth, and bad breath, which suggest **periodontitis;** x-rays may reveal some bone loss in the jaw area.
- extremely painful, inflamed gums coated with a gray-white mucus; sometimes accompanied by a mild fever, malaise, bad breath, excess saliva, and painful swallowing. These are signs of **Vincent's angina.**
- sudden and unexplained severe bone loss around molars and incisors, especially in young African American girls; this is indicative of **juvenile periodontitis.**
- extremely sore, swollen gums that bleed easily; perhaps accompanied by earaches, sinuslike infection, nosebleeds, fever, weight loss, and malaise. You may have **Wegener's granulomatosis,** a rare but potentially fatal disease.

CALL YOUR DENTIST IF:

- you have any of the groups of symptoms listed above; timely treatment can help prevent the spread of infection and potentially save teeth.

Periodontal disease (gum disease) is one of the most prevalent chronic diseases, with an estimated 98 percent of Americans over 60 affected by some form. A diet rich in refined sugars is largely to blame, but modern dentistry and good toothbrushes and toothpastes have helped offset some of the pernicious effects of our eating habits; as a result, just 8 percent of adults ever develop severe gum problems. That rate would be even lower if people made an effort to cut back on highly processed foods—notorious for the quantities of refined sugars they contain—and took dental hygiene more seriously. As it is, though, fewer than half of Americans see a dentist every year.

CAUSES

Periodontal disease is an infection of the gums and other tissues that support the teeth. The stage is set for problems when food particles, saliva, and bacteria are allowed to accumulate around the gum line, which encourages the formation of a soft bacterial mass known as plaque. Pockets can form as increasing amounts of plaque push between teeth and the surrounding membranes; these pockets and the decayed material in them create a good breeding ground for the bacteria already present. Excess sugar in the diet decreases saliva production (the body's best defense against bacteria in the mouth) and impairs disease-fighting white blood cells. The earliest stage of the resulting infection, known as **gingivitis,** is marked by painless inflammation, swelling, redness, and possibly bleeding. Certain vitamin deficiencies, medication, glandular disorders, and blood diseases may make you more susceptible to gingivitis; but in general, poor dental hygiene is the primary cause.

If the pockets around your teeth deepen and your gums turn an intense red, the problem may have become **periodontitis,** an inflammation of the periodontal ligament, which helps hold your teeth in their sockets of bone. If the infection worsens, it can cause bone and tooth loss. Periodontitis progresses slowly and often imperceptibly. Dentists used to think that bleeding gums

PERIODONTAL DISEASE

RECEDING GUM LINE
CALCULUS
ROOT
CROWN

A bacterial film called plaque can accumulate along the gum line at the base of the teeth if not brushed away. Plaque hardens into calculus, which irritates the gums and causes them to recede. Pockets that form between the gums and teeth collect more plaque and calculus, causing destruction of the bone and ligament supporting the tooth, eventually resulting in tooth loss.

were a reliable indicator of periodontitis, but current research suggests this is not the case. You are at no greater risk for periodontitis if routine brushing causes your gums to bleed than if your gums almost never bleed.

In those rare instances when periodontitis comes on suddenly, it may be another form of the disease—either **juvenile periodontitis** or **Vincent's angina.** Juvenile periodontitis, which can lead to severe bone loss around the permanent molars and sometimes the incisors, occurs most often in African American girls, for reasons that are not entirely clear to researchers but that suggest some sort of genetic link. As in other gum problems, poor dental hygiene seems to be a contributing factor.

Vincent's angina (also known as trench mouth, because a large number of World War I soldiers fighting in the trenches contracted it) is caused by a combination of poor diet, stress, and of course, bacteria. Particularly common in teenagers with poor dental hygiene and a high-sugar diet, Vincent's angina is characterized by extreme pain, some bleeding, and a distinctive gray-white mucus that covers the gums. It is

sometimes accompanied by a mild fever, malaise, bad breath, excess saliva, and painful swallowing.

A condition known as **strawberry gingivitis**—in which the gums become inflamed to the point of looking like overripe strawberries—can be the earliest sign of an uncommon though potentially fatal disease called **Wegener's granulomatosis.** The gums will be extremely sore and swollen, and they will bleed easily. Other symptoms include earaches, a sinuslike infection, nosebleeds, fever, weight loss, a cough, and malaise. Although the exact cause of the disease remains unknown, it progresses like a bacterial infection. It affects all ages and both sexes, although it is more prevalent in men; if left untreated, it can eventually damage the heart, lungs, and kidneys and cause renal failure.

In general, smokers are more than twice as likely to develop some kind of gum disease as nonsmokers. Other at-risk groups include people with diabetes, leukemia, and Crohn's disease, and pregnant women. Studies have shown that certain bacteria thrive on elevated hormone levels, which spells trouble not only for pregnant women but also for women taking oral contraceptives.

Chemotherapy and radiation treatments can also increase your risk for gum problems, as can exposure to toxic heavy metals such as mercury.

TREATMENT

The best treatment for periodontal disease is prevention. If you do develop gum problems, seek professional treatment and advice.

CONVENTIONAL MEDICINE

A proper daily dental regimen of thorough brushing and flossing—supplemented by regular trips to the dentist, who will clean areas you miss or perhaps can't reach—is the best way to prevent and to address most gum problems. Occasionally **gingivitis** is aggravated by an external factor that a dentist or orthodontist may be able to correct, such as poorly aligned teeth, excessive grinding, or ill-fitted crowns or bridges.

For aggressive forms of gingivitis, the dentist would first remove all plaque and calcified plaque (calculus) and then, perhaps, prescribe a chlorhexidine-based mouthwash. More effective than common commercial brands, such a mouthwash may have some unwelcome side effects, including staining the teeth or bringing on an allergic reaction.

Dentists typically follow a similar routine to treat **periodontitis,** though in some cases surgery is required to clean out the pockets of infection and to remove damaged bone. It's up to the patient to follow through with solid brushing, flossing, and rinsing.

For **Vincent's angina,** the dentist or periodontist will clear out damaged or dead tissue and usually also prescribe a painkiller. Occasionally an antibiotic is also necessary; but in most cases, a good diet, high fluid intake, plenty of rest, and good oral hygiene (including no smoking) should suffice.

In those rare instances when **Wegener's granulomatosis** develops, immediate treatment is crucial. Cytotoxic agents such as cyclophosphamide, when combined with corticosteroids, have dramatically cut the fatality rate (as high as 90 percent if left untreated) for this disease.

Some of the latest advances in technology have made dental visits a lot less painful and noisy, and more effective. Ultrasound lasers have not yet completely replaced scrapers and picks and other such implements, but they are more and more often the preferred cleaning tool for removing plaque and other material. And in the past, dentists often had difficulty identifying the exact bacteria responsible for any given case of periodontitis, but improved testing methods have made precise diagnosis and more effective treatment possible.

ALTERNATIVE CHOICES

Many alternative therapies exist for gum problems, including rinses and pastes that will reduce plaque, fight infection and inflammation, and slow bleeding. But these therapies are no better than conventional commercial products at reaching below the gum line to areas where periodon-

ATTENTION!

HEART DISEASE AND PERIODONTITIS

Young men who don't take care of their teeth and gums may be slipping into a lifestyle that places them at greater risk for heart disease. A 1993 study of nearly 10,000 subjects (men and women) found a 25 percent increase in heart disease among those with periodontitis. The connection was most remarkable in men under 50 with periodontitis, who had nearly double the risk of coronary heart disease as men who had little or no periodontal disease. Researchers could not determine if the gum problems were just a general indicator of poor hygiene and diet that led to other health problems or whether some direct correlation exists between heart problems and periodontitis. Either way, gum disease is a red flag.

titis blossoms. You still need to see a dentist regularly to ward off the risk of severe gum disease and tooth loss.

ACUPUNCTURE
A professional acupuncturist would work with the stomach and large intestine meridians to stimulate energy in the gum area.

AYURVEDIC MEDICINE
Massage bleeding gums with a mixture of lemon juice (half a lemon) and a cup of water; the acid can help reduce bacteria.

HERBAL THERAPIES
Massage gums with goldenseal (Hydrastis canadensis) or myrrh (Commiphora molmol) to fight infection. Gargle with bayberry (Myrica spp.) or prickly ash (Zanthoxylum americanum) to stimulate circulation, especially for bleeding gums. A combination of sage (Salvia officinalis) and chamomile (Matricaria recutita) makes an excellent mouthwash. Take echinacea (Echinacea spp.) to fight infection: Make a tea by boiling 1 to 2 tsp

of the root in 1 cup of water; simmer for 10 minutes, then drink three times a day. Or you can use 1 to 4 ml in tincture form. Or you can drink Roman chamomile *(Anthemis nobilis)* or myrrh *(Commiphora molmol)* tea to fight inflammation in the gums. CAUTION: Do not use myrrh if you are pregnant.

HOMEOPATHY
For tender, bleeding gums and excessive salivation try Mercurius vivus; take orally twice a day for three days. If you continue to have problems, see a professional homeopath.

MASSAGE
Massaging the gums can improve circulation and speed healing. Use the rounded part of your fingertips and move along your gum line or the outside of your jaw in small circular motions. A stimulator brush, which has only two rows of bristles and is used without toothpaste, can also be therapeutic.

NUTRITION AND DIET
Crucial for healthy gums is a diet low in refined sugars and high in fiber. (Fiber works much like a dog's bone or biscuit to help cleanse the teeth.) Other important nutritional elements include vitamins A (especially beta carotene), C, and E, as well as zinc, flavonoids (present in onions), and folic acid (particularly for pregnant women and women on oral contraceptives). Gingivitis is common in scurvy patients, a reflection of vitamin C's vital role in maintaining a healthy mouth.

AT-HOME REMEDIES
You can make a wide assortment of mouthwashes and toothpastes at home. Some of the most effective ingredients include:
◆ a combination of baking soda and hydrogen peroxide, for brushing your teeth or as a mouth rinse.
◆ a mixture of bayberry and prickly ash as a gargle.
◆ cashew oil, vitamin E oil, or poultices of goldenseal or myrrh massaged into the gums, to speed healing and protect against infection.

PREVENTION
Prevention of periodontal disease begins at home, with good routine dental hygiene. Too many of us give our teeth a quick brush twice a day and only occasionally a good flossing. For really proper care you need to floss daily, brush longer, rinse with a mouthwash, and massage your gum line. Always floss first, to loosen food particles and plaque, then brush your teeth gently but thoroughly with a soft brush using a circular motion. Rigorous horizontal brushing with hard bristles can cause your gums to recede. Mouthwashes combat bacteria, but they should not be substituted for brushing, which you should do two or three times a day.

The American Dental Association (ADA) recommends that you visit your dentist once or twice a year to get rid of intractable plaque and calculus, but some dentists believe that excellent at-home dental hygiene keeps the plaque and calculus from ever forming. To achieve "excellence" you have to spend at least 15 minutes twice a day working on your teeth, and another 15 minutes a day massaging your gums. If you don't think you can follow this rigorous a routine, take the ADA's advice.

If you plan to get pregnant, see a dentist for a good cleaning first. Women who have little or no plaque before their pregnancy rarely have the gum problems often associated with elevated hormone levels.

Diabetics and anyone undergoing chemotherapy or radiation treatments should see a dentist several times a year.

People with existing gingivitis or periodontitis should see their dentist every three months, or as needed to keep the condition under proper control and prevent recurrences. ■

H

- in men, thinning hair on the scalp, a receding hairline, or a horseshoe-shaped pattern that leaves the crown of the head exposed.
- in women, thinning of hair in general, but mainly at the crown; complete balding is rare.
- in children or young adults, sudden loss of patches of hair; known as **alopecia areata.**
- complete loss of all hair on the body; a rare disorder called **alopecia universalis.**
- especially in children, patches of broken hairs and incomplete hair loss, usually on the scalp but sometimes involving the eyebrows; the child is most likely rubbing or pulling out hair, a disorder called **trichotillomania.**
- excessive shedding of hair, but not complete baldness, associated with various illnesses and drug treatments, rapid weight loss, anemia, stress, or pregnancy; a condition known as **telogen effluvium.**

CALL YOUR DOCTOR IF:

- you suspect that you or your child has **alopecia areata,** or that your child has **trichotillomania;** both conditions should be evaluated by a doctor.
- you suffer an unexplained loss of hair on any part of your body; your doctor may want to check for an underlying disorder that might be responsible.

Human hair varies widely in color and texture, and people differ considerably in the amount of facial and body hair they have, depending on their age, sex, race, and genetic makeup. But in spite of the many differences that are found in hair, it's normal for all of us to have it on the top and back of our heads. When it starts to disappear there, it's considered **alopecia,** or baldness.

Hair grows everywhere on the body except the palms of our hands and the soles of our feet, but many hairs are so fine they're virtually invisible. Hair is made up of a protein called keratin, produced in hair follicles in the outer layer of skin; as follicles produce new hair cells, old cells are being pushed out through the surface of the skin at the rate of about six inches a year. The hair you can see is actually a string of dead keratin cells. The average adult head has about 100,000 hairs, and loses up to 100 of them a day; so finding a few stray hairs on your hairbrush is not necessarily cause for alarm.

Gradual thinning of hair with age is a natural condition known as **involutional alopecia.** More and more hair follicles go into a telogenic, or resting, stage, and the remaining hairs become shorter and fewer in number. **Androgenic alopecia** is a genetically predisposed condition that can affect both men and women. Men can begin suffering hair loss as early as their teens or early twenties, while most women don't experience noticeable thinning until their forties or later. In men, a receding hairline and gradual disappearance of hair from the crown is called **male pattern baldness.** In women, **female pattern baldness** is typically a general thinning over the entire scalp, with the most extensive hair loss at the crown.

Patchy hair loss in children and young adults, often sudden in onset, is known as **alopecia areata.** This disorder may result in complete baldness, but in about 90 percent of cases the hair returns, usually within a few years. With **alopecia universalis,** all body hair falls out and the likelihood of regrowth is slight, especially when it occurs in children. Tearing out one's own hair, a disorder known as **trichotillomania,** is seen most frequently in children.

CAUSES

Doctors do not know why certain hair follicles are programmed to have a shorter growth period than others. Although a person's level of androgens—male hormones normally produced by both men and women—is believed to be a factor, hair loss has nothing to do with virility. For that matter, the presence or absence of dandruff has no effect on balding either. An individual's genes, however—from both male and female parents—unquestionably influence that person's predisposition to male or female pattern baldness.

Temporary hair loss can occur in conjunction with a high fever, a severe illness, thyroid disorders, iron deficiency, general anesthesia, drug treatments, hormonal imbalance, or extreme stress, and in women following childbirth. In these conditions, collectively known as **telogen effluvium,** a large number of hair follicles suddenly go into a resting phase, causing hair to thin noticeably. Drugs that can cause temporary hair loss include chemotherapeutic agents used in cancer treatment, anticoagulants, retinoids used to treat acne and skin problems, beta-adrenergic blockers used to control blood pressure, and oral contraceptives.

Hair loss can also be caused by burns, x-rays, scalp injuries, and exposure to certain chemicals—including those used to purify swimming pools, and to bleach, dye, and perm hair. In such cases, normal hair growth usually returns once the cause is eliminated.

The causes of **alopecia areata,** a disorder that often strikes children or teenagers, remain unexplained. In most cases the hair grows back, although it may be very fine and possibly white before normal coloration and thickness return.

Although too-frequent washing, permanent waves, bleaching, and dyeing hair do not cause baldness, they can contribute to overall thinning by making hair weak and brittle. Tight braiding and using rollers or hot curlers can damage and break hair, and running hair picks through tight curls can scar hair follicles. In most instances hair grows back normally if the source of stress is removed, but severe damage to the hair or scalp sometimes causes permanent bald patches.

THREE TYPES OF HAIR LOSS

1 Male pattern baldness tends to run in families, affecting some men as early as the midteens. The hair begins to recede from the forehead and temples (*left*), and eventually from the crown, leaving a fringe of hair around the ears and across the back of the head (*right*).

2 Female pattern baldness affects only a small percentage of women, and usually only after menopause. The hair may thin out along the forehead, temples, and crown (*left*), and eventually the crown may become almost completely bald (*right*).

3 Alopecia areata is sudden, spotty balding in children and adults of either sex. Its cause is unknown. The bald spots may occur on the scalp, along the eyebrows, and in the beard, and they may be extensive. In most cases, the hair eventually grows back without treatment.

TREATMENT

Although remedies that promise to restore hair to balding heads have been around since ancient times, most men and women with thinning hair can do little to reverse the process. For cosmetic purposes, or after hair loss from surgical or drug treatments, many people turn to wigs, hairpieces, and hairweaving—even tattooing to simulate lost eyebrows and eyelashes. Some drugs may slow hair loss, and certain alternative treatments can relieve stress or bolster the health of remaining hair, but until recently no treatment could start hair growth where no hair exists.

CONVENTIONAL MEDICINE

Under certain circumstances, a preparation containing the drug minoxidil appears to provide moderate regrowth of hair on areas of the scalp that have gone bald. The effects are most promising in younger people who are just beginning to show signs of balding or who have small bald patches. The medication is applied to balding spots twice a day and must be continued daily; hair loss will recur if the application is stopped. More than 50 percent of users claim that it can thicken hair and slow hair loss, but it is not considered effective in men who already have extensive male pattern baldness. Side effects appear to be minimal, but in some users the drug may cause skin irritation. Oral minoxidil is reported to affect the heart rate in a small number of patients, so only the topical form should be used by people diagnosed with cardiovascular problems.

Hormone therapy may be prescribed for certain types of hair loss, but not without some risk. Although most cases of **alopecia areata** are resolved naturally, some doctors try to speed recovery with corticosteroids applied topically or injected in the scalp. The treatment may be painful and may cause permanent scarring in the scalp brought on by skin atrophy. Cortisone taken orally may stimulate new hair growth, but the effect is likely to be temporary. Prednisone, another orally administered steroid, has proved effective for **alopecia areata** patients, but its potential side effects include weight gain, metabolic abnormalities, acne, and menstrual problems. Hormone therapy in the form of birth-control pills may reverse baldness due to hormonal imbalances in young women.

Hair transplantation involves the relocation of plugs of skin from parts of the scalp containing active hair follicles to bald areas. A patient may need several hundred plugs—implanted 10

to 60 at a session. The transplanted hair may drop out, but new hair usually begins to grow from the transplanted follicles within several months.

A form of cosmetic surgery called scalp reduction involves tightening the scalp so that hair-bearing skin from the back and sides of the head is pulled toward the crown. Hair may then be transplanted to the remaining bald area at the top of the head. Like hair transplants, the process is painful and expensive, and it does nothing to retard genetic or age-related hair loss.

USE YOUR HEAD, SPARE YOUR HAIR

Shampoos and conditioners cannot prevent baldness, but overusing them can dry out the hair you have. Virtually all shampoos—even those touted as herbal, hypoallergenic, or vitamin-enhanced—are basically scented detergents with a lathering agent. Most brands are so concentrated that they actually work better when you dilute them. If your hair is very oily, you may want to wash it every day, but shampooing too often can strip your hair of its natural oil, which may lead to brittle, broken strands.

Claims that certain conditioners nourish and revitalize your hair have little merit. Hair—even the thickest, most vibrant-looking hair—is dead keratin. Hair conditioners contain waxes that give your hair a smooth feel, but they cannot alter its actual health. The bottom line: Count on shampoo to keep your hair and scalp clean, nothing more. Proper brushing will do more for the long-term health of your hair and scalp than will spending money on expensive shampoos, conditioners, dyes, and other questionable hair enhancers.

ALTERNATIVE CHOICES

Despite claims to the contrary, no alternative therapies can reverse normal balding, although some may encourage reversal of temporary hair loss and improve damaged hair. Certain relaxation techniques may stem shedding brought on by stress.

CHINESE MEDICINE

In Chinese medicine, hair is thought to be nourished by the blood, which is influenced by the liver and kidneys. Traditional tonics are intended to tone these organs and promote new hair growth; they include such herbs as polygonum (*Polygonum multiflorum*), lycium fruit (*Lycium barbarum*), Chinese foxglove root (*Rehmannia glutinosa*), Chinese yam (*Dioscorea opposita*), and cornus (*Cornus officinalis*).

HERBAL THERAPIES

For temporary or partial hair loss from a systemic disease, drug therapy, or some other known cause, herbalists recommend stimulating hair follicles and improving blood circulation in the scalp to encourage new hair growth. Try massaging your scalp using essential oil of rosemary (*Rosmarinus officinalis*) or rinsing your hair with tea made from sage (*Salvia officinalis*).

HOMEOPATHY

More than 20 homeopathic remedies are thought to be effective for hair loss, particularly thinning caused by pregnancy, stress, or emotional trauma. Look in your health food store for over-the-counter preparations, or consult a homeopathic professional for more advice.

MASSAGE

Whether it's visible or not, your scalp needs a steady supply of blood. Massage improves circulation, which in turn improves the health of your hair and scalp. A few drops of vitamin E oil massaged into the scalp is recommended to strengthen fragile hair and help prevent dry, flaky skin.

MIND/BODY MEDICINE

Emotional or physical stress may be a factor in some cases of hair loss. A regular exercise program or **relaxation** techniques such as **yoga, guided imagery,** or **meditation** can help relieve stress.

NUTRITION AND DIET

Hair loss can result from poor nutrition or a rapid drop in weight. In such cases, you should get back on a balanced diet and consult your doctor or a professional nutritionist about supplemental vitamins A, B complex, and C, as well as iron and zinc.

PREVENTION

Although you can't reverse natural balding, you can protect your hair from damage that may eventually lead to thinning. Some people, women in particular, put their hair under tremendous stress in the pursuit of beauty. Hair dryers, hot curlers, dyes, bleaches, hair straightening, permanent waves, and chemical-laden cosmetics may eventually result in dry, broken, and thinning hair. People who leave their hair its natural color and texture will end up with healthier hair. Use a basic shampoo designed for your hair type. If you must curl your hair, use sponge rollers and let it air-dry whenever possible.

Proper brushing can do as much for the condition of your hair as any over-the-counter product. Choose a moderately stiff, natural-bristle brush, which will not tear your hair. Use full strokes from the scalp to the tips of your hair, to distribute the hair's natural oil. Begin with 10 to 20 strokes a day and try to work up to 100. Be gentle, and avoid brushing your hair when wet, when it is especially fragile. Remember: Hair is not living tissue, so it cannot repair itself. ■

HAMSTRING INJURY

SYMPTOMS

- sharp pain in the back of the thigh, during or immediately after sports or other strenuous activity.
- swelling and loss of strength in the upper leg.
- difficulty walking or sitting, and inability to bend the leg.

CALL YOUR DOCTOR IF:

- you feel pain shooting down the back of your leg when you cough; you may have sciatica.
- you have chills or fever associated with the muscle pain; these may be symptoms of a bacterial or viral infection.
- your leg hurts when you walk and stops hurting when you are at rest; you may be developing a circulatory problem.

As the muscles that flex your knees and bend your legs, the hamstrings are involved in virtually every move you make. Each hamstring is actually a belt of three muscles that run along the back of your thigh from buttock to knee, where they connect to the bones of your lower leg. They are counterparts to the powerful quadriceps muscles at the front of your thighs and can be subject to great stress. Professional athletes and dancers are particularly prone to hamstring pulls, but anyone is susceptible, especially people who push themselves a little too far in weekend sports. The danger in a hamstring pull is giving in to the temptation to "play through the pain," which will aggravate and possibly complicate the injury. Recognizing pain as a warning to stop and let the body heal is the most important step in recovery.

CAUSES

A pulled hamstring is invariably the result of overstressing or tearing the muscle fibers, typically by suddenly twisting, straightening, or overextending the thigh. A minor hamstring pull is simply a case of stretching the muscle too far, but in some cases a crippling muscle spasm can result. Tearing the muscle belt itself, or separating the muscle from the connective tendons, is a much more serious injury.

DIAGNOSTIC AND TEST PROCEDURES
While the signs of a hamstring pull may seem obvious, you may want to confirm the nature and degree of the injury by seeing a family doctor or sports medicine specialist. Aching muscles and joints can sometimes mask more serious ailments such as viral infections, which can be accurately diagnosed only by experts.

TREATMENT

Like other strains, a hamstring pull generally heals itself. You can expect to regain full use of the leg in a few days or weeks, depending on your physical condition and the degree of the injury.

HAMSTRING STRETCH

1 Sit on the floor with your legs extended and slightly bent at the knees. Keeping your back as straight as possible, slowly bend from the hips and reach down your legs as far as you can without forcing the stretch. Hold in place for 15 seconds.

2 Without changing your position, reach toward your feet and try to touch your toes with your fingertips. Hold this position for 15 seconds, then slowly relax the stretch and sit back. Rest for 10 seconds, then repeat the exercise. Do 8 to 10 times.

CONVENTIONAL MEDICINE

The established recovery procedure for muscle strain is RICE: rest, ice, compression, and elevation. *(See Athletic Injuries.)* Your doctor may also recommend a painkiller such as aspirin or ibuprofen, which are also anti-inflammatory agents. Like all painkilling drugs, they should be used to relieve discomfort, not to mask pain in order to continue the activity.

Warm compresses, 10 minutes on and 10 off, will help relax the muscle after the initial pain subsides. Binding your thigh with an elastic bandage will support the injured muscle; you may want to use a crutch to keep weight off the leg.

ALTERNATIVE CHOICES

BODY WORK

If your body is overstressed and your muscles are stiff and contracted, **massage** by a trained therapist will help to relax and tone your muscles. In a typical treatment the therapist uses warm body oil or a cooling gel, sometimes followed by ultrasound to stimulate circulation, before loosening and manipulating the affected muscles.

HOMEOPATHY

Arnica is the homeopath's first-aid remedy for muscle injuries. It can be taken orally and applied as a salve to the painful area. Rhus toxicodendron and Ruta are also remedies for muscle strains.

NUTRITION AND DIET

Good natural sources of vitamin C, essential for tissue building, are citrus fruits and potatoes. Potassium and calcium for bones are found in bananas, leafy greens, and low-fat dairy products.

To help your muscles operate at their best, drink plenty of water or a sports beverage before and after every workout.

PREVENTION

The best way to avoid muscle strains is to keep your body in good condition and avoid pushing yourself too hard at work or play.

Before starting your favorite sport or physical activity, particularly those that put heavy demands on your legs, take a few minutes to warm up. Major muscles like your hamstrings work best if you stretch them gradually and let them relax. Once into the activity, don't overstress your muscles. They'll begin to tell you when they have had enough, and it's foolish—even dangerous—to push them past their limits. When the activity is over, stretch the muscles gradually so they don't tighten up and go into a muscle contraction, or cramp, which can be just as painful as a muscle pull—although shorter lived. The exercises above, left are specifically recommended to condition and strengthen your hamstring muscles. ■

HAND AND WRIST PAIN

Read down this column to find your symptoms. Then read across.

SYMPTOMS	AILMENT/PROBLEM
◆ painful swelling and stiffness in wrist and/or finger joints; possible chills or fever; wrist or fingers may feel hot.	◆ Inflammation of either the joint itself (arthritis or gout) or the bursa, a sac that surrounds the joint and encases it with lubricating fluid (bursitis)
◆ pain in the wrist or fingers when bending your fingers or moving your hand a certain way; no other symptoms.	◆ Tendonitis
◆ numbness, tingling, weakness, or burning in the hands; wrist pain that extends into the forearm and/or the palm; difficulty making a fist; symptoms worsen at night.	◆ Carpal tunnel syndrome
◆ intense pain in the wrist or hand after an injury; the painful area may also be swollen, misshapen, bruised, and/or stiff.	◆ Possibly a sprained ligament, a strained muscle or tendon, or a fractured bone
◆ a wrist or finger joint is painful, red, and swollen; temperature quickly rises to over 100°F; general sick feeling.	◆ A bone infection, called osteomyelitis, or a joint infection, called infectious arthritis
◆ a few days to six weeks after a streptococcus infection (such as a strep throat), joints (including wrists, fingers, or other joints) are swollen, red, and painful, and may feel warm; temperature is 100.4°F or higher.	◆ Rheumatic fever

H

WHAT TO DO	OTHER INFO
◆ Take nonsteroidal anti-inflammatory drugs (NSAIDs) or aspirin to reduce pain and swelling. With rest, bursitis usually heals itself in a few days. See your doctor for treatment of gout, which can cause kidney damage if left untreated.	◆ Gout symptoms may dissipate within a week if you avoid alcohol, caffeine, coffee (regular and decaffeinated), and foods containing purine.
◆ Follow the RICE regimen: rest, ice, compression, and elevation (see Tendonitis), and take aspirin or ibuprofen as needed for pain. If pain isn't relieved in a week or so, see your doctor.	◆ Usually the inflammation is caused by making repeated, stressful movements or overworking the joint.
◆ Take nonsteroidal anti-inflammatory drugs (NSAIDs) or aspirin to reduce pain. When working, take short exercise breaks: For two minutes, slowly move your hand in circles, rotating it around the wrist; then clench both hands into fists and extend your fingers, and repeat 20 times.	◆ Symptoms result when the swollen tendons press on the median nerve, which passes from your wrist into your hand. Wearing a soft wrist splint at night and, if possible, while working can help relieve the pressure and reduce the pain.
◆ For 48 to 72 hours after the injury, follow the RICE regimen: rest, ice, compression, and elevation. See Sprains and Strains. If the pain is severe, or you cannot move your wrist or hand or lift anything, **call your doctor now.** See Emergencies/First Aid: Fractures and Dislocations.	
◆ **Call your doctor now.** Without antibiotics, the stiffness of infectious arthritis can become permanent. For osteomyelitis, the painful joint is immobilized (sometimes with a plaster cast). If an abscess has formed, it may need to be surgically drained.	◆ Osteomyelitis is most common in growing children (under age 12).
◆ **Call your doctor now.** You need bed rest and antibiotics for at least five weeks. Early treatment is crucial to avoid possibly fatal heart damage.	◆ To prevent a recurrence, your physician may prescribe a daily antibiotic for five years or longer. You must also be vigilant about receiving treatment for every sore throat or infection you get.

H

H

SYMPTOMS

- headache, nausea, dizziness, irritability, thirst, and fatigue—usually on awakening—after drinking excessive amounts of alcohol.
- in some cases, tension, paleness, tremor, vomiting, heartburn, unsteady gait, and loss of appetite.

CALL YOUR DOCTOR IF:

- you are concerned that you have developed or are at risk of developing a dependency on alcohol; this can be triggered by trying to offset a hangover by drinking more alcohol. *(See also Alcohol Abuse.)*

When you drink to excess, you are likely to suffer the headache, nausea, and other disagreeable symptoms of a hangover. The most intense hangover occurs about 14 to 15 hours after drinking starts—in part, researchers believe, because of the accumulation in your system of products metabolized from alcohol, such as lactic acid.

CAUSES

Alcohol by-products called congeners seem to increase the severity of a hangover. Gin and vodka have few congeners and are thus least likely to produce a hangover, whereas brandy, champagne, and whiskey have the potential to cause the worst hangovers. Red wine can also bring on a hangover because it contains tyramine, a substance that can cause severe headaches.

TREATMENT

Time is the only cure for the occasional hangover. In almost all cases, however, you can ease hangover symptoms through the self-help suggestions offered below. If you suffer frequent hangovers, you may have an alcohol abuse or dependency problem; seek professional help.

CONVENTIONAL MEDICINE

Most doctors recommend taking aspirin, ibuprofen, or acetaminophen for the headache; drinking fluids to offset dehydration; and eating light foods

C A U T I O N !

Never take aspirin before drinking; when combined with alcohol, aspirin will make you drunker. Never treat a hangover with more alcohol; although you may temporarily offset a hangover's symptoms, you're at risk of developing a dependency on alcohol.

high in carbohydrates and fructose (a natural sugar in fruit juices and honey) to calm nausea.

ALTERNATIVE CHOICES

HERBAL THERAPIES
White willow *(Salix alba)* bark, which contains a natural form of salicylate, the active ingredient in aspirin, may help relieve a headache. Drink hot as a tea (1 cup water simmered with 2 tsp bark for 10 minutes) or chew the bark. Chamomile *(Matricaria recutita)* tea may counter nausea.

HOMEOPATHY
Some homeopathic medicines come in kits that include remedies for the occasional hangover. For nausea, try Nux vomica (6x to 30c) every hour, for up to three doses.

NUTRITION AND DIET
Nutritionists recommend fruit juices—said to help the body burn alcohol—diluted with water

▼ Hangover MYTHS AND FACTS

MYTH: *Coffee sobers you up or prevents a hangover.*
FACT: *Only time will sober you up. The caffeine in coffee may help get rid of a headache but cannot prevent a hangover. Coffee's stimulating effect might lull you into thinking your judgment or motor control hasn't been impaired.*
MYTH: *If you don't feel hung over, you haven't been impaired by alcohol.*
FACT: *Research shows that drinking affects next-day performance, even if all traces of alcohol are absent from your system. If you are preparing for any activity in which peak performance is required, don't drink the night before.*

ACUPRESSURE

1 Pressing Large Intestine 4 in the web between your thumb and index finger may help relieve hangover headaches. Use the thumb and index finger of your right hand to squeeze the web of your left hand for one minute. Repeat on the right hand. If you are pregnant, do not use LI 4.

2 To help calm nausea and vomiting, press Pericardium 6. Place your thumb in the center of your inner wrist, two finger widths from the wrist crease and between the two forearm bones. Press firmly for one minute, three to five times; then repeat on the other arm.

or seltzer and consumed at two times the volume of the amount of alcohol you have drunk; crackers and honey to ease nausea; and bouillon to restore salt and potassium levels. Vitamin C, taken before and after drinking, is thought to help your body clear the alcohol from your system.

AT-HOME REMEDIES
Drink several glasses of water to rehydrate your body. Drink water through the day. Cold compresses on your head or the back of your neck may also bring relief.

PREVENTION

Moderation is the key to preventing a hangover. By drinking slowly, you give your body time to get rid of the alcohol before it enters the blood and your brain. Drink on a full stomach to slow the rate at which alcohol is absorbed. Avoid drinks high in congeners, and avoid mixing alcohol with carbonated beverages: The bubbles speed the alcohol to your bloodstream. The less you weigh, the less alcohol you should consume. ■

SYMPTOMS

Attacks, often seasonal, of:
- prolonged, sometimes violent sneezing.
- itchy, painful nose, throat, and roof of mouth.
- nasal discharge.
- stuffy, runny nose.
- postnasal drip, resulting in coughing.
- watery, itchy eyes.
- head and nasal congestion.
- ear pressure or fullness.
- lethargy.

CALL YOUR DOCTOR IF:

- your condition becomes so severe that it interferes with your life and you're unable to control it with over-the-counter medications. Your physician may administer prescription drugs, such as nonsedating antihistamines, to help.
- a secondary infection develops in congested sinus cavities; signs are fever, pain, a yellow or green discharge, postnasal drip, and sinus or tooth tenderness.

Hay fever is an immune disorder characterized by an allergic response to pollen grains and other substances. Also known as **allergic rhinitis,** there are two types: **seasonal,** which occurs only during the time of year in which certain plants pollinate, and **perennial,** which occurs all year round. (A related problem, **nonallergic rhinitis,** shares symptoms with hay fever but doesn't result from an allergy. See Sneezing.)

Typically, if you suffer from hay fever in the spring, you're probably allergic to tree pollens. Grass and weed pollens may be causing your allergic reaction during the summer. In autumn ragweed may plague you, and fungus spores cause problems from late March through November.

People with **perennial** hay fever are usually allergic to one or more of these outdoor agents. Perennial hay fever can also be brought on by other allergy-causing substances, or allergens. These include house dust mites, feathers, and animal dander (the tiny skin flakes animals shed along with fur), all of which may be found in pillows, down clothing and bedding, shower curtains, heavy draperies, upholstery, and thick carpeting. Another common allergen, mold, is usually found in damp areas such as bathrooms and basements.

A hay fever attack can last between 15 and 20 minutes and may recur several times a day during your hay fever season. Although they can be exhausting, attacks cause no permanent damage.

CAUSES

If you suffer from hay fever, it's because your immune system views harmless inhaled pollen or other allergens as dangerous substances invading your body. Your system overreacts, flooding your bloodstream with a chemical known as histamine, which inflames the lining of your sinuses and eyelids and also sets in motion the other symptoms associated with hay fever, such as sneezing. All of these symptoms are meant to protect your body either by expelling the allergen or by swelling body orifices so it can't enter. As a result of congestion in the veins in the lining of your sinuses, dark circles, commonly known as allergic shiners, may appear under your eyes; if you have perennial allergic rhinitis, they may be present all year round. The swelling of your mucous membranes occasionally results in nasal polyps; nosebleeds are also common during hay fever attacks.

No one knows why some people's immune systems tend to overreact to pollen and other substances. Evidence points to the likelihood that hay fever is an inherited trait. People under age 40 with asthma or eczema are more likely to develop hay fever than those without these ailments.

DIAGNOSTIC AND TEST PROCEDURES

Your doctor may be able to make a diagnosis based on a physical exam and observation of your symptoms. Skin tests may be recommended to determine which pollens cause the most sensitivity. In a scratch or prick test, your physician makes tiny scratches or needle punctures in your back or arm and applies drops containing a small amount of possible allergy-causing substances. If your skin becomes red and itchy after 20 minutes, the test has pinpointed the offending allergens. A radioallergosorbent test, or RAST, may be used to check your blood for elevated levels of the antibodies produced by your immune system to guard against specific allergens. Your doctor may refer you to an allergist for further tests and treatment.

TREATMENT

Many medications are available to deal with the symptoms of hay fever, although the best approach appears to be prevention of attacks, or avoidance of known allergens, or both.

CONVENTIONAL MEDICINE

Medical treatment strategies typically begin with avoidance of allergens, then move on to drug therapy, and may finally resort to immunotherapy. Mild cases of hay fever can be controlled with over-the-counter antihistamines, such as chlorpheniramine, which have few side effects. These drugs must be taken regularly and over a long period of time to produce an effect. Phenylephrine and pseudoephedrine are decongestants that help unblock nasal passages. They can help during an acute attack but should be taken for a few days only since prolonged use can have the rebound effect of making congestion worse. If you're taking medication for a heart condition or are taking the antibiotic erythromycin or the antifungal drug ketoconazole, be sure to check with your doctor before taking a decongestant or antihistamine to avoid drug interactions. For severe cases your doctor may also prescribe a stronger antihistamine, such as loratadine, astemizole, or terfenadine.

Some over-the-counter nasal sprays contain both a decongestant and an antihistamine. These sprays help with pain and itching by opening clogged nasal passages and reducing inflammation. Regular use of the prescription spray cromolyn prevents the lining of the nasal passages from reacting to the allergen affecting you. More severe cases may benefit from a corticosteroid nasal spray such as beclomethasone.

Be aware that over-the-counter nasal sprays and drops may be addictive and should be used sparingly. Medications containing salicylates such as aspirin should also be avoided as they may worsen symptoms.

Another avenue to try is allergy shots, or immunotherapy. This treatment involves a series of injections of increasingly larger amounts of the allergen until your system becomes desensitized to it and no longer overreacts in response to it. Immunotherapy has shown positive results in up to 75 percent of sufferers with extreme cases of hay fever. Standard treatment lasts from one to three years.

ALTERNATIVE CHOICES

A number of alternative therapies can help with symptom control and as preventive measures.

AROMATHERAPY

Inhalations of eucalyptus *(Eucalyptus globulus)*, peppermint *(Mentha piperita)*, or hyssop *(Hyssopus officinalis)* may help to ease sinus irritation and pain.

H

CHINESE HERBS

Ephedra (Ephedra sinica) has a long history as a hay fever and allergy remedy. Chinese herbalists believe it loses its effectiveness over time and so is best used for short periods in combination with other herbs. An herbalist may combine ephedra with licorice (Glycyrrhiza uralensis), which is thought to have antiallergy and antiinflammatory properties. In some people, ephedra can produce side effects such as palpitations, insomnia, and high blood pressure. Ginseng (Panax ginseng) is another herb that's compatible with ephedra and may be especially effective when combined with herbal expectorants, which promote the expulsion of mucus. Commonly used expectorants include pinellia (Pinellia ternata), cynanchum (Cynanchum stautoni), and polygala (Polygala tenuifolia). Consult an herbalist specializing in Chinese medicine for more information.

HERBAL THERAPIES

The following mixture may prevent some symptoms. Infuse in 1 cup boiled water for 10 minutes: 2 parts elder (Sambucus nigra), 1 part ephedra (Ephedra sinica), 1 part eyebright (Euphrasia officinalis), and 1 part goldenseal (Hydrastis canadensis). Drink 1 cup of this tea three times a day during the two months before hay fever season begins. Be aware that ephedra may be too stimulating for children. Regular doses of parsley (Petroselinum crispum) may help with hay fever; it is thought to work by reducing your body's production of histamine.

You may be able to slow down your body's mucus production with goldenrod (Solidago virgaurea), garlic (Allium sativum), yarrow (Achillea millefolium), or agrimony (Agrimonia eupatoria). Bathe irritated eyes with compresses soaked in either eyebright (Euphrasia officinalis) or chamomile (Matricaria recutita); make a tea from the leaves and dilute it by 50 percent with water or saline solution before using to soak the compresses.

HOMEOPATHY

For watery, hot eyes, a burning nasal discharge with sneezing, and symptoms that feel worse late at night, try Arsenicum album. If your eyes feel inflamed and very watery, your nose is blocked at

ACUPRESSURE

1 Pressing Large Intestine 4 in the web between your thumb and index finger may help ease hay fever. Use the thumb and index finger of your right hand to squeeze the web of your left hand for one minute. Repeat this on the right hand. If pregnant, do not use LI 4.

2 Pressure on Governing Vessel 24.5 may also help relieve symptoms of hay fever. Place the tip of your middle finger at the top of the bridge of your nose, between your eyebrows. Press lightly for two minutes and breathe deeply. Do three to five times, at least twice a day.

night but has a watery discharge during the day, and you have a headache, consider using Euphrasia. Pulsatilla can help if your symptoms—thick, yellow mucus accompanied by a loss of taste and smell—are made worse by warm rooms but are better outdoors. If your watery, itchy eyes and sneezing, runny nose with a burning discharge become worse in a warm room, try Allium cepa. Consult a homeopathic practitioner for proper doses of these remedies.

NUTRITION AND DIET

Nutritionists believe that refined sugar and casein, the protein in dairy products, are mucusproducing substances that are best avoided during hay fever season. Taking a commercial preparation of the mineral dolomite, which contains calcium and magnesium, may help regulate histamine production.

Some researchers believe that honey has a desensitizing and antiallergic effect that may relieve some hay fever symptoms. Two months before the season starts, begin eating 2 tsp daily of raw honey that comes from a nearby hive. You can also try chewing a bite-sized piece of honeycomb for 5 to 10 minutes twice a day (but don't swallow it) or taking five tablets of pollen extract supplements every day beginning several weeks before hay fever season. Check with your doctor first to avoid potential allergic reactions.

Many people with hay fever are also allergic to certain foods and may experience symptoms as a result of eating allergy-triggering substances in such foods as eggs, nuts, fish, shellfish, chocolate, dairy products, wheat, citrus fruits, or food colorings or preservatives. To determine whether food allergies might be at the root of, or perhaps compounding, your hay fever problems, try an elimination diet. Stop eating all the suspected foods, including those mentioned above, as well as prepackaged or prepared foods, for 10 days. If your symptoms disappear or diminish, reintroduce one food at a time and see whether your symptoms recur. If they do, eliminate the offending food and all its by-products from your daily diet.

AT-HOME REMEDIES

The best way to combat the allergens that are assaulting you is to avoid them. Stay indoors between six and ten o'clock in the morning and on days when the pollen count is high. The pollen count drops on rainy days and climbs when it's hot, sunny, and windy outside. If you must go outdoors, wear protective glasses and hold a handkerchief over your nose and mouth or wear a dust mask with a filter for pollen. Resist the temptation to rub your eyes.

Keep windows—in your home and car—closed and the air conditioning turned on. Change ventilation system filters in your home once a month. Remove allergens from the air with ionizing air cleaners. Prevent mold in damp basements by using space heaters and dehumidifiers.

Avoid mowing your lawn or raking leaves since these activities stir up pollens and molds. However, try to keep your grass no more than an inch high in the spring and summer so as not to allow pollination. If you must do yard work yourself, wear a filtered mask and protective glasses. Wash your face, hands, and hair and rinse your eyes when coming in from outdoors to avoid leaving traces of pollen on your pillow.

Mites live in household dust and are impossible to get rid of entirely, but measures can be taken to minimize them: Remove thick carpeting, heavy drapes, and upholstered furniture; put plastic covers on mattresses and pillows; keep floors clean; avoid down (feathers) in comforters, clothing, sleeping bags, and pillows; and wear a mask when vacuuming.

PREVENTION

Although a tendency to develop hay fever could be in your genes, you may be able to avoid symptoms by taking preventive steps and being alert to the signals. If you have eczema or asthma, be aware that you may be more likely to develop hay fever. Consult an allergist or try the elimination or raw honey diets mentioned above. Strengthen your immune system with a healthful lifestyle including wholesome foods, exercise, vitamin supplements, and herbs. Cut down on environmental pollutants and toxins as much as possible by keeping your home clean and your yard neat.

SYMPTOMS

If your headache is:

◆ a dull, steady pain that feels like a band tightening around your head, you have a **tension headache.**

◆ throbbing, begins on one side, and causes nausea, you have a **migraine.** Visual disturbances, such as flickering points of light, may precede the headache.

◆ a throbbing pain around one red, watery eye, with nasal congestion on that side of your face, you have a **cluster headache.**

◆ a steady pain in the area behind your face that gets worse if you bend forward and is accompanied by congestion, you have a **sinus headache.**

CALL YOUR DOCTOR IF:

◆ a severe headache is accompanied by vomiting, limb weakness, double vision, slurred speech, or difficulty in swallowing; you may have a cerebral hemorrhage or an aneurysm—**get medical help now.**

◆ your headache is of a kind you've never had, occurs first thing in the morning, is persistent, brings on vomiting, and abates during the day; you may have high blood pressure or in very rare cases a brain tumor. See your doctor without delay.

◆ you have a high fever, light hurts your eyes, the pain is severe and is accompanied by nausea and a stiff neck; you may have meningitis—**get medical help now.**

◆ after a head injury, you are drowsy, with dizziness, vertigo, nausea, or vomiting; you may have a concussion. See your doctor without delay.

Although painful and troublesome, most headaches are minor health concerns and can be easily treated with aspirin or another analgesic. But if they are severe, recur frequently, or are attended by other symptoms, you may need to take additional steps, including consultation with your doctor.

Headaches are categorized according to their underlying causes. Muscle contraction, or **tension,** headaches make up one common group. Vascular (blood-vessel) headaches are a second common category; it includes both **migraine** and **cluster headaches.** A third group consists of headaches caused by **sinus** problems. *(See Sinusitis.)*

Tension headaches, which afflict almost everyone at one time or another, bring on a dull, persistent, nonthrobbing pain that can make your head feel as if it's gripped in a tight band. The muscles of your neck may seem knotted, and certain areas on your head and neck may be sensitive to touch. Nerve endings in the head and neck that have been irritated by taut muscles are the chief source of pain. Tension headaches can be short-lived and infrequent, or they can be enduring and chronic.

Migraines are the most debilitating of headaches; they can be completely incapacitating. With some sufferers—a minority—a migraine attack is preceded by a warning sign, called an aura; it may include visual disturbances such as flickering points of light, blind spots, or zigzag lines, or more rarely, numbness in a limb or the smelling of strange odors. Whether a warning occurs or not, a migraine will usually begin with an intense, throbbing pain on one side of the head. This pain may spread and is often accompanied by nausea and vomiting. A migraine can last from a few hours to three days and can cause oversensitivity to light, odors, and sound.

All the various symptoms of migraines seem linked to changes in the diameter of blood vessels in the head: The blood vessels constrict during the initial stage and dilate when the headache pain begins. These changes may be due to an imbalance in a brain chemical known as serotonin. Hormones, too, apparently can play a role; there is a strong correlation between changes in estrogen levels and migraines.

Cluster headaches are so named because they tend to come in bunches. Typically they begin several hours after a person falls asleep and are sometimes preceded by a mild aching sensation on one side of the head. The pain—severe, piercing, and usually located in and around one red, watery eye—is generally accompanied by nasal congestion and a flushed face. It lasts from 30 minutes to two hours, then diminishes or disappears altogether, only to recur perhaps a day later. A barrage of four or more attacks may occur in the course of the day, and cluster headaches can strike every day for weeks or months before going into long periods of remission. The vast majority of sufferers are men.

Sinus headaches are characterized by pain in the forehead, nasal area, eyes, and sometimes the top of the head; in some cases, they also produce a feeling of pressure behind the face. Inflammation or infection of the membranes lining the sinus cavities can give rise to such headaches. Also, the headache pain may stem from suction on the sinus walls, which occurs when nasal congestion creates a partial vacuum in the sinuses.

CAUSES

Headaches strike for many reasons. **Sinus headaches** typically result from hay fever and other seasonal allergies, or from a cold or the flu. With **tension headaches,** stress is the most common trigger; it may stem from anxiety about work or family life, or it may derive from some physical factor such as persistent noise. Eyestrain, poor posture, too much caffeine, or the grinding or clenching of teeth at night can also lead to tension headaches.

Migraines are somewhat more mysterious. Although much evidence indicates that constricting and swelling of blood vessels is involved, some researchers believe that the headaches are primarily neurological in origin. Because migraines often run in families, it seems likely that genetics can play a role. In any event, a wide range of factors can trigger an attack; among them are excessive caffeine, various foods or scents, naps, dry winds, changes in altitude or

COMMON SOURCES OF HEADACHE PAIN

AREA OF PAIN

NERVES

CLUSTER HEADACHE
Although their exact cause is unknown, cluster headaches may arise from pressure on nerves around the eyes. Swollen sinus tissue may press against portions of these nerves, causing these electrical pathways to short-circuit and emit pain signals.

MUSCLES

AREAS OF PAIN

TENSION HEADACHE
Of the various types of tension headaches, one is thought to be linked to disorders in certain muscles in the head and the neck. Pain can be localized around any of these muscles or can spread to affect a broad portion of the scalp.

SINUS CAVITIES

SINUS HEADACHE
With a sinus headache, congestion within the sinus cavities leads to swelling that puts pressure on surrounding tissue and nerves, causing pain to radiate across the face.

ACUPRESSURE

1 Sinus headaches may be relieved by pressing Stomach 3. While looking in a mirror, place the index fingers of both hands at the bottom of your cheekbones, fingertips directly under the pupils of your eyes. Press firmly for one minute. Repeat three times.

2 Pressure on Governing Vessel 24.5 may help ease headaches. Place the tip of your middle finger at the top of the bridge of your nose, between your eyebrows. Press lightly for two minutes and breathe deeply. Do three to five times, at least twice a day.

3 To reduce neck muscle stress that may be associated with tension headaches, try pressing Gall Bladder 20. Place the tips of the middle fingers in the hollows at the base of the skull, about two inches apart, on either side of the spine. Press firmly for one minute.

4 Pressing Large Intestine 4 may help relieve sinus headaches. Using the thumb and index finger of your right hand, squeeze the web of your left hand for one minute. Repeat this on the right hand. If pregnant, do not use LI 4.

5 Pressure to Liver 3 may provide headache relief. Place the index fingers at the top of each foot, fingertips next to the large knuckle of the big toe, between the big and second toes. Press for one minute, then release. Repeat two or three times, twice daily.

seasons, hormonal fluctuations or birth-control pills, missing a meal, or stuffy rooms. Migraines may also occur in the aftermath of intense emotions such as excitement or anger. Exercise, sexual activity, or very cold foods can also jump-start a migraine.

Cluster headaches are the most baffling of all. They are more common in heavy smokers than in nonsmokers, and alcohol consumption and certain foods seem to be involved in some cases, but the root cause is unknown.

DIAGNOSTIC AND TEST PROCEDURES

To rule out possible organic causes of headaches— for example, an aneurysm, tumor, or structural abnormality—a physician may employ vision tests, x-rays, a CT scan, a lumbar puncture, or an EEG.

TREATMENT

Both conventional and alternative medicine can be effective in dealing with headaches, and the two approaches may be combined. Almost all practitioners consider **relaxation** beneficial for **tension** and **migraine headaches,** for example.

CONVENTIONAL MEDICINE

Most **tension headaches** can be helped by analgesics such as aspirin, acetaminophen, or ibuprofen; antidepressants can help in chronic cases. **Sinus headaches** are relieved by antibiotics and decongestants.

A wide range of medications are prescribed for **migraines.** If you have three or more severe, prolonged migraines per month, your doctor may suggest using prophylactic, or preventive, medications on a continual basis. These include propranolol, a beta-adrenergic blocker that works by reducing constriction in blood vessels; a calcium channel blocker such as verapamil; or antidepressants. If your migraines are milder and occur less often than three times per month, your doctor may suggest drugs such as an isometheptene-containing combination or ergotamine (available as a suppository if the vomiting caused by your

H

migraines prevents you from keeping a pill down). The drug sumatriptan, available in tablet or injectable form, is designed to treat migraines and brings dramatic relief. A therapeutic nasal spray based on the serotonin-inhibiting drug dihydroergotamine (D.H.E. 45) acts quickly to constrict blood vessels and reduce inflammation. Even aspirin, if taken in effervescent form at the first sign of an attack, can be effective. Drink it 10 minutes after taking metoclopramide, which reduces nausea and improves absorption, to shorten an attack.

Simple analgesics do little for **cluster headaches,** because they do not act quickly enough. However, doctors have found that inhaling pure oxygen can be highly effective in providing relief. *(See At-Home Remedies, page 441.)* A short course of corticosteroids, methysergide maleate, and lithium carbonate can alleviate cluster headaches, as can some of the calcium channel blockers and vasoconstrictors that are used for migraines.

ALTERNATIVE CHOICES

The vast majority of alternative therapies attempt to address the underlying causes of headaches. Because tension and stress so often figure in headaches, relaxation techniques are a staple of therapeutic programs.

ACUPRESSURE

Follow the illustrations at far left to locate pressure points associated with headache relief. These techniques are often used in combination with one of the aromatherapy oils below.

AROMATHERAPY

The following herbal oils may aid relaxation, easing the pain of **tension** or **migraine** headaches. Moisten your fingertips with one or two drops of lavender *(Lavandula officinalis)* essential oil blended with a so-called carrier oil such as sunflower oil, then gently massage your temples with a circular motion; repeat in the hollows at the sides of your eyes, behind your ears, and over your neck. For a **sinus headache,** try the same techniques using eucalyptus *(Eucalyptus globulus)* or wintergreen *(Gaultheria procumbens)*. For any type of headache, inhale a blend of lavender, rosemary *(Rosmarinus officinalis),* and peppermint *(Mentha piperita).* Compresses applied to the affected area or a bath using these oils can relax muscles, easing pain.

CHIROPRACTIC

Some **tension headaches** are caused by posture that puts unnecessary strain on muscles. A chiropractor may be able to remove the strain through spinal or cervical manipulation and realignment. In some studies, spinal manipulation has been shown to produce fewer side effects and have longer-lasting results than conventional drug use.

HERBAL THERAPIES

Perhaps the most widely recommended herbal remedy for treating and preventing **migraines** is feverfew *(Chrysanthemum parthenium),* which is thought to work by blocking excessive secretion of serotonin, a neurotransmitter. When blood vessels constrict in the initial stage of a migraine, serotonin is released; feverfew may help counteract this by dilating those blood vessels. Chewing a leaf or two daily is one approach to prevention, but

C A U T I O N !

Although they can be effective against headaches when used on a temporary basis, painkillers—especially those containing caffeine or codeine—should not be taken over long periods of time. Studies show that the constant use of painkillers may have a rebound effect—actually causing headaches—or can block other medications, such as prophylactic drugs, that you may be taking on a regular basis to prevent migraine headaches. Dependence on painkillers may also hamper the effectiveness of endorphins, the body's natural painkillers. It also seems that dependence on painkillers may permanently alter the pain-control pathways in the brain and spinal cord.

this can occasionally cause mouth ulcers; as a substitute for the leaves, you can use 125-mg capsules. To offset an acute attack, take 3 or 4 capsules right away, then continue this dosage every four hours; but don't exceed 12 capsules in a day. Migraines brought on by stress may benefit from a combination of equal parts of hawthorn (Crataegus oxyacantha), linden (Tilia spp.), wood betony (Pedicularis canadensis), skullcap (Scutellaria lateriflora), and cramp bark (Viburnum opulus), taken three times a day as a tea or tincture. For migraines accompanied by nausea and vomiting, try taking 500 mg of dried ginger (Zingiber officinale) with water at the onset of the warning stage, if your headache pattern includes an aura; repeat every two hours if needed. Three daily doses of goldenseal (Hydrastis canadensis) in tincture, tea, or powdered form may help reduce **sinus headache** pain.

Tension headaches may respond to three daily infusions of valerian (Valeriana officinalis) when combined with skullcap and passionflower (Passiflora incarnata). **Cluster headaches** may get quick relief from several daily applications inside the nostrils of an over-the-counter ointment made from cayenne (Capsicum frutescens). The same ointment applied to the skin is also said to be effective in preventing **migraines.** Because cayenne is hot and can cause painful skin burns, it's best used under a doctor's care.

HOMEOPATHY

A range of homeopathic medicines are available to treat specific types of headaches. For a throbbing headache that is worse on the right side when lying down, try Belladonna. For severe, "splitting" headaches that feel worse with motion, noise, light, or touch, try Bryonia. For **sinus** pain with a thick, green nasal discharge, consider Kali bichromicum. For **migraines** or other chronic headaches, see a homeopathic practitioner.

LIFESTYLE

Regular **exercise** can release endorphins, the body's natural painkilling agents. Exercise may also help to dilate blood vessels, which increases blood flow and may counteract the constricting action that occurs at the onset of most **migraines.**

POURING PAIN AWAY

Your imagination can sometimes be the best medicine for a headache. Try this technique, which relies on your mind's own power to overcome pain. It helps to have a partner talk you through this exercise, but with practice you may be able to do it yourself.

Close your eyes and imagine that your headache is a liquid that fills a certain size of container—the more painful the headache, the bigger the container. Now imagine pouring your headache pain into a slightly smaller container, without letting any of the liquid overflow. Keep pouring the liquid into smaller and smaller containers; bit by bit, you should feel the pain reducing.

To nip a **tension headache** in the bud, try the following exercise while breathing deeply and thinking calm thoughts: While seated, inhale and gently tip your head back until you're looking up at the ceiling (be careful not to tip your head back too far, since this can compress the cervical spine); exhale and bring your head forward until your chin rests on your chest; repeat twice.

Keeping a headache diary can help you pinpoint the factors causing your specific headache patterns. The diary should provide answers to these 10 questions:

1. When did you first develop headaches?
2. How often do you have them?
3. Do you experience symptoms prior to the headaches?
4. Where is the pain exactly?
5. How long does it last?
6. At what time of day do the headaches occur?
7. Does the eating of certain types of food precede your headaches?

8. If you're female, at what time in your monthly cycle do they occur?
9. Are the headaches triggered by physical or environmental factors, such as odor, noise, or certain kinds of weather?
10. What words most accurately describe the pain of your headache: throbbing, stabbing, blinding, piercing . . . ?

MASSAGE
Massage therapy can relieve headache-producing tension in the muscles of your head, neck, shoulders, and face. Try giving yourself a 10-minute scalp massage: Place both middle fingers on your forehead at your hairline; using gentle pressure, gradually work them back to the crown of your head; tracing your hairline, repeat this motion in half-inch increments until you reach your temples; rotate your fingers on both sides for a few minutes; then bring both thumbs to the base of your skull along your hairline and massage both sides of your skull up to your crown to release any tightness.

MIND/BODY MEDICINE
Meditation and **progressive relaxation** therapies are effective in reducing stress, which can cause **tension headaches. Biofeedback** training methods can also be helpful in controlling stress. **Migraine headaches,** too, can be treated through a biofeedback method called thermal biofeedback, in which you learn to increase the temperature of your hands and feet. Warming these extremities involves dilating the vessels that carry blood to them—a process that, in turn, may reduce abnormal blood-vessel constriction in the skull and possibly result in diminished migraine frequency, intensity, and duration.

NUTRITION AND DIET
Among the foods sometimes associated with **migraine headaches** are chocolate, aged cheeses, citrus fruits, processed meats containing sodium nitrates or the food additive MSG, and red wine. Keeping a food diary can help you identify foods to eliminate.

Magnesium relaxes constricted blood vessels; low levels of magnesium may contribute to **mi-**graine and **cluster headaches.** Supplemental doses of 200 mg three times a day may be preventive. Taking 50 to 200 mg of niacin (vitamin B_3) and niacinamide at the first hint of pain may help keep blood vessels dilated, possibly reducing the initial constriction phase of **migraines** and avoiding an attack.

OSTEOPATHY
Osteopaths believe headache pain stemming from pressure on nerves or blood vessels can be eased by neuromuscular manipulation and soft-tissue massage of your head, neck, and upper back.

AT-HOME REMEDIES
◆ Holding an ice pack or a bag of frozen vegetables against your forehead while soaking your feet in hot water may stop a **migraine** if done right away.
◆ At the first sign of a headache, drink three glasses of very cold water, then retire with a cold compress to a dark, quiet room to sleep (without a pillow).
◆ Inhaling pure oxygen from a tank kept near your bed may offset nighttime attacks of a **cluster headache.** But be sure to consult a doctor on how to use the oxygen. ■

SYMPTOMS

People often do not recognize a hearing problem until it is brought to their attention by a relative or a friend. Symptoms can include:

◆ an inability to hear or distinguish some or all sounds in one or both ears.

◆ difficulty understanding conversation when many people are talking in the background.

◆ a need to turn up the volume on the television or radio louder than other people find comfortable.

Hearing problems are sometimes accompanied by dizziness, earache, discharge or bleeding from the ear, ringing noise in the ear, or in rare cases, weakness of facial muscles.

CALL YOUR DOCTOR IF:

◆ you notice any hearing problems; it is important that you receive a timely medical evaluation, because early treatment may enable you to avoid permanent damage and regain full hearing.

◆ you experience a sudden and total hearing loss in one or both ears; this may indicate a severe reaction to medication, a tumor on the auditory nerve, or a neurological problem. Seek medical care as soon as possible.

◆ you have some hearing loss and your ear secretes pus or fluid; this may indicate an ear infection or a perforated eardrum.

◆ your hearing loss is accompanied by dizziness and nausea; these may be signs of otitis media, Ménière's disease, or another condition that needs medical attention.

Some 28 million people in the United States have a hearing problem significant enough to interfere with their ability to understand conversations and communicate with others. As many as 2 million cannot hear at all and are considered profoundly deaf. Your chances of having a hearing problem increase dramatically with age: More than a third of people over the age of 75 experience difficulty hearing, a problem that often leads to frustration and social isolation.

One form of age-related hearing loss—known as **presbycusia**—usually begins between the ages of 40 and 50 and gets progressively worse. People with presbycusia often have trouble hearing higher frequencies and thus find it particularly difficult to understand women and children, who generally speak at a higher pitch than men. Presbycusia tends to afflict men more frequently and more severely than women.

Hearing problems are less common in children, but if left untreated, they can have a major impact on how well a child learns and makes friends. About 1 in 1,000 infants has a hearing problem severe enough to inhibit the child's ability to learn to speak.

Doctors divide hearing loss into two main categories. **Conductive** hearing loss occurs when something interferes with the transfer of sound waves from the outer to the inner ear. **Sensorineural** hearing loss results from damage to the inner ear or to the nerves that transmit sound impulses from the inner ear to the brain. Sounds may reach the inner ear, but they are not perceived because the necessary messages aren't sent correctly to the brain. Sometimes a person has a mixture of both types of hearing loss.

CAUSES

A hearing loss, whether partial or total, is not in itself an illness, but rather a symptom of an underlying disorder. A wide variety of conditions can lead to hearing problems. Common causes of **conductive** hearing loss include excessive earwax, ear infections, and a ruptured or perforated eardrum. Benign cysts, tumors, and objects lodged in the ear canal, such as an insect or a

THE MECHANICS OF HEARING

OUTER EAR CANAL
MALLEUS
BRANCHES OF AUDITORY NERVE
COCHLEA
STAPES

EARDRUM
INCUS

The ear picks up vibrations in the air, or sound waves, which resonate against the eardrum at the end of the outer ear canal. The eardrum transmits the vibrations to three tiny bones—the malleus, incus, and stapes—in the middle ear. The cochlea in the inner ear picks up the vibrations and transmits them as nerve impulses along the auditory nerve to the brain, which interprets the impulses as sound.

piece of a child's toy, can also block the transmission of sounds to the inner ear. In addition, several inherited conditions can cause conductive hearing loss. The most common of these is **otosclerosis,** a degenerative disease of the small bones in the middle ear. About 1 percent of the population is affected by otosclerosis, usually in both ears.

Genetics is also considered a major, if not the major, cause of **sensorineural** hearing loss, particularly in children. Experts estimate that half of the cases of profound deafness in children have a genetic source. A genetic predisposition is also an important factor in the development of **presbycusia.** People with presbycusia experience gradual destruction of the thousands of tiny hair cells that line the cochlea, the spiral-shaped cavity of the inner ear. Without the hairs, which help transfer sound vibrations into nerve signals that travel to the brain, perceiving sounds becomes difficult or impossible.

Prolonged exposure to loud noise, particularly if it is high pitched, can also destroy the sensitive hair cells of the cochlea and lead to partial or total sensorineural hearing loss. Workers whose jobs subject them to high-intensity noise, such as carpenters, construction workers, and rock musicians, are at increased risk, as are people with hobbies such as hunting or snowmobiling.

Several infectious diseases—most notably shingles, meningitis, syphilis, and cytomegalovirus—have been implicated in sensorineural hearing loss. In addition, if a woman contracts German measles during pregnancy, her child will be at increased risk of a permanent hearing disability. A child who receives inadequate oxygen during the birth process may also suffer some degree of irreversible damage to the hearing mechanisms of the ears.

Other causes of sensorineural hearing loss include Ménière's disease, tumors of the brain or auditory nerve, diabetes, and vascular disorders that lead to stroke, such as high blood pressure and atherosclerosis. High doses of aspirin, quinine, some types of antibiotics, and several diuretics used to treat high blood pressure may also lead to permanent damage of the inner ear. People with multiple sclerosis or other types of neurological diseases are prone to sensorineural hearing problems as well. In addition, a physical blow or penetrating injury to the ear may cause a permanent loss of hearing.

DIAGNOSTIC AND TEST PROCEDURES

To determine whether the underlying cause of your hearing problem is a medical condition for which you can be treated, your doctor will give you a general physical exam, including a careful examination of your ears. You may also be given some simple hearing tests. If the source of the problem remains unclear, you may be sent to an otologist or an otolaryngologist (both ear specialists) for formal hearing tests.

The most common of these tests is audiometry, which measures first how well you hear sounds conducted through the air (to determine **conductive** hearing loss) and then how well you hear sounds through the bones of your head (to determine **sensorineural** hearing loss). You will be put in a soundproof room and given earphones through which a series of sounds, ranging from low to high frequencies, will be played at increasing or decreasing loudness. You may also be given neurological tests, and the specialist may recommend an MRI or a CT scan to check for possible tumors.

TREATMENT

In most cases of **conductive** hearing loss, once the underlying cause of the problem has been treated, hearing returns. With **sensorineural** hearing loss, however, the damage tends to be permanent. Treatment can sometimes stop or slow down the progression of the loss, but the quality of hearing seldom returns to what it was before the damage occurred.

CONVENTIONAL MEDICINE

Treatment of your hearing problem will depend on its underlying cause. If it is a simple case of wax buildup, your doctor will clean out your ear with a cotton-tipped probe or a suction device. If your ear is infected, you may be treated with oral antibiotics or with ear drops containing an antibiotic and hydrocortisone to help relieve the itching. If fluid created by a middle ear infection does not drain away naturally, your doctor may perform a myringotomy, a procedure in which a small incision is made in the eardrum and the fluid is sucked out.

Repeated attacks of middle ear infections, as well as allergies, recurrent respiratory infections, and enlarged adenoids, can cause the eustachian tubes, which connect the pharnyx with the middle ear, to become blocked. The air pressure within the middle ear then drops, causing fluid to accumulate within the cavity and the eardrum to be sucked inward. This condition is relatively common among young children. Your child's doctor may recommend that a tiny plastic tube be inserted through the eardrum to balance the air pressure in the middle ear for six months or longer while the eustachian tubes recover.

Repeated middle ear infections can lead to other conditions that may require surgery to repair or replace damaged structures within the ear

GET THE WAX OUT

One of the most common causes of temporary hearing loss is excessive wax buildup. To remove the wax without damaging your ear, try this simple cleaning method:

Warm 1 tbsp of hydrogen peroxide by setting the jar in a sink full of hot water for a few minutes. Tilt your head to the side and put a dropperful of the warmed liquid in your blocked ear. Let it remain there for three minutes. Then tilt your head the other way and let the hydrogen peroxide run out onto a towel or tissue. The wax should be soft enough to be wiped away with a piece of cotton. Repeat if necessary.

If the wax is particularly stubborn and resists the hydrogen peroxide, try softening it first with several applications of 3 or 4 drops of castor oil or glycerin. If the wax has become firmly impacted, however, you may find it necessary to have the ear cleaned by your doctor.

and help return hearing to normal. For example, a middle ear infection in rare cases can spread to an area of the bone behind the ear called the mastoid process, and a special operation known as a mastoidectomy becomes necessary to remove the damaged bone and restore hearing.

If your hearing loss is caused by a ruptured eardrum, your doctor will probably prescribe an antibiotic to make sure that no infection develops in the middle ear. In some cases, a plastic patch is placed over the eardrum to protect it while it heals. If after a period of three months the eardrum has not responded to this treatment, your doctor may suggest a minor operation in which a tiny piece of tissue, often from a vein, is grafted onto the eardrum. This surgery is usually successful and returns hearing to normal.

If your hearing loss is caused by **otosclerosis,** your doctor will probably recommend a stapedectomy, an operation in which the diseased bones of the ear are replaced with tiny metal substitutes. Studies have shown that stapedectomies improve hearing in 90 percent of cases. However, the operation also has its risks: About 2 percent to 5 percent of people who undergo the surgery become totally deaf in the affected ear.

Because it usually involves damage to nerves or to the inner ear, **sensorineural** hearing loss cannot be treated successfully with either antibiotics or surgery. Some sensorineural losses can be prevented, however, with prompt medical care. A sudden hearing loss caused by a tiny blood clot in the artery that feeds the ear, for example, can be treated with anticoagulants. Your physician might also prescribe a vasodilator, which causes the blood vessels to expand and allows the clot to pass. If these drugs are taken within 24 hours of the first sign of the hearing loss and if the loss is partial, a full recovery is quite likely.

For **presbycusia** and other kinds of permanent hearing loss, the only method of treatment is a hearing aid, a device that contains a tiny microphone and amplifier to increase the volume of sound electrically. The hearing aid is powered by a tiny battery that lasts several months. Some hearing aids are worn behind the ear, although compact models that fit within the outer ear canal are now more common.

A hearing aid will not make your hearing problem go away, but it will improve your ability to hear. Be sure you are fitted by a qualified professional. Your doctor should be able to recommend a reputable audiologist or hearing-aid dealer, who will give you a hearing-aid evaluation and let you try several different kinds of devices. To ensure an exact fit and good performance, a mold will be made of your ear canal. Give yourself some time to get used to the aid, but if it is uncomfortable or does not seem to improve your hearing, take it back for a refund or an exchange. A reputable hearing-aid dealer should give you a trial period before the sale becomes final.

ACUPRESSURE

1 Pressing Gall Bladder 2 may help enhance hearing. Open your mouth and find the depression just in front of your ears. Place the tips of your middle fingers at the base of this depression, then slide them down a half-inch and close your mouth; your fingers should be on GB 2. Press for one minute, three to five times.

2 Hearing difficulty may also be eased by pressing Triple Warmer 17, located behind your earlobes. Using the tips of your index fingers, find the hollows behind the earlobes where your ears meet your jawbone—the TW 17 point. Press lightly for two minutes while breathing deeply, then release.

A small number of people with profound deafness have benefited from an operation known as a cochlear implant. Very thin wires, called electrodes, are implanted in the cochlea, the spiral-shaped area of the inner ear. One end of each electrode is connected to the auditory nerve, the other end to a small battery-powered speech processor and microphone, which are worn outside the ear. The microphone and processor convert sounds into electrical impulses that travel along the electrodes and stimulate the auditory nerve, which then sends the impulses to the brain. Although promising, cochlear implants have thus far had only limited success. Most people who have had the surgery report that the device improves their lipreading skills but does not enable them to understand speech without lipreading.

ALTERNATIVE CHOICES

As with conventional treatment, alternative therapies primarily address underlying problems that may be causing temporary hearing loss.

YOGA

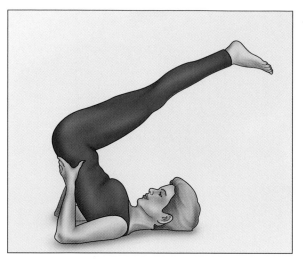

1 For the **Half Shoulder Stand,** lie on your back and bring your knees toward your forehead, supporting your hips with your hands. Inhale and extend your legs, keeping them at a right angle to your back *(above)*. Take a few deep breaths, then exhale and lower your legs.

2 To do the **Fish,** lie on your back with your arms along your sides, palms down. Inhale and arch your back and neck, keeping your buttocks on the floor. Support your weight with your hips and elbows *(above)*. Hold for 15 seconds, breathing deeply, then exhale and relax.

ACUPUNCTURE

Acupuncture cannot restore hearing lost as a result of permanent damage to the nerves or hearing mechanisms of the ear. However, in some cases it may help patients to discriminate better among the sounds they can hear. Acupuncture may also be used to help treat ear infections that may be causing temporary hearing problems. Consult a professional acupuncturist.

HERBAL THERAPIES

Several herbs may help heal ear infections that might lead to hearing problems. Garlic *(Allium sativum),* which has been shown to act as a natural antibiotic, is considered very effective. Put 1 to 3 drops of garlic oil in your ear three times daily. You can buy the oil in a health food store or make your own: Slice several garlic cloves and put them in 1 oz of olive oil for up to seven days; strain and store in the refrigerator, being sure to warm the oil before using.

Herbalists also recommend ginger *(Zingiber officinale),* another natural antibiotic, both in tincture and in tea form. To make ginger tea, put 1 tbsp of the fresh root in 1 cup boiling water; let simmer for 10 minutes. Drink several times a day.

The anti-inflammatory properties of either echinacea *(Echinacea* spp.) or goldenseal *(Hydrastis canadensis)* may help heal an ear infection. You can take either herb in tincture form (1 to 4 ml three times a day) or as a tea. To make the tea, pour a cup of boiling water over 1 to 2 tsp of the dried herb; let steep for 10 to 15 minutes. Drink three times a day.

Ginkgo *(Ginkgo biloba),* which has been shown to improve circulation, is sometimes recommended for inner ear disturbances and partial deafness. It is available in herb stores in a variety of forms; the recommended dosage is 40 mg of the dried herb or 1 to 2 tsp of the liquid extract three times a day.

HOMEOPATHY

For acute or chronic hearing problems, homeopaths recommend a variety of medications. Consult an experienced practitioner for specific remedies and dosages.

NUTRITION AND DIET

In some cases, hearing may be improved by reducing salt, which can cause fluids to be retained in the ear, where they can press against the hearing mechanism. If you are prone to repeated ear infections, avoid dairy products, which some alternative practitioners believe create excess mucus in the body. Some evidence indicates that vitamin A supplements (5,000 to 10,000 IU a day) may help hearing loss, particularly if the condition is accompanied by tinnitus, a ringing or roaring sensation in the ears.

YOGA

The Half Shoulder Stand and Fish positions *(opposite)* may help some forms of hearing loss by increasing the circulation of blood to the ears.

PREVENTION

◆ Wear earplugs if you are exposed to noise levels that may be harmful to your ears. Cotton balls are not sufficient, as they do not block enough sound; they can also become lodged deep in the ear canal.

◆ Do not listen to loud music with earphones.

◆ If you are at a concert and the music hurts your ears, put on earplugs or leave immediately. The overamplified sound may cause permanent damage.

◆ Educate your children about the danger of loud recreational noise.

◆ If you ride a subway, wear earplugs or cover your ears with your hands as the trains pass. The roar of the trains can damage your ears.

◆ To lower the risk of infectious diseases that may lead to permanent hearing loss, make sure your children receive all of their immunizations.

◆ If your ears tend to get severely blocked with wax frequently, clean them periodically with hydrogen peroxide *(box, page 444)*.

◆ Be sure to report any sudden hearing loss to your doctor immediately.

AIR TRAVEL DEAFNESS

If you fly with a stuffy nose, you may experience a condition known as aerotitis media, or barotrauma—a pushing in of the eardrum due to the sudden increase in air pressure in the plane's cabin as the plane descends. Any blockage in the eustachian tubes makes it impossible for air to pass through the tubes into the middle ear, where it would normally balance the air pushing on the eardrum from the outer ear canal. The condition is painful and usually results in some degree of temporary hearing loss. You may also feel dizzy and experience tinnitus, a ringing sensation in your ears. The symptoms usually go away completely in a few hours, but sometimes a myringotomy, a procedure that involves a small incision in the eardrum, becomes necessary.

If you must travel with a cold or sinus infection, take the following preventive steps:

◆ *Use a nasal decongestant or antihistamine an hour before takeoff and again an hour before landing.*

◆ *Suck on candy or chew gum to promote swallowing and help unblock the eustachian tubes.*

◆ *Take a deep breath through your mouth, hold your nose, and then blow out gently while keeping your mouth closed. This can help force air through your eustachian tubes.*

◆ *Take the homeopathic remedy Kali bichromicum in 6c or 30c potency at half-hour intervals during your flight, starting a half-hour before boarding the plane. This treatment is especially effective with young children.* ■

SYMPTOMS

Keep in mind that occasional, isolated disturbances of the heartbeat are common and usually harmless. Signs of more serious arrhythmias include the following:

For **tachycardia,** or abnormally rapid heartbeat:

- recurrent palpitations, defined as an uncomfortable awareness of your heartbeat. The palpitations may take the form of a strong pulse in the neck, a "flip-flopping" heart, or a fluttering, thumping, pounding, or racing beat in the chest.
- chest discomfort, weakness, fainting, sweating, shortness of breath, confusion, or dizziness.

For **bradycardia,** or abnormally slow heartbeat:

- fatigue, shortness of breath, lightheadedness, or loss of consciousness.

CALL YOUR DOCTOR IF:

- you experience irregular heartbeats that are recurrent or produce discomfort. Any sustained or intense arrhythmia should be investigated to determine its severity.
- while taking drugs to treat one form of arrhythmia, you notice a new pattern of irregular heartbeat. Some antiarrhythmic drugs may actually worsen the original heart condition.
- while taking antiarrhythmic medication, you experience side effects such as dizziness, vomiting, nausea, blurred vision, ringing in the ears, diarrhea, loss of appetite, or loss of consciousness. A new prescription will often correct the problem.

The healthy heart is a marvel of efficiency, pumping approximately five quarts of blood through the body every minute by means of regular, forceful contractions of its four chambers. Each perceived thump of the heart actually consists of two beats, one by the upper chambers, or atria, and one by the lower chambers, or ventricles. The contractions are triggered by electrical impulses originating in the sinus node, a specialized group of cells located in the heart's right atrium.

Any disturbance in the normal beating pattern of the heart is called an arrhythmia, or irregular heartbeat. Practically everyone experiences some version of an arrhythmia on occasion, usually in the form of a mild palpitation or a "skipped" heartbeat. (In fact, what feels like a skipped beat is really an early beat, weak enough not to be felt, then a one- or two-second pause, followed by a relatively forceful beat; the delay between beats feels like a skip.) Mild, isolated disturbances of this sort are normally harmless. A recurrent arrhythmia, on the other hand, should be checked by a physician.

There are two main categories of arrhythmia: **tachycardia,** meaning too fast a heartbeat, and **bradycardia,** meaning too slow a heartbeat. (Both conditions refer only to exceptional elevations or depressions of heart rate, not to the normal variance that occurs throughout the day depending on whether you are resting or active.) At rest, the heart beats somewhere between 60 and 100 times per minute. Tachycardia is defined as more than 100 beats per minute, while bradycardia is defined as fewer than 60 beats per minute. Both tachycardia and bradycardia can occur in surges or as persistent conditions.

Most arrhythmias fall into the tachycardia category. Some originate in the atria, some in the ventricles. Ventricular arrhythmias are typically more serious conditions. In fact, most cases of sudden cardiac death are due to ventricular arrhythmias, not heart attack, as was once thought. Particularly dangerous is **ventricular fibrillation,** in which activity within the ventricles is so uncoordinated that the ventricles are reduced to twitching, and virtually no pumping takes place. Ventricular fibrillation will cause death within a few minutes unless interrupted.

LEFT ATRIUM
RIGHT ATRIUM
SINUS NODE
ATRIOVENTRICULAR NODE
RIGHT VENTRICLE
LEFT VENTRICLE

Bradycardias can be due to problems with nerves that control heartbeat, with the sinus node, where the heart's electrical impulses originate, or with actual transmission of those impulses through the heart. In the latter condition, known as **heart block,** electrical signals fail to reach the ventricles from the atria because of some conduction problem. Signals may be blocked continuously or intermittently. In a worst-case scenario, electrical activity within the heart shuts down completely and beating stops.

CAUSES

Any condition that affects the structure of the heart muscle or its valves or that alters electrical activity within the heart is likely to interfere with regular heartbeat. As might be expected, many forms of heart disease cause arrhythmia. Severe coronary heart disease is a frequent trigger; it produces scar tissue in the heart that can disrupt the transmission of electrical signals. Congenital heart defects, heart muscle disease, heart valve disorders, and other diseases such as lung condi-

tions or hyperthyroidism may also produce arrhythmias. External forces such as electric shock or severe chest injury have also been known to trigger arrhythmias.

Ventricular arrhythmias most often stem from heart disease and are anticipated complications of heart attack. Atrial arrhythmias are also generally associated with heart disease, but may have other causes or no apparent cause. Atrial fibrillation is frequently associated with high blood pressure. Many bradycardias are associated with heart block.

A dysfunction in the autonomic nervous system (which regulates all involuntary bodily functions, including heartbeat) may also cause arrhythmias. Effective control by the autonomic nervous system depends on a fine balance between sympathetic nerves, which tell functions of the body to speed up, and parasympathetic nerves, which tell them to slow down. Sometimes stroke upsets the balance, and arrhythmia may result.

A sudden infusion of certain chemicals or hormones into the bloodstream can also disturb heart rate. Many drugs, including caffeine, nicotine, alcohol, cocaine, and inhaled aerosol propellants, can cause heart rate to race or become otherwise irregular. The same may occur in response to conditions that boost adrenaline (also known as epinephrine), such as shock, fright, and anxiety.

DIAGNOSTIC AND TEST PROCEDURES

An ECG reading of the heart's electrical activity provides the most accurate confirmation of arrhythmia. However, the ECG test is useful only when the arrhythmia occurs during testing, which often is not the case. To detect a suspected arrhythmia, a patient may be sent home wearing a Holter monitor. This portable device records the heart's electrical activity over a 24-hour period.

Tests that provoke arrhythmias make diagnosis easier. Exercising on a treadmill, for example, may induce an arrhythmia that is normally triggered by exertion.

Electrophysiologic testing is also useful in the diagnosis of arrhythmia. Tiny electrode catheters—introduced through veins or arteries and positioned at various points in the heart—record the transmission of electrical signals. The "electrical map" produced by the catheter readings diagrams the location, direction, and speed of signals, so that doctors can determine where the problem is originating or where signals may be getting blocked.

TREATMENT

Once an arrhythmia is confirmed, your doctor will decide whether the condition is serious enough to merit medical or surgical treatment. Treatment decisions depend not only on the type of arrhythmia but also on the patient's age, physical condition, and history of heart disease.

CONVENTIONAL MEDICINE

For mild conditions, your doctor will suggest some things that you can do to control the arrhythmia *(see At-Home Remedies)*. If necessary, medication is prescribed. A doctor bases the prescription on the type of arrhythmia, patient medical history, and the presence of other heart disease. Those drugs specifically categorized as antiarrhythmic—including quinidine, amiodarone, and also digitalis preparations—tend to be quite potent and can cause serious side effects, and thus are not prescribed routinely. They are often administered in conjunction with electrophysiologic testing to determine whether they will be effective and not cause an adverse reaction.

Application of electric shock to break an arrhythmia and restore normal heart rate is often used in emergencies; patients are then treated with drugs. Electric shock therapy might also be used if a patient fails to respond to medication or if a doctor anticipates an emergency because of another existing heart condition.

Sometimes, implantable devices are used to control arrhythmic conditions for the long term. People with symptomatic bradycardia usually wear implanted pacemakers. Anyone prone to ventricular tachycardias might wear a cardioverter defibrillator, an implantable electrode patch that provides automatic shock therapy when needed. People subject to both tachycardia

and bradycardia may be fitted with a pacemaker defibrillator, a device that can both restore normal heart rate by means of electric shock and maintain heart rate at a healthy, steady pace.

More invasive treatments are occasionally necessary. If a region of heart tissue is responsible for an arrhythmia, a technique known as catheter ablation may be used to correct the problem: Radio waves from a device inserted via a vein or artery literally zap the responsible area of heart tissue, putting it out of commission. In some cases, open-heart surgery to remove heart tissue may be called for.

ALTERNATIVE CHOICES

For emergency treatment and long-term prevention of severe arrhythmias, you should see a cardiologist. Alternative therapies may be able to complement, but should not replace, standard treatment of serious heart conditions. You may find that with the added support of alternative medicine, you are able to lessen your dependence on antiarrhythmic drugs. You may also discover that alternative options suffice in controlling mild arrhythmias.

AROMATHERAPY

Citrus oils, added to bathwater, may help quell minor palpitations. Try a few drops of orange flower oil, also called neroli oil.

CHINESE HERBS

Numerous Chinese herbal combinations treat symptoms of arrhythmia, but some herbs—such as ephedra *(Ephedra sinica)*—can actually worsen the condition. Be sure to consult a qualified herbalist, and tell your doctor of any herbs you may be taking for other problems.

HERBAL THERAPIES

Many herbs contain components that strengthen heartbeat and steady heart rate. Some, such as foxglove *(Digitalis purpurea)*, are too potent to be used by the layperson. Hawthorn *(Crataegus laevigata)*, a gentle yet effective herb for treating heart conditions, is most appropriate for home use. Hawthorn dilates vessels and stimulates the heart muscle, which can help stabilize arrhythmias. Steep 2 to 3 tsp of the herb in a cup of boiling water, and drink four cups a day.

HOMEOPATHY
Homeopathic medicine offers remedies for both immediate and long-term treatment of mild arrhythmias. Lachesis, Digitalis, and Aconite are among the remedies used to control palpitations. Consult a homeopathic physician for dosages.

LIFESTYLE
Heart rate rises in response to exercise, then typically resettles at a lower rate. Nonexercisers tend to have resting heart rates around 80 beats per minute, while exercisers average between 60 and 65 beats per minute. Exercise also helps get rid of excess adrenaline, a hormone that excites the heart along with the rest of the body.

Nicotine from smoking is a stimulant and may provoke arrhythmias in susceptible people. If you have been diagnosed with tachycardia and you smoke, you should quit.

MIND/BODY MEDICINE
Relaxation techniques can help prevent or control some arrhythmias by reducing stress, which elevates heart rate and can trigger certain heartbeat disturbances. Any number of activities, ranging from exercise to **meditation** and **yoga,** might help you relax. Find what works best for you and stick with it; the benefit of relaxation training takes time to be realized.

NUTRITION AND DIET
The minerals calcium, magnesium, and potassium play a crucial role in moderating heart activity. Too little of these minerals can cause arrhythmias. (And too much can also be a problem, especially with calcium.) Magnesium administered intravenously can correct tachycardia and many other arrhythmias. You can get magnesium from nuts, beans, soybeans, bran, dark green vegetables, and fish. Many fruits and vegetables supply potassium. Be aware that you can deplete your stores of magnesium and potassium by ingesting too much salt or saturated fat, as well as by overusing diuretics or laxatives.

A COLD SPLASH IN THE FACE

Have you ever wondered how sea lions survive the shock of diving into frozen waters? Like other mammals, they are protected by an automatic nervous response that immediately slows heart rate. Humans also have this nervous response, which may be particularly significant to you if you suffer occasional bouts of tachycardia. Next time an attack occurs, try plunging your face into a basin of cold water. Your heart rate will temporarily plummet, which may serve to break the tachycardia.

AT-HOME REMEDIES
◆ To control an attack of tachycardia, the best remedy is rest. Take a deep breath and relax.
◆ Gentle pressure to the prominent carotid artery on the right side of the neck may help break an attack of tachycardia. Ask your doctor to show you how and where to press.
◆ For atrial arrhythmias, try the "vagal maneuver." Sit down, bend forward at the waist, then hold your breath and strain as if blowing up a balloon. In so doing, you switch control from the sympathetic nervous system, which speeds bodily functions, to the parasympathetic nervous system, which slows them.

PREVENTION

Limit your use of caffeine, nicotine, alcohol, and stimulant drugs, all of which can speed heart rate. If you have a history of tachycardia, you should avoid these substances altogether. Reduce stress through exercise, meditation, or any other technique that works for you. If you have a heart condition, take proper steps to control it; this may also prevent or control arrhythmia. ■

SYMPTOMS

- a prolonged crushing, squeezing, or burning pain in the center of the chest. The pain may radiate to the neck, one or both arms, or the jaw.
- shortness of breath, dizziness, nausea, chills, sweating, weak pulse.
- cold and clammy skin, gray pallor, a severe appearance of illness.
- fainting. (In about 1 case in 10, this is the only indication that a heart attack is in progress.)

CALL YOUR DOCTOR IF:

- you or someone you are with manifests signs of a heart attack. **Seek emergency help without delay.**
- you suffer from angina (chest pain) and begin to experience pain that is similar but does not respond to medication; this may indicate that a heart attack is under way.
- your angina attacks become more frequent, prolonged, and severe; as angina worsens, the risk of heart attack increases.
- you are taking aspirin to prevent heart attack and your stool appears black and tarry. This could be a sign that aspirin has thinned your blood too much, a problem that can and should be corrected. *(See also Heart Attack, page 67, in Emergencies/First Aid.)*

In order to keep pumping, day in and day out, the heart requires its own constant supply of oxygen and nutrients. Two large, branching coronary arteries deliver oxygenated blood to the heart muscle. Should one of these arteries or branches shut down, a portion of the heart is starved of oxygen and fuel, a condition called **ischemia.** If an ischemic attack lasts too long, the starved heart tissue dies. This event defines heart attack, otherwise known as myocardial infarction—literally, "death of heart muscle."

Most attacks last for several hours. (But never wait to seek help if you think an attack is beginning.) The signs of the heart attack may be no more than shortness of breath, faintness, or nausea; and in some cases there are no symptoms. But most heart attacks produce some pain. The pain of a severe attack has been likened to a giant fist enclosing and squeezing the heart; if the attack is mild, it may be mistaken for heartburn. The pain may be constant or intermittent.

The majority of heart attack victims are warned of trouble well in advance by episodes of angina—chest pain that, like a heart attack, is provoked by ischemia. The difference is mainly one of degree: With angina, blood flow is quickly restored, pain recedes within minutes, and the heart is not permanently damaged; with heart attack, blood flow is critically reduced or fully blocked, pain lasts, and heart tissue dies.

About a third of all heart attacks occur without any previous warning signs. They are sometimes associated with a phenomenon known as **silent ischemia**—sporadic interruptions of blood flow to the heart that, for unknown reasons, are pain free, although they gradually damage the heart tissue. The condition can be detected by ECG testing. An estimated three to four million Americans may be afflicted with silent ischemia.

A third of all heart attack victims die before reaching a hospital; others suffer life-threatening complications while in the hospital. Serious complications include stroke, persistent heart arrhythmias, congestive heart failure, formation of blood clots in the legs or heart, and aneurysm in a weakened heart chamber. But those who survive the initial attack and are free from major problems a few hours later stand a better chance of full recovery.

Recovery is always a delicate process, because any attack weakens the heart to some degree. But generally, a normal life can be resumed within three months.

Heart disease remains the leading cause of death in the United States, with heart attack as the number one killer. But nothing is inevitable about those figures: Most forms of heart disease, including heart attack, are preventable.

CAUSES

Like earthquakes, many heart attacks occur as sudden catastrophes yet actually represent a culmination of events that have been proceeding beneath the surface for years. Most heart attacks are the end result of coronary heart disease, an atherosclerotic condition that clogs coronary arteries with fatty, calcified plaques. (As blood flow is gradually impeded, the body may compensate by growing a network of collateral arteries to circumvent blockages; the presence of collateral vessels may greatly reduce the amount of heart muscle damaged by a heart attack.) In the early

1980s, researchers confirmed that the precipitating cause of nearly all heart attacks is not the obstructive plaque itself, but the sudden formation of a blood clot on top of plaque that cuts off flow in an already narrowed vessel.

While the step-by-step process leading to heart attack is not fully understood, major risk factors are well-established. Some can be controlled. Of these, the main ones are high blood pressure, high cholesterol, obesity, smoking, and a sedentary lifestyle. Stress is also believed to raise the risk, and exertion and excitement can act as triggers for an attack.

Men over the age of 50 with a family history of heart disease are predisposed to heart attack. High levels of estrogen are thought to protect premenopausal women fairly well from heart attack, but risk increases significantly after menopause. Some women opt for hormone replacement therapy after menopause; the choice should be made with full knowledge that elevated estrogen levels also increase the risk for breast and uterine cancers. *(See Menopausal Problems.)*

DIAGNOSTIC AND TEST PROCEDURES

A cardiologist relies on various tests and scans to diagnose a heart attack and to identify sites of arterial blockage and tissue damage. ECG recordings of electrical activity within the heart, supported by blood tests, provide data for an initial assessment of the patient's condition. Images of the heart and coronary arteries supplied by angiograms and radioisotope scans locate specific areas of damage and blockage. With such data, the attending physician can pursue proper treatment and anticipate potential complications.

TREATMENT

Heart attack is a medical emergency that must be quickly addressed by conventional medicine. Alternative medicine cannot compete with standard drug and surgical therapy during the emergency and follow-up phases of heart attack treatment. However, alternative medicine can make valuable contributions to prevention and recovery.

WHERE THE PAIN MAY BE

Heart attack pain can strike any of the areas shown at left. On the front of the body *(top)*, the most likely sites are the center and left side of the chest, the neck, and the inside of the left arm *(blue)*. Pain sometimes develops in the jaws *(green)*, in the right chest and arm *(pink)*, the shoulders, and in the area between the navel and breastbone *(yellow)*. On the back *(bottom)*, pain can occur between the shoulder blades *(blue)*.

CONVENTIONAL MEDICINE

Heart attack victims are usually hospitalized in special coronary care units for at least 36 hours. Standard drug therapy includes a painkiller such as morphine, beta-adrenergic blocker drugs to calm the heart, and aspirin to reduce clotting activity. In some cases, clot-dissolving drugs like t-PA or streptokinase are also administered. These drugs are most effective if given within a few hours of heart attack onset. Emergency angioplasty, and possibly surgery, might be performed to remove a clot, reopen a clogged artery, or bypass blocked arteries.

Once past the critical phase, patients continue to receive beta blockers to calm the heart, nitrates to increase heart blood flow, and anticoagulants such as heparin, warfarin, or aspirin to prevent further clotting.

While hospitalized, heart attack patients are hooked to ECG machines for constant monitoring, in case heart rhythm abnormalities develop. If the heart starts beating too fast or too slow, various medications may be given. Some patients may be fitted with pacemakers. If a patient experiences a dangerous arrhythmia known as ventricular fibrillation, an electric shock to the chest is administered. Patients who show signs of congestive heart failure are given a variety of medications to decrease strain on the heart and to encourage the heart to beat more forcefully.

People recovering from a heart attack are urged to get back on their feet as quickly as possible, which reduces the chances of blood clots forming in the deep veins of the legs; the clots could travel through the circulatory system and lodge in the lung, creating a blockage. Gentle exercise is recommended, but nothing that requires significant exertion. Long-term recovery from heart attack requires psychological and lifestyle adjustments: Habits such as smoking, heavy drinking, and eating high-fat foods have to go.

As a preventive measure, most heart attack survivors take a daily aspirin tablet to thin the blood. Other drugs may also be prescribed, depending on the individual case.

Some patients require invasive procedures to improve blood flow to the heart over the long term. The two most common procedures are angioplasty—a catheter technique that widens clogged arteries by splitting plaques— and coronary bypass surgery, which diverts blood flow around clogged arteries.

ALTERNATIVE CHOICES

HERBAL THERAPIES

Of the many herbs used to treat chronic heart conditions, hawthorn (*Crataegus laevigata*) is

---

TROUBLE FOR TYPE A

In 1964 Dr. Meyer Friedman and Dr. Ray Rosenman published an article in JAMA, the Journal of the American Medical Association, that launched a provocative and ongoing debate about personality and heart disease. They contended that people with certain personality traits are more likely to have heart attacks. These people fit a behavior pattern described as Type A: impatient, competitive, driven, achievement oriented, and quick-tempered. Their Type B counterparts are less hurried, more easygoing, and less easily riled.

Over the years, researchers have continued to test the theory. Some studies confirm Type A personality as a major risk factor for heart disease, while others conclude just the opposite. On balance, the data seem to favor a link between Type A personality and heart disease. The task now is to identify those traits that are most responsible for increased risk. Two traits seem particularly significant: the tendency to react with hostility to even minor irritations, and consistently high levels of stress-related hormones.

perhaps most valuable; it dilates coronary arteries and is said to improve metabolic function within the heart. Hawthorn not only may help prevent heart attacks but also is thought to speed recovery from an attack. Numerous other herbs are used to treat conditions that increase the risk of heart attack. For more information, see High Blood Pressure, Blood Clots, and Cholesterol Problems.

LIFESTYLE
Regular aerobic exercise greatly enhances efforts to prevent or recover from heart attack. If you already have a heart condition, schedule a stress test before beginning an exercise program in order to determine how much exertion is safe. Heart attack survivors are advised to exercise with other people rather than alone during the first months of recovery. Many community health and recreation centers offer physician-supervised cardiovascular rehabilitation programs.

MIND/BODY MEDICINE
Reducing stress by training the mind and body to relax may help prevent heart attack and can aid in recovery. Many techniques promote relaxation—among them, **meditation, biofeedback,** and **yoga.** Relaxation has also been shown to provide relief from pain, which may be encountered during the recovery period.

State of mind is another important consideration in heart attack recovery. People with a positive attitude about recovery tend to do much better than people who view themselves as "cardiac cripples." You may find that a particular mind/body technique helps you to focus on positive thoughts. You may also find, as many others have, that sharing thoughts and emotions with a support group is extremely beneficial.

NUTRITION AND DIET
The basic goals of a heart-healthy diet are to keep salt, sugar, and saturated fat to a minimum so as to reduce cholesterol, control blood pressure, and hold weight in check. Eating magnesium-rich foods such as nuts, beans, bran, fish, and dark green vegetables may help prevent heart attack. Magnesium protects the heart directly and indirectly, by stabilizing heart rate, reducing coronary artery spasm, and combating such conditions as atherosclerosis and high blood pressure.

Much evidence suggests that unstable chemical compounds known as free radicals make the body more vulnerable to heart attack by striking the heart and coronary arteries and promoting atherosclerosis. Free radicals can be neutralized by antioxidants like vitamins A, C, and E. Fruits, vegetables, and grains supply many of the antioxidant vitamins.

Eating root vegetables such as carrots may also help prevent heart attack. These vegetables lower cholesterol over the long term and reduce blood-clotting activity.

AT-HOME REMEDIES
◆ Remember: Having a heart attack does not make you an invalid. You can best heal your heart by remaining active.
◆ Do not take birth-control pills if you have had a heart attack; they are linked to increased blood-clotting activity.
◆ Get a pet. Pet owners recover more quickly from heart attacks—probably because of reduced stress levels—and tend to live longer than people without pets.

PREVENTION
◆ Stay in touch with friends and family. Research shows that people with poor social support are more vulnerable to heart disease. Also, seek ways to control feelings of anger and hostility; these emotions may add to heart attack risk.
◆ Assess your heart attack risk profile and make appropriate changes to diet and lifestyle early.
◆ If you are at high risk for heart attack, have yourself tested regularly for silent ischemia.
◆ Talk with your doctor about taking an aspirin daily. Studies have shown that this regimen significantly reduces the risk of heart attack. ■

SYMPTOMS

◆ a burning feeling in the chest just behind the breastbone (the sternum) that occurs after eating and lasts a few minutes to several hours.

◆ chest pain, especially after bending over or lying down.

◆ burning in the throat—or hot, sour, or salty-tasting fluid at the back of the throat.

◆ belching.

H

CALL YOUR DOCTOR IF:

◆ you experience heartburn along with any of the following: difficulty swallowing, shortness of breath, sweating, dizziness, vomiting, diarrhea, extreme abdominal pain, fever, or black or bloodstained bowel movements. You may have a strangulated hiatal hernia, pancreatic problems, gastritis, stomach ulcers, or cancer. Or it could be a heart attack; **call for medical help now.**

◆ you take an antacid to relieve heartburn and do not feel relief within 15 minutes. This may also be a sign of a heart attack; **call for medical help now.**

◆ your heartburn is aggravated by exercise and relieved by rest. You may have heart disease.

◆ you have chronic heartburn (daily or almost daily). Your esophagus is being repeatedly burned by stomach acid, which can lead to esophagitis, esophageal scarring, stomach ulcers, or cancer.

Despite its name, heartburn has nothing to do with the heart. (Some of the symptoms, however, are similar to those of a heart attack or heart disease.) It is an irritation of the esophagus that is caused by stomach acid. With gravity's help, a muscular valve called the lower esophageal sphincter, or LES, keeps stomach acid in the stomach. The LES is located where the esophagus meets the stomach—below the rib cage and slightly left of center. Normally it opens to allow food into the stomach or to permit belching; then it closes again. But if the LES opens too often or too far, stomach acid can reflux, or seep, into the esophagus and cause a burning sensation.

Occasional heartburn isn't dangerous, but chronic heartburn can indicate serious problems. Heartburn is a daily occurrence for 10 percent of Americans and 50 percent of pregnant women. It's an occasional nuisance for another 30 percent of the population.

CAUSES

The basic cause of heartburn is an underactive LES that doesn't tighten as it should. Two excesses often contribute: too much food in the stomach (overeating) or too much pressure on the stomach (frequently from obesity or pregnancy). Certain foods commonly relax the LES, including tomatoes, citrus fruits, garlic, onions, chocolate, coffee, alcohol, and peppermint. Dishes high in fats and oils (animal or vegetable) often lead to

CAUTION!

Antacids can mask or aggravate some ailments. Do not take antacids without consulting your doctor if you have high blood pressure, an irregular heartbeat, kidney disease, chronic constipation, diarrhea, colitis, any kind of intestinal bleeding, or any symptoms of appendicitis. Pregnant or nursing mothers should consult a physician before taking any medication, including antacids.

heartburn, as do certain medications, especially some antibiotics and aspirin. Stress, which strains the nerves controlling the LES, can cause heartburn. And smoking, which relaxes the LES and stimulates stomach acid, is a major contributor.

DIAGNOSTIC AND TEST PROCEDURES

Your description of your symptoms may be all a doctor requires, but sometimes additional procedures are necessary. The esophagus can be viewed through an endoscope, a long, thin, flexible tube inserted through the mouth, or by x-ray. To determine if your heart is the cause of your symptoms, an electrocardiogram (ECG), a recording of the heart's electrical activity, may be taken.

TREATMENT

Most physicians advocate antacids for occasional heartburn. Alternative practitioners rely on herbal remedies to reduce acid and relaxation therapies to lessen stress.

CONVENTIONAL MEDICINE

The primary objective is to identify the cause of the heartburn, so it can be avoided in the future. Over-the-counter antacids or bismuth subsalicylate is commonly prescribed to neutralize stomach acid. If antacids don't quell the symptoms, your doctor may prescribe cimetidine, ranitidine, or omeprazole to reduce the stomach's production of acid, or cisapride or metoclopramide to make the stomach empty itself faster. When all else fails, surgery may be required to repair the LES, but this is relatively rare.

ALTERNATIVE CHOICES

For additional therapies, see Hiatal Hernia, a condition often accompanied by heartburn.

CHINESE HERBS

Taken once or twice, a tea made from 10 grams orange peel, 4 slices fresh ginger (*Zingiber officinale*), 10 grams poria (*Poria cocos*), 10 grams

agastache (*Agastache rugosa*), and 3 grams licorice (*Glycyrrhiza uralensis*) may alleviate heartburn. If it doesn't, call your physician. This mixture should not be taken daily.

HERBAL THERAPIES

Ginger (*Zingiber officinale*) tea can diminish heartburn quickly, and chamomile (*Matricaria recutita*) tea's calming effects are especially helpful for stress-related heartburn.

HOMEOPATHY

Specific heartburn symptoms often respond well to homeopathic remedies. The dosage is 6c, taken every 15 minutes; repeat up to three times, then repeat the series once if needed. After eating spicy foods, take Nux vomica; after rich foods take Carbo vegetabilis; and for burning pain, take Arsenicum album.

PREVENTION

Heartburn is often preventable. The keys are maintaining a reasonable weight, avoiding things that cause stomach acid to reflux into your esophagus (*see Causes, opposite*), getting adequate rest and exercise, and minimizing stress.

If you must lie down after eating, lie on your left side; your stomach is lower than your esophagus in this position. ∎

SYMPTOMS

The symptoms listed below apply to several types of heart condition. Bear in mind, however, that each type of heart disease has its own set of indicators; that most symptoms associated with heart disease could be caused by other conditions; and that some forms of heart disease may have no noticeable effects.

- tight, suffocating chest pain, often associated with angina and heart attack.
- sharp, piercing chest pain, a common sign of **pericarditis.**
- sensations of fluttering, thumping, pounding, or racing of the heart, known as **palpitations.**
- shortness of breath.
- fluid retention in the legs, ankles, abdomen, lungs, or heart.
- lightheadedness, weakness, dizziness, or fainting spells.

CALL YOUR DOCTOR IF:

- you experience unusual chest pain, particularly if it persists or recurs. It may be heartburn, but it could also indicate a heart attack.
- you experience recurrent disturbances of heartbeat (heart arrhythmias). If frequent or persistent, irregular heartbeats may signal a serious heart condition.
- you become suddenly dizzy, light-headed, weak, or faint. Even if the cause is not heart disease, it could be serious.

See also Emergencies/First Aid entries on heart attack and cardiac and respiratory arrest.

The human heart is built for amazing endurance—billions of beats in an average lifetime—but, like any other part of the body, it is vulnerable to breakdowns. Heart problems vary widely in their nature and severity. They may be transient or chronic, slow-developing or sudden, inconvenient or deadly. Some types of heart disease, closely linked to diet and lifestyle choices, are preventable; others are due to genetic inheritance, infections, or other uncontrollable factors. Two of every five Americans will ultimately die of heart disease; the daily toll is approximately 2,500 people. Fortunately, the death rate is declining steadily, thanks largely to improved medical care and widespread public education about risk factors.

Following is a list of the most common types of heart disease; see also individual entries for more specific information.

HEART ARRHYTHMIAS
Arrhythmias are disturbances in the heart's normal beating pattern. The irregularities occur in many forms, each with its own potential causes and treatments. Serious arrhythmias are a frequent consequence of other heart diseases but may also occur independently. (See Heart Arrhythmias.)

CORONARY HEART DISEASE
Coronary heart disease, the most common of all heart problems, is characterized by blockages in the coronary arteries that result in a reduction in blood flow to the heart muscle, depriving it of vital oxygen. Usually, the disease stems from atherosclerosis, an inflammatory condition sometimes called hardening of the arteries.

Severe coronary heart disease can lead to **congestive heart failure,** a general weakness of the heart that results in ineffective pumping action. Coronary heart disease can also result in painful episodes of angina or a heart attack or, in the worst case, sudden cardiac death.

While the exact causes of coronary heart disease are imperfectly understood, certain major risk factors have been identified. People with family histories of heart disease are at risk. Men are more apt to be affected than women, although neither sex is immune. Age is important:

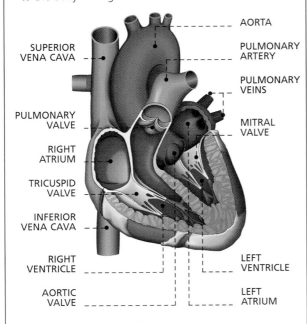
For both men and women, the likelihood of heart disease increases significantly after the age of 65. Diabetics are also more prone to heart disease. *(See Diabetes.)*

A number of risk factors can be mitigated or eliminated. People with high blood pressure and high blood levels of "bad" (LDL, or low-density lipoprotein) cholesterol are inclined to develop atherosclerosis and related conditions; but both blood pressure and cholesterol levels can often be moderated through proper diet and lifestyle choices. Smoking—also obviously a matter of choice—greatly increases the risk of heart disease because of the damaging effect that toxins in the smoke have on blood vessels. Nicotine also boosts heart rate, which takes a direct toll on the heart by forcing it to work harder; additionally, the chemical causes blood vessels to constrict, elevating blood pressure.

Obese people have a greater-than-average likelihood of developing heart disease. Their extra weight places added strain on the heart and blood vessels. In addition, obese people tend to have high cholesterol; this may be due partially to dietary choices, but is also tied to the fact that obesity is associated with abnormal fat metabolism.

Being sedentary increases risk, since exercise has a protective effect on the heart and blood vessels. People who exercise regularly tend to be trimmer and to have lower blood pressure and higher levels of "good" (HDL, or high-density lipoprotein) cholesterol. For many people, exercise also acts to reduce stress—another risk factor.

Medical researchers define stressful situations as those that arouse a fight-or-flight response—the body's physiological preparations to deal with a threat—yet allow for neither, thus generating feelings of anxiety, helplessness, and loss of control. Because stress is intangible, its effect on heart disease is difficult to quantify, but there is much evidence to suggest that persistent internalized stress—no matter what the cause—increases the chances of developing heart disease and may aggravate an existing heart condition.

HEART VALVE DISEASE

The heart has four valves: the pulmonary, mitral, tricuspid, and aortic. The valves open and close to permit blood flow between the heart's four chambers and connected blood vessels. A defective valve may fail either to open properly, obstructing blood flow, or to close properly, allowing blood leakage. Congenital heart disease and various inflammatory conditions are among the causes of valve disorders.

Valve disorders frequently involve the mitral and aortic valves, which control blood flow on the left side of the heart. The most common valve disorder is called **mitral valve prolapse:** Excess valve tissue interferes with the normal closing of the valve, causing leakage. In most people this is not a serious problem, but some individuals require medication or, in rare cases, surgery to prevent infection of the valve or excessive stress on the heart.

H

Endocarditis is an inflammatory condition that affects heart valves. This disease is an infection or inflammation of the endocardium, the innermost layer of heart tissue that lines the chambers and valves. It is usually caused by bacterial infection, with the staphylococcus and streptococcus bacteria as most likely culprits. Bacteria may enter the blood and take root in the heart during illness, after surgery, or as a result of intravenous drug use. Endocarditis tends to strike people with preexisting valve problems. The disease can be fatal if left untreated, but it can generally be cured with antibiotics. If heart valves are seriously damaged as a result of endocarditis, valve replacement surgery may be needed.

Rheumatic heart disease, another type of heart disease affecting valves, was very common earlier in this century but is now largely preventable with antibiotic treatment, although it still occurs. The disease stems from damage to the heart muscle and valves caused by rheumatic fever, which itself is associated with strep throat. Symptoms of rheumatic heart disease are usually delayed for many years, but if valves were damaged severely enough by the fever, they will eventually leak or impede proper blood flow.

Rheumatic heart disease generates characteristic heart murmurs that can be detected upon examination. Congestive heart failure and atrial fibrillation, a particular type of arrhythmia, are also common complications. In cases of severe rheumatic heart disease, valves must be either reopened or replaced surgically.

PERICARDIAL DISEASE

Any disease of the pericardium, the membranous sac surrounding the heart, is classified as pericardial disease. One of the more common is an inflammatory condition called **pericarditis.** It is usually caused by viral infection, a connective-tissue disease such as lupus or rheumatoid arthritis, or trauma to the pericardium. Pericarditis often follows open-heart surgery. Excess fluid buildup within the pericardium is a frequent symptom of the disease. Listening with a stethoscope, a doctor might detect the disease upon hearing a characteristic scratching sound called a pericardial rub. Acute cases are marked by

fever and sharp pain in the center of the chest. Pericarditis often subsides on its own, but it also responds to anti-inflammatory drugs such as aspirin or, in severe cases, corticosteroid hormones. Occasionally, fluid must be drained from the pericardium.

PRIMARY MYOCARDIAL DISEASE

Diseases of the heart muscle, or myocardium, are collectively referred to as primary myocardial disease, or **cardiomyopathy.** When diseased, the myocardium becomes abnormally stretched, thickened, or stiff. Among the many potential causes of cardiomyopathy are connective-tissue diseases, genetic heart conditions, metabolic disorders, reactions to certain drugs or toxins such as alcohol, and viral infections. Often, the precise cause of cardiomyopathy is unknown. In any event, either the myocardium becomes too weak to pump efficiently, or stiffening prevents filling of the heart. Symptoms can include chest pain, shortness of breath, swelling of the feet and ankles, and light-headedness. When cardiomyopathy progresses to the point of causing serious arrhythmias or congestive heart failure, the outlook for long-term survival is poor. Sudden death is another outcome associated with some cardiomyopathies, including **idiopathic hypertrophic subaortic stenosis,** which has claimed the lives of a number of prominent young professional athletes. If cardiomyopathy can be detected and treated early enough, either with drugs or with transplant surgery, symptoms can often be controlled and heart failure averted for many years.

CONGENITAL HEART DISEASE

Should anything go awry in the formation of the heart during prenatal development, a baby will be born with one or more congenital heart defects. Such defects are quite common, occurring in about 7 of every 1,000 babies.

The exact causes of defects are generally hard to pin down; genes and environmental factors inside the mother's body may both contribute. Chromosome abnormalities, including the one that causes Down syndrome, have been linked to many congenital heart defects. Infections contracted during pregnancy by the mother, such as German measles, may also result in congenital heart disease for the child.

Congenital heart defects range widely in their effects. Some are apparent immediately, but others do not produce noticeable symptoms until adulthood. Minor conditions often clear up on their own, while the most severe conditions cannot be corrected and are fatal. Fortunately, many congenital heart defects can be treated surgically, if necessary.

Among the most common types are **septal defects,** or holes in the wall dividing the left and right sides of the heart. If a septal defect is big enough to cause problems, it can be patched surgically. Another frequently seen defect is **pulmonary stenosis,** a condition in which one of the four heart valves—the pulmonary valve—is so narrow that blood flow to the lungs is restricted; with surgery, the valve can be pried open or replaced. In some babies, a small blood vessel known as the ductus arteriosus fails to close at birth as it should. This condition, known as **patent ductus arteriosus,** allows some blood that is headed for the body via the aorta to leak back into the pulmonary artery, placing the heart under added strain. This problem can also be corrected surgically.

Some so-called blue babies are born with a combination of four heart defects, which basically results in oxygen-poor blood flow to body tissues. The excess of deoxygenated blood gives the baby a bluish tinge. Unless treated, most people with this condition would not survive to middle age. However, surgery successfully corrects the condition 90 percent of the time.

THE RISKS
FOR WOMEN

A 50-year-old woman arrives in the emergency room complaining of severe chest pain and difficulty breathing. The attending physician orders tests and eventually finds that the patient's coronary arteries are smooth and free of clots. In medical parlance, this patient is said to have Syndrome X—a condition that presents the classic symptoms of angina or heart attack without the classic cause, coronary artery blockage.

Until recently, cardiologists had done little to explain Syndrome X. (It is still under study, but one theory holds that it is caused by circulation problems in small vessels of the heart.) Lack of interest stemmed in part from lack of concern: Nearly two-thirds of Syndrome X patients are women, and traditionally women were thought to get heart disease only rarely. However, statistical evidence is challenging that notion—and changing attitudes about women and heart disease.

Among other things, the evidence indicates that heart disease is the number one killer of American women. Half of all American women eventually die of heart disease, and six times as many die of heart attacks annually as succumb to breast cancer.

Women tend not to display the textbook symptoms of heart disease—most likely a result of the fact that most of the textbooks are based on all-male studies. It also turns out that some traditional diagnostic and treatment tools (such as exercise stress tests) do not work as well for women as for men. And the death rate for women who have undergone coronary bypass surgery is twice as high as that for men, probably because women's blood vessels are smaller. However, the same risk factors (such as smoking and high blood pressure) apply to both sexes.

Syndrome X, then, is but one of the challenges confronting doctors in their efforts to address the special problems women face when it comes to heart disease.

DIAGNOSTIC AND
TEST PROCEDURES

In diagnosing heart disease, a doctor first asks a patient for a description of symptoms. The patient's general physical condition is assessed through a standard medical examination and history taking. Listening to the heart for swishing or whooshing sounds, collectively known as **heart murmurs,** may provide important clues about heart trouble. If heart disease is suspected, further tests are done to find out what is actually happening inside the heart. An electrocardiogram, or ECG, is usually the first test to be performed. By recording electrical activity within the heart, the ECG quickly reveals any electrical abnormalities in the heart that may be a source of trouble. Further details can be garnered by imaging the heart, using x-rays, a variety of scans, or angiography, a special technique that allows for x-rays of blood vessels.

TREATMENT

With heart disease, conventional and alternative medicines each have their own strengths. When used as complements to each other, they can provide the best possible prevention and treatment of heart disease.

CONVENTIONAL MEDICINE

Conventional medical care—discussed above and in specific entries elsewhere in this book— is essential once heart disease begins to produce noticeable symptoms. Conventional care aims to stabilize the condition immediately, to control symptoms over the long term, and to provide a cure when possible. While appropriate changes to diet and lifestyle are always recommended, the mainstays of conventional care are drugs and surgery.

ALTERNATIVE CHOICES

The strong suit of alternative medicine is prevention. Natural therapies that focus on diet, nutrition, herbalism, and purification of the body through exercise, stress reduction, and detoxification can significantly reduce the body's vulnerability to certain types of heart disease, although some cannot be prevented. Several alternative therapies are also beneficial complements to the conventional treatment of heart disease.

BODY WORK

Since all forms of body work help the body to relax, any of them might be applicable to prevention and control of heart disease. The reason is simple: Relaxation reduces stress, and stress has been identified as a likely risk factor for coronary heart disease. You can put yourself in the hands of a body work therapist, or you can teach yourself **yoga** or **qigong.** See also Mind/Body Medicine, opposite.

YOGA

Use the **Sphinx** to reduce stress. Lie on the floor. Place both forearms on the floor with your palms down and your elbows directly under your shoulders. Inhale and push your chest away from the floor as far as comfortably possible without lifting your elbows. Hold for a few deep breaths, then relax and exhale.

CHELATION THERAPY

Chelation therapy is sought annually by thousands of Americans who suffer from angina and atherosclerosis. Advocates claim that it is safer and cheaper than, and as effective as, many conventional drug or surgical treatments. Critics contend that while chelation therapy is useful in treating certain conditions, cardiovascular disease is not necessarily one of them. See Atherosclerosis for a fuller explanation of chelation therapy.

CHINESE MEDICINE

Practitioners of traditional Chinese medicine generally view heart disease as arising from heart weakness or blocked energy flow. Depending on the symptoms, standard treatment would involve prescribed herbal remedies plus massage, **acupuncture,** and dietary recommendations.

CHIROPRACTIC

While chiropractic medicine is inappropriate for acute care of heart conditions, it shares with conventional medicine many long-term treatment aspects. A chiropractic physician would recommend suitable diet and lifestyle changes, and would also perform skeletal manipulation

H

when appropriate. Some studies indicate that regular chiropractic manipulation can reduce hypertension.

HERBAL THERAPIES

The plant world is full of herbs that can affect the heart. The therapeutic properties of some have been rigorously documented. The effects of others, such as motherwort (Leonurus cardiaca) and yarrow (Achillea millefolium), are not as well researched yet perhaps no less valid. Certain herbs, such as foxglove (Digitalis purpurea) and lily of the valley (Convallaria majalis), contain compounds called cardiac glycosides that make them particularly potent. Because of their potentially dangerous side effects, they should be administered only by a qualified medical herbalist. Many of the gentler "heart" herbs do not contain cardiac glycosides yet still improve cardiovascular function. The most noteworthy of these is hawthorn (Crataegus laevigata). Any herbal treatment of the heart should be supervised by a medical herbalist and approved by your doctor. For further herbal recommendations, see Atherosclerosis, Cholesterol Problems, Circulatory Problems, and High Blood Pressure.

HOMEOPATHY

Homeopathic remedies may complement, but should not replace, prescribed medication for chronic heart conditions. A homeopath would provide a constitutional remedy based on the manifest symptoms of heart disease, plus other characteristic symptoms such as food preferences, sleep patterns, mood, and temperament.

LIFESTYLE

If you smoke, quit. You should also get in the habit of exercising, since exercise strengthens the heart and blood vessels, reduces stress, and has been shown to reduce blood pressure while also boosting HDL cholesterol levels. Numerous studies done in recent decades indicate that drinking alcohol in moderation may actually reduce the risk of heart disease. But more than one drink a day, and a few drinks per week, is not recommended.

MIND/BODY MEDICINE

For many people, learning to relax can help prevent and treat heart disease. While success varies from person to person, stress-reduction techniques have been shown to moderate high blood pressure, heart arrhythmias, and emotional responses such as anxiety, anger, and hostility that have been linked to coronary heart disease, angina, and heart attack. The choice of relaxation technique is up to you. Some that have proved beneficial are **meditation,** progressive relaxation, prayer, and **biofeedback** training.

NUTRITION AND DIET

Even modest changes in diet and lifestyle can significantly reduce the risk of heart disease. Most people now know that eating foods low in cholesterol, saturated fat, and salt will help keep blood pressure low and decrease the formation of plaques—calcified fatty deposits—in blood vessels. Less known to the general public are those specific vitamins, minerals, and nutrients, such as magnesium, potassium, niacin (vitamin B$_3$), many other B-complex vitamins, vitamin E, coenzyme Q10, L-carnitine (an amino acid), and the fatty acids in fish oils, that specifically protect against heart and arterial disease. For more information concerning these and other heart-related nutrients, see Atherosclerosis, Cholesterol Problems, Heart Attack, and High Blood Pressure.

PREVENTION

◆ To stabilize both blood pressure and cholesterol levels and to keep your weight in check, try to eat more fruits, vegetables, and grains, and fewer foods that are salty, high in fat, or fried.

◆ Exercise regularly, in order to tone your heart and blood vessels—and to shed excess pounds.

◆ Drink alcohol in moderation, if you do drink.

◆ Don't smoke.

◆ Learn to control stress rather than letting it control you.

◆ If you feel you are at risk, ask your doctor about taking an aspirin a day to prevent heart attack. ∎

SYMPTOMS

- bright red anal bleeding that may streak the bowel movement or the toilet tissue.
- tenderness or pain during bowel movements.
- painful swelling or a lump near the anus.
- anal itching.
- a mucous anal discharge.

CALL YOUR DOCTOR IF:

- you experience any anal bleeding for the first time, even if you believe you have hemorrhoids. Colon polyps, colitis, Crohn's disease, and colorectal cancer can also cause anal bleeding. An accurate diagnosis is essential.
- you have been diagnosed with hemorrhoids, and you have anal bleeding that is chronic (daily or weekly) or more profuse than the streaking described above. Though rare, excessive hemorrhoidal bleeding can cause anemia.

Hemorrhoids are essentially varicose veins of the rectum. The hemorrhoidal veins are located in the lowest area of the rectum and the anus. Sometimes they swell, so that the vein walls become stretched, thin, and irritated by passing bowel movements. When these swollen veins bleed, itch, or hurt, they are known as hemorrhoids, or piles. Hemorrhoids are classified into two general categories: internal and external.

Internal hemorrhoids lie far enough inside the rectum that you can't see or feel them. They don't usually hurt, because there are few pain-sensing nerves in the rectum. Bleeding may be the only sign of their presence. Sometimes internal hemorrhoids prolapse, or enlarge and protrude outside the anal sphincter. If so, you may be able to see or feel them as moist, pink pads of skin that are pinker than the surrounding area. Prolapsed hemorrhoids may hurt, because the anus is dense with pain-sensing nerves. They usually recede into the rectum on their own; if they don't, they can be gently pushed back into place.

External hemorrhoids lie within the anus and are usually painful. If an external hemorrhoid prolapses to the outside (usually in the course of passing a stool) you can see and feel it. Blood clots sometimes form within prolapsed external hemorrhoids, causing an extremely painful condition called a thrombosis. If an external hemorrhoid becomes thrombosed, it can look rather frightening, turning purple or blue, and possibly bleeding. Despite their appearance, thrombosed hemorrhoids are usually not serious and will resolve themselves in about a week. If the pain is unbearable, your doctor can remove the thrombosis, which stops the pain, during an office visit.

Anal bleeding and pain of any sort is alarming and should be evaluated; it can indicate a life-threatening condition, such as colorectal cancer. Hemorrhoids are the most common cause of anal bleeding and are rarely dangerous but a definite diagnosis from your physician is a must.

CAUSES

About half of the people in the U.S. will suffer from hemorrhoids at some point in life; for most,

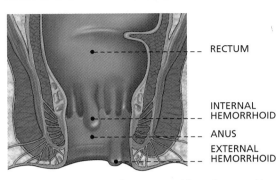

RECTUM

INTERNAL
HEMORRHOID

ANUS

EXTERNAL
HEMORRHOID

Veins in the rectum and anus are subjected to considerable pressure whenever a stool is passed. Pushing or straining may cause veins in the rectal wall to bulge, creating clusters of swollen, or dilated, veins called hemorrhoids. Internal hemorrhoids can form anywhere inside the anal canal, while external hemorrhoids are visible at, or just below, the opening of the anus.

this will happen between ages 20 and 50. Researchers are not certain what causes hemorrhoids. "Weak" veins—leading to hemorrhoids and other varicose veins—may be inherited. It's likely that extreme abdominal pressure causes the veins to swell and become susceptible to irritation. Sources of this pressure include obesity, pregnancy, standing or sitting for long periods, liver disease, straining from constipation or diarrhea, coughing, sneezing, vomiting, and holding one's breath while straining to do physical labor.

Diet has a pivotal role in causing—and preventing—hemorrhoids. People who consistently eat a high-fiber diet are unlikely to get hemorrhoids, whereas those who prefer a diet high in refined foods can expect them. A low-fiber diet or inadequate fluid intake causes constipation, which contributes to hemorrhoids in two ways: It encourages straining to have a bowel movement, and it also aggravates the hemorrhoids by producing hard stools that further irritate the swollen veins.

DIAGNOSTIC AND TEST PROCEDURES

Your doctor will first visually examine the anal area, perhaps by inserting a lubricated gloved finger or an anoscope (a hollow, lighted tube for viewing the lower few inches of the rectum) or a proctoscope (which works like an anoscope but provides a more thorough rectal examination). More procedures may be needed to identify internal hemorrhoids or rule out other ailments that frequently cause anal bleeding, such as anal fissure, colitis, Crohn's disease, and colorectal cancer. To see further into the anal canal (into the lower colon, or sigmoid), sigmoidoscopy may be used, or the entire colon may be viewed with colonoscopy. For both procedures, a lighted, flexible viewing tube is inserted into the rectum. A barium x-ray can show the entire colon's interior. First a barium enema is given, then x-rays are taken of the lower gastrointestinal tract.

TREATMENT

Once you have them, hemorrhoids don't usually go away completely unless you undergo one of the procedures below. They can get better, however, so that living with them is tolerable. Both conventional and alternative practitioners consider diet the best tool for treating hemorrhoids. A diet rich in high-fiber foods and low in refined and junk foods is essential. Probably half of all hemorrhoid sufferers find relief with dietary changes alone.

Most hemorrhoid treatments aim to minimize pain and itching. Warm (but not hot) sitz baths are the most time-honored and oft-suggested therapy: Sit in about three inches of warm water for 15 minutes, several times a day, especially after a bowel movement. If you are pregnant, discuss any treatment, including dietary changes, with your doctor before proceeding.

CONVENTIONAL MEDICINE

If you have been diagnosed as having hemorrhoids, a high-fiber diet combined with sitz baths and acetaminophen should reduce discomfort within two weeks. If symptoms persist, your physician may suggest one of the following procedures. All except laser coagulation and surgery can be performed in your doctor's office.

Injection. An internal hemorrhoid can be in-

H

jected with phenol in oil, quinine, and urea, or morrhuate sodium, which creates a scar and closes off the hemorrhoid. The injection hurts only a little, as any injection does. With a success rate of 90 percent, this is many physicians' first choice. Results are not permanent, however; repeat injections may be needed every two or three years.

Banding. Prolapsed hemorrhoids are often removed using rubber-band ligation. A special tool secures a tiny rubber band around the hem-

---

Over-the-Counter Relief

Controversy continues to rage about the efficacy of hemorrhoid medicines. In the United States., we annually spend roughly $200 million on creams, ointments, and suppositories that promise to relieve inflammation and pain.

The basic ingredient in all these medicines is a lubricant, such as lanolin, cocoa butter, vegetable oil, or one of many others. Some also include an anesthetic such as benzocaine or lidocaine, or an astringent such as tannic acid or zinc compounds, purported to reduce swelling by constricting capillaries. Hemorrhoids, however, are not capillaries; they're veins, and astringents may have no effect on them. Anesthetics may provide short-term relief, but only in cream or ointment form: Suppositories usually go too far up into the anal canal to help the hemorrhoids below.

Lubrication is the greatest benefit of most over-the-counter hemorrhoid medications. Plain petroleum jelly works as well and can be applied with your finger. For pain relief, try acetaminophen and sitz baths.

---

orrhoid, shutting off its blood supply almost instantly. Within a week, the hemorrhoid shrivels and falls off. This painless method is successful about 75 percent of the time.

Coagulation or **cauterization.** Using either an electric probe, a laser beam, or an infrared light, a tiny burn painlessly seals the end of the hemorrhoid, causing it to close off and shrink. This is most useful for prolapsed hemorrhoids.

Surgery. For large internal hemorrhoids or extremely uncomfortable external hemorrhoids (such as thrombosed hemorrhoids that are too painful to live with), your physician may elect traditional surgery, called hemorrhoidectomy. In the hospital, under general anesthesia, the hemorrhoid is removed. After the operation, expect a week or so of bed rest, with analgesics prescribed for discomfort.

The success rate for hemorrhoid removal approaches 95 percent, but unless dietary and lifestyle changes are made, hemorrhoids are likely to recur.

ALTERNATIVE CHOICES
Try one or several of these therapies to alleviate hemorrhoid discomfort. If symptoms persist despite your efforts at relief, contact your physician.

ACUPUNCTURE
The most responsive point for relieving hemorrhoid pain is Governing Vessel 20. Others that may augment it are Stomachs 25 and 36, Governing Vessel 14, and Large Intestine 11. See a licensed practitioner for treatment; see pages 22–23 for point locations.

HERBAL THERAPIES
Applied twice daily, pilewort (*Ranunculus ficaria*) ointment can reduce the pain of external hemorrhoids: Simmer 2 tbsp fresh or dried pilewort in 7 oz petroleum jelly for 10 minutes. Allow to cool before using; store leftover ointment in a closed container. Pilewort may also be taken as a tea.

HOMEOPATHY
More than a dozen remedies, each taken at 12x, can help hemorrhoid pain. Choosing the right one

requires attention to your symptoms and, usually, a homeopath's help. For a sore, bruised, and perhaps bleeding anus, try Hamamelis. Aesculus can ease sharp, spiking rectal pain that is worsened with bowel movements, and Sulphur can reduce burning and itching aggravated by warmth.

MASSAGE

This technique moves matter through the intestines, helping to prevent the constipation that contributes to hemorrhoids. Lie on your back, and use your fingers or your palm to make long, sweeping strokes. Repeat each stroke three to six times. Begin on your left side. Just below your ribs, stroke toward your feet; then stroke across your abdomen from the right to left just below your rib cage. Finally, point your fingertips toward your feet, and drag your hand up your right side from pelvis to ribs.

NUTRITION AND DIET

Prevent constipation by following a high-fiber diet. Meals and snacks should consist primarily of vegetables, fruit, nuts, and whole grains, and as few refined foods and meats as possible. If this is a big change for you, introduce the new foods slowly, to avoid gas. If you aren't able to eat enough high-fiber food, supplement your diet with psyllium stool softeners or bulk-forming agents. (Avoid laxatives, which cause diarrhea that can further irritate the swollen veins.) Drink at least eight glasses of water each day; if your life is especially active or you live in a hot climate, you will need more. It's almost impossible to drink too much water.

Monitor your sodium intake. Excess salt in the diet causes fluid retention, which means swelling in all veins, including hemorrhoids.

YOGA

Yoga can encourage blood flow away from hemorrhoids, reducing pain, inflammation, and bleeding. Try the Half Shoulder Stand, Shoulder Stand, Plow, and Bridge, holding each posture for a few minutes each day. A good complement for these postures is lying on a slant board with your head down for 15 minutes each day.

AT-HOME REMEDIES

◆ Try not to sit for hours at a time, but if you must, take breaks: Once every hour, get up and move around for at least five minutes. A doughnut-shaped cushion can make sitting more comfortable and ease hemorrhoid pressure and pain.

◆ Insert petroleum jelly just inside the anus to make bowel movements less painful.

◆ Dab witch hazel (Hamamelis virginiana), a soothing anti-inflammatory agent, on irritated hemorrhoids to reduce pain and itching.

◆ Resist the temptation to scratch hemorrhoids, as it makes everything worse: The inflamed veins become more irritated, the skin around them becomes damaged, and the itching itself intensifies. Instead, to help stop the itching, apply an over-the-counter 0.5 percent hydrocortisone cream to the skin (not inside the anus—on the outside only) and a cold pack.

◆ If you need a pain reliever, try acetaminophen. Avoid ibuprofen and aspirin, which foster bleeding.

◆ Bathe regularly to keep the anal area clean, but be gentle: Excessive scrubbing, especially with soap, can intensify burning and irritation.

◆ Don't sit on the toilet for more than five minutes at a time, and when wiping, be gentle. If toilet paper is irritating, try dampening it first, or use cotton balls or alcohol-free baby wipes.

◆ When performing any task that requires exertion, be sure to breathe evenly. It's common to hold your breath during exertion, and if you do, you're straining, and contributing to hemorrhoid pain and bleeding.

PREVENTION

A healthful diet and lifestyle are good insurance for preventing hemorrhoids, whether you already suffer hemorrhoid symptoms or are intent on never experiencing them. Regular exercise is also important, especially if you work a sedentary job. Exercise helps in several ways: keeping weight in check, making constipation less likely, and enhancing muscle tone. ■

H

SYMPTOMS

Many cases of hepatitis go undiagnosed because the disease is mistaken for the flu or because there are no symptoms at all. The most common symptoms of hepatitis are:
- loss of appetite.
- fatigue.
- mild fever.
- muscle or joint aches.
- nausea and vomiting.
- abdominal pain.

Less common symptoms include:
- dark urine.
- light-colored stools.
- jaundice.
- generalized itching.
- altered mental state, stupor, or coma.

CALL YOUR DOCTOR IF:

- your flulike symptoms persist or you notice any of the more serious signs; chronic hepatitis can lead to cirrhosis and even death.
- a friend or family member comes down with hepatitis; you may be infected with the organism that causes the disease.
- your symptoms follow a visit to a country where hepatitis is common; you may have contracted the disease during your travels.

Hepatitis, a general term that means inflammation of the liver, applies to a group of viral disorders commonly known as hepatitis A, B, C, D, and E. Another type of hepatitis is brought on through alcohol abuse or the use of drugs, or by ingestion of toxins in the environment.

Hepatitis is the most common of all serious contagious diseases. About 70,000 cases are reported to the Centers for Disease Control and Prevention each year, but researchers estimate that the number of people in the United States who actually have the disease is closer to 500,000. Many hepatitis cases go undiagnosed because they are mistaken for the flu. Hepatitis is serious because it interferes with the liver's many functions. Among other things, the liver produces bile to aid digestion, regulates the chemical composition of the blood, and screens potentially harmful substances from the bloodstream.

The five viruses that cause hepatitis can be transmitted in different ways, but they all have one thing in common: They infect the liver and cause it to become inflamed. Generally, the acute phase of the disease lasts from two to three weeks; complete recovery takes about nine weeks. Although most patients recover with a lifelong immunity to the disease, a few hepatitis victims (less than 1 percent) die in the acute phase. Others may develop chronic hepatitis, in which the liver remains inflamed for six months or more. This condition can lead to cirrhosis and possibly death.

CAUSES

Although their effects on the liver and the symptoms they produce can be similar, the various forms of hepatitis are contracted in different ways. In the case of viral hepatitis, the severity and duration of the disease are largely determined by the organism that caused it.

Hepatitis A, which is generally contracted orally through fecal contamination of food or water, is considered the least dangerous form of the disease because it does not lead to chronic inflammation of the liver. The hepatitis A virus commonly spreads through improper handling of food, contact with household members, sharing toys at day-care centers, and eating raw shellfish taken from polluted waters.

Hepatitis B, the most widespread of the hepatitis viruses, infects an estimated 300,000 people every year in the United States alone. The virus can pass from mother to child at birth or soon afterward; the disease organism can also travel between adults and children to infect whole families. Hepatitis B can also spread through sexual contact, blood transfusions, and needle sharing by intravenous-drug users. In a third of all hepatitis B cases the source cannot be identified.

The majority of hepatitis B patients recover completely, but a small percentage of them can't shake the disease and may develop chronic hepatitis and possibly cirrhosis. People with chronic hepatitis become carriers, meaning they can transmit the disease to others even when their own symptoms have vanished. Only 1 or 2 percent of hepatitis B patients die from the disease.

Hepatitis C is usually spread through contact with blood or contaminated needles. Although hepatitis C may cause only mild symptoms or none at all, 20 percent to 30 percent of chronic carriers develop cirrhosis within 10 years. The disease can be passed on through blood transfusions, but a recently developed test has greatly reduced the number of such cases. In a third of all hepatitis C cases, the source of the disease is unknown.

Hepatitis D occurs only in people infected with hepatitis B and tends to magnify the severity of that disease. It can be transmitted from mother to child and through sexual contact. Rarest among the five hepatitis viruses, hepatitis D is also the most dangerous because it involves two forms of the disease working at once.

Hepatitis E occurs mainly in Asia, Mexico, and Africa; only a few cases are reported in the United States, mostly among people who have returned from a country where the disease is widespread. Like hepatitis A, this type is usually spread through fecal contamination, and it does not lead to chronic hepatitis. This form is considered slightly more dangerous than hepatitis A, especially in pregnant women.

Alcoholic, toxic, and **drug-related hepatitis** can produce the same symptoms and liver inflammation that result from viral hepatitis. This form is caused not by invading microorganisms but by excessive and chronic consumption of alcohol *(see Alcohol Abuse),* ingestion of environmental toxins, or misuse of certain prescription drugs and over-the-counter medications such as acetaminophen.

DIAGNOSTIC AND TEST PROCEDURES

When the patient's symptoms suggest hepatitis, the doctor normally takes blood samples and runs tests to check for the presence of a disease organism. More blood samples may be necessary later—even after the symptoms have vanished—to check for complications and determine if the patient is a carrier of the disease.

The doctor may also require a liver biopsy, or tissue sample, in order to determine the extent of the damage. A biopsy is commonly performed by inserting a needle into the liver and drawing

CAUTION!

Beware of Hidden Dangers

Because the liver plays a key role in processing drugs, alcohol, and toxins in the bloodstream, a patient with hepatitis may find that some medications, alcoholic beverages, and herbs that are normally tolerated can aggravate the condition. If you have hepatitis, do not attempt to treat the disease on your own; consult a physician or licensed practitioner. Avoid alcoholic beverages and ask your doctor if it is all right to use birth-control pills, antibiotics, or over-the-counter medicines. Be sure to tell your physician or practitioner all the medications that you are taking, including even seemingly innocuous over-the-counter drugs such as aspirin or acetaminophen.

out a fragment of tissue, which is then sent to a laboratory to be analyzed.

TREATMENT

There are only a few specific remedies for most types of hepatitis. The conventional approach in each case is to treat the disease with rest and proper diet and to make efforts to contain its spread. Some alternative remedies, when administered by a trained professional, can be used to complement a doctor's care and may help relieve symptoms.

CONVENTIONAL MEDICINE

Although your doctor may recommend bed rest, you may find that simply restricting physical activity is enough to make you feel better. The general rule is this: If you feel well, get up; if you don't, take it easy or lie down. Avoid contact with others to keep the virus from spreading.

Good nutrition is an important part of treatment for all types of hepatitis. In most cases, eating properly means a simple regimen of nutritious, well-balanced meals that supply adequate calories. Many hepatitis patients like to eat a hearty breakfast because their appetites wane and nausea intensifies as the day progresses. Patients who have trouble eating larger meals may prefer to eat smaller amounts at each sitting and snack frequently throughout the day.

Treatment for alcoholic, toxic, and drug-related hepatitis is generally the same as that for viral hepatitis, although hospitalization is more common for nonviral hepatitis, and severe cases tend to be more life-threatening. As is often the case, simply removing the offending drink, toxin, or drug goes a long way toward helping patients recover from nonviral hepatitis.

If your hepatitis, either viral or nonviral, is in the acute stage, avoid alcoholic beverages, as the body's efforts to process alcohol put an added strain on the already injured liver. Also be aware that the sexual partner of an infected person, particularly if he or she has hepatitis B, may run the risk of contracting the disease.

A primary-care physician can usually provide

WHAT'S BEST TO EAT

The right kind of diet can play a very important part in how your body handles a case of hepatitis. If you have acute or chronic hepatitis, you should increase your intake of fiber, including whole-grain cereals, fruits and vegetables, and cooked dried beans and peas. These foods encourage the elimination of bile acids and toxins that can accumulate in the liver and gallbladder.

Some nutritionists contend that massive doses of vitamin C, perhaps taken intravenously, can improve viral hepatitis by reducing inflammation in the liver. Studies also suggest that large doses of vitamin B_{12} and folic acid may reduce the time that it takes a patient to recover from the disease. Ask your doctor or a licensed nutritionist for the vitamins and dosages that are right for you.

adequate care for patients with all types of hepatitis. However, severe cases may require treatment by a hepatologist or gastroenterologist—specialists in diseases of the liver. Hospitalization is normally unnecessary unless the patient cannot eat or drink, or is vomiting.

Most people recover completely from hepatitis. Mild flareups may occur over a period of several months as the disease is subsiding, but each flareup is usually less severe than the one before it, and a relapse doesn't mean you won't make a full recovery.

Hepatitis in pregnant women usually does not increase the risk of birth defects or other pregnancy problems, and infection of the baby in the uterus is rare. If the mother has hepatitis B, however, the baby is likely to contract the disease at birth. A hepatitis B vaccine now available will reduce these chances significantly if administered to the infant immediately after delivery. If you are pregnant, your doctor will test you for hepatitis B; if you are infected with the virus, your baby will be given immune serum globulin shots and a hepatitis vaccination.

Doctors sometimes recommend drug therapy for patients with certain types of hepatitis. The drug interferon is commonly used to treat chronic cases of hepatitis B and hepatitis C. Interferon has been shown to help rid the body of the virus and reduce inflammation and liver damage in 15 percent to 20 percent of people with these forms of the disease, thus reducing the risk of cirrhosis. For some hepatitis cases doctors prescribe corticosteroids to suppress inflammation. Use of these drugs to control hepatitis is controversial, however, because they may have side effects that harm the immune system.

Almost every known drug has at one time or another been implicated as a cause of liver damage. If you currently have hepatitis, or if you have a history of liver disease or other liver problems, tell your doctor before taking any medication.

Regardless of what kind of hepatitis you have or what treatment you receive, you should continue seeing your doctor for checkups until blood tests indicate the virus is gone. A person can remain a carrier of hepatitis B or hepatitis C as long as the virus is present in the blood, even if all symptoms have disappeared.

ALTERNATIVE CHOICES

Nonconventional therapies, when taken properly, may help reduce inflammation in the liver and alleviate symptoms of hepatitis. Used improperly, however, some of these treatments can inflict further damage on the liver or lead to other complications. In general, hepatitis does not lend itself to self-medication. Don't take chances with this disease. If you want to supplement a doctor's care with an alternative remedy, consult a licensed practitioner for help in choosing the right medications and determining exact dosages.

HOMEOPATHY

Homeopaths sometimes prescribe Phosphorus to reduce liver inflammation and relieve the symp-

toms of hepatitis. Other remedies include Taraxacum officinale, Lycopodium, and Chelidonium majus, depending on the individual symptoms. Consult a professional homeopath for exact preparations and dosages.

PREVENTION

The keys to avoiding hepatitis are vaccinations, good hygiene, and informed common sense. Adequate sanitation and clean personal habits will help reduce the spread of hepatitis A and hepatitis E. In areas where sanitation is questionable, boil water. Cook all food well and peel all fruit.

Healthcare workers involved in the treatment of patients with hepatitis B, C, or E should wash their hands, utensils, bedding, and clothing with soap and hot water, especially in the first two weeks of illness, when the patient is most contagious.

People planning to travel to countries where hepatitis is widespread are advised to have immune serum globulin shots or vaccinations before leaving. Immune serum globulin may prevent infection from some types of hepatitis after exposure if administered within 48 hours.

To prevent the spread of hepatitis B, avoid exposure to infectious blood or body fluids. Do not have intimate contact or share razors, scissors, nail files, toothbrushes, or needles with anyone who has the disease. If you suspect that you have been exposed, you should receive immune serum globulin and vaccinations for hepatitis A and hepatitis B as soon as possible. ∎

H

- an obvious swelling beneath the skin in the abdomen or the groin; it may disappear when you lie down and may or may not be tender.
- a heavy feeling in the abdomen that is sometimes accompanied by constipation.
- discomfort in the abdomen or groin when lifting or bending over.

CALL YOUR DOCTOR IF:

- you suspect that you have a hernia. Sometimes hernias require urgent medical care; an accurate diagnosis is important.
- you know you have a hernia, and you are nauseated and vomiting or are unable to have a bowel movement or pass gas. You may have a strangulated hernia or an obstruction, which are emergencies. **Seek medical care immediately.**

A hernia occurs when an organ or tissue squeezes through a hole or a weak spot in a surrounding muscle. The most common types are inguinal, incisional, femoral, and umbilical.

In an **inguinal hernia,** the intestine or the bladder protrudes through the abdominal wall or into the inguinal canal, in the groin. About 80 percent of all hernias are inguinal, and most occur in men because of a natural weakness in this area.

In an **incisional hernia,** the intestines push through the abdominal wall at the site of previous abdominal surgery. This type is most common in elderly and overweight people who are inactive after abdominal surgery.

A **femoral hernia** occurs when the bladder or intestine enters the canal carrying the femoral artery into the upper thigh. Femoral hernias are most common in women, especially those who are pregnant or obese.

In an **umbilical hernia,** part of the small intestine passes through the abdominal wall near the navel. Common in newborns, it also afflicts obese women or those who have had many children.

CAUSES

Ultimately, all hernias are caused by a combination of muscle weakness and strain: A weak spot in the muscle tears under the pressure of strain, and an internal organ or tissue then pushes through the tear. Sometimes the muscle weakness is present at birth; more often, it occurs later in life. Poor nutrition, smoking, and overexertion all can weaken muscles and make hernias more likely. Anything that causes muscle strain can then induce hernia, including obesity, lifting heavy objects, diarrhea or constipation, or persistent coughing.

DIAGNOSTIC AND TEST PROCEDURES

A doctor's physical examination is often enough to diagnose a hernia. Sometimes hernia swelling is visible when you stand upright; usually, the hernia can be felt if you place your hand directly over it and then bear down. Ultrasound may be used to see a femoral hernia, and abdominal x-rays may be ordered to identify a bowel obstruction.

INGUINAL HERNIA

An inguinal hernia occurs in the thin band of muscles at the inguinal canal, where a man's spermatic cord runs from the testicles through the abdominal wall. If the muscle wall is weakened, part of the small intestine can protrude through it, creating a bulge in the groin *(below)*. An inguinal hernia can restrict blood flow or cause a bowel obstruction and is considered a medical emergency.

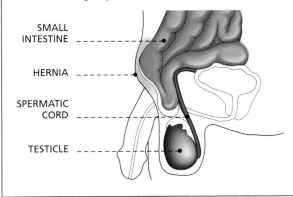

SMALL INTESTINE

HERNIA

SPERMATIC CORD

TESTICLE

TREATMENT

In babies, umbilical hernias frequently heal themselves within four years, making surgery unnecessary. For all others, the standard treatment is conventional hernia-repair surgery (called herniorrhaphy). If left untreated, the protruding organ may become strangulated (have its blood supply cut off), and infection and tissue death may occur as a result. A strangulated intestinal hernia may result in intestinal obstruction, which can lead to infection, gangrene, intestinal perforation, shock, or even death.

CONVENTIONAL MEDICINE

Your doctor may manually press your hernia back into place and advise you to wear a special belt, known as a truss, that holds a hernia in place until surgery. Over-the-counter analgesics can help ease discomfort.

Hernia surgery is performed under either local or general anesthesia. The surgeon repositions the herniated tissue and, if strangulation has occurred, removes the oxygen-starved part of the organ. The damaged muscle wall will then be repaired. Increasingly, inguinal herniorrhaphy is performed using a laparoscope, a thin telescope-like instrument that requires a smaller incision and involves a shorter recovery period.

Patients often walk around the day after hernia surgery. There are usually no dietary restrictions, and work and regular activity may be resumed in a week. Complete recovery takes four to six weeks, with no heavy lifting for at least three months. Hernias often return after surgery, so preventive measures are especially important to avoid a recurrence.

ALTERNATIVE CHOICES

If you have—or believe you have—a hernia, you need to be under a doctor's care. Alternative therapies cannot cure hernia; they can, however, relieve the discomfort.

CHINESE HERBS

To make a compress that may help relieve the pain of an umbilical hernia, crush ⅓ tsp wood sorrel *(Oxalis corniculata)* and ¼ tsp Asian pennywort *(Hydrocotyle rotundifolia)* and add to ½ cup warm cooked rice. Place the compress over the navel for three to four hours; repeat two or three times.

LIFESTYLE

Gentle exercise on a regular basis tones and strengthens stomach muscles. One good choice to do daily: Lie on your back with knees bent and feet on the floor. Keeping your shoulders on the floor, lift your buttocks and your lower back; gently lower yourself. Repeat 10 times.

PREVENTION

Avoid obesity and physical strain; practice good nutrition (both to avoid constipation and to enhance muscle strength); and maintain toned abdominal muscles. When lifting heavy objects, always bend from the knees, not the waist. If something is too heavy, don't lift it at all. ∎

SYMPTOMS

The majority of people who have hiatal hernias don't even realize it. Those who do know typically find out when visiting a doctor because of chronic heartburn. Symptoms may include the following:

- heartburn; regurgitation.
- difficulty swallowing.
- chest pain radiating from below the breastbone (the sternum).
- a bloated feeling after eating.
- shortness of breath.

CALL YOUR DOCTOR IF:

- radiating chest pain is not relieved by taking an antacid. You may have angina, or you may be having a heart attack. **Get medical care immediately.**
- you are being treated for heartburn or hiatal hernia, and you feel sudden chest or stomach pain, have difficulty swallowing, and are vomiting. You may have a hernia that has strangulated, which is a medical and surgical emergency. **Seek medical help without delay.**
- your hiatal hernia is accompanied by chronic heartburn. Stomach acid is repeatedly burning your esophagus, which can lead to esophagitis (an inflamed and ulcerated esophagus), esophageal scarring, stomach ulcer, or cancer. See a physician soon.

The hiatus is an opening in the diaphragm (a muscle separating the abdomen and chest) that the esophagus passes through to reach the stomach. If the hiatus weakens and stretches, part of the stomach and/or the esophagus can squeeze into the chest cavity, producing a hiatal hernia.

Essentially, there are three types of hiatal hernias. In a **sliding hernia,** the lower esophagus and stomach move upward, bringing the top part of the stomach into the chest cavity. In a **paraesophageal hernia,** the stomach moves through the hiatus and rests beside the esophagus. **Mixed hernias** have features of both sliding and paraesophageal hernias.

Although typically small, some hiatal hernias expand until a large portion of the stomach is squeezed through the hiatus. Slow bleeding, from the compressed stomach or from esophagitis, can eventually cause anemia. Sometimes a hernia will become strangulated, or so tightly constricted that blood flow is cut off to the squeezed part of the stomach and the nearby esophagus. This is unlikely in mixed and sliding hernias but common in paraesophageal hernias. Generally, sliding and mixed hiatal hernias show no symptoms and pose no threat to good health.

CAUSES

All ages are susceptible, but frequency increases with age: More than half of those over age 50 have a hiatal hernia. Sliding hernia is by far the most common type. Like other hernias, hiatal hernias are probably caused by excessive pressure in the abdomen related to pregnancy, obesity, injury, or straining to have a bowel movement. Risk factors include constipation, heavy lifting, and persistent coughing or vomiting.

Usually, hiatal hernias cause no symptoms, but when they do, symptoms are worsened by wearing tight clothing, eating foods that cause heartburn, and bending over or lying down after eating.

DIAGNOSTIC AND TEST PROCEDURES

A physical examination for hiatal hernia is similar to that for heartburn, with two additions:

X-rays may be ordered to show the hernia, and if anemia is a concern, a blood sample may be taken to check your red blood cell count.

TREATMENT

Heartburn or other symptoms that occur with **sliding** or **mixed hernias** may be treated by both conventional and alternative therapies. **Paraesophageal hernias,** however, should be repaired by conventional surgery because the danger of strangulation is high.

CONVENTIONAL MEDICINE

Often, alleviating heartburn is all that is required. Surgery is indicated, however, if a paraesophageal hernia exists, or when sliding or mixed hernias bleed or become large, strangulated, or inflamed. In surgery, the hiatus is reinforced and the stomach is repositioned. This surgery is now commonly done using a laparoscope, a thin telescope-like instrument for viewing inside the abdomen. Typically, a two-night hospital stay is required and regular activity may be resumed in two weeks.

ALTERNATIVE CHOICES

The therapies for hiatal hernia symptoms are similar to those for heartburn.

ACUPRESSURE

To relieve heartburn, use deep thumb pressure to massage these points for at least one minute: Stomach 36, Spleen 6, Pericardium 6, and Liver 14. *(See pages 22–23 for point locations.)*

HERBAL THERAPY

Slippery elm *(Ulmus fulva)* tea is soothing and is reputed to have strong anti-inflammatory qualities. Mix 1 part powdered bark in 8 parts water, simmer for 10 minutes, and drink ½ cup, three times daily.

LIFESTYLE

Refrain from eating large meals; instead, eat four or five small meals each day, and eat slowly. This, along with maintaining a weight in proportion to your height, will minimize abdominal pressure—and heartburn. Reducing fat in your diet may also substantially reduce symptoms. Smoking is an intense heartburn generator; if you smoke, stop.

PREVENTION

To prevent symptoms:
◆ Wear loose clothing. Anything that presses on the stomach can aggravate hiatal hernia symptoms.
◆ When your stomach is full, avoid bending over or lying down. This increases abdominal pressure and makes gravity work against you, so heartburn is more likely.

To prevent hiatal hernia:
◆ Maintain a reasonable weight.
◆ Don't smoke. ■

TWO TYPES OF HIATAL HERNIAS

ESOPHAGUS

STOMACH

DIAPHRAGM

The esophagus passes through the hiatus—a small opening in the diaphragm separating the chest and abdominal cavities *(left)*. A sliding hiatal hernia *(inset, below, left)* occurs when the lower esophagus and a small part of the stomach push through the hiatus into the chest cavity. In a paraesophageal hiatal hernia *(inset, below, right)*, part of the stomach balloons up beside the esophagus.

SLIDING HIATAL HERNIA

PARAESOPHAGEAL HIATAL HERNIA

SYMPTOMS

◆ repeated, involuntary contractions of the diaphragm that cause air to rush suddenly into the lungs and close the glottis—the part of the larynx containing the vocal cords—creating the "hic" sound; hiccups generally are of short duration and often follow a big meal or too much alcohol. Occasionally, a prolonged episode of hiccups can last days or weeks.

CALL YOUR DOCTOR IF:

◆ your hiccups persist for more than a day; prolonged hiccups can result from irritation of the nerves of the diaphragm or of the diaphragm itself from pneumonia, esophagitis, pancreatic problems, alcohol abuse, or hepatitis.

◆ hiccups and fever occur after major surgery in the upper abdomen and lead to a loss of appetite; under these conditions the hiccups may be indicative of an abscess under the diaphragm or over the liver.

Hiccups—involuntary spasms of the diaphragm—are usually a minor annoyance and last only for a short time. They can affect anyone, and most pregnant women will tell you that they have even felt their unborn child hiccup in the womb.

CAUSES

No one knows why the diaphragm sometimes contracts involuntarily, causing hiccups. But the condition can be related to nerves or to having had too much food or drink; rarely is it a secondary complication of a disease, but it has been associated with both appendicitis and diabetes.

TREATMENT

Most cases of hiccups resolve spontaneously, although sufferers can try to hasten this resolution with various home remedies.

CONVENTIONAL MEDICINE

Medical intervention is rarely needed; but if a case of hiccups fails to stop after a day, a visit to the doctor's office may be warranted to rule out disease-related causes. Drugs that have given relief in cases of prolonged hiccups include baclofen and chlorpromazine. If your hiccups arise from esophagitis, a condition caused by stomach acid backing up into the esophagus, your doctor may prescribe cimetidine, ranitidine, or omeprazole, drugs that suppress acid production in the stomach at the cellular level. See Heartburn for more information.

ALTERNATIVE CHOICES

ACUPRESSURE

Acupressure exercises seek to trigger a relaxation response in the throat, lungs, or diaphragm to stop the hiccups. Deep breathing is an important part of the exercise. Try the following exercises in succession to relieve the hiccups. *(See pages*

ACUPRESSURE

1 To stop an attack of hiccups, try palm pressure. Place the palms of your hands over both eyes, with the heels resting on your cheekbones. Gently massage around your eyes for one minute by pressing the pads below your thumbs inward toward your palms.

2 Follow the palm treatment with a short series of light presses with the end of your finger to Governing Vessel 25, at the tip of your nose. The combination of palm and finger pressure should make your hiccups go away.

22–23 for more information on point locations.)

◆ Lightly press Triple Warmer 17 (in the indentation behind the earlobes) with your middle and index fingers. Hold lightly for one minute.

◆ Curve your fingers to hold the base of your rib cage directly below your nipples (Spleen 16). Press up, into the indentations at the base of your ribs, and breathe deeply for one minute.

◆ Place your right middle finger in the hollow at the base of your throat (Conception Vessel 22) and gently direct pressure downward. At the same time, use all the fingers of your left hand to firmly hold the center of your breastbone (Conception Vessel 17). Close your eyes and breathe deeply for one minute.

ACUPUNCTURE

Acupuncturists report effective relief of prolonged hiccups by stimulating points on the hands, feet, and back; seek help from a professional.

HERBAL THERAPIES

To stop the hiccups, herbalists recommend warm chamomile *(Matricaria recutita)* tea, which is said to act as an antispasmodic agent. Another reme-dy that might bring relief is a tea that combines ½ tsp of tinctures of peppermint *(Mentha piperita)* and boneset *(Eupatorium perfoliatum)* with a few drops of cayenne *(Capsicum frutescens)* and the juice of a quarter lemon in 1 cup hot water.

HOMEOPATHY

Spasming of the diaphragm may be eased by Ignatia, Cuprum metallicum, or Nux vomica. Seek help from a practitioner.

OSTEOPATHY

In cases of prolonged hiccups, an osteopath might adjust the painful areas around the vertebrae at the level of the diaphragm to bring relief.

AT-HOME REMEDIES

The goal of any of these cures is either to override or to disrupt the nerve impulses that cause the hiccups. Here are some suggestions that may help you stop the hiccups:

◆ Place a tsp of sugar under the tongue and let it dissolve slowly; or swallow the sugar dry; or take the sugar with a glass of water.

◆ Bend forward from the waist and drink water from the opposite side of the glass.

◆ Tickle the roof of your mouth with a cotton swab at the point where the hard and soft palates meet.

◆ Hold your breath and swallow at the same time you feel the urge to hiccup. You may need to repeat this two or three times until your hiccups cease.

◆ Place a brown paper bag over your mouth and breathe forcefully and rapidly into it at least 10 times. Be sure the seal around your mouth is tight so no air gets in.

◆ Suck on a lemon wedge soaked in angostura bitters or sprinkled with cayenne, or swallow 1 tsp vinegar.

◆ If your child has the hiccups, tickle him gently while instructing him to hold his breath and not to laugh. ■

SYMPTOMS

In the vast majority of cases, there are no clear warning signs of hypertension (high blood pressure). If symptoms do occur, they may include:

◆ headaches, chest pain or tightness, nosebleeds, and numbness and tingling; you may have severe hypertension.

◆ excessive perspiration, muscle cramps, weakness, palpitations, and frequent urination; you may have secondary hypertension, possibly caused by a tumor or an adrenal gland disorder.

CALL YOUR DOCTOR IF:

◆ while taking antihypertensive drugs you experience worrisome side effects, such as drowsiness, constipation, dizziness, or loss of sexual function. Your doctor may need to prescribe a different drug.

◆ you are pregnant and develop hypertension; high blood pressure can affect not only your health but also that of your unborn child.

◆ you are experiencing severe headaches, nausea, blurred vision, and confusion or memory loss; you may have **malignant hypertension,** which can result in stroke or heart attack if left untreated.

◆ your diastolic pressure—the second number in a blood pressure reading—suddenly shoots above 130; you may have **malignant hypertension.**

If someone were to take your blood pressure immediately after you'd delivered a speech or jogged five miles, the reading would undoubtedly seem high. This is not necessarily cause for alarm: It's natural for blood pressure to rise and fall with changes in activity or emotional state. It's also normal for blood pressure to vary from person to person, even from one area of your body to another. But when blood pressure remains consistently high, corrective steps should be taken.

High blood pressure, or hypertension, is the most common of all cardiovascular diseases in the industrialized world. It is the leading cause of stroke and a major cause of heart attack. In the United States alone, approximately 40 million people have high blood pressure. This figure includes more than half of all Americans over the age of 60, and about 64 percent of those over 70.

Blood pressure refers to the force of blood pushing against artery walls as it courses through the body. Like air in a tire, blood fills arteries to a certain capacity. Just as too much air pressure can damage a tire, so can too much blood pressure threaten healthy arteries.

A blood pressure reading appears as two numbers. The first and higher of the two is a measure of systolic pressure, or the peak force of blood as it is actually being pumped by the heart. The second number measures diastolic pressure, or the force of blood when the heart is filling for the next beat. Normal blood pressure rises steadily from about 90/60 at birth to about 120/80 in a healthy adult. People with blood pressure as high as 140/90 on at least two occasions are said to have high blood pressure. If the levels remain high, the doctor will probably begin treatment. Patients with blood pressure readings as high as 200/120 should receive treatment immediately.

Consistently high blood pressure forces the heart to work far beyond its capacity. Besides injuring blood vessels, it can damage the brain, eyes, and kidneys. Even so, many hypertensives do not realize they have the condition. Indeed, hypertension is often called "the silent killer" because it rarely exhibits symptoms even as it inflicts serious damage on the body. Left untreated, high blood pressure can lead to vision problems, such as swelling of the optic nerve or hemor-

H

rhaging in the retina, as well as to heart attack, stroke, and other potentially fatal conditions, including kidney failure (see Kidney Disease). Hypertension may also lead to congestive heart failure, a common disorder of the elderly that can result in breathing problems. Fortunately, high blood pressure can be controlled effectively. The first step is discovery, so have your blood pressure checked regularly.

CAUSES

In as many as 95 percent of reported hypertension cases in the United States, the underlying cause cannot be determined. This type of high blood pressure is called **essential hypertension.** Patients who suffer organ damage as a result of high blood pressure are said to have **malignant hypertension;** the diastolic pressure in such cases usually exceeds 130. Malignant hypertension is a dangerous condition that develops rapidly and requires immediate medical attention.

When a direct cause can be identified, the condition is described as **secondary hypertension.** Among the known causes of secondary hypertension, kidney disease ranks highest. The condition can also be triggered by tumors or other abnormalities that cause the adrenal glands to secrete excess amounts of the hormones that elevate blood pressure. Birth-control pills (specifically those containing estrogen) and pregnancy can boost blood pressure, as can medications that constrict blood vessels.

Though **essential hypertension** remains somewhat mysterious, it has been linked to certain risk factors. High blood pressure tends to run in families, for example, and it is more likely to affect men than women. Age and race also play a role. In the United States, African Americans are twice as likely as Caucasians to become hypertensive, although the gap begins to narrow at around age 44. After age 65, African American women have the highest incidence of high blood pressure.

Essential hypertension is also greatly influenced by diet and lifestyle. The link between salt and high blood pressure is especially compelling. People living on the northern islands of Japan eat more salt per capita than anyone else in the world and exhibit the highest incidence of essential hypertension. By contrast, people who add no salt to their food show virtually no traces of essential hypertension. The majority of all hypertensives are "salt sensitive," meaning that anything more than the minimal bodily need for salt is too much for them and leads to an increase in blood pressure. Other factors that have been associated with essential hypertension include obesity; diabetes; stress; insufficient intake of potassium, calcium, and magnesium; lack of physical activity; and chronic alcohol consumption.

TREATMENT

While **essential hypertension** cannot be cured, it can be treated effectively, and **secondary hypertension** can often be cured by addressing the underlying cause. You can do a number of things to control your high blood pressure—but consult a physician before you get started. Together, you and your doctor can design a treatment program that's just right for your condition.

CONVENTIONAL MEDICINE

If you have high blood pressure, you'll probably find out about it during a routine checkup. (You may also have noticed a problem while taking your own blood pressure, but be sure to check with your doctor for a diagnosis.) Take the opportunity to learn what you can do to bring your pressure under control. Most doctors prefer to suggest lifestyle changes before prescribing drugs. A comprehensive lifestyle program will include dietary changes that promote nutrition and lower salt intake, regular aerobic exercise, weight loss, and a ban on smoking. These days, many conventional physicians recommend **yoga, meditation,** or other relaxation techniques to reduce stress.

Some hypertension cases require drug therapy, either because of their severity or because they have failed to respond to self-help measures. A number of drugs have proved effective for high blood pressure—among them diuretics, which rid the body of salt and excess fluids, and beta-adrenergic blockers, drugs that make the heart beat more slowly and with less force. Other medications—including calcium channel blockers, angiotensin-converting enzyme (ACE) inhibitors, alpha$_1$-adrenergic blockers, and centrally acting agents—lower blood pressure by relaxing and dilating arteries. Warning: Do not stop taking prescribed medication until you have consulted your physician; abrupt cessation can be harmful.

ALTERNATIVE CHOICES

Many alternative therapies for high blood pressure focus on relaxation techniques. Others are attempts to get closer to the physiological roots of the problem, either by changing the patient's habits or lifestyle, or by influencing the operation of the heart and blood vessels.

ACUPRESSURE

Applying gentle pressure to several key points on the body *(right)* may help improve circulation and reduce high blood pressure.

BODY WORK

Regular sessions of **massage** or **shiatsu** can help lower blood pressure by promoting relaxation. Both therapies employ touch and manipulation to reduce tension in the body. While massage treats the entire body, shiatsu emphasizes special pressure points, such as those on the backs of the legs and on the inner wrist.

CHINESE MEDICINE

Traditional Chinese healers treat high blood pressure by coupling **acupuncture** with **herbal** and **massage** therapy. Acupuncture may benefit people with moderate hypertension, but it is not recommended for those with severe cases. Chrysanthemum flower *(Chrysanthemum indicum)*, peony *(Paeonia lactiflora)* root, eucommia bark *(Eucommia ulmoides),* and prunella *(Prunella vulgaris)* are among the many Chinese herbs that might be prescribed for high blood pressure.

HERBAL THERAPIES

Hawthorn *(Crataegus laevigata),* used to treat many circulatory disorders, may help reduce high

ACUPRESSURE

1 Pressing Pericardium 3 may help relax the nervous system. Locate the point along your biceps tendon at the elbow crease, in a direct line with your ring finger. Using your thumb, apply firm pressure for one minute, then repeat on the other arm.

2 Pressure on Spleen 6 may help regulate blood pressure. The point is four finger widths up from the inner anklebone, near the edge of your shinbone. Press gently with your thumb for one minute, then switch legs. Do not use this point if you are pregnant.

blood pressure. Over time, the herb may help dilate blood vessels while also moderating heart rate. Hawthorn tea can be prepared at home by steeping the dried flowers and berries in hot water for 10 to 15 minutes. Research indicates that ample consumption of garlic *(Allium sativum)* and onion *(Allium cepa)* can help reduce blood pressure. Valerian *(Valeriana officinalis),* used only when needed, may work as a relaxant for people experiencing undue stress. *(See also Anxiety.)*

MIND/BODY MEDICINE

A number of methods, including **biofeedback**, **meditation**, and **hypnotherapy**, call on the mind to relax the body and, practiced over time with guidance from trained professionals, may help lower blood pressure. Positive imagery—picturing yourself floating in calm water, for instance—can also work well for some people.

NUTRITION AND DIET

Adjusting the foods you eat will help keep your blood pressure in check. Your diet should be high in fiber, low in fat and salt. With these pointers in mind, emphasize fruits, vegetables, and whole grains. Enhance the flavor of your food with seasonings other than salt, and avoid processed foods, which tend to be high in sodium. You should also watch what you drink. Studies suggest that caffeine elevates blood pressure, at least in the short term, while moderate use of alcohol may lower it. Keep cocktails to a minimum, though; more than two ounces of alcohol per day can aggravate hypertension.

Of the vitamins and minerals that help lower blood pressure, potassium has one of the best track records. To get the 3,000 to 4,000 mg per day that researchers recommend, start eating more fresh vegetables and fruits, especially bananas. (Ask your doctor before taking potassium supplements, as too much of the substance can be dangerous.) Fish is a good source of fatty acids, which help relax arteries and thin the blood. Although it does contain sodium, celery is especially beneficial because it also contains ingredients believed to relax blood vessel walls.

Several studies have demonstrated that hypertensives benefit from daily doses of calcium (800 mg) or magnesium (300 mg). Patients sometimes respond better to one than to the other. After checking with your doctor, try calcium supplements for a month. If you do not notice improvement, try magnesium. You can also get calcium naturally from nonfat or low-fat milk, yogurt, and cheese. Many types of seeds, nuts, beans, peas, and dark green leafy vegetables contain both calcium and magnesium.

YOGA
Mainly because of its relaxing effects, yoga is highly recommended for hypertension.

AT-HOME REMEDIES
◆ Adopt a healthful diet. Eat lots of fruit, vegetables, and whole grains. Give up salty foods and add seasonings other than salt to your meals. Consume alcohol and caffeine sparingly.
◆ Exercise regularly to shed extra pounds and get your blood flowing. Activities such as walking, jogging, cycling, and swimming lower blood pressure over the long term.
◆ You can't always avoid stress, but you can learn better ways to cope with it. Researchers believe that stress does not come simply from having too much to do. Rather, it arises from situations that leave you feeling you have no control over matters. Next time you feel stressed, ask yourself why, then concentrate on solving the problem.
◆ If you smoke, quit.

PREVENTION

You can help keep your blood pressure at a healthful level and reduce your risk of heart disease by making a few changes in your lifestyle.
◆ Watch what you eat. Stay away from salt and fat, concentrating instead on foods that are high in fiber, calcium, and magnesium.
◆ Get plenty of exercise. Regular aerobic workouts condition the heart and keep blood vessels dilated and working properly.
◆ If you are overweight, try to trim down. Even a small weight reduction can make a big difference.
◆ If you smoke, now is the time to stop. ■

H

SYMPTOMS

◆ raised, whitish, usually itchy welts of varying size, surrounded by a red rash. *(See the Visual Diagnostic Guide.)*

◆ swelling below the surface of the skin that burns rather than itches, often around the eyes and lips, less frequently on the hands and feet, and rarely inside the throat, on mucous membranes, or on the genitals; these symptoms indicate an allergic reaction known as **angioedema.**

CALL YOUR DOCTOR IF:

◆ burning or itchy welts begin to develop in your throat. You may be at risk of suffocation.

◆ you develop hives accompanied by dry throat, cough, cold sweats, nausea, dizziness, difficult breathing, or a sharp drop in blood pressure after a bee sting or insect bite. This may be a severe allergic reaction known as anaphylaxis. *(See Emergencies/First Aid: Shock.)*

◆ you have recurring bouts of hives lasting a month or more. You may have a chronic condition that needs professional treatment.

◆ you develop symptoms of **angioedema,** particularly in the head and neck. This requires medical attention before the condition spreads to the throat or tongue and blocks the air passage to the lungs.

◆ you develop hives after a blood transfusion. You may be having an allergic reaction to donor blood.

Hives, or urticaria, is a common allergic reaction in which a rash or welts appear on the skin. Hives are typically quite itchy and can last just a few minutes or several days before going away. Occasionally, however, these annoying blotches can signal more serious problems, especially when accompanied by symptoms such as difficult breathing.

In **angioedema,** hives develop beneath the skin and can cause disabling swelling of internal organs, life-threatening blockage of air passages, or severe, uncontrollable intestinal contractions. If the swelling occurs in the throat, it can cause suffocation. Chronic cases of hives that do not itch but are accompanied by abdominal pain or diarrhea may be the result of **hereditary angioedema.**

People who simultaneously develop hives and such symptoms as fever, nausea, abdominal cramps, and shortness of breath immediately after a bee sting, insect bite, or drug injection are in the throes of **anaphylaxis.** This severe shock to the immune system requires prompt medical attention. In rare cases, failure to get help quickly can be fatal.

CAUSES

When an allergen invades or irritates your body, it unleashes chemicals known as histamines. *(See Allergies.)* Some people react to a high histamine level by developing the rash we call hives. Common allergens that can provoke hives include certain milk products, fish, and nuts; drugs such as penicillins and aspirin; and various food additives, emulsifiers, flavorings, or preservatives. Extreme cold or heat, stress, and pressure on the skin may induce an attack of hives, as can insect bites, infections such as strep throat in children and hepatitis B in adults, and—in very rare cases—blood transfusions.

TREATMENT

The first step in controlling hives is to identify the cause, if possible. Once you have identified the source of the problem, try to avoid exposure to it in the future. To relieve itching, apply calamine lotion or a cold compress to the area.

A mild case of hives often disappears on its own after a few hours. A longer-lasting case should respond to the manufacturer's recommended dosage of an over-the-counter oral antihistamine. If your hives don't disappear in a few days, see a doctor. If you develop symptoms of **angioedema** or **anaphylaxis** get medical help immediately. *(See Emergencies/First Aid: Shock.)*

CONVENTIONAL MEDICINE

For chronic or especially troublesome outbreaks of hives, your doctor will probably order a course of prescription antihistamines. Treatment with oral corticosteroids will reduce swelling faster than antihistamines but is usually reserved for severe cases in which suffocation or other complications are indicated. Ultraviolet light treatments are effective for hives caused by exposure to cold. If you have the subsurface welts of **angioedema,** you may require hospitalization.

ALTERNATIVE CHOICES

Herbal, homeopathic, and other alternative therapies offer various ways to relieve the itching of hives. Relaxation techniques and special diets may provide answers for chronic cases that may be rooted in stress or allergies.

ACUPRESSURE

Pressure points that may help counteract an attack of hives are Gall Bladder 20, at the back of the head on either side of the spinal column, and Large Intestine 4, in the web between thumb and forefinger. Massage these points firmly for 60 seconds several times a day. CAUTION: Do not press Large Intestine 4 during pregnancy. *(See pages 22–23 for more information on point locations.)*

HERBAL THERAPIES

To combat itchy hives, apply a chickweed *(Stellaria media)* poultice or add a few teaspoons of the dried herb to your bathwater. A tincture or infusion of valerian *(Valeriana officinalis)*, passion-flower *(Passiflora incarnata)*, or peppermint *(Mentha piperita)* may help relieve stress-related hives; valerian should be taken in doses up to 10 ml to be effective.

HOMEOPATHY

If your hives sting and itch, try Urtica urens (12x). Apis (12x), derived from the honeybee, is especially good when you have considerable redness and swelling. Either remedy is available over the counter and should be taken every two to three hours up to four doses, or until symptoms ease.

MIND/BODY MEDICINE

Stress can raise histamine levels in some people just as easily as a bee sting. Several relaxation techniques, such as **hypnotherapy**, **guided imagery,** and **qigong**, may be helpful in relieving chronic hives.

NUTRITION AND DIET

Food additives, as well as natural toxins in certain foods, are prime suspects in tracing the cause of mild to moderate cases of hives. Some of the most likely irritants are found in milk products, nuts, fish, eggs, flour, beans, chocolate, strawberries, and tomatoes. You may be able to identify the food responsible for your hives by process of elimination: For a few days eat foods that you think will not make you break out, then gradually start eating suspect foods, keeping a careful record of how your body responds to each one. If your hives persist, consult an allergy specialist for more intensive testing.

AT-HOME REMEDIES

One of the best remedies for hives is a soothing bath. Add 5 or 6 tbsp of oatmeal, 3 tbsp of cornstarch or sodium bicarbonate, or a strong infusion of chickweed to your bathwater. If you are allergic to bee stings or other insect bites, ask your doctor about prescribing an emergency kit containing epinephrine, which is a potent bronchodilator. ■

SYMPTOMS

- weakness.
- hunger.
- nervousness.
- dizziness.
- trembling.
- heavy or cold perspiration.
- pale or ashen skin.
- tingling in hands and feet.

For diabetics, symptoms might also include:
- headache.
- nausea.
- rapid heartbeat.
- uncooperative behavior, suggesting confusion or drunkenness.
- unconsciousness, coma, or convulsions.

CALL YOUR DOCTOR IF:

- you are diabetic and experience symptoms of hypoglycemia several times within a few days; your doctor may need to adjust your dosages of insulin or oral hypoglycemia medication.
- you feel faint and think you might become unconscious; if you have diabetes, you need immediate treatment for your blood sugar levels. If you are not diabetic, you should have a professional evaluation of your overall health to pinpoint the underlying cause of your blood sugar imbalance. For diabetics on insulin, untreated hypoglycemia can result in a coma or irreversible brain damage.

H

In most cases, hypoglycemia—literally, low blood sugar—can be treated easily without professional intervention when the symptoms are recognized early enough. Although the condition most often occurs in people with diabetes, non-diabetics can, in rare cases, also experience hypoglycemia attacks. Whether you are diabetic or not, if these episodes become frequent, you need to consult a professional about how to keep your blood sugar levels under control.

CAUSES

The body draws on glucose, the sugar circulating in your bloodstream, for energy. When glucose levels fall below normal, the body cannot meet its energy requirements. The symptoms and complications of hypoglycemia develop as your system tries to extract energy from body fat and muscle.

To convert glucose into energy, the body relies on the pancreatic hormone insulin, whose levels normally rise and fall with energy demand. When there is too much insulin in the bloodstream, available supplies of glucose are burned up too quickly, resulting in hypoglycemia.

Insulin levels can rise sharply after a meal, when the sudden rise in blood sugar levels triggers increased production by the pancreas. By the same token, glucose levels may drop as a result of a missed meal or vigorous exercise. Hypoglycemia can also be brought on by stomach surgery, some types of cancer, liver disease, alcohol, high fevers, and reactions to food or drugs.

In some people, excess insulin production is caused by small tumors that develop on the pancreas. Certain foods, especially simple sugars, can also boost insulin production. To avoid bringing on an attack of hypoglycemia, diabetics who administer their own insulin thus need to monitor their dosages and their diet carefully.

DIAGNOSTIC AND TEST PROCEDURES

If you have several attacks of hypoglycemia, you need to find out if diabetes is the underlying cause. Your doctor can determine this through a glucose tolerance test, which measures your body's ability to process glucose, or through a blood test two hours after eating. If you have diabetes, the physician may induce an attack of hypoglycemia to help you learn to recognize and respond to the symptoms.

TREATMENT

Most remedies for hypoglycemia concentrate on regulating the content and timing of your diet to make sure you receive sufficient blood glucose and insulin supplies at appropriate times.

CONVENTIONAL MEDICINE

If you are diabetic and become unconscious during a hypoglycemia attack, it is essential that you receive immediate medical treatment. A doctor can inject glucose directly into your bloodstream, but if that is not possible, a friend or family member trained in the procedure can give you an injection of glucagon, a hormone that helps your body regulate blood sugar levels. Diabetics should always wear a Medic Alert bracelet or tag identifying their condition so that medical personnel can give appropriate treatment if the patient becomes disoriented or unconscious during a hypoglycemia attack. People with diabetes also should always have some hard candy on hand to eat if they start feeling hypoglycemic.

For diabetics, conventional long-term treatment for hypoglycemia aims to regulate blood levels of glucose and insulin to maintain the proper balance between the two. In many cases, this equilibrium can be achieved through diet modification alone. The recommended diet for alleviating hypoglycemia includes small, frequent meals (at least six a day) made up of foods with lots of complex carbohydrates (such as beans, pasta, bread, and potatoes); fiber (vegetables) and fat; and only limited amounts of simple sugars (such as candy or cookies), alcohol, and fruit juices.

If necessary, your doctor may also treat your diabetes with medications such as streptozocin or diazoxide to limit your body's insulin production or to improve your blood glucose levels. If your hypoglycemia is caused by small pancreatic

tumors that secrete too much insulin, the doctor may recommend having the tumors removed.

ALTERNATIVE CHOICES

Nonconventional remedies emphasize nutrition and diet, with supplements of vitamins, minerals, and herbs.

HERBAL THERAPIES

A decoction made from gentian (Gentiana lutea) helps to stimulate the endocrine, or hormone-producing, glands. Boil ½ tsp of shredded gentian root in a cup of water for 5 minutes and drink warm, 15 to 30 minutes before a meal. It must taste bitter to be effective.

NUTRITION AND DIET

◆ Small, frequent meals of whole foods, especially whole grains, fermented dairy products (such as cheese), and lean meat and fish will boost your blood sugar; fruit juice may also help during a hypoglycemia attack.

◆ Supplements of chromium—a mineral found in brewer's yeast, whole-grain breads and cereals, molasses, cheese, and lean meats—may help improve blood sugar levels. If you are diabetic, check with your healthcare practitioner before beginning to supplement your diet with brewer's yeast.

◆ Avoid alcohol (a simple sugar), caffeine, and cigarette smoke, since they can create large swings in your blood sugar levels.

AT-HOME REMEDIES

Whether you are diabetic or not, if you take action immediately in response to the symptoms of hypoglycemia, you can ward off a more serious attack and avoid any lingering aftereffects. Treatment is as easy as eating or drinking any substance containing simple sugar, such as a soft drink (nondiet), candy, or even a sugar cube. Sugar combined with a protein source, like a piece of cheese or a glass of milk, may help slow the absorption of glucose into your blood and prevent the disorienting "seesaw" effect caused by rapidly changing blood sugar levels. *(See Diabetes.)* ■

SYMPTOMS

In general, problems with your immune system manifest themselves as a tendency to catch colds, the flu, and various other infections more frequently than usual; to get easily tired; or to develop allergies. For specific symptoms of immune system disorders, see AIDS, Allergies, Arthritis, Asthma, Chronic Fatigue Syndrome, Diabetes, Hay Fever, Lupus, and Multiple Sclerosis.

CALL YOUR DOCTOR IF:

◆ you suspect you have an immune system disorder; you need to be properly diagnosed so that you can be properly treated.

The job of the immune system is to seek out, recognize, and destroy pathogens—disease-causing substances or organisms, such as bacteria and viruses. In fighting off these trespassers, your body produces such symptoms of illness as fever and malaise.

When a pathogen enters the bloodstream, a type of immune cell called a macrophage absorbs it, then calls up two other types of immune cells—B cells and T cells. B cells produce antibodies to fight the invader directly. T cells help in various other ways. So-called helper T cells activate the immune response by alerting other immune system cells that an invader is present; killer T cells destroy the intruder; and suppressor T cells regulate and switch off immune activity when the job is done. The immune system then remembers the chemical signature of that particular pathogen and can respond much more rapidly with antibodies should the same pathogen ever attempt another invasion.

In most people, most of the time, the immune system does its job efficiently, but problems in its response to the environment are common. An overactive immune system, for example, results in **autoimmune disorders.** In these cases, for reasons that aren't clear, the immune system mistakes normal, healthy tissues for foreign invaders and attacks them. Examples of autoimmune disorders include rheumatoid arthritis, multiple sclerosis, lupus, Type 1 diabetes, scleroderma (skin hardening), and myasthenia gravis (destruction of muscle proteins). Researchers suspect that chronic fatigue syndrome and Lou Gehrig's disease may be autoimmune diseases as well.

Another type of immune error occurs when the system overreacts to something harmless, as with allergies. In the case of hay fever, for example, the immune system mistakes pollen for a dangerous invader and marshals a powerful and sometimes deadly response.

The opposite occurs when the immune system fails to respond adequately, resulting in **immunodeficiency** diseases. AIDS is perhaps the best-known example; other immunodeficiency disorders are inherited, extremely rare, and potentially fatal.

For people who are generally healthy, it's

possible for the immune system to become temporarily depressed. When this happens, fighting pathogens becomes more difficult, and as a result, your body becomes more susceptible to infections, which hit you harder and stay with you longer than they would otherwise.

CAUSES

Among the things that can temporarily weaken the immune system are environmental toxins, stress, poor diet, lack of exercise and sleep, and abuse of alcohol and tobacco. Over time, these factors can have a long-lasting debilitating effect on your immunity. Studies have also shown that emotional stress, ranging from such everyday events as a disagreement to such dramatic ones as the death of a spouse, can affect immune functioning. Certain medications (especially corticosteroids and anticancer drugs), radiation therapy, and—some researchers believe—an overdependence on antibiotics can also adversely affect your immune system.

Scientists believe that **autoimmune diseases** may result from a combination of genetic, molecular, cellular, and environmental factors. Any enduring illness, but particularly cancer, diabetes, or kidney disease, can weaken your body's immune defenses.

People born with inherited defects in their immune systems, such as a decreased number of lymphocytes (a type of white blood cell that produces antibodies), suffer from serious **immunodeficiencies** that make them extremely vulnerable to infection. Diminished immune functioning can also result from such events as having your spleen surgically removed or having to take immune-suppressing medication following organ transplant surgery.

DIAGNOSTIC AND TEST PROCEDURES
To check for impaired immune functioning, your doctor may administer a number of tests. An immunoelectrophoresis test detects lower-than-normal levels of various antibodies. Another test, known as antigenic stimulation, determines whether your body is able to produce certain antibodies. Your doctor may also test for the effects of an impaired immune system: A thyroid function test, for example, will reveal an underactive thyroid, and x-rays can reveal pneumonia or sinusitis.

TREATMENT

Boosting your immunity may involve altering your eating and exercise habits. Your doctor may refer you to a nutritionist and a physical therapist for specific guidelines.

CONVENTIONAL MEDICINE
Your doctor may discuss with you any stressful events or situations that are adversely affecting your health and suggest making necessary lifestyle changes. The first step your doctor may suggest is to actively stimulate your immune system with vaccines; if that fails, he may try gamma globulin, a blood derivative product that may also work to normalize your immune system.

For people with serious, inherited **immunodeficiencies,** antibody injections, tissue or bone marrow transplantation, and long-term courses of antibiotics may control the problem.

Medical researchers are uncertain of exactly how the malfunctioning of your immune system known as autoimmunity works. For **autoimmune disorders** your doctor may suggest nonsteroidal anti-inflammatory drugs (NSAIDs), corticosteroids, or other, more powerful, immunosuppressive medications, depending on your particular ailment and its severity.

If you suffer from allergies, your doctor may suggest a variety of environmental controls to avoid the substances causing your system to overreact. If that proves insufficient to relieve your symptoms, medications such as antihistamines, decongestants, or inhaled corticosteroids may be advised. The third step in controlling overactive immunity is a series of allergy shots, or immunotherapy, to desensitize your system so it can react normally.

YOGA

1 The **Child** may help strengthen your immune system. Sit on your heels, thighs together. Exhale slowly while bending for-ward from your hips. Bring your forehead to the floor. Breathe deeply for 20 seconds, then inhale as you arise. Do once.

2 For vitality, do the **Bridge.** Lie on your back, knees bent and palms on the floor. Inhale and tense your buttocks, then slowly raise your pelvis. Clasp your hands underneath your body and arch upward as you press your shoulders to the floor. Hold the position for 15 to 20 seconds as you breathe deeply. Then unclasp your hands and ex-hale as you slowly lower your pelvis back down to the floor. Do once.

3 For stamina, try the **Half Moon.** Raise your arms as you inhale. Clasp your hands and exhale as you push your right hip out and stretch to the left. Breathe deeply for 20 sec-onds, keeping your shoul-ders and hips in line. Inhale as you return to center. Do once on each side.

ALTERNATIVE CHOICES

A number of alternative therapies are available for various autoimmune disorders. Consult the entries on multiple sclerosis, arthritis, lupus, and diabetes for possible remedies. The alterna-tive choices suggested in the sections on aller-gies and hay fever may be helpful for those problems. Always consult your healthcare prac-titioner before embarking on alternative treat-ments. In addition to the remedies mentioned below, you might want to consider **acupuncture, massage,** or **homeopathy,** which may help with your specific symptoms. For each method, con-sult a specialist in the field.

CHINESE HERBS

Dried slices of the Chinese remedy known as polyporus, from the mushroom *Polyporus umbel-latus,* can be made into a tea and drunk for a ton-ic effect on the immune system. Astragalus *(As-tragalus membranaceus)* tea or tincture may help combat viral infections and enhance the func-tioning of immune cells. The traditional Minor Bupleurum Combination, taken as a tea or in tablet form, may strengthen the immune system. Ginseng *(Panax ginseng)* may improve immune functioning by protecting against the damage caused by free radicals.

HERBAL THERAPIES

Echinacea *(Echinacea* spp.), long thought to be a potent immunostimulant, may have antiviral and antibacterial properties as well. Garlic *(Allium sativum)* may have anti-infective and immune-enhancing qualities. Shiitake *(Lentinus edodes),* enokidake *(Flammulina velutipes),* and reishi *(Ganoderma lucidum)* mushrooms may promote production of antibodies.

MIND/BODY MEDICINE

Research into the mind's effect on the immune system, called psychoneuroimmunology, has pro-duced some findings on the relationship between happiness and health. One study has confirmed earlier reports that stress depresses immunity, and feeling good boosts it. Moreover, the data turned up an unexpected discovery: It seems that the impact of positive experiences such as expressions of love or feelings of accomplishment continues for two days, whereas the effects of negative events such as criticism or arguments last only one day. This suggests that the affirming consequences of happiness are more powerful and longer lasting than the negative effects of sadness—by 2 to 1.

Progressive relaxation techniques such as **meditation, yoga,** and **qigong** can promote a deep sense of relaxation and reduce stress. Regular exercise is considered to be another effective way to relieve stress.

Researchers are exploring how **guided imagery** or visualization techniques may help boost immune systems that have become depressed from tension buildup or illness. Athletes have long employed guided imagery to picture themselves winning a race or performing a difficult maneuver. One visualization exercise, called palming, involves summoning up a particular mental image to reduce stress and enhance your mental focusing abilities. To try this technique, close your eyes and cover them with your hands. Concentrate on filling your visual field completely with blackness, then invite yourself to see a color you associate with stress; next, substitute that color in your mind's eye with one you perceive as soothing—replace red with blue, for example. A variation on this technique might be to picture a tense scene, such as a traffic jam, and replace the image with a calmer one, such as a lake or meadow.

NUTRITION AND DIET

Nutritionists may recommend a diet high in fresh vegetables and fruit, whole grains, brown rice, low-fat dairy products, fish, and poultry, and low in refined sugars, white flour, junk foods, red meats, and saturated fats. A daily antioxidant multivitamin containing the U.S. recommended daily allowance of vitamins A, B complex, C, and E, with zinc, selenium, and other trace minerals, can play a role in shoring up immunity. *(See Atherosclerosis for more information on antioxidants.)*

One theory holds that juice or water fasts may release a hormone that enhances the immune system. Fasts also cut down on the system's work load, because less energy is expended to process food allergens. Fasts are best attempted under the care of a doctor or nutritionist who will advise you on how to safely begin and end one, as well as about some of the side effects to expect. Don't fast if you're pregnant or diabetic, or if you have a heart condition or an ulcer.

AT-HOME REMEDIES

◆ Any of the herbal teas mentioned under **Chinese Herbs** or **Herbal Therapies** can easily be made at home and used for self-treatment.

◆ Identify the stressors in your life and try to avoid them, or else reduce their toll by practicing one of the relaxation therapy techniques mentioned at left under Mind/Body Medicine.

PREVENTION

Change your habits to include things that actively promote good health.

◆ Avoid overeating and overindulging in alcohol, caffeine, and tobacco. Get plenty of rest, exercise regularly, and eat a balanced diet.

◆ Don't assault infections with antibiotics right away unless your physician deems it necessary. The immune system grows stronger with every battle won, so helping it fight with remedies less powerful than antibiotics—such as analgesics, vitamins, and herbal therapies—will allow the immune system to do its job.

◆ As much as possible, avoid radiation exposure, harmful chemicals, and prolonged use of immunosuppressive drugs such as corticosteroids, all of which can damage immunity. ■

SYMPTOMS

◆ a small patch of blisters that after a few hours breaks into a red, moist area that oozes or weeps fluid; appears mainly on the face, but also on exposed areas of the arms and legs.

◆ in a few days, formation of a golden or dark-yellow crust resembling grains of brown sugar. The infection may continue to spread at the edges of the affected area.

See also the Visual Diagnostic Guide.

CALL YOUR DOCTOR IF:

◆ you have sores on your face that do not go away in 48 hours after starting treatment. An impetigo infection needs prompt medical attention.

◆ small, very itchy, pus-filled ulcers form, with a dark brown crust. This indicates **ecthyma,** an ulcerated form of impetigo that penetrates deep into the skin. If left untreated, it may cause scarring and permanent changes in pigmentation.

◆ symptoms of impetigo appear on a baby. Any persistent skin disorder in infants requires medical attention.

◆ a child suffering from impetigo develops nausea, headaches, low urine output, or puffiness around the face and on limbs. These are signs of **glomerulonephritis,** a kidney disease caused by bacterial toxins.

Note: Sores associated with impetigo may be mistaken for herpes, a viral infection. Impetigo spreads faster, never develops inside the mouth, and is rarely confined to one area of the body. If in doubt, see a doctor for an accurate diagnosis.

Impetigo is a highly contagious bacterial infection. It can appear anywhere on the body but usually attacks exposed areas. Children tend to get it on the face, especially around the nose and mouth, and sometimes on the arms or legs. The infected areas appear in patches ranging from dime- to quarter-sized, starting as tiny blisters that break and expose moist, red skin. After a few days the infected area is covered with a grainy, golden crust that gradually spreads at the edges.

In extreme cases the infection invades a deeper layer of skin and develops into **ecthyma,** an ulcerated form of the disease. Ecthyma forms small, pus-filled ulcers with a crust much darker and thicker than that of ordinary impetigo. Ecthyma can be very itchy, and scratching the irritated area spreads the infection quickly. Left untreated, the ulcers may cause permanent scars and pigment changes.

The gravest potential complication of impetigo is **glomerulonephritis,** a severe kidney disease that occurs in about 1 percent of cases, mainly in children. With antibiotic treatment and dietary restrictions, most patients recover from this disease without lasting effect.

CAUSES

Impetigo is an infection caused by either streptococcus or *Staphylococcus aureus* bacteria. These bacteria lurk everywhere—in unclean bathrooms, in spoiled food, and in our own bodies. If a child with an open wound or fresh scratch bathes in an unscrubbed basin or tub, for example, he may contract impetigo. Using a towel or even a bar of soap previously used by a person infected with impetigo can spread the infection. Other skin-related problems, such as body lice, fungal or strep infections, boils, or various forms of dermatitis, can make a person susceptible to impetigo.

Most people get this highly infectious disease through physical contact with someone who has it, or from sharing the same clothes, bedding, towels, or other objects. The very nature of childhood, which includes lots of physical contact and large-group activities, makes children the primary victims and carriers of impetigo. Excessive sweating, malnutrition, and poor hygiene can aggravate the condition.

TREATMENT

The key to treating—and preventing—impetigo is good personal hygiene and a clean environment. Once the infection occurs, prompt attention will keep it under control and prevent its spread.

CONVENTIONAL MEDICINE

Even if only one family member has impetigo, everyone in the household should follow the same sanitary regimen. Regular washing with soap and water can clear up mild forms. If the sores don't clear up in 48 hours, or if the infected person is a small child, see a doctor. To break the chain of contagion, the doctor may prescribe antibacterial baths for the entire household as well as for the infected patient.

A topical mupirocin ointment, available only by prescription, is highly successful in treating routine cases. Don't try over-the-counter antibacterial ointments; they are too weak to kill strep and staph infections, and applying the ointment carelessly may actually spread the impetigo. If mupirocin does not help in 48 hours, ask your doctor about an oral antibiotic such as penicillin or erythromycin. Penicillin injections protect against complications of severe infections, shorten healing time, and reduce the chance of recurrence.

ALTERNATIVE CHOICES

As a superficial bacterial infection, impetigo may respond to various alternative treatments, particularly herbal ointments. Be wary of further irritating the skin with products you've never tried before, and see a doctor if the sores do not improve markedly in 12 to 24 hours.

HERBAL THERAPIES

Goldenseal *(Hydrastis canadensis)* is recommended for staph infections. Mix 1 tbsp of goldenseal powder with enough water or egg white to make a paste; apply it to your sores, which should clear in two to three days. Goldenseal may stain the skin, temporarily making the impetigo look worse.

Another recommended herbal remedy is myrrh *(Commiphora molmol).* Place 5 to 10 drops of tincture directly on the impetigo three times a day. Tea tree oil *(Melaleuca* spp.) is cited specifically for its antibacterial properties. Applied topically to impetigo, it soothes the itch and promotes healing.

HOMEOPATHY

Treat impetigo with Mezereum when there are thick scabs with pus underneath. Graphites may be helpful when there is an oozing, honeylike discharge. Try Rhus toxicodendron to relieve extreme itchiness and Arsenicum album when burning or rawness is present. Take the suggested remedy in 12x potency every four to six hours, stopping when you see improvement. See a doctor if sores persist after 48 hours of treatment or if they spread.

NUTRITION AND DIET

Since vitamin A is crucial for skin growth and maintenance, impetigo sufferers should eat plenty of yellow and leafy green vegetables, or add 50,000 IU of beta carotene (vitamin A) to their daily diet. Zinc, said to boost the immune system, is also recommended at up to 45 mg a day. Do not take megasupplements for more than a few weeks, or give them to a child, without medical supervision.

AT-HOME REMEDIES

◆ If you have only a few small impetigo sores, simply bathing them regularly with soap and warm water, using the medications mentioned above, and exposing them to air will soothe the itchiness and should clear them up. For more severe cases, wash the infected area with antibacterial soap and follow up with an appropriate medical treatment.

◆ Anyone in a household who develops impetigo should use a clean towel with each washing. Be sure to launder those towels separately. ∎

SYMPTOMS

Being unable to have or keep an erection is the defining mark of impotence. The problem may manifest itself in several ways. If impotence
- is transient or appearing only occasionally, the problem is not likely to be serious; all men experience impotence at some time.
- develops gradually and persistently, there is probably a physical cause; this is generally the case with chronic impotence.
- develops abruptly but you still have early-morning erections and are able to have an erection while masturbating, the problem is likely to have a psychological cause.

CALL YOUR DOCTOR IF:

- impotence is linked with anxiety or threatens your sexual relationship. At a minimum, your physician can help clear up misinformation, which commonly exacerbates sexual problems.
- impotence persists. Physical causes of impotence can be harbingers of more-general, potentially dangerous conditions; for example, narrowing of the penile artery may indicate coronary artery disease (see Atherosclerosis; Heart Disease). For the impotence itself, a physician may be able to suggest a procedure that can alleviate the problem, or might advise the use of a mechanical device if there is no cure.

Impotence—the inability to attain or maintain an erection of the penis adequate for the sexual satisfaction of both partners—can be devastating to the self-esteem of a man and of his partner. It afflicts as many as 20 million American men on a continuing basis, and transient episodes affect nearly all adult males. But nearly all men who seek treatment find some measure of relief.

CAUSES

As recently as two decades ago, physicians tended to blame impotence on psychological problems or, with older men, on the normal aging process. Today, the pendulum of medical opinion has swung away from both notions. While arousal takes longer as a man ages, chronic impotence warrants medical attention. Moreover, the difficulty is often organic in origin. Today, urologists believe that physical factors underlie perhaps 90 percent of cases of persistent impotence in men over age 50.

Because erection is primarily a vascular event, it is not surprising that the most common causes in this age group are conditions that block blood flow to the penis, such as atherosclerosis or diabetes. Another vascular cause may be a faulty vein, which lets blood drain too quickly from the penis. Other physical disorders, as well as hormonal imbalances and certain operations, may also result in impotence.

The vascular processes that produce an erection are controlled by the nervous system, and certain prescription drugs may have the side effect of interfering with necessary nerve signals. Among the possible culprits are a variety of stimulants, sedatives, diuretics, antihistamines, and agents to treat high blood pressure, cancer, or depression. In addition, alcohol, tobacco, and illegal drugs, such as marijuana, may contribute to impotence.

With younger men, psychological problems are the likeliest reason for impotence. Tension and anxiety may arise from poor communication with the sexual partner or a difference in sexual preferences. The sexual difficulties may also be linked to depression, feelings of inadequacy, personal sexual fears, rejection by parents or peers, or sexual abuse in childhood.

TREATMENT

If you are troubled by occasional impotence, remember that arousal takes longer as you get older and that satisfaction should not be equated with performance. If your impotence is severe and persistent, you should seek medical help. The number of treatment options has increased in recent years.

CONVENTIONAL MEDICINE

For safety and efficacy, the first choice of many urologists in cases of chronic, severe impotence is a vacuum inflation device, especially for elderly men. This instrument draws blood into the penis by creating negative pressure around it; a rubber ring is then slipped over the base of the penis to maintain erection. The ring should be removed after 30 minutes to restore circulation.

An erection can also be produced by self-injection of papaverine or prostaglandin before sex; these drugs may also improve long-term potency and penile blood flow. Medically administered testosterone shots help some men, but no specific level of the hormone guarantees potency.

Taking the drugs pentoxifylline or yohimbine an hour or two before intercourse may help in cases of poor vascular flow. Other sexual stimulants may be psychologically helpful to some men.

For blood-vessel problems, vascular surgery to open arteries leading to the penis benefits up to half the patients who opt for this treatment. The effectiveness of such surgery was oversold when it was first developed in the 1970s, but techniques have been improved.

When none of these therapies work, some men choose a penile implant. The least expensive is a semirigid type that produces a permanent erection. More-sophisticated and -expensive implants are inflated by a pump mechanism placed beneath the skin of the scrotum.

If the cause is judged to be psychological, it is crucial to review your relationship with your partner and to examine other possible sources of stress or tension in your life. A trained therapist can aid in these matters and may help unearth problems such as unreasonable guilt, performance anxiety, or inhibiting attitudes toward sex that were learned at an early age.

ALTERNATIVE CHOICES

Many alternative therapies promote the good health and relaxation needed for a satisfying sex life. In addition to trying the choices listed below, you may want to consider consulting a professional, such as an **acupuncturist** or a **homeopath.**

AROMATHERAPY

Essential oils of clary, sandalwood, and ylang-ylang encourage relaxation and feelings of sensuality. Add 2 drops of each to 4 tsp of massage oil or to a warm bath.

CHINESE HERBS

Practitioners believe that too much anxiety can cause energy stagnation in the liver. Golden chamber, a combination of herbs, sometimes with cibot root added, is often prescribed.

HERBAL THERAPIES

Ginkgo, damiana, and Asian ginseng are sold in many formulations as sexual stimulants. Keep in mind, however, that claims that they act as aphrodisiacs are misleading at best.

AT-HOME REMEDIES

◆ Practice different kinds of intimacy and touching; try not to focus only on the erection. Partners who proceed with patience and learn to enjoy each other in a variety of ways often return to full potency. (See Sensate Focus Exercises in the Sexual Dysfunction entry.)

◆ Moderate (not excessive) exercise helps relax the body, boost energy levels, increase physical awareness, and stimulate sexuality.

◆ Stress or anxiety diverts blood from the sexual organs. Try relaxation techniques, including **yoga, meditation,** and **massage.** Mutual massage slows down lovemaking and opens up communication. ■

- inability to control urination.
- involuntary urination when coughing, laughing, sneezing, running, or performing other physical activity.

CALL YOUR DOCTOR IF:

- you have become unable to control your urination after an illness such as a bladder infection or after taking a new medication. Sudden loss of urinary control may also indicate neurological damage.
- self-help remedies for controlling your urination are not working.

Although it is typically age related, incontinence—the involuntary loss of urine—is not, as commonly believed, an inevitable consequence of aging. The condition often reflects an underlying disorder and is usually treatable, even in the elderly. With proper care, about 70 percent of cases can be improved or cured.

If left untreated, however, the condition will not improve and may actually worsen. Incontinence can lead to bladder or urinary tract infections. And the presence of leaked urine on the skin may cause uncomfortable rashes or other skin disorders. In those instances where treatment doesn't work, patients can avoid such complications by using special absorbent pads and other aids designed to help manage the problem.

An estimated 10 million American adults are incontinent. Women are more prone to the condition than men, in part because they have a pelvic floor (a group of tissues and muscles) that weakens and sags with age or after childbirth, making leakage more likely.

CAUSES

Normal urinary control involves the entire urinary system—the kidneys, ureters, bladder, urethra, and pelvic muscles—as well as the central nervous system. When the bladder fills, it sends a message to the nerves in the spinal cord, which then initiates what is known as the voiding reflex, the contraction of the bladder muscles that forces urine into the urethra and out of the body. Incontinence can occur when any part of this complex process is disrupted.

Medical professionals group incontinence into three major categories, although many people—women especially—experience symptoms of more than one. With **stress incontinence,** the muscles surrounding the urethra are so weakened that they can no longer resist a sudden increase in bladder pressure. Coughing, sneezing, laughing, exercising, or otherwise moving in a way that puts sudden pressure on the bladder can cause leakage—but usually only a few drops.

With **urge incontinence,** the bladder, like that of an infant or toddler, simply contracts whenev-

KEGEL EXERCISES

PELVIC FLOOR
MUSCLES
VAGINA
BLADDER
URETHRA

Women with stress incontinence can use Kegel exercises to strengthen the pelvic floor muscles that support the uterus and bladder and control contractions of the vagina and urethra. While urinating, slowly contract the pelvic floor muscles, halting the flow of urine. Hold for up to 10 seconds and repeat several times. You can also do the exercises at other times, while standing, sitting, or lying down.

er it is full; the patient has no control over the sudden urge to void. This is a common type of incontinence among healthy people, but it can also occur in people with illnesses involving the central nervous system, such as stroke, Alzheimer's disease, Parkinson's disease, and multiple sclerosis. The leakages typically involve copious amounts of urine, because the bladder empties.

Overflow incontinence occurs when a patient can no longer feel the sensation that signals when it is time to go. The bladder never empties normally and remains at least partially full; excess urine just spills out, usually in relatively small amounts. Overflow incontinence is associated with diabetes or, in men, with an enlarged prostate that blocks the flow of urine (see Prostate Problems); in women, a fibroid or ovarian tumor can be at fault. Medicines or neurological disorders affecting the bladder nerves can be a cause.

Surgery on or near the urinary tract can sometimes leave scars or other damage that causes incontinence. Even a slipped spinal disk can trigger leakages by pressing on the nerves that send messages to and from the bladder.

In women, pregnancy and childbirth, which stretch and weaken many of the muscles that support urinary control, can result in incontinence. Studies have shown that the more vaginal births a woman has had, the more likely she is to leak urine while exercising. After menopause, falling levels of the hormone estrogen cause the tissues of the urinary tract system to thin, which may weaken the pelvic floor, leading to incontinence.

Incontinence is a potential side effect of many diuretics, sedatives, antidepressants, antihistamines, and other medications. Sometimes curing the condition can be as simple as switching to a different drug. Talk to your doctor.

DIAGNOSTIC AND TEST PROCEDURES

To determine the cause of your condition, your doctor will ask for a detailed medical history, including questions about your symptoms—for example, how frequently you urinate or how much urine you are able to pass each time you urinate. You will then be asked for a urine sample, which will be checked for infection. The doctor will also examine the rectum, genitals, and abdomen to rule out such problems as a tumor or an enlarged prostate. You may be asked to cough to see if that triggers a leakage—a sign of **stress incontinence.** To test for **overflow incontinence,** the doctor may insert a catheter into your bladder after you have urinated to see if any residual urine remains.

If standard treatments have failed to resolve your incontinence, or if your doctor believes surgery may help, you may be referred to a specialist, usually a urologist, for additional tests. A common one is uroflowmetry, in which you will be given fluids to fill your bladder and then be asked to urinate into a special machine that records the rate of flow. Another useful test is cystometry, a somewhat uncomfortable procedure in which narrow tubes are inserted into the bladder and rectum to measure how much pressure the muscles in the bladder exert.

TREATMENT

Most cases of incontinence can be cured or, at the very least, greatly improved with treatment.

Both conventional and alternative medicine have effective strategies for dealing with the problem. Indeed, many conventional practitioners routinely recommend two nonmedical approaches—**Kegel exercises** and **biofeedback**—for patients suffering from stress incontinence. If you wish, you can try alternative methods first. However, if the condition persists or worsens, see a doctor for a full evaluation and diagnosis.

CONVENTIONAL MEDICINE

Many physicians prefer that their patients try behavior modification techniques before taking any medication. Such treatments are safer than drugs and are often just as effective. Two of the most commonly prescribed are the muscle-strengthening exercises known as **Kegels** *(page 495)* and **biofeedback.**

Bladder retraining is another useful technique. For seven days you will keep a written record of how much you drink, how often you urinate, and how much urine you produce. You will then start urinating at scheduled intervals, usually every 30 or 60 minutes. Gradually, over a period of several weeks, you will increase the length of time between visits to the toilet.

If your doctor decides you need medication for your condition, the drug he or she prescribes will depend on the cause of the incontinence. If your urine test reveals signs of an infection, you will be given antibiotics. If you are a post-menopausal woman, you may be given hormone replacement therapy to increase your estrogen levels (although the benefits of this treatment are unconfirmed). If you have **stress incontinence,** you may receive pseudoephedrine, ephedrine, or phenylpropanolamine, drugs that tone the sphincter, the circular muscle around the urethra that helps control urination. To help reduce the involuntary bladder contractions that characterize **urge incontinence,** you may be given propantheline bromide, imipramine, or oxybutynin chloride, drugs that also help muscles involved in urination work properly.

Special devices called pessaries, which are inserted into the vagina to support the pelvic muscles, can help some women with **stress incontinence.** A doctor must fit you for a pessary and give you a prescription for it.

A newer treatment for stress incontinence in women is the use of small, cone-shaped vaginal weights that train weakened pelvic muscles by exercising them in much the same fashion as other muscles are trained using barbells. You insert the lightest cone into your vagina, pointed end down, and contract the muscles for several minutes to keep it from falling out. When you can keep the cone in place for 20 to 30 minutes, you then try a heavier weight—and so on over a period of weeks, progressively toning and conditioning your pelvic muscles until they are working at full strength once more.

If none of these treatments work, your doctor may recommend surgery. In women whose incontinence is the result of pregnancy and childbirth, operations to repair damaged muscles and ligaments or to reposition the bladder can be very effective, particularly in cases of **stress incontinence.** In another procedure an artificial sphincter is implanted; by manually opening and closing this device, you can control the flow of urine and prevent leakages.

If your incontinence cannot be cured or controlled, you can learn to manage the problem with the help of some specially designed aids, including absorbent and odor-neutralizing undergarments and devices that catch urine and drain it into a concealed plastic bag. Talk to your doctor about these options.

ALTERNATIVE CHOICES

Most alternative methods for dealing with incontinence are aimed at building up the pelvic floor to give the bladder more support—and therefore more control.

ACUPUNCTURE

Acupuncturists believe that incontinence results from a deficiency of kidney and spleen chi. To restore the balance of chi in the affected parts, practitioners stimulate the specific points related to these organs and their channels. Consult a professional acupuncturist.

BIOFEEDBACK

Studies have shown that biofeedback techniques can lead to complete bladder control in up to 25 percent of incontinent patients and to substantial improvement in another 30 to 50 percent. Treatment sessions typically involve inserting a catheter through the urethra into the bladder and then slowly filling the bladder with fluid while the patient uses biofeedback techniques to control the urge to urinate.

CHINESE HERBS

Golden lock tea, a mixture of several herbs that traditional Chinese herbalists believe helps the body retain fluids, is sometimes recommended as a treatment for incontinence.

CHIROPRACTIC

Adjustment of the bones and joints around the pelvis can help strengthen the muscles of the urinary system, leading to increased bladder control. An **osteopath** can provide a similar form of this treatment.

HOMEOPATHY

Depending on the cause of the condition, homeopaths have numerous remedies to treat incontinence. Some that are often prescribed include:

◆ for **stress incontinence,** particularly in the elderly, Causticum, which is said to restore vitality to aging tissue.

◆ for both **stress** and **urge incontinence,** particularly when a person is rising from a prone position, Pulsatilla, thought to relieve irritation of the lining of the urinary tract system and restore it to proper functioning.

Consult a homeopathic practitioner for additional remedies.

NUTRITION AND DIET

Try to keep your weight down. Excess body weight puts pressure on your bladder muscles, weakening them.

The straining that accompanies constipation can also weaken bladder muscles. Avoid constipation by increasing the amount of fiber in your diet; eat more whole-grain foods and fruits and vegetables.

Avoid alcohol, caffeine, sugar, spicy foods, and acidic fruits and juices—all of which can irritate the bladder and trigger leaks.

REFLEXOLOGY

Reflexologists manipulate those areas on the foot that are said to stimulate the ureters, bladder, kidneys, adrenal glands, and lower spine. *(See Bladder Infections.)*

AT-HOME REMEDIES

◆ Avoid constipation: Eat plenty of whole grains, fruits, and vegetables.

◆ Do Kegel exercises daily *(page 495).*

◆ Retrain yourself to urinate at longer intervals. Aim for three to six hours between trips to the bathroom.

◆ Don't smoke. Nicotine can irritate your bladder.

◆ Double void: After urinating, wait a few seconds, then try again.

◆ If you are a woman with **stress incontinence,** try crossing your legs when sneezing or coughing. A recent study showed that this simple practice can be very effective in stopping leakage.

◆ If all else fails, buy special supplies. A variety of highly absorbent and odor-neutralizing underpants, pads, and shields are available. Try different brands until you find the ones that suit your needs. ■

INDIGESTION

- heartburn.
- gas or belching.
- abdominal pressure and/or pain, which can radiate toward the chest.
- mild nausea.
- vomiting.

CALL YOUR DOCTOR IF:

- any abdominal pain continues for more than six hours; this may indicate appendicitis, stomach ulcer, gallstones, or other disease. You may need emergency care.
- you experience indigestion with any of the following: prolonged vomiting, vomiting of blood, black or bloody bowel movements, severe upper abdominal pain, pain radiating into your neck and shoulder, shortness of breath, or feeling weak or faint. Your indigestion may be part of a larger problem, such as gallstones, gastritis, pancreatic problems, stomach ulcer, or possibly cancer. Or you might be having a heart attack; **get medical help immediately**.
- you have repeated bouts of indigestion accompanied by abdominal pain, fever, or dark urine. Your discomfort may indicate gallstones, stomach ulcer, or liver disease.
- your indigestion consistently follows your eating dairy products. You may suffer from lactose intolerance.

Indigestion is a catchall term for assorted stomach discomforts. Symptoms of indigestion are cues that normal digestion has been interrupted for one or more reasons. If stomach acid enters the esophagus, for example, you may feel heartburn. Swallowing too much air while eating or drinking can induce a distended stomach and cause excessive belching. Stomach infections or inflammation can bring on gastritis. Sufferers of irritable bowel syndrome may regularly experience abdominal pain, bloating, and diarrhea.

Indigestion may be occasional or chronic (daily or almost daily). Though uncomfortable, indigestion itself is not life-threatening. It can accompany serious problems, however, and should not be ignored.

CAUSES

Everyone—all ages, men and women alike—feels occasional indigestion. The likelihood increases with age, as the digestive system gradually becomes less efficient.

Occasional or chronic indigestion may be brought on by overeating; overindulging in alcohol; frequently using analgesics—such as aspirin—and other pain relievers; eating while under stress; or eating food that does not agree with your system. For a list of common "trigger foods," see Heartburn.

The two most common causes of chronic indigestion are obesity, which increases pressure in the abdomen, and smoking, which increases production of stomach acid and relaxes the sphincter between the esophagus and stomach. Also, about half of all chronic indigestion sufferers are infected with the bacterium *Helicobacter pylori*. This bacterium is known to cause stomach ulcers, and researchers are trying to determine if it causes other kinds of indigestion as well.

DIAGNOSTIC AND TEST PROCEDURES
Your own description of your symptoms and a physical examination may be all your doctor requires for a diagnosis. Tests that may be necessary include those used to diagnose heartburn.

Depending on your symptoms, your doctor may order other procedures to identify or rule out more serious disorders.

TREATMENT

Indigestion can result from a number of causes, so no single remedy will help everyone. Fortunately, there are many choices for relief. For indigestion with heartburn, also read the treatment suggestions for heartburn and hiatal hernia.

CONVENTIONAL MEDICINE

During a physical examination, your doctor will discuss your symptoms and try to determine what caused the indigestion. If there is no serious underlying disorder, the doctor will treat the symptoms and suggest ways to avoid indigestion in the future. Heartburn remedies—antacids and other medications that alter the stomach's production of acid—are often the first line of defense. If excess stomach acid makes ulcer a threat, sucralfate, which coats and protects the stomach lining, may be prescribed. Extremely painful indigestion may warrant a combination of antacid and the anesthetic lidocaine. If *H. pylori* is detected, antibiotics will be given to treat the infection.

ALTERNATIVE CHOICES

Because indigestion sufferers may have several disorders at once, healers suggest diverse therapies. With most alternative treatments, patience is essential. Quelling persistent indigestion may take weeks or even months.

ACUPRESSURE

To reduce symptoms of indigestion, massage the following for at least one minute: Large Intestine 4 and Stomach 25, 36, and 37. If gas is also a problem, add Bladder 20 and 60, and Spleen 6. See pages 22–23 for information on point locations.

AYURVEDIC MEDICINE

Shatavari *(Asparagus racemosus)* may speed up digestion and alleviate many indigestion symptoms. Ayurvedan bitters may also enhance digestion, including those from *Picrorhiza kurrooa* rhizomes and the trunk wood and bark of the common teak tree *(Tectona grandis)*. Visit an Ayurvedic healer to select a remedy and dosage.

HERBAL THERAPIES

Various teas may calm digestive distress. To reduce stomach acidity, drink meadowsweet *(Filipendula ulmaria)* tea once or twice daily, before meals (add 1 tsp to 1 cup boiling water, steep for 10 minutes, then filter). If you also feel stressed, add lavender *(Lavandula officinalis)* or chamomile *(Matricaria recutita)*. If bloating or gas is a problem, try a tea of peppermint *(Mentha piperita)*, chamomile, or lemon balm *(Melissa officinalis)*.

Certain herbs are reputed to promote digestion and soothe and heal the esophagus, making them particularly appropriate for indigestion with heartburn. About 30 minutes before eating, drink ½ cup of tea made from goldenseal *(Hydrastis canadensis)*, barberry *(Berberis vulgaris)* bark, gentian *(Gentiana lutea)* root, or Oregon grape *(Mahonia aquifolium)* root.

AT-HOME REMEDIES

◆ Refrain from smoking, especially before eating.
◆ For occasional indigestion with heartburn, use antacids or bismuth subsalicylate.
◆ Try one or several of the herbal teas above to relieve your specific symptoms.
◆ Relax after eating. Exercise diverts blood from the stomach, making digestion less efficient.
◆ If you frequently chew gum, stop for a while to see if your symptoms dissipate. It's common to swallow air when chewing gum, which can cause indigestion.

PREVENTION

Indigestion is universal; it's almost impossible to avoid it forever. You can encounter it less often, however, if you watch your weight; avoid overeating (especially foods rich in fat) or overindulging in alcohol; avoid your "trigger" foods; and abstain from smoking. ∎

SYMPTOMS

Fever, chills, sweating, headaches, muscle aches, and fatigue are symptoms common to many infections.

◆ Diarrhea, vomiting, nausea, abdominal cramps, gas pains, and dehydration may result from an **intestinal infection**.

◆ Coughing, sneezing, chest pain, sore throat, congestion, and watery eyes are signs of a **respiratory infection**.

◆ Painful and frequent urination, bloody or foul-smelling urine, or vaginal itching may occur with a **bladder infection**.

◆ Rash, sores, inflammation, itching skin, redness, blisters, or pimples may develop because of a **skin infection**.

◆ Localized pain, irritation, or tenderness may occur with infections of the ears, eyes, mouth, teeth, or gums.

◆ Intense anal itchiness may accompany a **worm infection** in the lower intestines.

◆ Arthritic pain and inflammation, often localized, may signal a **joint infection**.

CALL YOUR DOCTOR IF:

◆ you or your child develops a fever over 101°F or that lasts more than 24 hours. If your ability to breathe, swallow, see, speak, or move is impaired, **get emergency medical help now.**

◆ diarrhea, vomiting, sore throat, or other symptoms persist or worsen after several days. Your infection needs medical diagnosis and treatment.

◆ a bite or other injury penetrates the skin. Bite and puncture wounds need immediate medical attention.

The human body is at constant war against disease-causing pathogens, or germs, which can enter the body through inhaled air, ingested food and water, broken skin, insect or animal bites, and sexual contact. Once on or inside the body, pathogens try to survive and reproduce. Most do not succeed. Many succumb to the body's internal heat or chemical environment, or to "friendly" bacteria; others are expelled in mucus, urine, sweat, and feces. Those that survive do so by preying on healthy cells and tissue. Some pathogens can live only in certain types of tissue; others can spread through the body. The three-part process of invasion, growth, and the body's reaction constitutes infection, and though most infections are minor and short-lived, some evolve into serious—even life-threatening—diseases.

Once a pathogen invades, the body's immune system counterattacks. Proteins called antibodies team up with special white blood cells to neutralize and destroy pathogens. The immune system also is able to "remember" contacts with a particular pathogen so it can suppress repeat invasions. This cellular memory—sometimes aided by vaccines—gives the body immunity against countless disease-causing pathogens.

Rapid immune system response stops or weakens most—but not all—infections. Sometimes immune cells fail to recognize and attack pathogens, especially unfamiliar ones. At other times, the body's counterattack isn't enough. People whose immune systems are weakened by fatigue, poor nutrition, certain medical treatments, or illnesses such as AIDS are more susceptible to infection than are people in good general health.

CAUSES

The pathogens that cause infections are bacteria, fungi, animal parasites, and viruses. **Bacteria, fungi,** and **parasites** generally invade body tissue, steal nutrients from healthy cells, and release toxins; some parasites—which can range in size from single-celled protozoa to visible worms—actually kill healthy cells. **Viruses** are really sub-life forms that survive only by invading living cells and multiplying inside them.

Understandably, the parts of the body that are most accessible to pathogens are those most vulnerable to infection. Pathogens readily infect the eyes, ears, mouth, genitals, and the skin itself. **Skin infections** are extremely common and can be caused by any type of pathogen. Ear infections are usually bacterial; eye infections may be viral or bacterial. Other pathogens can enter the body through broken skin and infect the bloodstream.

Any type of pathogen can invade the gastrointestinal tract, usually through contaminated food or water. Most cases of food poisoning are caused by bacteria, while giardiasis, an intestinal affliction dreaded by hikers, results from drinking water contaminated by parasitic protozoa.

Most respiratory infections, including common colds, flu, and mild forms of pneumonia, are caused by inhaling or ingesting viruses. Severe cases of pneumonia are usually bacterial, as are whooping cough and strep throat. Many lesser-known respiratory ailments are fungal infections.

The urinary tract usually flushes out pathogens but is prone to infection when it is swollen, irritated, or obstructed. Ailments ranging from common bladder infections to serious kidney infections are usually bacterial.

Although many infections are confined to a body part or system, some infectious diseases spread through the body. Malaria, for example, is caused by a mosquito-borne parasite; tuberculosis is bacterial. AIDS, the deadliest infectious disease of recent times, is a viral disorder.

DIAGNOSTIC AND TEST PROCEDURES

Many common infections are recognizable from their symptoms, but to treat infections that persist or whose potential severity is unknown, a doctor needs to determine the specific cause. Diagnosis usually is accomplished by lab analysis of blood, urine, feces, or infected tissue samples.

TREATMENT

Minor infections are of short duration and usually clear up on their own, but serious infectious diseases require medical treatment.

CONVENTIONAL MEDICINE

Bacterial infections are cured by killing the bacteria with antibiotics, such as penicillin and its derivatives. Many fungal and parasitic infections also respond to antibiotics or antimicrobial drugs. The only downside is that overuse or misuse of antibiotics can suppress the body's own natural immune reactions.

Antibiotics are useless against viral infections. Although some antiviral drugs can reduce symptoms, it's difficult or impossible to develop more effective treatment because viruses mutate, or change forms, so often. Standard therapy for most viral infections is simply to relieve symptoms, prevent secondary bacterial infection, and allow the body to heal itself.

Over-the-counter and prescription medications can relieve typical symptoms and speed recovery from minor infections. Preventive vaccines are by far the best medicine against viral infection, and they are available for many infectious diseases.

ALTERNATIVE CHOICES

Proper nutrition, rest, and stress-reducing activities can help prevent and combat infection. Various herbal, Chinese, and other alternative therapies can relieve symptoms and promote healing. See the entries for specific ailments for more information.

PREVENTION

◆ Be sure you and your children are vaccinated against infectious diseases, especially before starting school or traveling abroad.

◆ To prevent the start of infection, refrigerate meat, seafood, and dairy products; wash raw vegetables and fruit thoroughly; keep a clean kitchen; wash your hands before and after handling food.

◆ Practice good personal hygiene: Bathe regularly; wash your hands after using the toilet; sterilize cuts and wounds with antiseptic soap. ■

SYMPTOMS

Infertility is defined as an inability to conceive after a year of regular, unprotected intercourse. The male partner, female partner, or both may account for the condition. It is an impairment; it is not the same as sterility, which means that reproduction is physically impossible.

CALL YOUR DOCTOR IF:

you desire a child but have not conceived after a year of trying ("trying" means unprotected intercourse averaging three times a week). Begin by seeing your regular doctor before approaching a specialized clinic. The cause may be a simple one, such as not having intercourse near the time of ovulation.

For many couples, infertility is a crisis, often accompanied by feelings of guilt or inadequacy. But a diagnosis of infertility is not a verdict of sterility. While about 15 percent of all couples are infertile (that is, they are unable to conceive after a year of trying), only 1 or 2 percent are sterile (meaning that conception is physically ruled out). Of couples who seek help, about half can eventually bear a child, either on their own or with medical assistance.

In cases of infertility, about 40 percent are caused by a problem in the man, and another 40 percent by a problem in the woman. Both the man and the woman are contributors in the remaining 20 percent of cases.

CAUSES

In men, the most common reasons for infertility are sperm disorders, such as a low count (the number of sperm in the ejaculate), low motility (impaired swimming ability of sperm), malformation of the sperm, or blocked sperm ducts. Sperm output can also be temporarily reduced by high temperature in the sperm-manufacturing testicles—a result of spending long periods in a hot tub, for example, or wearing tight underwear. A temperature problem may also have an organic origin: If a vein around a testicle gets twisted—a fairly common condition called a varicocele—cooling of the testicle by blood is diminished.

In women, infertility can often be traced to a lack of ovulation or an impeded journey of the egg from the ovary to the uterus via the fallopian tubes. A failure to ovulate may be caused by hormonal imbalances or by cysts in the ovary. Interruption of an egg's progress through the fallopian tube from ovary to uterus may result from endometriosis, tumors, adhesions, infection, or prior surgery. In the uterus, implantation of the egg may be prevented by fibroid growths, endometriosis, tumors, cervical problems, or irregular uterine shape. Fertilization may not take place if the cervical mucus damages sperm or impedes their progress.

Age is a factor: In women, fertility declines after 35, and conception after 45 is rare. Being overweight, or underweight, can also play a role.

In both men and women, fertility can be diminished by psychological factors, such as anxiety and depression, and by environmental agents, such as radiation, pesticides, and other chemicals *(see Environmental Poisoning)*.

DIAGNOSTIC AND TEST PROCEDURES

In tracing the cause of infertility, a physician generally begins by interviewing the partners about their health histories, use of medications, and sexual histories and practices. The man undergoes a physical examination first, since male infertility is usually related to sperm health or function, which can be readily tested.

For the woman, testing generally begins with a full physical exam and cervical smear. A physician will then determine whether the ovaries are producing and releasing eggs normally. Blood tests can measure hormone levels.

The ovaries and uterus may be examined by ultrasound, and a specific test can check for tubal blockage or abnormality in the uterus. A postcoital test, done two to five hours after intercourse, can determine whether the man's sperm and woman's cervical mucus are compatible.

TREATMENT

Many couples once pronounced barren can now produce their own child. Some may be helped by common-sense steps that raise the chances of conception *(see At-Home Remedies)*.

Couples are often advised to have intercourse just before ovulation, which occurs 13 to 15 days before menstruation and may be indicated by a slight rise in body temperature or by chemical changes detectable with an over-the-counter urine-testing kit. A new device is able to detect ovulation from a single drop of saliva.

A more aggressive strategy is to induce ovulation with hormones or fertility drugs. Such drugs have a good record of success, but they also increase the chance of multiple births.

In men, disorders of the prostate gland, seminal vesicles, testicles, or urethra can often be treated. A varicocele can be tied off, allowing testicle temperature to return to normal.

The small percentage of couples whose infertility cannot be corrected can try artificial fertilization. In the procedure known as IVF (in vitro fertilization), the egg is fertilized outside the woman's body, then placed in the womb or fallopian tube. In another procedure, called GIFT (gamete intrafallopian transfer), egg and sperm are brought together in a fallopian tube. Both methods are difficult and seldom succeed on the first attempt; they are also costly.

ALTERNATIVE CHOICES

A variety of alternative treatments may enhance fertility. Among professionals you may want to consult are **acupuncturists** and **homeopaths.**

MIND/BODY MEDICINE

Relaxation techniques can reduce psychological stress, which sometimes contributes to infertility. Behavior therapy may help, as can **massage, yoga,** or **meditation.**

NUTRITION AND DIET

Zinc is important for fertility in both sexes; a supplement of 15 mg a day may help (take 2 mg of copper if taking zinc). Vitamin C has been shown to aid men whose sperm clump together, and it may improve sperm count. The amino acids arginine and carnitine may be of benefit to men whose sperm count or sperm motility is low.

AT-HOME REMEDIES

For women:
◆ Don't douche; it makes the vagina less hospitable to sperm.
◆ After intercourse, remain supine for a few minutes; this holds your organs in the best position for sperm to enter the cervix.

For men:
◆ Avoid excessive alcohol.
◆ Stay healthy; a bad cold or flu can depress sperm count for up to three months.
◆ Keep testicles cool; avoid saunas, hot tubs, and close-fitting underwear. ■

INFLAMMATION

Read down this column to find your symptoms. Then read across.

SYMPTOMS	AILMENT/PROBLEM
◆ a scratch, cut, or break in the skin anywhere on the body that becomes painful, red, swollen, and/or oozes pus; may be accompanied by fever and swollen lymph nodes.	◆ Infection; skin abscess
◆ cuticle or nail fold becomes swollen, red, painful; cuticle may lift away from the base of the nail; pus may ooze out if the inflamed area is pressed.	◆ Paronychia (infection of the cuticle or nail fold)
◆ rim of eyelid becomes inflamed and the skin scales; may itch; often seen in people with dandruff.	◆ Blepharitis (inflammation of the eyelids)
◆ redness, burning, and itching in one or both eyes; your eye may become bloodshot and have a sticky discharge.	◆ Conjunctivitis
◆ swollen, red vulva and itching, irritated vagina; may have an unusual, thick, white discharge; sexual intercourse may be painful; urinating may sting and be more frequent.	◆ Yeast infection
◆ in men whose partners use contraceptive jelly or douches, the foreskin or glans (head of the penis) becomes inflamed after sexual intercourse; in women, the area around the vaginal opening (labia, urethra, clitoris) becomes inflamed after using contraceptive foam or gel, douching, spraying deodorant, or washing with soap.	◆ Genital allergic reaction
◆ sore, swollen foreskin; may have difficulty cleaning under the foreskin without pain.	◆ Balanitis (inflammation of the foreskin)

- See Cuts, Scratches, and Wounds; Infections.

- **Call your doctor now** if you develop an infected cut on the palm or web of your hand; such infections spread quickly and can lead to permanent loss of function.

- See Nail Problems. Warm soaks can help cleanse the wound and soothe the pain.

- Infection often starts under a hangnail or after some trauma to the nail bed, so keep your nails cut and clean, and avoid polishes and cuticle trimmers.

- Bathe eyelids with warm saline solution to remove crusts; your doctor may recommend an antibiotic or sulfonamide-based ointment.

- Your eyelid may invert and lashes may fall out; sties often develop.

- Conjunctivitis usually resolves itself on its own, although in some cases you may need an antibiotic ointment; consider a boric acid eyewash to soothe the irritation or an eyewash solution of the herbal remedy eyebright *(Euphrasia officinalis).*

- Bacteria, viruses, allergies, stress, eyestrain, and poor nutrition can all cause forms of conjunctivitis.

- Use over-the-counter or prescription medications for a vaginal yeast infection. See also Vaginal Problems.

- Diabetics and people who have HIV infection are more prone to all types of yeast infections.

- See Allergies; Penile Pain; Vaginal Problems.

- Wash your genitals with plain water; harsh or perfumed soaps (especially shampoos) can irritate sensitive tissue.

- See Penile Pain.

- Young boys may develop balanitis from inadequate washing; see a doctor if the inflammation persists.

I

◆ pain, swelling, and redness around a toenail, usually the big toe. The sharp end of the nail will be pressing into the flesh on one or both sides of the nail bed.

CALL YOUR DOCTOR IF:

◆ the ingrown nail becomes infected (severe pain and pus develop), the pain doesn't go away after attending to the nail, or your nails are so hard or thick that you cannot relieve the condition. Medical intervention is needed, especially in diabetics, who are at risk for complications from foot infections.

I ngrown nails—when the nail grows into the flesh instead of over it—usually affect the toenails, particularly the big toe. People with curved or thick nails are most susceptible, although anyone can suffer from ingrown nails as a result of an injury or because of improper grooming of the feet. Diabetics need to be aggressive in treating and preventing minor foot ailments because they can develop into serious medical problems.

CAUSES

Ingrown nails are most frequently caused by cutting your toenails too short or rounding the nail edges, or by wearing ill-fitting shoes or tight hosiery that presses the nail into your toe. You can also develop an ingrown nail after an injury such as stubbing your toe.

TREATMENT

Most ingrown nail problems can be prevented with proper grooming of the toes and by wearing better-fitting shoes and hosiery *(see Prevention, opposite)*. Seek help from a healthcare professional if home management techniques do not relieve your symptoms or if the nail becomes infected.

CONVENTIONAL MEDICINE

If you seek medical help because your ingrown nail has become infected, your doctor will probably prescribe an oral antibiotic such as erythromycin and may prescribe a topical corticosteroid ointment or inject a corticosteroid solution into the area around the inflammation. In some cases your doctor may recommend partial removal of a severely ingrown nail. Permanent removal of the entire nail may be advised if ingrowth occurs repeatedly.

ALTERNATIVE CHOICES

Alternative therapies focus on relieving symptoms and healing any infection.

DIGGING IN

SITE OF
INFECTION
INGROWN
NAIL

A damaged or improperly trimmed nail can become ingrown, burrowing into the skin at the side of the nail bed. The site can become painful and infected and may not heal until the nail is removed. If a nail is ingrown, soften the area with water or lotion; lift the nail away from the skin and trim the ingrown portion. To avoid ingrown nails, always trim nails straight across.

HERBAL THERAPIES

Medical herbalists may suggest soaking the toe in a warm solution of calendula (*Calendula officinalis*)—1 tbsp tincture to 1 pt water—to soften and cleanse the nail. Dry the foot and insert a thin strand of sterile cotton under the nail to lift it away from the skin until it grows out. Change the cotton daily. Calendula tincture (10 drops) may also be applied directly to the toe as an antiseptic and to encourage new skin growth.

HOMEOPATHY

If home management doesn't bring relief, consult your homeopathic physician. When pus is present and the toe is sensitive, the remedy usually prescribed is Hepar sulphuris (12c), three times daily for one to two days. For minor pain and inflammation a homeopath may recommend Silica (12c) three times a day for two or three days.

AT-HOME REMEDIES

Trim the excess nail and put a thin strand of sterile cotton under the corner of the nail to lift it away from the skin until it grows out. Change the cotton daily. If you can't ease the nail out of the skin, try first soaking your foot in warm salt water and then applying an over-the-counter topical solution for ingrown nails or a cream containing 10 percent urea. Lemon is said to act as a natural softening agent. If you want to try a natural remedy, tie a fresh lemon slice around the toe and leave it on overnight. When the nail is pliable enough to ease out of the flesh, trim it, and then apply the cotton as directed above.

PREVENTION

Proper grooming is the first step in preventing ingrown nails. An elderly relative may need assistance, because nails get thicker and wider with age and because older people often have impaired vision and greater difficulty reaching their feet. Parents should groom young children's nails.

Soak the feet first to soften the nails. Always cut the nail straight across using nailclippers, and leave enough nail to cover the toe to protect it. (Do not use scissors, which are difficult to manipulate in the corners of the nail.) Smooth sharp edges with an emery board.

Wear socks and shoes that fit properly. Women especially need to be aware that tight, pointed, high-heeled shoes and tight stockings can cause ingrown nails by putting pressure on the toes.

Don't TRY IT!

Never try to correct an ingrown nail by cutting a V into the top edge of your toenail. This old wives' tale developed from the mistaken idea that the ingrown nail was caused by the nail being too big and that the sides could be encouraged to grow toward the center by cutting away some of the existing nail. Nails grow only from the base of the nail bed to the top of the toe. ■

Most insect bites produce only minor irritation and such symptoms as:
- swelling at the site of the bite.
- itching or burning.
- local numbness or tingling.

Bites of poisonous spiders and scorpions may produce the following symptoms:
- intense pain.
- stiffness; joint pain.
- muscle spasms.
- abdominal pain.
- fever or chills.
- difficulty breathing or swallowing.
- spreading, ulcerated wound.
- impaired speech, convulsions.

Sometimes, an insect or spider bite causes a potentially fatal allergic reaction known as **anaphylactic shock.** Its symptoms include:
- rapid swelling around the eyes, lips, tongue, or throat.
- difficulty breathing.
- wheezing or hoarseness.
- severe itching or cramping, or numbness.
- dizziness.
- a reddish rash, or hives.
- stomach cramps.
- loss of consciousness.

CALL YOUR DOCTOR IF:

- you think you have been bitten by a poisonous spider or scorpion.
- you experience any of the symptoms of anaphylactic shock. It is a very severe, possibly life-threatening condition. **Call 911 or your emergency number now.**

See Emergencies/First Aid: Shock.

The bites of most spiders and insects, including mosquitoes, fleas, flies, bedbugs, and chiggers, are similar in appearance and pose little danger. Typically, the injection of salivary fluid or venom into the skin provokes a small itchy swelling that lasts a few hours or days. The bites are seldom dangerous; however, mosquitoes in certain areas may transmit diseases such as malaria and encephalitis.

For people allergic to insect or spider bites, such bites can cause severe trauma and even life-threatening **anaphylactic shock.** Also, the bites of a few spiders, ticks, and insects are poisonous or associated with specific diseases.

Ticks. While most tick bites are harmless, several species can cause life-threatening diseases; see Rocky Mountain Spotted Fever and Lyme Disease. Ticks may also transmit tularemia, relapsing fever, and a newly identified and potentially fatal ailment called ehrlichiosis. Rarely, a bite may trigger tick paralysis, which starts with numbness and pain in the legs and can result in respiratory failure.

Spiders. Bites are seldom fatal; infants, the elderly, and people with allergies are at greatest risk. Most dangerous is the **black widow,** found throughout the country and especially in warmer areas. The bite itself often passes unnoticed, but within hours, intense pain and stiffness may begin, occasionally followed by muscle spasms, abdominal pain, chills, fever, and difficulty in swallowing or breathing. About 4 percent of bites end in death.

The bite of the **brown recluse spider** is painless but may cause a spreading, ulcerated wound. Infrequently, reactions include fever, chills, joint pain, and convulsions; death is rare.

Scorpions. Stings cause a sharp, burning pain, followed by numbness. Rarely, scorpion neurotoxin produces shock, or even a life-threatening syndrome of rapid breathing, impaired speech, and muscle spasms. Fewer than 1 percent of stings are fatal, usually to very young and elderly victims.

Fire ants. Recent arrivals from Mexico, fire ants produce small, fluid-filled bites that may ulcerate. The ants bite into the skin, then sting repeatedly in an arc around the bite. The venom is capable of causing severe reactions and even, in some cases, death.

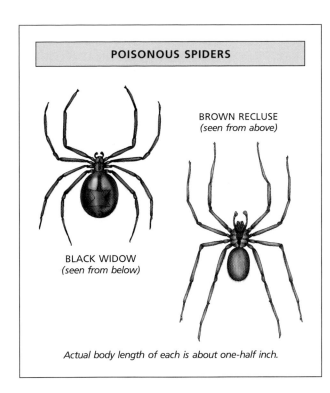

POISONOUS SPIDERS

BROWN RECLUSE
(seen from above)

BLACK WIDOW
(seen from below)

Actual body length of each is about one-half inch.

TREATMENT

For insect bites that aren't serious, the goal of treatment is simply to relieve discomfort. In the rare cases of bites that cause a severe reaction, it is essential to get medical help immediately.

CONVENTIONAL MEDICINE

The discomfort of many insect bites can be soothed by an ice cube, a cold washcloth, calamine lotion, a paste of baking soda, or an over-the-counter hydrocortisone ointment.

If you think you've been bitten by a **black widow spider,** seek medical help. A doctor may prescribe cold compresses, calcium gluconate for muscle pain, and an antianxiety drug for spasms. A spreading, ulcerated wound from a **brown recluse spider** bite should be surgically cleaned and repaired; a corticosteroid injection can ease pain. Do not apply ice. For any spider bite, be sure your tetanus immunization is current.

If you find a **tick** embedded in your skin, remove it carefully without crushing; grip it near the head with tweezers or gloved fingers and pull gently and steadily. If you think you've been infected, watch for a rash at the site of the bite, which may indicate tularemia, relapsing fever, ehrlichiosis, or other disease.

For a **scorpion** sting, seek medical help if symptoms are severe. You may receive antivenin to neutralize the poison, or calcium gluconate or phenobarbital to relieve muscle spasms.

Some relief for the itchy pustules caused by **fire ants** is provided by anti-itching cream.

For **mosquito** or other minor bites, apply calamine lotion.

ALTERNATIVE CHOICES

For minor bites, some doctors suggest rubbing the bite with an aspirin that has been crushed and moistened with water. Others recommend calendula *(Calendula officinalis)* ointment every four to six hours.

HOMEOPATHY

Pyrethrum tincture may help relieve pain. For allergic reactions, Apis (6c) every 10 minutes may help before medical care arrives.

NUTRITION AND DIET

Large doses of B-complex vitamins, including 50 mg vitamin B_1 (thiamine), taken orally may act as an insect repellent. Use with caution; in some people this approach may cause itching or rash. Zinc, taken daily (60 mg), is also said to be a natural repellent; because it is a copper antagonist, it should not be taken for more than one month unless copper supplements are included. Garlic *(Allium sativum)* may also repel insects; try one 400-mg capsule three times a day.

PREVENTION

Essential oil of eucalyptus *(Eucalyptus globulus)* is a natural insect repellent. Make a solution by adding 5 drops to a cup of water, and dab on your skin. Essential oil of citronella discourages insects when placed on exposed skin. A few dabs of calendula *(Calendula officinalis)* ointment on the face, arms, and legs may keep insects away. ■

SYMPTOMS

- ◆ persistent trouble falling asleep.
- ◆ failure to sleep through the night.
- ◆ waking up earlier than usual.

CALL YOUR DOCTOR IF:

- ◆ you experience disturbed sleep for more than a month without apparent cause. You may need referral to a sleep-disorder specialist to monitor your sleep patterns and test for underlying physical ailments.
- ◆ your insomnia is associated with a life-changing event, such as the loss of a job or a loved one. You may need sleep medication for a brief period.
- ◆ your sleep medication is no longer effective, or you have been taking medication for more than a few nights without success. You may be at risk of becoming addicted to the medication.
- ◆ you never seem to get enough sleep and fall asleep without warning during the day. You may be suffering from **narcolepsy.**

After infancy, humans function the way the world turns—on a natural cycle that repeats itself about every 24 hours. During this daily cycle—known as the circadian rhythm—most adults sleep between 6 and 8 hours, usually at night and without interruption. A few nights of poor sleep do us no harm, but prolonged insomnia can have serious consequences. Insomnia is one of the most commonly reported health problems: About 1 in 3 people encounters sleep problems in a given year, and twice as many women as men. Because sleep patterns change as we age, most sleep disorders are reported by the elderly.

Insomnia can be described in terms of both duration and severity. **Transient insomnia** is associated with a temporary disturbance of one's normal sleeping pattern—caused, perhaps, by travel or relocation—and usually lasts no more than several nights. **Short-term insomnia,** lasting two or three weeks, can accompany worry or stress and typically disappears when the apparent cause is resolved. **Chronic insomnia** is a more complex disorder with potentially serious effects, including immune disorders: When people are deprived of sleep over long periods, the body's production of natural killer cells—an important part of the immune system—becomes depressed, potentially lowering resistance to disease.

The rare disorder called **narcolepsy** is characterized by attacks of irresistible drowsiness during the day, disrupting the pattern of a person's normal activity. A narcoleptic may not sleep well at night but suffer sleep attacks during the day, while talking, working, and even when driving a vehicle—a potentially life-threatening event.

CAUSES

Insomnia may be caused by physical illness, a stress-filled lifestyle, excessive caffeine consumption, or chronic pain; or it may simply be the result of poor sleeping habits, such as napping during the day and going to bed at irregular hours. It is often linked to alcohol or drug abuse and to misuse of certain medications. Psychological factors alone account for about half of all insomnias evaluated by sleep therapists. For example, stress brought on by situations like a troubled marriage, a chronically ill child, or an unrewarding job can disrupt sleep. Depression is one of the most common causes of insomnia, and people with anxiety, schizophrenia, and other psychiatric disorders may also sleep poorly.

Certain physical illnesses interfere with sleep, especially disorders of the heart, lungs, kidneys, liver, pancreas, and digestive system. Other important physical causes include heartburn, chronic pain, and breathing disorders such as sleep apnea *(see Snoring)*. Insomnia often accompanies menopause, when sleep is disrupted by hot flashes or night sweats. Abnormal blood sugar levels can cause people suffering from diabetes or hypoglycemia to wake up during the night.

Your own habits and lifestyle may be impeding your sleep pattern. Sedentary behavior and keeping an erratic schedule can contribute to insomnia, as can overconsumption of caffeine and other stimulants, or alcohol and other depressants. Over-the-counter drugs and prescription medications—from beta-adrenergic blockers to thyroid preparations—can interfere with sleep, as can the accidental or deliberate misuse of sleeping pills, to say nothing of illegal drugs *(see Drug Abuse)*. There is even some evidence that using electric blankets can disrupt normal sleep.

Many illnesses are disturbing enough to the body that the normal sleep pattern is disrupted. Among them is the mysterious ailment called restless leg syndrome (RLS). Sufferers describe an unpleasant, creepy-crawly sensation when they lie still, causing an irresistible urge to move their limbs, even during sleep.

A common cluster of causes known as **circadian rhythm sleep disorders** include jet lag and shift-work sleep disorder. Airplane travel over several time zones disrupts the body's biological clock, which may not adjust itself to the time change for several days. An irregular work schedule or changing from day work to a night shift can also cause insomnia until a person adjusts to the new sleep pattern; some people never adjust completely. Environmental factors such as noise, light, and stale air can cause insomnia or reduce the quality of sleep, even when they don't actually keep you awake.

Transient insomnia, while not physically harmful, can become habitual and very difficult to resolve. The cause of **narcolepsy** is unclear. It may follow an injury to the head or brain, but most cases show no evidence of medical abnormality. The disorder may have its basis in a neurological malfunction of sleep-wake mechanisms in the brain.

TREATMENT

Transient insomnia, which may occur during travel, usually disappears when you return to a regular sleep pattern. **Short-term insomnia,** which may be caused by a family illness or by job stress, may be treated with natural sleep aids *(see Nutrition and Diet, page 513)* or, in some cases, with medication. **Chronic insomnia,** which disrupts sleep for extended periods of time, may call for a thorough physical examination, alteration of some life habits, and perhaps psychotherapy to identify a hidden cause.

Treatment for **narcolepsy** is limited by inadequate understanding of its cause. A physician or professional sleep therapist may advise 10-minute naps when you feel drowsy so you will feel rested when you need to be awake. Caffeine, used in moderation, may be helpful, and sometimes medications such as amphetamines are prescribed. For **circadian rhythm sleep disorders,** most people will readjust after a few days on a new schedule. If you have to sleep during the day, keep the bedroom as quiet and dark as possible. If insomnia is due to a physical ailment or condition such as diabetes or menopause, treating that underlying condition should correct the insomnia.

CONVENTIONAL MEDICINE

Persistent or severe insomnia is something you should discuss with your doctor in order to rule out an underlying ailment and possibly to try an appropriate medication. If you suspect that your sleeplessness is caused by depression, ongoing anxiety, or stress, your doctor may want you to consult a psychiatrist or psychologist. You may be referred to a sleep evaluation center, where experts will conduct physical and psychological tests and monitor your sleep pattern in order to evaluate your situation in depth.

Each year about five million people use sleep medications, but doctors no longer prescribe them as freely as they once did. Barbiturates, in particular, are to be avoided whenever possible because of their addictive power, the danger of overdose, and their toxicity when combined with alcohol. If you take barbiturates, do so only for a day or two at a time and only as prescribed for your particular condition. (See Drug Abuse.) Benzodiazepines such as triazolam and temazepam are safer than barbiturates, but even they can cause dependence, and they can be fatal if taken with alcohol or other drugs that depress the central nervous system. Benzodiazepines gradually lose their effectiveness and may even worsen insomnia as people develop tolerance to them. It is difficult to stop using benzodiazepines, because abrupt withdrawal may cause distressing symptoms, including renewed insomnia. An anti-insomnia drug called zolpidem is said to be less addicting than benzodiazepines.

ALTERNATIVE CHOICES

Many poor sleepers simply need help relaxing. If you're a habitual insomniac, and trying to get to sleep just makes you more awake, the following alternative choices may help reduce your worry about sleep while relaxing your body and mind. If the root cause of insomnia is stress, any treatment must address the underlying problem.

AROMATHERAPY

A relaxant effect may be provided by oils of chamomile (*Matricaria recutita*), lavender (*Lavandula officinalis*), neroli, rose, and marjoram. Add a few drops to your bathwater or sprinkle a few drops on a handkerchief and inhale.

BODY WORK

Massage can promote relaxation and better sleep. While this may not be possible on a daily basis, it is a good complement to full-body exercises that may have caused stiff, tight muscles.

TIPS FOR A GOOD NIGHT'S SLEEP

- ◆ *Go to bed only when you are sleepy.*
- ◆ *Get up at about the same time every morning, no matter when you go to bed.*
- ◆ *Use relaxing presleep rituals: Try a warm bath with Epsom salt, an excellent muscle relaxant.*
- ◆ *Have a light snack—a piece of toast or an apple—or read for 10 minutes before you turn out the light.*
- ◆ *Keep a regular schedule for vigorous exercise during the day. If possible, exercise at the time of day that helps you sleep best. For most people, this means in the morning or afternoon, not close to bedtime.*
- ◆ *Avoid alcohol and caffeine for several hours before bedtime. Remember that caffeine is present not just in coffee but in chocolate, tea, and many soft drinks and over-the-counter remedies.*
- ◆ *For children, avoid overstimulation, such as loud games or exciting TV shows, just before bedtime.*

HERBAL THERAPIES

Half an hour before bedtime, drink a calming herbal tea made with chamomile (*Matricaria recutita*), St.-John's-wort (*Hypericum perforatum*), lime blossom, passionflower (*Passiflora incarnata*), or hops (*Humulus lupulus*); for insomnia from nervous tension, use vervain or skullcap (*Scutellaria lateriflora*). Valerian (*Valeriana officinalis*) is effective and seldom causes morning sleepiness: Brew valerian tea or take about 20 drops of tincture in water at bedtime; experiment to find the dosage that suits you best. Note that valerian, like any sleeping aid, acts as a central nervous system depressant and should not be used every night.

HOMEOPATHY

A homeopathic practitioner may prescribe Nux vomica for insomnia caused by anxiety or restlessness, Ignatia for grief, or Muriaticum acidum for emotional problems. Other remedies are available, depending on the nature of the insomnia.

LIFESTYLE

Moderate exercise—a 20- to 30-minute routine three or four times a week—will help you sleep better and give you more energy. Tailor the routine to your physical condition, and exercise in the morning or afternoon, not close to bedtime. Breathing exercises can promote relaxation; here's a routine you can do anywhere, anytime:

◆ Exhale completely through your mouth.
◆ Inhale through your nose to a count of four.
◆ Hold your breath for a count of seven.
◆ Exhale through your mouth for a count of eight. Repeat the cycle three times.

MIND/BODY MEDICINE

Meditation, yoga, and **biofeedback** can reduce tension and promote better sleep. Visualization or **guided imagery** is an effective path to relaxation: Hold a peaceful image in your mind before bedtime. You can learn these techniques from an instructor, a how-to book, or an instructional tape.

NUTRITION AND DIET

Melatonin, a hormone secreted naturally by the pineal gland, is said to induce sleep without negative side effects; try a 5-mg capsule nightly for two weeks at bedtime. Because experience with this hormone is limited, consult your doctor.

Calcium and magnesium taken 45 minutes before bedtime have a tranquilizing effect. Use a 2:1 ratio, such as 500 mg of calcium and 250 mg of magnesium in tablet or capsule form.

High or low blood sugar can disrupt sleep patterns. To help stabilize blood sugar, avoid sweets and fruit juices. To actuate the brain's sedative neurotransmitters, eat starchy food—a plain baked potato, a slice of bread, or an apple—half an hour before bedtime.

Warm milk, a traditional sleep aid, may provide more psychological than physiological benefit. It does contain tryptophan, a sleep-inducing amino acid, but it also contains many other amino acids that compete to enter the brain.

AT-HOME REMEDIES

Be sure your bedroom is quiet and dark. Earplugs and eye shades may help; light comes in even through closed eyelids.

Both children and adults may have trouble sleeping if they are overstimulated by activity or watching television just before bedtime. A quarter hour of quiet conversation, light reading, or soft music may make all the difference.

If you wake up at night and can't go back to sleep, remain quiet and relaxed. Sleep is normally punctuated by periods of restlessness, or even waking. Be patient; sleep usually returns.

Remember, a few nights of poor sleep do no long-term harm. Even if you toss and turn trying to get to sleep, you are probably getting more periods of sleep than you think.

PREVENTION

If your bedroom is too noisy or too bright, do what you can to create a quiet, dark environment with adequate ventilation and humidity; excessively dry air can cause nasal passages to contract and make you uncomfortable. Wearing earplugs and eye shades will help to keep out distractions.

If you're working nights and simply can't sleep well during the day, ask your employer about changing back to a regular daytime job. A strategy that works for some people who must work at night involves installing lights much brighter than normal during the night shift and then wearing dark glasses as they go home and prepare for sleep. This helps to shift their circadian rhythm so they sleep better in the daytime and remain more alert at night.

Try not to be rigid about when and how much you sleep. Worrying about a sleep schedule can just make it harder to fall asleep. If you prefer taking a nap during the day and sleeping less at night, do so. The total amount of sleep you get in a 24-hour period is more important than your daily schedule. ■

IRRITABILITY

Read down this column to find your symptoms. Then read across.

SYMPTOMS	AILMENT/PROBLEM
Persistent irritability, combined with the following symptoms, events, or situations:	
◆ pessimistic attitude; lack of self-esteem; poor appetite; lethargy; insomnia; loss of interest in normal activities, including sexual relations.	◆ Depression
◆ depression alternating with elation, hyperactivity, or continuous talking.	◆ Manic-Depression
◆ inability to sleep; periods of wakefulness at night.	◆ Insomnia
◆ in women, changes in behavior—along with fatigue and anxiety—up to 10 days before a menstrual period, with changes disappearing a few hours after the onset of menstruation.	◆ Premenstrual Syndrome
◆ in women, a noticeable change of behavior at about age 50.	◆ Menopausal Problems
◆ eliminating caffeine or alcohol from your diet, stopping smoking, or discontinuing a drug or medication.	◆ Withdrawal symptoms
◆ a change in family, work, or other routine activity or lifestyle.	◆ Stress
◆ dizziness, headache, fatigue, anxiety, nausea, or shortness of breath not related to any other known ailment.	◆ Environmental Poisoning
◆ during winter months, depression.	◆ Seasonal Affective Disorder

WHAT TO DO	OTHER INFO
◆ See Depression. Consult a doctor, psychotherapist, member of the clergy, or friend. If symptoms are accompanied by thoughts or threats of suicide, see your doctor immediately.	◆ Depression often goes undiagnosed because symptoms vary among individuals. For example, some people sleep or eat more, not less, than usual when they become depressed.
◆ See Manic-Depression. Exercise or relaxation activities may help to reduce or counter the symptoms.	◆ Mood swings may occur frequently or years apart. Family or spouse should be involved in any treatment.
◆ See Insomnia. Try to identify and correct the underlying cause of sleeplessness. Exercise or relaxation activities may be helpful.	◆ Transient insomnia associated with travel or relocation usually lasts only a few nights.
◆ See Premenstrual Syndrome. When symptoms are present, try to avoid irritating or stressful situations at home and at work.	◆ Premenstrual Syndrome (PMS) may share symptoms of depression, but the conditions are not the same. No specific cause of PMS has been identified, but some authorities cite hormonal imbalances.
◆ See Menopausal Problems. Ask your doctor about hormone replacement therapy.	◆ Men also experience more irritability as they age. If behavioral changes seem extreme, or there are other persistent symptoms, consult your physician about an underlying ailment.
◆ See Alcohol Abuse, Drug Abuse, Nicotine Withdrawal.	◆ Severity of withdrawal symptoms is related to the duration of substance abuse. During any withdrawal period, work closely with a therapist.
◆ See Stress. Try exercise and relaxation techniques. Family dysfunctions are best treated by a family therapist.	◆ Persistent conflict between parents can raise the likelihood of behavioral and emotional problems in children.
◆ See Environmental Poisoning. Discuss symptoms with your employer or doctor to determine the precise cause.	◆ If you think a chemical, persistent noise, or other environmental agent is making you ill, change surroundings or otherwise avoid contact with it.
◆ See Seasonal Affective Disorder. Exposure to sunlight or other full-spectrum light.	◆ Seasonal affective disorder is linked to short days and periods of low sunlight.

SYMPTOMS

- constipation or diarrhea shortly after meals, over a period of several months, usually accompanied by abdominal cramps or bloating and increased intestinal gas.
- bowel movements different in frequency or consistency from your normal pattern.

CALL YOUR DOCTOR IF:

- you have pain in the lower left abdomen, fever, and sometimes a change in the frequency of bowel movements; you may have diverticulitis.
- you discover blood in your stools; you could have colon polyps or colorectal cancer.
- you have a fever, or you have been losing weight unexpectedly; such symptoms may signal disorders such as ulcerative colitis or Crohn's disease.
- your stools are different from their usual frequency and consistency and may be passed with mucus; these may be warning signs of colorectal cancer.

Your digestive system seems totally out of control. Either you can't stay out of the bathroom, or your stomach is tied in knots. Your bowel movements may be loose and runny, or unusually hard. One likely explanation is that you may be having a bout of irritable bowel syndrome, sometimes called **spastic colon** or **spastic colitis.**

Irritable bowel syndrome (IBS) is the most common of all digestive disorders. The most frequently encountered symptom is abdominal pain with diarrhea or soft, frequent stools. In other cases, IBS comes with abdominal cramps and painful constipation, usually following meals. Whatever the specific symptoms, your digestion seems normal but your bowel movements become abnormal and stay that way for several weeks or longer.

Twice as many women as men report IBS symptoms to their physicians, but many people experience IBS without recognizing it and never seek medical assistance. Only a small percentage of the general population has chronic symptoms, yet IBS is estimated to affect 10 to 15 percent of adults at some time in their lives, often during periods of significant change or stress. The onset of IBS is usually in early adulthood, although it can affect children.

CAUSES

As part of the digestive process, the intestines move food through the intestinal tract by synchronized wavelike contractions called peristalsis. Irritable bowel syndrome occurs when peristalsis becomes irregular and uncoordinated, disrupting the normal digestive process. IBS usually strikes without warning, and most sufferers have bowel movements more frequently than normal, although some become constipated.

There is no known cause of IBS. Many authorities consider it a stress-induced illness, while others lean toward food sensitivities, especially as people age. Overeating, or binge eating, is known to aggravate IBS, as is too much fat in the diet. Lactose intolerance, eating irregularly or too quickly, and smoking may all be factors in IBS. The sugar substitutes sorbitol and aspartame can induce diarrhea in some people. Certain antibiotics alter the population of bacteria in the intestines, causing diarrhea, fever, and abdominal pain. Morphine and codeine, the aluminum salts of antacids, and the prescription drug methotrexate can cause constipation and intestinal upset. Tricyclic antidepressants may cause constipation, yet newer serotonin uptake inhibitors do not have this effect. Certain antihistamines, mineral supplements, diuretics, antipsychotics, and sedatives can also result in constipation in some people.

DIAGNOSTIC AND TEST PROCEDURES

No specific medical test diagnoses IBS, but your doctor will probably send stool samples for lab testing to rule out more serious diseases. Since stress is a potential element in IBS, you may be asked about your personal history, including factors that may be causing emotional or psychological problems. The diagnosis may also include a sigmoidoscopy, in which a flexible tube is inserted into the rectum to allow the doctor to examine the inside of the colon. Other procedures may include a barium enema, which coats the intestinal lining so it can be seen on an x-ray.

TREATMENT

Since irritable bowel syndrome does not have a specific underlying cause, treatment is directed mainly at relieving the symptoms.

CONVENTIONAL MEDICINE

The first line of conventional medical therapy involves an assessment of the quality of your diet—especially your fat and fiber intake. Your doctor may then recommend an appropriately balanced nutritional program. You may be told to cut fat consumption and to take a bulk-forming, soluble fiber dietary product like psyllium *(Plantago psyllium)*. If that doesn't help, your doctor may prescribe loperamide to slow the movement of food through the intestines, dicyclomine to calm the

gastrointestinal tract, or atropine or belladonna to relieve stomach cramps.

Reassurance that IBS is not a psychosomatic or an imaginary illness may help reduce or alleviate many symptoms and reduce stress. If you appear depressed or under excessive strain, from either past or present experiences, you may be referred to a mental health practitioner for further evaluation. Counseling or psychotherapy may help you relieve concerns that are aggravating your condition.

ALTERNATIVE CHOICES

Various herbal and dietary remedies may be effective in preventing or soothing the discomfort of diarrhea and constipation. Relaxation techniques may be particularly effective in coping with stress-related aspects of the problem.

ACUPUNCTURE

An acupuncturist will determine an appropriate approach by asking you questions about stresses in your life that may be at the root of the problem. Treatment for IBS typically involves 10 to 12 sessions in which needles are inserted along the liver, spleen, and kidney meridians. For symptomatic relief of diarrhea, the acupuncturist will probably insert the needles near the navel and left knee. If you are experiencing a bad bout of diarrhea, the practitioner may employ moxibustion, in which heat is applied near the points, for quick relief.

EXERCISE

Walking at an aerobic pace for 20 to 30 minutes gets the heart pumping, stimulates the digestive process, and relaxes the body. Vigorous exercise is also recognized as an effective way of combating and controlling stress. **Yoga** *(see illustration page 518)* not only conditions the muscles and connective tissue but also is thought to tone the internal organs, including the digestive tract.

HERBAL THERAPIES

For diarrhea, make a carob *(Ceratonia siliqua)* tea: Pour 1 cup of hot water over 1 tsp of roasted carob powder. Drink three times a day.

YOGA

1 To ease bowel spasms, try abdominal massage. Sit on your heels, thighs together. Place your left fist on the right side of your abdomen, press your right elbow over it, and cup your left elbow in your right hand. Exhale, bend forward, and bring your forehead to the floor. Breathe deeply. Relax and gently massage the area with your fist 15 to 20 seconds. Rise and massage your abdomen with your fingers. Repeat on your left side. Do twice daily.

2 **Standing Angle** may help release bowel tension. Inhale and step wide to the right, with your arms outstretched. Exhale, bend forward at the hips, and grasp your feet *(above)*. Breathe deeply for 15 to 20 seconds, then inhale and rise slowly. Do once.

To calm an overactive gastrointestinal tract, try a European favorite: Take one or two enteric-coated peppermint *(Mentha piperita)* oil capsules between meals, three times daily. Reduce the dose if you have a burning sensation when you move your bowels. If you can't locate the capsules, try peppermint tea: Steep 1 tsp of dried peppermint leaves in a cup of boiling water for 30 minutes, and drink three to four cups a day. Infusions of chamomile *(Matricaria recutita)*, marsh mallow *(Althaea officinalis)* root, bayberry *(Myrica* spp.), or slippery elm *(Ulmus fulva)* also are soothing to the intestinal tract and can be made the same way.

Sometimes the bacteria in your digestive tract are killed when you take certain antibiotics, or they become overwhelmed by other types of intestinal flora. To make sure that your digestive tract contains healthy bacteria, eat a cup of plain yogurt daily or ask your doctor about taking *Lactobacillus acidophilus* supplements.

HOMEOPATHY
A homeopathic practitioner will determine which remedy is appropriate to get at the root cause of the IBS. For relief of occasional diarrhea, try prepared remedies available in health food stores. Ignatia may be helpful if you are having spasms of pain and diarrhea after emotional upsets. If you are passing offensive-smelling gas and mucus in the stools, take Mercurius vivus. If sudden cramplike pains are relieved by bending over, take Colocynthis. If your stools are soft but you have to strain to pass them, try Nux vomica.

LIFESTYLE
A number of techniques have been found helpful for IBS, including training in muscle **relaxation.** After four to six weeks of daily practice, you will learn how to relax your previously tense muscles and relieve symptoms brought on by stress.

Biofeedback training is another technique that has become accepted by more and more conventional doctors and often is covered by insurance. In one form of biofeedback, painless electrodes are placed on the forehead to monitor muscle tension as an indicator of stress. Patients are taught to relax their muscles by actuating audio or visual signals that indicate the level of tension in the muscle.

Of all the relaxation techniques, the most familiar may be **hypnotherapy.** A practitioner uses the power of suggestion to teach a patient in a hypnotic state how to relax the smooth muscles of the intestines. **Guided imagery,** often taught by yoga instructors and massage therapists, can also teach you new ways to relax yourself.

NUTRITION AND DIET

Certain foods may contribute to IBS by irritating your gastrointestinal tract. Most things that people say taste good—from hamburgers and fries to ice cream and chocolate—are made with lots of fat. Whether it's vegetable oil or animal fat, or saturated or unsaturated, dietary fat overload is something many people simply can't handle, no matter how much they love the taste. Other known irritants to some people's digestive tracts are eggs and dairy products, spicy foods, and coffee—especially decaffeinated. To check for food sensitivities, try an elimination diet: Stop eating a suspected food for 10 to 30 days, then try it again. If you get an adverse reaction, avoid that food in the future.

If you are like most Americans, you are not eating enough fiber. To correct a dietary fiber imbalance:

- gradually increase the amount of fresh fruits and vegetables, whole grains, and bran in your diet, or
- take 1 tbsp of bran stirred into a glass of fruit juice or water every day, or
- take a soluble fiber, like psyllium *(Plantago psyllium)* seed. Stir 1 tbsp into a glass of cold water and drink once a day.

When you are taking supplemental fiber, be sure to drink several extra glasses of plain water a day. You may experience a certain amount of intestinal gas at first, but it should subside as your body adjusts.

To stop diarrhea, try two capsules of activated charcoal three or four times a day. Be aware, however, that charcoal can interfere with the body's absorption of any other medications you may be taking.

ACUPRESSURE

To ease bowel pain caused by IBS, place the index fingers of both hands on points ST 25, two finger widths from your navel on either side. Press down firmly for one minute while breathing deeply, then release. Do three to five times.

PREVENTION

Whether your own case of IBS is characterized by diarrhea or constipation, making sure you have enough fiber in your diet is a must. The average American adult ingests less than 20 grams of fiber a day, although the recommended amount is 30 grams. It makes no difference whether you eat more fiber-rich foods or take dietary supplements, as long as you get your fiber allowance up to par. If you smoke, quit; and avoid excessive amounts of caffeine.

For coping with stress, you have lots of options. If you practice yoga, include Cobra and knee-to-chest postures *(see Constipation),* which help the abdominal organs as well as enhance overall relaxation. Purchase or make a guided imagery tape that you can listen to at home. Get regular exercise—anything from a brisk 20-minute walk, to a round of golf or tennis or a half-hour's worth of swimming laps. Healthy outlets for stress are great preventives to many gastrointestinal problems, including IBS. ∎

ITCHING SKIN

Read down this column to find your symptoms. Then read across.

SYMPTOMS	AILMENT/PROBLEM
For itching accompanied by a rash, see also Rashes.	
◆ bloodstains, pain, and itching when you have a bowel movement; most common in middle-aged women.	◆ Anal fissure
◆ intensely itchy, dry, thickened skin that usually appears on the wrist, face, behind the knees, and in the crook of the arm; can be aggravated by food allergies, stress, and weather conditions.	◆ Eczema
◆ itching and a feeling of fullness around the anus, possibly accompanied by a mucus discharge, some pain, and constipation.	◆ Hemorrhoids
◆ an itchy, ring-shaped lesion that extends from the groin to the upper thigh and, possibly, includes the genitals; most common in men. Aggravated by tight clothes, obesity, and warm weather.	◆ Jock itch
◆ severe itching on your head or pubic area; you may see small white specks. General itching, possibly accompanied by lesions on the shoulders, buttocks, and stomach.	◆ Lice
◆ threadlike streaks in your stools, sometimes accompanied by extreme itching around the anus and possible swelling; insomnia and stomach pains.	◆ Pinworms
◆ unexplained localized body itch that precedes an outbreak of extremely painful small blisters, usually on one side of the face or torso.	◆ Shingles
◆ unexplained general body itch.	◆ Any of a number of diseases and conditions, including diabetes, Hodgkin's disease and non-Hodgkin's lymphoma, jaundice and other liver problems, kidney failure, liver or pancreatic cancer

I

WHAT TO DO	OTHER INFO
◆ Use a hydrocortisone or anesthetic cream for pain and swelling. See your doctor about any anal bleeding.	◆ Ice compresses will reduce swelling. Two or three warm baths a day can provide relief.
◆ Apply corticosteroid cream to the affected areas, then cover them with plastic wrap overnight.	◆ Eczema is also called atopic dermatitis.
◆ Take acetaminophen for pain. Drink at least eight glasses of water a day and eat plenty of fiber. See your doctor for persistent or recurring cases.	◆ Whole-grain breads, vegetables, fruits, and nuts help prevent constipation, which can lead to hemorrhoids or make them worse.
◆ Use an over-the-counter antifungal medication.	◆ Herbalists recommend swabbing lemon juice on the affected area to soothe and dry up the lesion.
◆ Use over-the-counter shampoo or medication containing a pediculicide (an insecticide for use on the skin to kill mites and lice).	◆ Never use pediculicides around the eyes; rub petroleum jelly onto eyelashes and eyelids and then pluck trapped lice off with tweezers. Combing hair with a fine-toothed comb can work for head lice.
◆ The entire household needs to see a doctor for treatment (even those not infected). Mebendazole is commonly prescribed. See Worms.	◆ Most patients have no symptoms. If you have shared clothes or bedding with someone with pinworms, get treated as a precaution.
◆ See your doctor. Take analgesics for pain; you may be prescribed an antiviral drug.	◆ Shingles on the face, especially around the eyes, can scar and impair vision. **Call your doctor now.**
◆ Call your doctor without delay if you suspect you have one of these conditions. See Kidney Disease and entries for the other diseases listed at left.	

SYMPTOMS

- a yellowish or greenish tinge to the skin.
- yellowing of the whites of the eyes; this is usually a more reliable sign of jaundice than yellowing of the skin.
- dark-colored urine.
- in some cases, generalized itching.

CALL YOUR DOCTOR IF:

- you notice jaundice in your infant; though jaundice in newborns is common, it may indicate a more serious condition.
- you notice jaundice in yourself, in another adult, or in a school-age child; jaundice may be a sign of gallstone-related problems or liver failure, both of which can be serious if left untreated.

J

aundice, a yellowing of the skin and whites of the eyes, is not a disease itself but a symptom of an underlying disorder. The discoloration occurs when excessive amounts of the body pigment bilirubin accumulate in the bloodstream. Normally bilirubin—a natural by-product of the breakdown of red blood cells in the liver—mixes with the digestive juice bile and passes harmlessly out of the body through the digestive tract. But if the liver is not functioning properly or the passage of bile is obstructed (perhaps by gallstones), bilirubin backs up into the blood. Jaundice in newborns and very young children, in most cases, is relatively benign. But in older children and adults it can be a sign of a more serious ailment.

CAUSES

More than half of all newborn infants experience what is called **physiological jaundice,** the consequence of an inexperienced liver suddenly being required to function on its own. In the womb, a fetus's blood passes through the mother's liver, which disposes of any excess bilirubin. After birth, however, the newborn's liver has to handle the job alone, and sometimes it takes time for the new organ to get up to speed. In rare cases, excessive amounts of bilirubin can damage the child's brain. For this reason, and because it may be a symptom of a serious underlying problem, jaundice should never be ignored.

Premature infants and those with a family history of jaundice stand a slightly higher than normal chance of developing it, as do some breast-fed infants. Physicians can't predict which infants will get jaundice and which will not.

Some cases of jaundice in newborns stem from an incompatibility between the mother's and child's blood types. The mother's immune system attacks blood cells in the fetus, resulting in the development of jaundice in the child after birth. Infant jaundice can also come as a result of some other illness or disorder, such as blocked bile ducts, bowel obstructions, hepatitis, mononucleosis, herpes infections, or even bruises sustained at birth. *(See also Bowel Movement Abnormalities and Genital Herpes.)*

Illness-related jaundice is generally a more serious concern in older children and adults. Frequently the underlying cause in such cases is cirrhosis, caused when liver cells are damaged and replaced by scar tissue. The damaged liver cannot process and dispose of bilirubin effectively, so the pigment backs up into the bloodstream.

Other factors or conditions that can disrupt liver function and lead to jaundice include hepatitis, certain drugs and toxins, pregnancy, and congestive heart failure. In some cases, gallstones become lodged in a duct carrying bile from the liver and gallbladder to the small intestine. Its path blocked, the bile backs up and seeps into the bloodstream.

DIAGNOSTIC AND TEST PROCEDURES

You can perform a simple test to check for jaundice in your infant. Using your finger, press gently on the tip of the baby's nose or forehead. If the skin looks white when you pull your finger away, the baby is fine. (This is true regardless of the child's race.) If the spot has a yellowish tinge, the baby is developing jaundice. It's best to perform this test in natural daylight, as artificial light can give the skin a yellow cast. Note: Dark orange or tea-colored urine may indicate jaundice even when the skin appears normal.

If jaundice shows up in school-age children or adults, the doctor may take a blood sample to check for liver damage. The physician may also recommend an examination with ultrasound or x-rays to check for bile duct obstructions.

TREATMENT

Generally, the best way to treat jaundice is to correct the underlying cause; the exact remedy, conventional or alternative, will depend on the nature and severity of the case.

CONVENTIONAL MEDICINE

Most cases of **physiological jaundice** in an infant can be treated through carefully timed exposure to early-morning, late-afternoon, or indirect sunlight.

The light will mimic the function of the liver, changing the bilirubin in the child's body to a form that can be excreted through the digestive tract.

If blood tests show that the newborn has high levels of bilirubin, the physician may recommend phototherapy, in which the infant is placed under a special high-intensity lamp until the bilirubin levels drop. Some hospitals rent lamps that are designed to hang over the crib, or fiberoptic blankets that allow light to penetrate to the baby's skin.

Infants whose jaundice is caused by an illness or other disorder may have to be hospitalized while doctors care for the underlying condition. Treatment for illness-related jaundice in older children and adults will depend on the cause. *(See Cirrhosis, Gallstones, and Hepatitis.)*

ALTERNATIVE CHOICES

Since jaundice is a symptom and not a disease in itself, the underlying disease must be diagnosed before a course of treatment can be established. Alternative remedies should be regarded as complementary care, used to supplement conventional medical treatment.

CHINESE HERBS

A Chinese practitioner may treat jaundice with various combinations of herbs. These remedies must be prepared only by a trained professional.

HERBAL THERAPIES

Various herbs, including dandelion *(Taraxacum officinale)*, vervain *(Verbena officinalis)*, and milk thistle *(Silybum marianum)*, are used in the treatment of jaundice. Consult a practitioner for the proper amounts and methods of use.

HOMEOPATHY

A number of homeopathic remedies are appropriate for treating jaundice; the exact prescription will depend on the underlying cause. Consult a professional homeopath for the preparations and dosages that are appropriate for you. ■

SYMPTOMS

◆ itchy red bumps in the groin area and on the external genitalia; the rash may extend to the buttocks and inner thighs.

CALL YOUR DOCTOR IF:

◆ over-the-counter remedies fail to work after a week or two.
◆ the rash spreads or gets worse.
◆ you develop a chronic condition, in which the rash keeps coming back.

Jock itch is the common name for a fungal infection of the groin known technically as tinea cruris. If you're a man, you've probably had it at some time in your life. But women can get jock itch too; although the fungus is different, the symptoms are the same. The culprit in women is a yeast infection called candidiasis, which begins in the vagina and may spread to external skin if left untreated. Men and women who perspire a lot or who are obese and are likely to have folds of skin that rub against each other are particularly prone to developing rashes in the groin area.

CAUSES

Jock itch is caused by a fungus known as *Trichophyton rubrum*, which is from the same family of organisms responsible for athlete's foot. The fungus thrives in moist, warm areas. Wearing an athletic supporter, or jockstrap, can promote it.

You will probably be able to tell on your own that you have jock itch. If you are in doubt, though, see your doctor, who will almost certainly be able to confirm a diagnosis by visual examination alone.

TREATMENT

You will usually not need to seek professional care for jock itch, unless the rash is severe or widely spread. In the vast majority of cases, you will be able to treat the problem with over-the-counter medications.

With proper treatment, the cure rate for jock itch is very high, but about 20 percent of people develop a chronic condition. If this turns out to be the case for you, seek help from your doctor, who will be able to prescribe stronger medications.

CONVENTIONAL MEDICINE

Most ointments for jock itch contain antifungal agents such as miconazole and clotrimazole.

BEST TREATMENT TIPS

- ◆ *Keep your groin area clean and dry.*
- ◆ *Change your athletic supporter and underwear every day, and wash them in hot water.*
- ◆ *Wear clean cotton shorts under your jockstrap.*
- ◆ *If you have been prone to jock itch in the past and normally wear briefs, consider switching to boxer shorts, which can help keep the groin area drier by allowing better air circulation.*
- ◆ *Use baby powder to prevent the moisture that can lead to jock itch.*
- ◆ *Shower with antibacterial soaps; rinse well to prevent the buildup of potentially irritating soap remnants.*
- ◆ *Do not use someone else's towel at the gym; jock itch is mildly contagious.*
- ◆ *Dry your groin well with a towel or with a hair dryer on its lowest setting.*
- ◆ *Change your clothes as soon as you finish working out.*

These ointments are available in drugstores without a prescription. If you're not sure what to buy, ask the pharmacist to recommend something.

Apply the medicine to the affected area every day as directed until the rash goes away; keep using it for at least a month longer to make sure you have killed the fungus. Keep the area dry and wear loose-fitting clothing until the rash clears up.

To prevent the rash from getting worse or coming back, change your underwear every day and wash it in hot water. If the rash comes back or if you develop an infection, consult your doctor, who can prescribe an antibiotic.

ALTERNATIVE CHOICES

In addition to prescription and over-the-counter medicines, a number of alternative therapies may help speed the healing process.

AROMATHERAPY

A common aromatherapy treatment for a variety of skin conditions involves applications of tea tree oil (*Melaleuca* spp.). Dilute it with a carrier oil such as almond oil and apply to your rash several times a day.

Other oils recommended by aromatherapists to relieve itching are cedarwood (*Juniperus virginiana*) and jasmine (*Jasminum officinale*). Apply these oils in a similar fashion, several times a day.

HERBAL THERAPIES

Herbalists say that one of the best remedies for jock itch is to swab your groin area with diluted freshly squeezed lemon juice. Lemon juice soothes the skin and will help to dry up the rash.

AT-HOME REMEDIES

- ◆ Wash the affected area with an antibacterial soap.
- ◆ Use a hair dryer on the lowest setting after showering to dry the affected area as thoroughly as possible.
- ◆ Apply over-the-counter antifungal creams or drying powder two or three times a day until the rash goes away.
- ◆ Take a warm bath to relieve itching.
- ◆ Apply diluted lemon juice (*see Herbal Therapies, above*).
- ◆ Apply oils of tea tree, cedarwood, or jasmine. ■

JOINT PAIN

Read down this column to find your symptoms. Then read across.

SYMPTOMS	AILMENT/PROBLEM
◆ joint pain after an injury; the joint is mis-shapen and can't be moved.	◆ Dislocation
◆ joint and muscle pain; fever, chills, headache, weakness, malaise, nasal congestion, cough; possibly, vomiting and diarrhea.	◆ Flu
◆ chronic joint pain and stiffness; limited joint movement; symptoms worse after sitting or sleeping; more common in people over 50 and those who overexert their bodies.	◆ Osteoarthritis
◆ pain, swelling, redness, warmth, and stiffness in more than one joint.	◆ Rheumatoid arthritis
◆ sharp, intense pain, swelling, redness, warmth, and stiffness in one joint, often affecting the joint at the base of the big toe, or sometimes the ankle or knee.	◆ Gout
◆ pain, warmth, and stiffness in one or more joints, and possibly redness and swelling, especially when stretching or extending the joint; restricted range of movement.	◆ Bursitis
◆ pain, swelling, redness, warmth, and stiffness; possibly, chills, fever, weakness, sore throat, rash.	◆ Infectious arthritis
◆ pain, swelling, redness, and warmth in joints; abdominal pain and diarrhea; cramps or pain after eating; chronic low-grade fever; loss of appetite, fatigue, weight loss.	◆ Inflammatory bowel disease (Crohn's disease or ulcerative colitis)
◆ joint and muscle pain; headache, fatigue, malaise, fever; several months earlier, circular or oval-red rash with white center, preceded by a tick bite.	◆ Lyme disease

J

◆ **Call your doctor or obtain emergency care now.** See Emergencies/First Aid: Fractures and Dislocations.

◆ If a joint appears misshapen, do not move the patient or the joint unless absolutely necessary.

◆ See Arthritis. Your doctor may prescribe analgesics, exercises, heat treatment, and physical therapy.

◆ The usual treatment is a nonsteroidal anti-inflammatory drug (NSAID) and/or the drug colchicine.

◆ Following a low-purine, vegetarian diet may help prevent attacks. Eating cherries, strawberries, or blueberries may help ease the pain.

◆ **Call your doctor now.** The usual treatment is anti-inflammatory drugs, intravenous antibiotics if the cause is bacterial, and drainage of excess fluid from joint.

◆ This type of arthritis is usually a complication of a recent injury or disease.

◆ **Call your doctor now.** The usual treatment is with antibiotics.

◆ The disease always starts with the bite of a deer tick. Joint pain may occur in a later stage of the disease, several months or more after the bite.

SYMPTOMS

- reddish or cloudy urine, although microscopic traces of blood may be evident in routine urine analyses before the urine changes color. While blood in the urine is usually a sign of kidney infection, it can also be associated with cancer.
- dull pain in the abdomen, lower back, or side.
- a detectable mass in the lower back that feels smooth and firm, but not tender.
- with advanced kidney cancer, fatigue, intermittent low-grade fever, vomiting, appetite and weight loss, and a general sense of ill health.

CALL YOUR DOCTOR IF:

- you experience any symptoms of kidney cancer. The most likely symptoms will be discolored urine, pain in the back or side, and sometimes a mass in the kidney region.

The kidneys are a pair of bean-shaped organs located just above the waist on either side of the spine. The outer portion of each kidney is actually a web of nephrons (capillaries and tubules), which cleanse the blood and produce urine. Benign cysts that resemble fluid-filled sacs commonly develop in the nephron web; much less often, a malignant tumor forms.

Renal cell carcinoma, the most common type of adult kidney cancer, starts in a kidney's outer portion. The next most common type, **transitional cell carcinoma,** originates in the interior of the kidney, where urine collects. Cancer cells may eventually spread to blood vessels, lymph nodes, fat, nearby organs such as the liver or adrenal glands, and ultimately the lungs or bones.

Adult kidney cancer accounts for about 2 percent of cancers in the U.S., but its incidence is steadily rising. It is twice as common in men as in women, and it usually begins after age 40. If diagnosed early, patients have a 60 to 80 percent chance of surviving at least five years; the five-year survival rate for advanced cases drops substantially, depending on how far the cancer has spread beyond the kidney. Of children with kidney cancer, 95 percent have **Wilms' tumor;** if treated early enough, almost all cases are curable.

CAUSES

Kidney cancer is strongly associated with a number of other health problems: congenital defects of the kidney or bladder, frequent urinary tract infections, kidney disease requiring long-term dialysis, and von Hippel-Lindau disease—a rare condition affecting the brain capillaries. A specific genetic defect has been found to cause **Wilms' tumor.**

Smokers are twice as likely to develop kidney cancer as nonsmokers. The disease is also associated with exposure to industrial agents such as asbestos, naphthalenes, aniline dyes, and benzidines, and to phenacetin, a painkiller no longer marketed in the U.S. Diets high in fat and protein may increase risk, as does obesity. Aflatoxins—molds that grow in milk, grains, nuts, and seeds—have also been linked to kidney cancer.

DIAGNOSTIC AND TEST PROCEDURES

If your doctor detects a mass in the abdominal or kidney region or—using a stethoscope—hears an unusual noise over the renal artery, he will check for kidney cancer. (Less commonly, high blood pressure, abnormal liver function, high red blood cell count, or a high level of calcium in the blood may raise suspicions.) The doctor will use ultrasound, a CT scan, or a special x-ray test called an intravenous pyelogram (IVP) to identify and locate a kidney tumor. If the tumor proves malignant, other imaging tests help to determine whether the cancer has spread.

TREATMENT

If it is caught early, a kidney tumor will be removed surgically. The surgeon tries to remove only the cancerous area but may have to take out the entire kidney along with surrounding fat, lymph nodes, and possibly the adrenal gland. Radiation therapy and chemotherapy can reduce tumor size but are not consistently effective in preventing the spread of kidney cancer. Chemotherapy after surgery cures local **Wilms' tumor** in 9 out of 10 cases.

Neither radiation nor chemotherapy is particularly successful in treating advanced kidney cancer. Hormonal therapy is sometimes prescribed, and new therapies are being tested constantly in the hope of improving cure rates. Immunotherapy using either interferon or interleukin 2 to boost the body's natural cancer-killing powers has shown promise. After remission, patients must be checked regularly for recurrence or delayed complications. *(See Cancer for more information about therapies.)*

PREVENTION

If you smoke, quit now. Keep trim, cut back on high-fat foods, and limit your consumption of red meat. Throw out any foods that become moldy or rancid, including nuts, seeds, or rice.

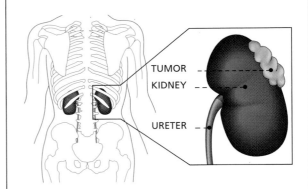

CANCER IN THE KIDNEYS

TUMOR

KIDNEY

URETER

The kidneys are a pair of fist-sized organs that filter waste from the blood at the amazing rate of 1½ qt a minute. Early detection of kidney cancer is difficult, because small kidney tumors produce very few symptoms. The cancer tends to start near the top of the organ *(inset)*. The kidneys' waste-processing efficiency is affected only in the late stages of the disease.

PLANTS AND CANCER TREATMENT

Researchers at the National Cancer Institute have tested thousands of plant samples in the hope of isolating specific chemical compounds that may help treat or prevent cancer. Occasionally a promising compound is identified. For example, tests show that a compound called coumarin, found in certain nontoxic herbs, can enhance the effects of the chemotherapy agent cimetidine; treatment combining coumarin and cimetidine induced significant regression in several kidney cancer patients.

Nevertheless, active plant constituents interact in complex ways that are neither predictable nor fully understood. Herbal specialists warn against taking herbs in the hope of benefiting from one of their constituents; cancer patients should never take any herbal remedy without an oncologist's explicit approval. Taking toxic herbs is dangerous under any circumstances. A knowledgeable physician may be able to recommend herbs that improve overall health by stimulating the immune system, but no herbal remedy has been shown to cure cancer. ∎

K

SYMPTOMS

- frequent thirst and urge to urinate.
- the passing of very small amounts of urine.
- swelling, particularly of the hands and feet, and puffiness around the eyes.
- unpleasant taste in the mouth and urinelike odor to the breath.
- persistent fatigue or shortness of breath.
- loss of appetite.
- increasingly higher blood pressure.
- pale skin.
- excessively dry, persistently itchy skin.
- in children: increased fatigue and sleepiness; decrease in appetite; and eventually, poor growth.

CALL YOUR DOCTOR IF:

- you are experiencing any of the symptoms listed above. Although any of them may indicate another disorder, each is one of the warning signs of kidney disease, which is a life-threatening illness. Consult your doctor without delay.

The kidneys, two fist-sized organs located on either side of the spine just above the waist, perform a life-sustaining role. They cleanse the blood by removing waste and excess fluids, maintain a healthful balance of various body chemicals, and help regulate blood pressure.

When the kidneys become diseased or damaged, they can suddenly or gradually lose their ability to perform these vital functions. Waste products and excess fluid then build up inside the body, causing a variety of symptoms, particularly swelling of the hands and feet, shortness of breath, and a frequent urge to urinate. If left untreated, diseased kidneys may eventually stop functioning. Loss of kidney function is a very serious and potentially fatal condition.

CAUSES

Kidney disease is classified as either **acute** (when loss of function occurs suddenly) or **chronic** (when deterioration takes place gradually, perhaps over a period of years). The chronic form can be particularly insidious: It may not show any symptoms until considerable, often irreparable damage has been done.

The causes of **chronic kidney disease** are often difficult to pinpoint. Most are the result of another disease or condition, such as diabetes, high blood pressure, or atherosclerosis—all of which impede the flow of blood inside the kidneys. Lupus and other diseases of the immune system that affect blood vessels may also trigger kidney disease by causing the kidneys to become inflamed.

Some chronic kidney diseases, most notably polycystic kidney disease (in which cysts form on the kidneys), are inherited. Others are congenital—the result of some sort of urinary tract obstruction or malformation that the person was born with and that predisposes the victim to kidney infections and diseases.

Chronic kidney disease may also result from long-term exposure to toxic chemicals or to drugs, including certain illegal drugs, such as heroin. Researchers also suspect that excessive amounts of vitamin D and protein, particularly in the diets of the elderly or the very ill, may harm the kidneys. But in many chronic cases, the precise cause remains unknown.

Acute kidney disease can occur within a matter of days following the onset of any medical condition that suddenly and dramatically reduces the flow of blood to the kidneys. Examples are a heart attack, a traumatic injury such as one sustained in an automobile accident, a serious infection, or a toxic reaction to a drug.

Inhaling or swallowing certain toxins, including methyl, or wood, alcohol; carbon tetrachloride; antifreeze; and poisonous mushrooms, can also cause the kidneys to suddenly malfunction. Marathon runners and other endurance athletes who do not drink enough liquids while competing in long-distance athletic events may suffer acute kidney failure due to a sudden breakdown of muscle tissue, which releases a chemical called myoglobin that can damage the kidneys.

DIAGNOSTIC AND TEST PROCEDURES

For a diagnosis, your physician will have you undergo blood and urine tests and, if your kidneys can tolerate it, a special x-ray, known as an intravenous pyelogram (IVP), for viewing them. If the diagnosis remains unclear, your doctor may also do a needle biopsy, using a special needle device to remove a small sample of kidney tissue for microscopic examination.

TREATMENT

Kidney disease is a life-threatening condition that requires medical care. Alternative treatments may be used to supplement that care, but before trying them you should discuss them thoroughly with your doctor.

Medications, especially those that control diabetes and high blood pressure, can sometimes help slow the progress of chronic kidney disease. Some medical practitioners have found that certain restrictive diets are useful, particularly if the condition is caught early. But if these measures fail, and the kidneys deteriorate to the point where they can no longer function at all, there are only two treatments: dialysis, in which artifi-cial devices clean the blood of waste products, or a kidney transplant.

CONVENTIONAL MEDICINE

If you are diagnosed with one of the more serious forms of kidney disease, your doctor may prescribe several medications. Because high blood pressure is both a cause and a symptom of the condition, you will probably receive a prescription for angiotensin-converting enzyme (ACE) inhibitors to slow the rate of injury to the kidneys or a diuretic to keep your blood pressure down. To balance your body's chemicals, which can be thrown dangerously out of kilter by malfunctioning kidneys, you may also be given drugs such as sodium polystyrene sulfonate, which lowers potassium levels, and calcium citrate, which blocks the stomach's absorption of phosphorus.

If a blood test reveals that the level of your red blood cells has fallen, your doctor may prescribe a medication with an iron supplement to rebuild your body's stores of erythropoietin, a natural blood-building substance. Your doctor may also recommend that you take calcium supplements to keep your bones from weakening, an occasional side effect of chronic kidney disease. Because many drugs are excreted through the kidneys, you will also need to consult with your doctor before taking any over-the-counter medications. You may be told to avoid ibuprofen and acetaminophen, which have been implicated as possible contributors to kidney disease.

Although the approach remains controversial in conventional medical circles, a growing number of physicians now encourage dietary changes to help manage chronic kidney disease. *(See Nutrition and Diet.)* Some studies have shown that rigid adherence to a diet that severely restricts protein can delay or even prevent continued kidney deterioration. This is especially true of people whose kidney disease is the result of diabetes. Studies have shown that diabetics who follow a diet that keeps their blood glucose levels within a tight range can help retard the progress of kidney disease.

Dialysis treatment, which uses artificial devices to perform the kidneys' functions, is necessary for cases of advanced kidney disease. Two types of dialysis are commonly used today. **Hemodialysis** involves a mechanical filter that cleans the blood. A surgeon implants a shunt, a small tube that connects an artery and a vein in the patient's arm or leg. Several times a week, for three or four hours at a time, another tube is connected to the shunt and the patient's blood is pumped out of the body into the hemodialyzer and then pumped back.

Another method, called **peritoneal dialysis,** makes use of the inner lining of the abdomen, or peritoneal membrane—which has many of the kidneys' filtering characteristics—to help clean the blood. A plastic tube is surgically implanted in the patient's abdomen. Then, during each treatment, a fluid called dialyzate is infused through the tube into the abdomen. Waste products carried by the blood circulating through tiny vessels in the peritoneal membrane filter into the dialyzate, which is drained out after several hours. This process is repeated three to five times a day. While the fluid is in the abdomen, the patient can go about normal daily activities.

Both types of dialysis present possible complications and risks, most notably that of infection. The stress of having to continually do the procedure can also take its toll on a patient's emotional well-being. For these reasons, people with advanced kidney disease often opt for a **kidney transplant.** New antirejection drugs and improved follow-up care have greatly increased the success rate for such surgery. Today, the three-year survival rate for patients who receive a donor kidney from a living relative is about 75 percent; for those whose transplanted kidney comes from an unrelated deceased donor, the rate is about 60 percent.

Not every person with kidney disease is a candidate for a transplant; a patient may have an underlying condition or other medical factor that rules out such an operation.

ALTERNATIVE CHOICES

Because kidney disease is a serious illness, you should try alternative therapies only after talking them over with your physician.

CHINESE HERBS
Traditional Chinese health practitioners use several herbs in the treatment of kidney disorders. However, because many herbs can be harmful to the kidneys, you should always consult your physician before taking the advice of an herbalist or ingesting any herbal remedies.

HOMEOPATHY
Homeopathic remedies are generally safe for the treatment of chronic kidney conditions. However, the remedies should be prescribed by a practitioner skilled in both conventional and alternative medicine, and they should never be used as a substitute for conventional medicine.

NUTRITION AND DIET
A special restricted diet can decrease the workload on diseased kidneys, keep body fluids and chemicals in balance, and fend off a buildup of waste products in the body. Although such diets should be specifically tailored to each patient's individual needs, they all typically incorporate the following general restrictions:
◆ protein: no more than 1 gram per kilogram of body weight per day.
◆ potassium: no more than 2 grams per day.
◆ phosphorus: no more than 1 gram per day (usually accomplished by adhering to protein restrictions).
◆ sodium: in advanced cases of kidney disease, no more than 2 grams per day.

Calcium supplements (1,500 mg per day) are frequently recommended in order to counteract the bone weakening that frequently accompanies kidney disease.

CHEMICALS THAT CAN DAMAGE THE KIDNEYS
Several of the chemicals found in common household products have been linked to both acute and chronic kidney disease. By reading product labels carefully and taking a few simple precautions, you can limit your exposure to these harmful toxins.

Cadmium. This rare, naturally occurring metal is used in the manufacture of pesticides, rub-

K

ber tires, plastics, paints, and other products. Because of its industrial uses, it is now widely found in water and food supplies. Some precautions:

◆ Limit your intake of foods with high levels of cadmium, most notably liver and kidney products, flounder, mussels, scallops, oysters, and vegetables grown with sewage sludge fertilizers.

◆ Be sure any paints, dyes, or ceramic glazes you use for arts and crafts projects are cadmium-free.

◆ Do not use antique cookware or serving dishes; they may contain cadmium-based pigments.

◆ Avoid tobacco smoke.

Carbon tetrachloride (methane tetrachloride; tetrachloromethane; perchloromethane). A clear, colorless liquid with an etherlike smell, carbon tetrachloride was once a common household solvent until questions were raised about its toxicity. To avoid:

◆ Dispose of any old cans or bottles of cleaning products in your home during your community's next hazardous waste roundup program.

◆ Use a carbon filter on faucets to remove the chemical from your drinking and cooking water.

Chloroform (trichloromethane; methenyl chloride; methane trichloride; methyl trichloride; formyl trichloride). This sweet-smelling and sweet-tasting chemical is found in drinking water as a by-product of chlorination and found in the air as the result of automobile and industrial pollution. Chloroform is also still used as an ingredient in some cough syrups, toothpaste, liniments, glues, pesticides, and other consumer products. To avoid:

◆ Be sure your shower stall is well ventilated. Chloroform evaporates from chlorinated hot water, and levels can rise quickly inside an enclosed shower.

◆ To further reduce your exposure to chloroform while showering, put an activated charcoal filter on the cold-water pipe going into your hot-water heater.

◆ Read product labels carefully, and exercise

extreme caution when using any product listing chloroform among its ingredients.

Ethylene glycol (1,2-dihydroxyethane; 1,2-ethanediol; ethylene alcohol; ethylene dihydrate). This clear, sweet-tasting chemical is found primarily in automobile antifreeze and brake fluid and in cosmetics, particularly those with a creamy texture. To avoid:

◆ Read cosmetics labels carefully; avoid those products containing the chemical.

◆ Do not allow children, who are sometimes attracted to the sweet taste of products containing ethylene glycol, to play in garages or other areas where cars and their supplies are kept. Promptly clean up any fluids that leak from your car.

Oxalic acid (oxalic acid dihydrate; ethane dioic acid). Used in both powder and liquid form, oxalic acid is found in some heavy-duty household cleaning products. Several freckle-fading and skin-bleaching cosmetics contain this chemical. It is also found in the leaves of some plants. To avoid:

◆ Read the labels of heavy-duty household cleaners and polishes carefully; avoid those that contain oxalic acid.

◆ Do not use any bleaching agents on your skin that contain the chemical.

◆ Never eat rhubarb leaves, which contain high concentrations of oxalic acid.

Tetrachloroethylene (PCE; carbon dichloride; perchloroethylene; PERC; 1,1,2,2-tetrachloroethylene). This colorless, heavy liquid is the most widely used dry-cleaning chemical in the United States. Some precautions:

◆ Keep your car windows open when bringing clothes home from the dry cleaner.

◆ Air dry-cleaned clothes outside or on a well-ventilated porch for at least six hours before bringing them inside.

◆ Air dry-cleaned sleeping bags for several days before using them.

◆ Avoid spot removers, rug and upholstery cleaners, and paint strippers that contain tetrachloroethylene. ■

- continuous pain that usually begins in the back above the waist and spreads down into the groin.
- rapidly rising fever—often to 104°F.
- frequent urge to urinate, even though the bladder is empty.
- cloudy or bloody urine.
- severe nausea or vomiting.

CALL YOUR DOCTOR IF:

- you have symptoms that lead you to think you have a kidney infection, which is a serious ailment requiring immediate medical attention.
- you notice blood in your urine; this may also indicate kidney disease, a kidney stone, a bladder or kidney tumor, a bladder infection, or a prostate infection *(see Prostate Problems)*. See your doctor without delay.
- you are experiencing any pain or difficulty with urination; this may also be a sign of a sexually transmitted disease, a vaginal problem, a kidney stone, or a bladder or prostate tumor. See your doctor without delay.

Kidney infections occur when infectious organisms—usually bacteria—enter the body and travel to the kidneys, where they cause swelling and inflammation. A kidney infection can be acute (coming on suddenly) or chronic (recurring periodically over the course of many years).

Kidney infections are very serious. Left untreated, they can lead to permanent kidney damage and result in chronic kidney disease. The infection can also spread into the blood, causing blood poisoning. Anyone can develop a kidney infection, but pregnant women are at increased risk, in part because the pressure of the fetus on the bladder makes it more difficult to empty the bladder completely (urine left in the bladder is a potential medium for bacterial growth).

CAUSES

Like bladder infections, kidney infections are most often caused by the bacterium *Escherichia coli (E. coli)* or other bacteria that normally reside harmlessly in the intestines. Indeed, the infection typically begins in the bladder—having entered through the urethra—and then spreads to the kidneys.

In addition, the use of catheters—tubes that are inserted into the bladder to empty it—can trigger a kidney infection. Catheters may be inserted during the recovery period after a surgical procedure and are also sometimes used with nursing home residents or for people who have certain types of neurological conditions that affect bladder control.

DIAGNOSTIC AND TEST PROCEDURES

You will need a thorough medical evaluation to find out if you have a kidney infection and to determine the infectious agent causing it. The evaluation will include blood and urine tests. If you have had frequent infections, or if your doctor suspects that an underlying structural abnormality is to blame, more tests may be suggested. Your doctor may order an intravenous pyelogram (IVP), an x-ray technique for viewing the kidneys; a cystoscopy, a procedure in which a lighted tube

K

inserted through the urethra is used to examine the bladder; or an ultrasound scan, which produces a detailed image of the kidneys.

TREATMENT

Kidney infections require immediate medical treatment; delay in clearing the body of infection can lead to serious complications. Advocates of alternative medicine stress that their treatments should be used only as a supplement to conventional medical care.

CONVENTIONAL MEDICINE

Antibiotics and bed rest are often all that is required to bring an acute kidney infection under control within 48 hours. Your physician will also ask you to drink large quantities of water—at least 3 qt a day—to help flush out the bacteria from your urinary tract. Young children, the elderly, or people who are very weakened by the illness are sometimes hospitalized to ensure that they get enough fluids and antibiotics.

Chronic kidney infections are also treated with antibiotics and large quantities of fluids. Because a chronic infection is sometimes caused by urine flowing back from the bladder into the kidneys, surgery to repair this structural problem may also be necessary.

Kidney infections sometimes return without manifesting any overt symptoms, so your doctor may also ask you to come in for follow-up blood tests and checkups.

ALTERNATIVE CHOICES

Because kidney infections are so serious, most alternative practitioners will insist that you seek conventional medical care. If you decide to use alternative treatments in addition to conventional ones, be sure your caregivers are in communication with one another. Once the kidney infection has cleared up, alternative therapies may help prevent a recurrence.

HOMEOPATHY

Homeopaths use treatments known as drainage remedies or European-combination remedies to help rid the body of a kidney infection. Be sure to seek out a practitioner familiar with these remedies. One combination sometimes prescribed includes Apis, Phosphorus, and Teribinthina.

NUTRITION AND DIET

Until you are cured of the infection, avoid foods that might irritate the urinary tract and put undue stress on the kidneys. Alcohol, coffee, salt, black tea, chocolate, carbonated beverages, citrus fruits, tomatoes, spicy foods, vinegar, artificial sweeteners, and sugar are all considered potential irritants.

PREVENTION

Because most kidney infections start in the bladder, prevention begins with keeping bacteria out of the entire urinary tract.

◆ Practice good bathroom hygiene. Clean yourself thoroughly after using the toilet. Women should wipe from front to back to avoid spreading fecal bacteria to the opening of the urethra.

◆ Urinate as soon as possible when you feel the urge and empty your bladder completely.

◆ Wear cotton underwear and loose clothing that does not trap heat and moisture in the crotch.

◆ Drink plenty of liquids.

◆ Drink at least 12 fl oz of cranberry juice a day. Research suggests that cranberries have properties that help fight off urinary tract infections. (See Bladder Infections.)

Women:

◆ Empty your bladder after intercourse to flush any bacteria that may have been pushed in.

◆ If you use a diaphragm, make sure that it fits properly and don't leave it in too long.

◆ Avoid using scented soaps, bubble baths, and vaginal deodorants, all of which have chemicals that can irritate the urinary tract and make it more vulnerable to infection. ■

SYMPTOMS

- waves of sharp pain that start in the side and move toward the groin.
- nausea and vomiting.
- profuse sweating.
- blood in urine.

Sometimes an infection is present and may cause these additional symptoms:

- fever and chills.
- frequent urge to urinate.
- painful or excruciating urination.
- cloudy or foul-smelling urine.

CALL YOUR DOCTOR IF:

- you think you have kidney stones; a medical evaluation is essential to diagnosis and treatment.
- you are experiencing waves of sharp pain in your side or abdomen; such pain may also be a sign of another serious condition, such as gallstones, pelvic inflammatory disease, or an intestinal obstruction. **Seek immediate medical help.**
- you are experiencing any pain or difficulty with urination; this could also be a sign of a bladder infection, a sexually transmitted disease, a vaginal problem such as vaginitis, an enlargement of the prostate *(see Prostate Problems),* or a bladder or prostate tumor. See your doctor without delay.
- you notice blood in your urine; it may also indicate kidney disease, a bladder or kidney tumor, or a urinary or prostate infection *(see Prostate Problems).* See your doctor without delay.

Kidney stones usually form in the center of the kidney, where urine collects before flowing into the ureter, the tube that leads to the bladder. They are created when certain substances in urine—including calcium and uric acid—crystallize and the crystals clump together. Small stones are able to pass out of the body in the urine and often go completely unnoticed. But larger stones irritate and stretch the ureter as they move toward the bladder, causing excruciating pain and blocking the flow of urine. Sometimes a stone can be as large as a golf ball, in which case it remains lodged in the kidney, creating a more serious condition.

Kidney stones are more common in young and middle-aged adults than in the elderly, and they are much more prevalent in men than in women. People living in hot climates are sometimes prone to kidney stones because their bodies become dehydrated, concentrating the minerals in their urine.

If you've had a kidney stone once, you are likely to get one again. So it's important to determine as best you can what caused the stone to form and to take steps to prevent a recurrence.

CAUSES

Why some people form kidney stones and others don't is not always clear. In 90 percent of cases, the cause remains unknown. The condition appears to run in families, and people who suffer from gout, inflammatory bowel diseases, and chronic urinary tract infections also seem to be predisposed to it. Medical evidence suggests that drinking too few fluids can cause stones, as can prolonged bed rest.

Chronic use of antacids containing calcium has also been linked to kidney stones. Dietary deficiencies, especially of vitamin B_6 and magnesium, and excessive amounts of vitamin D also may be factors in the formation of stones. An imbalance of these vitamins and minerals can increase the amount of calcium oxalate in the urine; when the levels become too high, the calcium oxalate does not dissolve, and crystals may begin to form. In genetically susceptible people, eating foods that are themselves rich in calcium oxalate—such as chocolate, grapes, spinach, and strawberries—may also promote stones.

DIAGNOSTIC AND TEST PROCEDURES

Because many of the symptoms of kidney stones also indicate other disorders, a doctor must confirm the presence of a stone. An evaluation will include blood and urine tests and probably an intravenous pyelogram (IVP), a special x-ray technique for viewing the kidneys, or an ultrasound scan to reveal the stone's size and location.

TREATMENT

CONVENTIONAL MEDICINE

Because 90 percent of kidney stones pass out of the body on their own within three to six weeks, your doctor will most likely at first prescribe only plenty of water—at least 3 qt a day—and a pain medication, such as aspirin or acetaminophen with oxycodone. A hot-water bottle can also help ease the inevitable discomfort. You may be asked to urinate through a strainer so the stone can be recovered and analyzed. Once the stone's composition is known, your doctor can prescribe drugs or suggest dietary changes to prevent your developing another one. The vast majority of kidney stones consist of calcium oxalate, so doctors often prescribe a thiazide diuretic to prevent recurrences.

If complications develop, such as an infection or total blockage of the ureter, the stone must be surgically removed. Depending on its size, type, and location, the stone is taken out either by conventional surgery or, more commonly, with a thin telescopic instrument called an endoscope. The surgeon passes the endoscope through the urethra into the bladder or ureter and then either pulls the stone out or bombards it with sound waves or laser beams, breaking it up into tiny pieces. If the stone is lodged in the kidney, the instrument is inserted into the kidney through an incision in the patient's side. A new method, known as extracorporeal shock wave lithotripsy, uses high-energy shock waves to break up kidney stones without surgery.

ALTERNATIVE CHOICES

In addition to the Chinese herbal remedy below, you might want to consider **acupuncture** or **homeopathy;** both therapies may help ease pain, and acupuncture may help facilitate the passing of a stone. In all cases, advocates stress that you should be monitored by a health professional.

CHINESE HERBS

Practitioners of Chinese medicine sometimes prescribe star fruit *(Averrhoa carambola)* to help relieve pain and promote urination. Place three fresh star fruit in a pan with 2 tsp of honey. Boil the fruit until it is soft, then eat the fruit and its juice. Repeat every day until the stone has passed and you are pain free.

PREVENTION

You can do many things, mainly dietary, to prevent a recurrence of stones. But always check with your doctor first; the stone's composition will determine which preventive steps you should take.

◆ Drink at least 3 qt of liquid every day, more in hot weather.
◆ Avoid or eat sparingly foods containing calcium oxalate (chocolate, celery, grapes, bell peppers, beans, strawberries, spinach, asparagus, beets, black tea). You may need to limit your overall intake of calcium, but do not do so without your doctor's advice.
◆ Take daily supplements of vitamin B_6 (10 mg) and magnesium (300 mg), both of which reduce the formation of oxalates.
◆ Avoid foods that raise uric acid levels: anchovies, sardines, organ meats, brewer's yeast.
◆ Reduce uric acid by eating a low-protein diet.
◆ Avoid antacids; they are often high in calcium.
◆ Reduce salt to no more than 3 grams per day; higher amounts may raise the level of calcium oxalate in your urine.
◆ Avoid vitamin D supplements, which can increase calcium oxalate levels.

■

KNEE PAIN

Read down this column to find your symptoms. Then read across.

SYMPTOMS	AILMENT/PROBLEM
◆ knee pain following an injury; knee is not misshapen.	◆ Soft-tissue injury
◆ knee pain following an injury; possibly, popping and the inability to bear weight or move the knee; knee may "catch" or give way or may be misshapen.	◆ Ligament or cartilage damage
◆ knee pain in athletes or active people, or after you bang or twist your knee; possibly, swelling.	◆ Overuse injury such as runner's or biker's knee; water on the knee (synovitis); or jumper's knee (patellar tendonitis)
◆ pain and swelling below the kneecap in an active adolescent undergoing a growth spurt.	◆ Growing pains (Osgood-Schlatter disease)
◆ pain, swelling, redness, warmth, and stiffness in your knee and other joints.	◆ Rheumatoid arthritis
◆ pain, warmth, and stiffness in your knee, especially if you frequently kneel on a hard surface; pain is felt mainly upon bending your knee.	◆ Housemaid's knee (bursitis)
◆ chronic aching and stiffness in your knee; limited movement; may improve with rest; more common in people over 50 and those who overexert their bodies.	◆ Osteoarthritis
◆ knee pain with redness, warmth, and swelling; fever, general feeling of illness; possibly, recent illness.	◆ Bone or joint infection

K

◆ Try RICE: rest, ice (cubes wrapped in a thin cloth), compression (not-too-tight bandage), elevation (with pillows). *(See Sprains and Strains.)* Take an anti-inflammatory painkiller such as ibuprofen.

◆ When swelling subsides, consider taking hot baths with Epsom salt, and choose an exercise that strengthens the muscles near the injured area without stressing the injury.

◆ Call your doctor. Apply ice and take an anti-inflammatory painkiller such as ibuprofen if needed. Keep the leg raised to reduce swelling.

◆ Surgery may be recommended, especially in young people; physical therapy is usually needed. Severe knee pain after an injury may also indicate a dislocation or fracture. *(See Emergencies/First Aid: Fractures and Dislocations.)*

◆ See Athletic Injuries. Try RICE: rest, ice (cubes wrapped in a thin cloth), compression (not-too-tight bandage), elevation (with pillows). Call your doctor. Bracing or taping may be needed.

◆ Massage can be especially helpful for tendonitis. Runners should run on soft surfaces and wear quality running shoes to prevent overuse injuries. Start any exercise program gradually.

◆ Have the affected person avoid exercise that strains the knee, such as jumping and squatting, until symptoms are gone (6 to 12 months). Muscle-stretching exercises, ice, and anti-inflammatory painkillers such as ibuprofen may be helpful.

◆ You may be able to feel a tender bump below your child's kneecap. If pain is severe, your doctor may recommend taping or a knee immobilizer.

◆ See Arthritis. Take an anti-inflammatory painkiller such as ibuprofen.

◆ Take an anti-inflammatory painkiller such as ibuprofen. Your doctor may inject your knee with anti-inflammatory and local anesthetic drugs.

◆ Pain may be alleviated by acupuncture; chiropractic may help restore active range of motion.

◆ See Arthritis. Your doctor may prescribe analgesics and exercises.

◆ The cause may be wear and tear on joint tissue from aging, from being overweight, or possibly, from overuse in work or sports activities.

◆ **Call your doctor now.** The usual treatment is with antibiotics. *(See Infections.)*

◆ Both infectious arthritis and bone infection can result in permanent damage if they are not treated.

K

SYMPTOMS

You may be lactose intolerant if you experience some of the following symptoms after consuming milk products:

- abdominal cramps.
- bloating.
- frothy diarrhea.
- vomiting.
- flatulence.

CALL YOUR DOCTOR IF:

- you have the above symptoms in response to even tiny amounts of high-lactose foods, such as milk, ice cream, or soft cheese. This may indicate **primary lactose intolerance.**
- you develop symptoms after an illness or after taking medication. This may indicate **secondary lactose intolerance.**
- your newborn infant has symptoms from birth. This probably signifies **congenital lactose intolerance.**

In all three cases, you should seek an evaluation and treatment advice from your doctor.

Lactose is the primary sugar found in mammalian milk. Digestion of lactose requires the enzyme lactase, produced in the small intestine, which breaks lactose into two simpler sugars. When the intestine produces little or no lactase, milk sugar is not digested. It moves into the colon, where bacteria ferment it, producing hydrogen, carbon dioxide, and organic acids. The results of this fermentation are diarrhea, flatulence, and abdominal discomfort.

Newborns require high intestinal lactase levels for survival. Later in life, though, about two-thirds of all people lose the ability to produce lactase. Most of the people who keep producing it throughout adulthood are those of northern and middle European ancestry, the major population group that has herded milk animals for thousands of years. In other populations—Mediterranean, African, Asian, and Native American—75 to 100 percent of adults are lactose intolerant. It is believed that more than 30 million Americans have some degree of lactose intolerance.

Primary lactose intolerance may begin at any time but usually develops between the ages of 3 and 13 and continues throughout life. **Secondary lactose intolerance** may occur if the intestinal lining is temporarily damaged by diarrhea or medications such as nonsteroidal anti-inflammatory drugs (NSAIDs), aspirin, and antibiotics, which can halt lactase production for several weeks.

More unusual is **congenital lactose intolerance,** in which the small intestine produces no lactase. Consumption of any amount of lactose is intolerable and even dangerous, especially for infants, in whom diarrhea quickly leads to dehydration. This disorder is apparent in the first week of life; the infant must be fed a lactose-free diet.

While lactose intolerance has been investigated as a cause of colic in infants, the evidence is inconclusive. Often, a child who does not seem to tolerate lactose as an infant can consume dairy products without difficulty by age 10 or 12.

CAUSES

In people with **primary lactose intolerance,** the production of intestinal lactase declines steadily from early childhood until adolescence, when levels are less than 10 percent of those present at birth. This is the norm in areas of Asia, Africa, and the subtropics where people historically consume little or no milk after infancy.

Secondary lactose intolerance is caused by illness, side effects of medication, or other environmental change and is usually temporary.

Congenital lactose intolerance, which is present at birth, is caused by a faulty gene for lactase production.

DIAGNOSTIC AND TEST PROCEDURES

Lactose intolerance is traditionally diagnosed by comparing your health history with the symptoms of lactose intolerance. Diagnosis can also be made by a simple breath test. After lactose enters the large intestine, bacteria in the colon attack it and give off large quantities of hydrogen, which is eliminated by the respiratory system. Your doctor can detect this by means of a breath analyzing device.

If you have some of the symptoms listed above, you can check your own level of lactose tolerance by abstaining from all milk products for two weeks. If your symptoms disappear and then reappear when you try milk again, you are probably lactose intolerant. Even so, you will probably be able to eat or drink small amounts of lactose-containing foods, and there is no harm in doing so. *(See At-Home Remedies, right.)*

TREATMENT

There is no treatment for the underlying mechanism of lactose intolerance. For **primary lactose intolerance,** the recommended approach is to reduce or eliminate lactose-containing foods from the diet. Often, however, small amounts of lactose—or the symptoms themselves—can be tolerated. Another option is to use lactose-reduced dairy products or to take lactase tablets with any dairy products you consume. For **secondary lactose intolerance** adults can abstain from dairy products and infants can be given soy formula until the underlying illness or condition passes.

AT-HOME REMEDIES

◆ If your lactose intolerance is severe, read labels carefully; avoid any product that contains lactose, especially milk (including nonfat milk), soft cheeses, and ice cream. Instead, look for special lactose-reduced cottage and American cheeses. Hard cheeses, such as cheddar, Swiss, and Jarlsberg; buttermilk; and sour cream are also generally low in lactose.

◆ Yogurt with live and active cultures is a good source of calcium and protein for those who are lactose intolerant. The bacteria found in active cultures help digest the lactose in the yogurt.

◆ Try slowly increasing the amount of lactose you eat; symptoms may decrease. Or try eating some yogurt before drinking milk or eating ice cream.

◆ For most people intolerance is not the same as an allergy. Even a lactose-intolerant person can assimilate a cup or so of milk, especially when it is accompanied by foods high in fat, which slows digestion. A low-lactose diet is much easier to achieve than a truly lactose-free diet and may be sufficient.

◆ Look for milk products that contain the enzyme betagalactosidase. Such lactose-reduced milks are easier to digest.

◆ Lactase produced from a yeast or fungus is commercially available and may be added to milk or taken in capsule or tablet form before consuming milk products.

◆ Soy protein formulas are effective milk substitutes for lactose-intolerant infants, and soy products (including milk, yogurt, cheese, and ice cream) can be substituted for milk products in adult diets.

◆ Acidophilus milk, which contains *Lactobacillus acidophilus* (the bacteria found in yogurt), helps break down lactose and is beneficial for digestion in general.

◆ If you do have to give up dairy products, be sure to get enough **calcium** from other sources, such as dark-green leafy vegetables, canned fish, tofu, beans, apricots, and sesame seeds. ■

LARYNGITIS

SYMPTOMS

- hoarseness and loss of voice.
- pain when speaking.
- tickling and rawness in the throat.
- a constant need to clear the throat.
- loss of voice accompanied by the flu, a cold, or pneumonia.
- fever (occasionally).

CALL YOUR DOCTOR IF:

- hoarseness and discomfort last more than a week; this could signal a bacterial infection or more serious disorder.
- you develop laryngitis after being exposed to environmental toxins, such as poisonous fumes or noxious odors; such exposure might have caused more damage than just a simple inflammation of your vocal cords.
- laryngitis occurs along with or as a result of alcohol abuse or chronic bronchitis, which require a doctor's care.
- a child's hoarseness turns into a sharp, barking cough, which could indicate a severely restricted airway or, possibly, croup.

If you lose your voice, or the sounds coming out of your mouth sound several notes higher—or lower—than normal, you may have laryngitis. Specifically, this disorder is an inflammation of the mucous membrane of the larynx, or the part of your windpipe that contains the vocal cords. Your vocal cords open and close during the course of normal speech *(right)*. If your vocal cords are swollen, the sounds you make become distorted. You'll be hoarse, or you may lose your voice altogether.

CAUSES

Anything that makes your vocal cords swell can result in laryngitis. Viruses are the number one culprit, although bacteria are frequently responsible. Allergies and exposure to certain harsh chemicals or toxins can also cause the vocal cords to swell. Overuse is another common cause, to which many rock stars and overexcited football fans can attest. In rare instances laryngitis comes as a result of growths or tumors (called nodules or nodes) that develop on or around the vocal cords.

TREATMENT

Viral laryngitis usually goes away by itself in a few days without any treatment. For this reason, persistent laryngitis is a warning sign that something other than a pesky virus may be causing your hoarseness and tickly throat.

CONVENTIONAL MEDICINE

If the diagnosis is viral laryngitis, you can alleviate symptoms until your body rids itself of the virus. However, if a physician determines that a bacterial infection has set in, you'll most likely be given antibiotics. Take the entire course—usually 7 to 10 days—even if you feel better right away. Stopping the treatment prematurely can result in a worse infection later on.

For most allergies, doctors usually prescribe antihistamines, which reduce swelling and in-

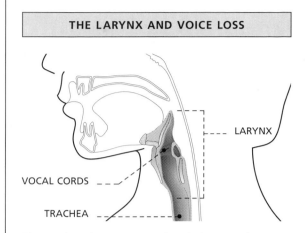

flammation. For serious allergic reactions, during which you find it hard to breathe, your physician may prescribe a systemic steroid medication. No medication is necessary if your laryngitis is caused by simple overuse; in that case, the best solution is to rest your voice.

ALTERNATIVE CHOICES

To treat laryngitis, alternative practitioners often prescribe methods to soothe the raw throat or boost the immune system, or they encourage rest.

ACUPUNCTURE

A recent study of traditional Chinese remedies found that many patients with laryngitis or tonsillitis benefited from acupuncture. Consult a licensed acupuncturist for proper treatment.

HERBAL THERAPIES

To help restore the voice, try gargling with a tea made from red sage *(Salvia officinalis* var. *rubia)*, bayberry *(Myrica* spp.), or white oak *(Quercus alba)* bark. A tincture of echinacea *(Echinacea* spp.) every hour for two days is thought to help

boost the immune system. Mix 10 drops of the tincture in a glass of water and swallow.

HOMEOPATHY

If laryngitis is a result of overuse or trauma to the vocal cords, use Arnica (6x or 12x) every hour; if you notice no improvement after four or five hours, try another preparation. For laryngitis that is accompanied by dryness of the throat and the feeling of a plug in the larynx, use Spongia tosta (12x) four times a day. For laryngitis accompanied by a dry, croupy cough that comes on suddenly after exposure to cold weather or with the first signs of a cold, use Aconite (6x or 12x) every two hours. If these remedies don't work, consult a practitioner.

NUTRITION AND DIET

Drinking plenty of fluids, eating lots of raw fruits and vegetables, and reducing your intake of refined carbohydrates may help speed your recovery from laryngitis. To boost your immune system, supplement your diet with vitamin C, 20,000 to 80,000 IU a day of beta carotene (vitamin A), and garlic.

AT-HOME REMEDIES

◆ Rest your body as well as your voice—completely. If you must speak, whisper; do not engage the vocal cords at all.
◆ Drink plenty of liquids, such as water or tea mixed with a little honey or lemon.
◆ Inhale steam from a pot of boiling water.
◆ Apply warm compresses to your throat.

PREVENTION

The best way to prevent laryngitis is to avoid straining your voice and to give it proper rest after overuse. If you're prone to laryngitis, try to stay away from cigarette smoke or other environmental toxins. If you think your laryngitis stems from an allergic reaction to a certain kind of food, experiment by removing suspected items from your diet, then reintroduce them one by one while monitoring the effect. *(See Allergies.)* ■